Science of Flexibility

Second Edition

Michael J. Alter, MS

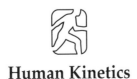

Human Kinetics

Library of Congress Cataloging-in-Publication Data

Alter, Michael J., 1952-
    Science of flexibility / Michael J. Alter. -- 2nd ed.
        p.   cm.
    Rev. ed. of: Science of stretching. c1988.
    Includes bibliographical references and index.
    ISBN 0-87322-977-0
    1. Stretch (Physiology)   2. Joints--Range of motion.   I. Alter,
    Michael J., 1952-   Science of stretching.   II. Title.
    QP310.S77A45   1996
    612.7'6--dc20   95-50410
                                                                                       CIP

ISBN: 0-87322-977-0
Copyright © 1996, 1988 by Michael J. Alter

This book is a revised edition of *Science of Stretching*, published in 1988 by Human Kinetics.

Acquisitions Editor: Richard Frey, PhD; **Developmental Editor:** Julie Rhoda; **Assistant Editors:** Jacqueline Blakley, Sandra Merz Bott, Lynn Hooper, Susan Moore, and Hank Woolsey; **Editorial Assistants:** Jennifer J. Hemphill and Andrew T. Starr; **Copyeditor:** Karen Bojda; **Proofreader:** Pam Johnson; **Typesetter:** Kathy Boudreau-Fuoss; **Text Designer:** Robert Reuther; **Layout Artist:** Denise Lowry; **Photo Editor:** Boyd LaFoon; **Cover Designer:** Jack Davis; **Photographer (cover):** David Black; **Illustrators:** Beth Young, Jennifer Delmotte, Michael Richardson and Keith Blomberg; **Printer:** Braun-Brumfield

Printed in the United States of America   10 9 8 7 6 5 4 3 2 1

Human Kinetics
Web site: http://www.humankinetics.com/

United States: Human Kinetics, P.O. Box 5076, Champaign, IL 61825-5076
1-800-747-4457
e-mail: humank@hkusa.com

Canada: Human Kinetics, Box 24040, Windsor, ON N8Y 4Y9
1-800-465-7301 (in Canada only)
e-mail: humank@hkcanada.com

Europe: Human Kinetics, P.O. Box IW14, Leeds LS16 6TR, United Kingdom
(44) 1132 781708
e-mail: humank@hkeurope.com

Australia: Human Kinetics, 57A Price Avenue, Lower Mitcham, South Australia 5062
(08) 277 1555
e-mail: humank@hkaustralia.com

New Zealand: Human Kinetics, P.O. Box 105-231, Auckland 1
(09) 523 3462
e-mail: humank@hknewz.com

Blessed are You, L-rd our G-d, King of the universe, who has formed man in wisdom and created within him holes and holes[1] and spaces and spaces.[2] It is revealed and known before your glorious throne that if but one of them were to be closed when it should be opened, or one of them should be opened when it should be closed, it would be impossible to exist even for a short while. Blessed are You L-rd, who heals all flesh and performs wonders.

**A loose English rendition of the
Traditional Jewish Morning Blessings**

---

[1] openings or orifices

[2] cavities, ducts, or tubes

To Steve, Nadine, and Bob

Contents

Preface

Many professionals are concerned about the limitations of flexibility and with techniques for its optimal development. This text, written primar-ily for these professionals, provides readers with an up-to-date survey of knowledge on flexibility, including the factors that affect the quality and extent of flexibility, range of motion (ROM), and various methods to maintain and enhance it. Recent research in basic and clinical sciences has substantiated and explained many theories and exercise procedures from a variety of disciplines. Accordingly, this second edition of *Science of Flexibility* is much more extensive in scope than its predecessor. I have reorganized and revised many of the chapters, more than doubling the text: It has five new chapters, many new illustrations and tables, and a reference list that has almost tripled in entries.

One major change from the first edition is having fewer stretching exercises and warm-up drills. Readers who want an extensive presentation of stretching exercises can refer to *Sport Stretch* by this author, which provides 311 stretching exercises arranged by muscle group and level of difficulty.

Among the additions to this edition, chapter 14 discusses joint play, mobilization, and manipulation. A growing number of people receive services from chiropractors, osteopaths, and massage therapists, and I have explored the philosophy and techniques of these practitioners whose practices are devoted in large measure to maintaining and enhancing their patients' range of motion. In developing this chapter, I visited ten chiropractic colleges, three osteopathic colleges, and two massage therapy schools. Chapter 15 explores controversy regarding stretching itself, in particular eight commonly cited stretching exercises. This chapter clearly discloses the lack of consensus among the "experts" on this subject. Chapter 16 deals with the relationship of stretching and special populations: seniors, pregnant women, and people who have physical disabilities or impairments. This chapter is significant because of the growing senior population and the importance of recognizing that flexibility and stretching benefit more than the young, active, and healthy populations. Lastly, chapter 20 analyzes the functional aspects of stretching and flexibility for a variety of sports and health conditions.

What you will find in this text is a general overview. Publishers have devoted entire books and journals to a single concept you will read about in this survey. Scientists are continually developing knowledge of the body's workings, and professionals are responsible for keeping abreast of new information in an array of related disciplines. *Science of Flexibility* will contribute to your appreciating the wonder of the human body and understanding the subject of flexibility and its relationship to the body's optimal development.

Acknowledgments

Producing this text was a cumulative team effort, and, hence, I wish to express deep gratitude to the many people who made it possible. First, I wish to acknowledge Rick Frey, division director for the Human Kinetics Academic Division. Rick was responsible for initially approving the project, and he shouldered the burden of guiding me in making those dreaded "cuts and deletions" necessary to produce a viable final product of appropriate length.

Second, I wish to acknowledge the patience, skill, loyal support, and assistance of my developmental editor, Julie Rhoda, who had the task of directing and managing the project. It was always a pleasure to hear her soft-spoken, warm, and encouraging voice. Julie helped smooth the process of this mini marathon.

I am also indebted to the external reviewers. In particular, I wish to extend my appreciation to Marjorie Moore whose contributions were substantial. If the text outline appears logical and sequential, it is due in great measure to her input. She also helped me realize that key ideas needed additional clarification, pointing out discrepancies so that the book manuscript could be improved.

Another person deserving special recognition is the copyeditor Karen Bodja. Copyeditors are usually thought to merely check the mechanical details of the author's writing, such as spelling, punctuation, and grammar. However, Karen went beyond this narrow job description and in a literal sense assumed the role of "co-ownership." She raised insightful questions, assisted in reordering the flow of logic, and enhanced the readability and clarity of the text.

I am once again indebted to the excellent work of artist Michael Richardson, who illustrated the 60 stretching exercises found toward the end of the text. A reviewer of the first edition wrote, "[It is] remarkable in that from such a simple presentation so much about the complex motions of the body can be expressed." These drawings indeed reflect the highest degree of craftsmanship.

In addition, I wish to thank the publishers and authors who granted permission to quote passages and reproduce drawings, photographs, and other illustrative material. In particular, my thanks go to Anne E. Atwater, PhD; Rene Cailliet, MD; Jerome V. Ciullo, MD; M.H. Gladden, PhD; S. Gracovetsky, PhD; Professor Sir Andrew Huxley; Dr. I.A. Kapandji; Florence P. Kendall, PT; C.D. Nordschow, MD, PhD; Barry W. Oakes, MD; Gerald H. Pollack, PhD; Bob Pritchard; J. Sachse, MD; Raymond W. Sandoz, DC; Kuan Wang, PhD; Gretchen Ward Warren; and James E. Zachazewski, PT. They added greatly to the content, clarity, and usefulness of the text.

Last, I wish to acknowledge the efforts of the production director Ernie Noa, production manager Judy Rademaker, typesetter Kathy Fuoss, text designer Robert Reuther, layout artist Denise Lowry, assistant editors Hank Woolsey, Lynn Hooper, Susan Moore, and Sandra Merz Bott, and all of the other members of the Human Kinetics staff for their helpfulness throughout the production of this text.

Credits

Figure 2.1 from *Range of Motion Exercise* (pp. 6-7) by J. Loeper, 1985, Minneapolis: Sister Kenny Institute. Copyright 1985 by Sister Kenny Institute. Reprinted by permission.

Figures 3.1, 3.3, 3.6, 3.7, 3.8, 3.11, 5.11, and 5.12 from *Muscles & Molecules: Uncovering the Principles of Biological Motion* (p. 4) by G.H. Pollack, 1990, Seattle: Ebner & Sons. Copyright 1990 by G.H. Pollack. Reprinted by permission.

Figure 3.5 from "Scarcomere-Associated Cytoskeletal Lattices in Striated Muscles" In *Cell And Muscle Motility* (Vol. 6) (p. 318) by J.W. Shay (Ed.), 1985, New York: Plenum Press. Copyright 1985 by Plenum Press. Reprinted by permission.

Figure 3.9 from *A Textbook of Histology* (11th ed.) (p. 281) by D.W. Fawcett, 1986, Philadelphia: W.B. Saunders. Copyright 1986 by D.W. Fawcett. Reprinted by permission of D.W. Fawcett.

Figure 3.10 from "The Variation in Isometric Tension With Sarcomere Length in Vertebrate Muscle Fibres" by A.M. Gordon, A.F. Huxley, and F.J. Julian, 1966, *Journal of Physiology* (London), 184, pp. 185-166. Copyright Cambridge University Press. Reprinted by permission.

Figure 3.12 from "Regulation of Skeletal Muscle Stiffness and Elasticity by Titin Isoforms: A Test of the Segmental Extension Model of Resting Tension" by K. Wang, R. McCarter, J. Wright, J. Beverly, and R. Ramirez-Mitchell, 1991, *Proceedings of the National Academy of Science*, 88(6), p. 7104. Copyright 1991 by K. Wang. Reprinted by permission of the National Academy of Science.

Figure 3.13 from *Applied Kinesiology: Vol. 1. Basic Procedures and Muscle Testing* (p. 10) by D.W. Walther, 1981, Pueblo, CO: Systems DC. Copyright 1981 by Systems DC. Reprinted by permission.

Figure 3.14 and 10.6 from "Repair of Injured Skeletal Muscle: A Molecular Approach" by B. Russell, D.J. Dix, D.L. Haller, and J. Jacobs-El, 1992, *Medicine and Science in Sports and Exercise* 24(2), p. 193. Copyright 1992 by the American College of Sports Medicine. Reprinted by permission.

Figure 4.1 from "The Multicomposite Structure of Tendon" by J. Kastelic, A. Galeski, and E. Baer, 1978, *Connective Tissue Research*, 6(1), p. 21. Copyright 1978 by Gordon and Breach Science Publishers, Inc. Reprinted by permission.

Figure 4.2 from "The Microfibrils of Connective Tissue: I. Ultrastructure" by S. Inoue and C.P. Leblond, 1986, *The American Journal of Anatomy*, 176(2), p. 136. Copyright © 1986 by Alan R. Liss, Inc. Reprinted by permission of Wiley-Liss, a division of John Wiley and Sons, Inc.

Figure 4.3 reprinted with permission. D.J. Prockop and N.A. Guzman. "Collagen Diseases and the Biosynthesis of Collagen." *Hospital Practice* volume 12, issure 12, page 62. Illustration by Bunji Tagawa.

Figure 4.4 reprinted by permission of VCH Publishers, Inc., 220 East 23rd St., New York, N.Y., 10010 from: Hukins: *Connective Tissue Matrix*, 1984.

Figure 4.5 from "Electromechanical Transcution and Transport in the Extracellular Matrix" by A.J. Grodzinsky, 1987, *Advances in Microcirculation*, **13**, p. 37. Copyright 1987 by S. Karger AG. Reprinted by permission of S. Karger AG.

Figure 6.11 from "Neural Factors Versus Hypertrophy in the Time Course of Muscle Strength Gain" by T. Moritani and H.A. de Vries, 1979, *American Journal of Physical Medicine*, 58(3), p. 117. Copyright 1979 by Williams & Wilkins. Reprinted by permission.

Figures 7.2, 7.3, 7.4, 7.5, and 7.6 from Burns Kattenburg collection, Harvard Theatre Collection. Reprinted by permission.

Figures 8.1 and 10.2 from *Clinical Anatomy for Medical Students* (4th ed.), by R.S. Snell, 1992, Boston: Little, Brown, and Company. Copyright 1992 by Little, Brown, and Company. Reprinted with permission.

Figure 8.2 from "Biomechanics of the Pelvis" by B.H. Faucret. In *A Collection of Monographs on the Biomechanics of the Pelvis* (p. 49, Des Moines, IA: American Chiropractic Association. Copyright 1980 by B.H. Faucret. Reprinted by permission.

Figure 8.3, 8.4, 8.5, and 8.6 from "Cervical Mobilization Induced by Eye Movement" by J. Sachse and M. Berger, 1989, *Journal of Manual Medicine*, 4(4), p. 155. Copyright 1989 by Springer-Verlag. Reprinted by permission.

Figure 9.2 from "The Cytoskeleton of Skeletal Muscle: Is It Affected by Exercise? A Brief Review" by C.M. Waterman-Storer, 1991, *Medicine and Science in Sports and Exercise*, 23(11), p. 1244. Copyright 1991 by the American College of Sports Medicine. Reprinted by permission.

Figure 9.3 and 9.4 from "Acute Soft Tissue Injuries: Nature and Management" by B.W. Oakes, 1981, *Australian Family Physician* 10 (Suppl.) pp. 3-16. Copyright 1981 by the Australian Family Physician. Reprinted by permission.

Figure 10.1 from "Normal Flexibility According to Age Groups" by H.O. Kendall and F.P. Kendall, 1948, *Journal of Bone and Joint Surgery*, 30A(3), pp. 690-694. Copyright 1948 by the Journal of Bone and Joint Surgery [A]. Reprinted by permission.

Figure 10.3 from "Mid-Forceps Delivery: A Vanishing Art?" by D.N. Danforth and A.H. Ellis, 1963, *American Journal of Obstetrics and Gynecology*, 86(1), pp. 29-37. Copyright 1963 by Mosby-Year Book. Reprinted by permission.

Figures 10.4, 17.13, and 18.7 from *Muscles Testing and Function* (2nd ed.) (p. 233) by H.O. Kendall, F.P. Kendall, and G.E. Wadsworth, 1971, Baltimore: Williams and Wilkins. Copyright 1971 by Williams and Wilkins. Reprinted by permis-

sion.

Fgure 10.5 is reprinted with permission from the *Research Quarterly for Exercise and Sport*, vol. 63, no. 2. The *Research Quarterly for Exercise and Sport* is a publication of the American Alliance for Health, Physical Education, Recreation and Dance, 1900 Association Drive, Reston, VA 22091.

Figures 10.7 and 10.8 Tables 10.1and 10.2 from "Diurnal Variations in the Stresses on the Lumbar Spine" by M.A. Adams, P. Dolan, and W.C. Hutton, 1987, *Spine*, 12(2), p. 136. Copyright 1987 by J.B. Lippincott Co. Reprinted by permission.

Figure 12.1 from the personal collection of Dr. Jerome V. Ciullo. Reprinted with permission.

Figure 13.1 and Table 13.1 from "Flexibility for Sports" by J.E. Zachazewski. In *Sports Physical Therapy* (pp. 201-238) by B. Sanders (Ed.), 1990, Norwalk, CT: Appleton & Lange. Copyright 1990 by Appleton & Lange. Reprinted by permission.

Figure 13.2 from "Rehabilitation" by J.J. Irrgang. In *Sports Injuries: Mechanisms, Prevention, and Treatment* (2nd ed.) (p. 82) by F.H. Fu and D.A. Stone (Eds.), 1993, Baltimore: Williams and Wilkins. Copyright 1993 by Williams and Wilkins. Reprinted by permission.

Figures 13.5 and 13.6 from *Facilitated Stretching* (p. 82) by R.E. McAtee, 1993, Champaign, IL: Human Kinetics. Copyright 1993 by R.E. McAtee. Reprinted by permission.

Figure 13.7 and Tables 13.3 and 14.1 from *Rehabilitation Techniques in Sports Medicine* (p. 75) by W.E. Prentice, 1990, St. Louis: Times Mirror/Mosby. Copyright 1990 Times Mirror/Mosby. Reprinted by permission.

Figure 13.10 reprinted with permission from the *Journal of the American Osteopathic Association* 81 (4) pp. 67-72. Copyright 1981 by the American Osteopathic Association.

Figure 13.11 from Stretch Mate. Courtesy of Fred Dolan, 24 Water St., Holliston, MA 01746. Reprinted with permission.

Figure 14.1 from *Mobilisation of the Spine: A Primary Handbook of Clinical Method* (5th ed.) (p. 182) by G.P. Grieve, 1991, London: Churchill Livingstone. Copyright 1991 by Longman Group Ltd. Reprinted by permission.

Figure 14.3 from "Chiropractic Treatment of Low-Back Pain" by K.C. Kranz, 1988, *Topics in Acute Care and Trauma Rehabilitation*, 2(4), p. 54. Copyright © 1988 Aspen Publishers, Inc. Reprinted by permission.

Figure 14.4 and 14.5 from "Some Physical Mechanisms and Effects of Spinal Adjustments" by R.W. Sandoz, 1976, *Annals of the Swiss Chiropractors' Association*, 6, p. 92. Copyright 1976 by the Swiss Chiropractors' Association. Reprinted by permission.

Figure 14.6 from "The Physics of Spinal Manipulations. Part IV. A Theoretical Consideration of the Physician Impact Force and Energy Requirements Needed to Produce Synovial Joint Cavitation" by M. Haas, 1990, *Journal of Manipulative and Physiological Therapeutics*, 13(7), p. 381. Copyright 1990 by the Journal of Manipulative and Physiological Therapeutics. Reprinted by permission of the Journal of Manipulative and Physiological Therapeutics.

Figures 15.1, 15.2, 15.3, and 15.6 from *The Rejuvenation Strategy* (p. 34) by R. Cailliet and L. Gross, 1987, Garden City, NJ: Doubleday. Copyright 1987 by R. Cailliet & Magilla, Inc. Reprinted by permission.

Figure 15.4, 15.7, 15.8, 15.9, 15.10, and 16.1 from *Sport Stretch* (pp. 67 and 77) by M.J. Alter, 1990, Champaign, IL: Human Kinetics. Copyright 1990 by M.J. Alter. Reprinted by permission.

Figure 15.5 from "The Importance of Pelvic Tilt in Reducing Compressive Stress in the Spine During Flexion-Extension Exercises" by S. Gracovetsky, M. Kary, I. Pitchen, S. Levy, and R.B. Said, 1989, *Spine*, 14(4), p. 415. Copyright 1989 by J.B. Lippincott. Reprinted by permission.

Figures 17.1, 17.3, 17.4, 17.5, 17.6, 17.7, 17.8, 19.8, 19.9, 19.10, and 19.11 from *Living Anatomy* (p. 139) by J.E. Donnelly, 1982, Champaign, IL: Human Kinetics. Copyright 1982 by J.E. Donnelly. Reprinted by permission.

Figure 17.2 from *Classical Ballet Technique* (p. 11) by G.W. Warren, 1989, Tampa, FL: University of South Florida Press. Photo by Juri Barikin. Reprinted by permission of University Presses.

Figures 17.10, 17.11, 17.14, and 17.15 reprinted from *Anatomy of Movement* by Blandine Calais-Germain with permission of Eastand Press, Inc., P.O. Box 12689, Seattle, WA 98111. Copyright 1993. All rights reserved.

Figures 17.12 and 18.11 from *Joint Motion: Method of Measuring and Recording* (p. 55), 1965, Chicago: American Academy of Orthopaedic Surgeons. Copyright 1965 by the American Orthopaedic Association. Reprinted by permission. (Out of print. The information found in this publication is presently being revised and updated

by the American Academy of Orthopaedic Surgeons.)

Figure 17.16 from *Coaching Women's Gymnastics* (p. 80) by B. Sands, 1984, Champaign, IL: Human Kinetics. Copyright 1984 by B. Sands. Reprinted by permission.

Figure 17.17 from "The Pathogenesis of Dance Injury" by W.T. Hardaker, L. Erickson, and M. Myers. In *The Dancer as Athlete* (pp. 12-13) by C.G. Shell (Ed.), 1984, Champaign, IL: Human Kinetics. Copyright 1986 by C.G. Shell. Reprinted by permission.

Figures 18.2 and 18.3 from *The Physiology of the Joints: Vol. 3. The Trunk and the Vertebral Column* (p. 29) by I.A. Kapandji, 1978, Edinburgh: Churchill Livingstone. Copyright. I.A. Kapandji. Reprinted by permission.

Figures 18.4 and 18.5 from *A Practical Guide to Management of the Painful Neck and Back* (p. 37) by J.W. Fisk and B.S. Rose, 1977, Springfield, IL: Charles C Thomas. Copyright 1977 by Charles C Thomas, Publisher. Reprinted by permission.

Figures 18.8, 18.9, 18.10, 18.12, 18.14, 18.15, 19.3, 19.4, and 19.6 from *Shoulder Pain* (p. 2) by R. Cailliet, 1966, F.A. Davis. Copyright 1966 by F.A. Davis Company. Reprinted by permission.

Figures 19.1, 19.5, and 19.7 from *Low Back Pain Syndrome* (3rd ed., p. 65) by R. Cailliet, 1981, Philadelphia: F.A. Davis. Copyright 1981 by F.A. Davis Company. Reprinted by permission.

Figure 19.2 from *Manual of Orthopaedic Surgery* (p. 130) by the American Orthopaedic Association, 1985, Park Ridge, IL: Author. Copyright by the American Orthopaedic Association. Reprinted by permission.

Figure 20.1 from *Lower Extremity Injuries in Runners Induced by Upper Body Torque (UBT)* by B. Prichard, 1984, presented at the Biomechanics and Kinesiology in Sports U.S. Olympic Committee Sports Medicine Conference January 8-14, 1984, in Colorado Springs, CO. Copyright 1984 by Bob Prichard/SOMAX Posture & Sport. Marin Medical Center 711 D Street #208, San Rafael. CA 94901. Reprinted by permission.

Figures 20.2 and 20.3 from *Training Distance Runners* (p. 17) by D. Martin & P. Coe, 1991, Champaign, IL: Human Kinetics. Copyright 1991 by D. Martin and P. Coe. Reprinted by permission.

Figure 20.4 from "What Film Analysis Tells Us About Movement," by A. Atwater. Paper presented at the *Annual Meeting of the Midwest Asso-*

ciation for Physical Education of College Women, French Lick, IN, October 1967. Copyright 1967 by A. Atwater. Author can be contacted at the university of Arizona. Reprinted by permission.

Figure 20.5 from *Winning Wrestling Moves.* (p. 151) by M. Mysnyk, B. Davis, and B. Simpson, 1994, Champaign, IL: Human Kinetics. Copyright 1994 by Mark Mysnyk. Reprinted with permission.

Table 4.2 from "Relative Importance of Various Tissues in Joint Stiffness," by R.J. Johns and V. Wright, 1962, *Journal of Applied Physiology* 17(5), pp. 824-828. Copyright 1962 by American Physiological Society.

Table 4.4 from "Collagen Metabolism," by P. Bornstein and P.H. Byers, 1980, *Current Concepts.* Copyright 1980 by The Upjohn Company. Reprinted with permission.

Tables 5.1, 5.2, and 5.3 from "Biophysical Factors of Range-of-Motion Exercise," by A.A. Sapega, T.C. Quendenfeld, R.A. Moyer, and R.A. Butler, 1981, *The Physician and Sportsmedicine* 9 (12), pp. 57-65. Copyright 1981 by McGraw-Hill. Reprinted with permission.

Table 6.1 from "Articular Neurology and Manipulative Therapy," by B.D. Wyke. In *Aspects of Manipulative Therapy* (p. 73) by E.F. Glasgow, L.T. Twomey, E.R. Scull, and A.M. Kleynhaw (Eds.), 1985, London: Churchill Livingstone. Copyright 1985 by Churchill Livingstone. Reprinted with permission.

Table 11.1 from *Communicating with Patient: Improving Communication, Satisfaction, and Compliance* (p. 180), by P. Ley, 1988, London: Croom Helm Ltd. Copyright 1988 by Croom Helm Ltd. Reprinted with permission.

Table 12.1 is reprinted with permission from the *Research Quarterly for Exercise and Sport*, vol. 51, no. 4. The *Research Quarterly for Exercise and Sport* is a publication of the American Alliance for Health, Physical Education, Recreation and Dance, 1900 Association Drive, Reston, Va 22091.

Table 13.2 is reprinted with permission from the *Research Quarterly for Exercise and Sport*, vol. 58. no. 2. The *Research Quarterly for Exercise and Sport* is a publication of the American Alliance for Health, Physical Education, Recreation and Dance, 1900 Association Drive, Reston, VA 22091.

Chapter 1

A Modern Overview of Flexibility and Stretching

The outcome of any flexibility program can be made more predictable and less haphazard if certain biological and biomechanical principles are understood and applied. In evaluating one's flexibility and formulating a flexibility training program, one must consider not only the benefits of increased flexibility, but also the potential for injury and impairment of function and performance if training occurs under suboptimal conditions. Everyone—including coaches, instructors, trainers, therapists, physicians, dancers, and professional and recreational athletes—should take advantage of every opportunity to develop optimal flexibility.

Historical Overview

Since antiquity, stretching and the development of flexibility have been employed to achieve various purposes. Historically and geographically widespread examples of the uses of flexibility are found in paintings and carvings. These purposes can be viewed as being on a continuum. At one end, flexibility can be used constructively to improve one's well-being. At the opposite end of the continuum, it can be used to the detriment of the individual's well-being and ultimately cause death. These detrimental uses include torture (for the purposes of interrogation, intimidation, and punishment) and execution.

Constructive Historical Uses of Stretching

According to Egan (1984), the origin of flexibility as a training method is unknown. However, it is thought that the ancient Greeks used some type of flexibility training that enabled them to dance, perform acrobatic stunts, and wrestle with greater ease. In addition, flexibility training must have been incorporated into the three kinds of ancient Greek gymnastics: the medical, comprising the prophylactic (to prevent disease and maintain one's health) and the therapeutic (the application of remedies to cure conditions and diseases); the warlike (military training); and the athletic.

Stretching postures called *asanas* have been a part of Near Eastern and Far Eastern traditions for thousands of years. Today, asanas are commonly thought of as just physical postures; however, this was not their original purpose. In his *Yoga Sutras* (one of the earliest Yoga texts, written in the second century A.D.) Patanjali succinctly discusses the method and purpose of the asanas. In Aphorism II, 46 Patanjali defines these postures in just two words: "*sthira-sukha*," which is defined as being in a "stable and easy posture" or "firm and relaxed posture" (Woods 1914) from which one can obtain a higher state. Stretching, another part of the Near and Far Eastern tradition, has been a vital component in developing defensive and offensive survival skills in various martial arts (e.g., karate and the modern tae kwon do).

Detrimental Historical Uses of Stretching

Historically, stretching has been used to people's detriment. For example, Beccaria (1764) in his classic essay identified five purposes that torture has historically served during an interrogation: (1) to make one confess to a crime, (2) to clear up contradictory statements, (3) to discover accomplices, (4) to purge one of infamy, and (5) to discover other crimes of which one might be guilty but not accused. Besides interrogation, stretching forces can be employed as a means of punishment. Punishment "involves the intentional infliction of unpleasantness or pain upon human beings by other human beings" (Wasserstrom 1977). The purposes or functions usually ascribed to formal punishment are deterrence, reformation, revenge, retribution, and protection of society by incapacitation of the offender. Well-known methods of torture, interrogation, and punishment include the hoist and the rack.

The ultimate form of punishment is death. Since ancient times it has been known that stretching forces, if applied to the proper part of the body and with sufficient force, are capable of initiating death, either slowly or quickly. One of the oldest and cruelest traditional methods of execution is being *drawn and quartered*. As described by Parry (1975), this entails having the four limbs tied to horses that are made to gallop in different directions. Ultimately, the body becomes dismembered. In contrast, if properly executed, a modern hanging can result in a relatively fast and painless death, as opposed to a slow strangulation.

Defining Flexibility

The word *flexibility* means different things to different people depending on their point of reference. For example, it may be applied to both animate and inanimate objects. Hence, the term can be defined in several different ways depending on the discipline or the nature of the research. The word flexibility is derived from the Latin *flectere* or *flexibilis*, "to bend." *The New Shorter Oxford English Dictionary* (1993) defines flexibility as the "ability to be bent, pliable."

There appears to be little agreement about the definition of so-called "normal" flexibility. In the disciplines of physical education, sports medicine, and allied health sciences, perhaps one of the simplest definitions of flexibility is the range of motion available in a joint or group of joints (Corbin et al. 1978; de Vries 1986; Hebbelinck 1988; Hubley-Kozey 1991; Liemohn 1988; Stone and Kroll 1986). For others, flexibility also implies freedom to move (Goldthwait 1941; Metheny 1952), the capacity of a joint to move fluidly through its full range of motion (Heyward 1984), the ability of a person to move a part or parts of the body in a wide range of purposeful movements at the required speed (Galley and Forster 1987), the total achievable excursion (within limits of pain) of a body part through its potential range of motion (Saal 1987), normal joint and soft tissue range of motion in response to active or passive stretch (Halvorson 1989), the ability of a muscle to relax and yield to a stretch force (Kisner and Colby 1990), and the ability to move a joint through a normal range of motion without undue stress to the musculotendinous unit (Chandler et al. 1990).

The Differences Among Flexibility, Hypermobility, and Joint Laxity

Flexibility, hypermobility, and joint laxity are not synonymous terms. *Flexibility* refers to the extensibility of periarticular tissues to allow normal or physiologic motion of a joint or limb. In contrast, *laxity* refers to the stability of a joint (Saal 1987). Excessive joint laxity can be a result of a chronic injury or a congenital or hereditary condition, such as *Ehlers-Danlos syndrome* (EDS). Throughout this text, the term *flexibility* will refer to the degree of normal motion; *laxity* will refer to the degree of abnormal motion of a given joint; and in general, *hypermobility* will refer to the range of motion in excess of the accepted normal motion in most of the joints.

The Nature of Flexibility

Goniometry is the measurement of joint range of motion. Range of motion (ROM) may be measured in two ways. First, it can be quantified in *linear units* (e.g., inches or centimeters). Second, it can be evaluated in *angular units* (degrees of an arc). Regardless of the method, the data should be clear, simple, and understandable.

One important part of total development is physical fitness. Physical fitness is multidimensional and includes flexibility, cardiorespiratory endurance, strength, and muscular endurance. Since the early 1900s a battery of tests have been developed to assess physical fitness. Although it may be common to think of flexibility as being a very general characteristic, more or less uniform throughout the body (i.e., to consider people generally very flexible or inflexible in the body joints), research studies do not substantiate this point (Holland 1968; Holland and Davis 1975). In fact, there is unanimous agreement that flexibility does not exist as a general characteristic but is *specific* to a particular joint and joint action (S. Bryant 1984; Corbin and Noble 1980; Harris 1969a, 1969b; Holland 1968; Merni et al. 1981; Munroe and Romance 1975; Sigerseth 1971). For example, adequate ROM in the hip does not ensure adequate ROM in the shoulder. Similarly, sufficient ROM in one hip may not indicate adequate ROM in the other hip. In short, measurement of one or several body joints cannot validly be used to predict ROM in other body parts (Holland 1968). These differences reflect genetic variation, personal activity patterns, and the specialized mechanical strains that the individual has imposed on his or her connective tissue (Holland and Davis 1975).

There are three basic types of flexibility. *Static flexibility* relates to ROM about a joint with no emphasis on speed (Fleischman 1964; Heyward 1984). Two examples of static flexibility are slowly bending to touch the floor or performing a "split." *Ballistic flexibility* is usually associated with bobbing, bouncing, rebounding, and rhythmic motion. Another term somewhat related to the latter is *dynamic flexibility*. This term refers to the ability to use a range of joint movement in the performance of a physical activity at either a normal or rapid speed (Corbin and Noble 1980; Fleischman 1964). Hence, dynamic flexibility does not necessarily denote ballistic or fast types of movement. However, it should be pointed out that a rigorous definition of dynamic flexibility has not been universally accepted (Hubley-Kozey 1991). An alternative term is *functional flexibility* (Clippinger-Robertson 1988). An example of "slow" dynamic flexibility is the ability of a ballet dancer to slowly raise and hold her leg at a

60° angle, whereas a split leap is an example of "fast" dynamic flexibility. Obviously, most athletic events involve dynamic flexibility. Here too, the type of flexibility is specific to the type of movement (i.e., its speed and angle) of a given discipline and thus not necessarily related to just ROM.

Flexibility is specific to a given group of sports as well as to a given joint, a given side, and a given speed. Furthermore, even within sports groups, particular patterns of flexibility are related to frequent or unique joint movements in those activities, events, or positions. Those joints demanding flexibility are characteristic of a given sport and of each subgroup within a sport. For example, research has shown that a number of sports and arts require the development of specific flexibility patterns to achieve success in the chosen discipline. These disciplines include ballet (DiTullio et al. 1989; Hamilton et al. 1992), baseball (Fleisg et al. 1995; Gurry et al. 1985; Magnusson, Gleim, and Nicholas 1994; Tippett 1986), ice hockey (Agre et al. 1988; Song 1979), power lifting (Chang, Buschbacher, and Edlich 1988), swimming (Bloomfield et al. 1985; Oppliger et al. 1986), and tennis (Chandler et al. 1990). Therefore, flexibility training should be prescribed accordingly (Zernicke and Salem 1991; this will be reviewed in chapter 20).

The Flexibility Training Program

To obtain maximum benefits from a training program to enhance ROM, you must know and understand what can and cannot be achieved by using it properly. Before examining the supposed value of such programs, we need to differentiate between various types of flexibility training programs. In the arena of athletics, *training* in general has been defined as "a multi-sided process of the expedient use of aggregate factors (means, methods and conditions) so as to influence the development of an athlete and ensure the necessary level of preparedness" (Matveyev 1981, 22). An essential component of any training program is a flexibility training program.

A *flexibility training program* is defined as a planned, deliberate, and regular program of exercises that can permanently and progressively increase the usable range of motion of a joint or set of joints over a period of time (Aten and

Knight 1978; Corbin and Noble 1980). According to Evjenth and Hamberg (1984), stretching can be divided into two categories: self-stretching and therapeutic muscle stretching. The former is commonly used in fitness exercises, athletic training, and dance. Related, but more specific in design, is *therapeutic muscle stretching* (TMS). TMS can be defined as specific muscle stretching performed, instructed, or supervised by a therapist for patients with dysfunctions of the musculoskeletal system (Mühlemann and Cimino 1990). Such patients may or may not be athletes. Needless to say, therapeutic muscle stretching and self-stretching may supplement each other (Evjenth and Hamberg 1984).

A common and distinct entity that should be employed in most exercise regimens is a *flexibility warm-up/cool-down program*, which is defined as a planned, deliberate, and regular program of exercises that is done immediately before and after an activity to improve performance or to reduce the risk of injury in the activity. (The term *cool-down* is synonymous with *warm-down*.) A flexibility warm-up/cool-down program alone will not improve flexibility during weeks following the program (Aten and Knight 1978; Corbin and Noble 1980). In contrast, self-stretching and TMS have been demonstrated to retain improved flexibility during weeks following activity (Zebas and Rivera 1985).

The Benefits of a Flexibility Training Program

When one begins a flexibility training program, the potential benefits are virtually unlimited. The quality and quantity of these benefits are ultimately determined by two factors. The first of these factors is the individual's *ends*—an individual's goals or objectives, the context of which may be biological, psychological, sociological, or philosophical. The second factor, the *means*, is the methods and techniques used to attain one's goals. If one's ends are purely emotional or psychological, as opposed to biological or physiological, then certain stretching techniques would be employed and others would not. What, then, can one expect from a flexibility training program? In light of the recent proliferation of material on the subject, we will now examine the purported benefits of flexibility training.

Union of the Body, Mind, and Spirit

From a purely esoteric point of view, a flexibility training program can serve to unify one's body, mind, and spirit. Of the many disciplines that claim to seek the perfection and harmony of the body, mind, and spirit, yoga is probably the most widely known. The word *yoga* is derived from the Sanskrit root *yuj*, meaning "to bind, attach, and yoke" (Iyengar 1979). An equivalent idea is conveyed by the English phrase "getting into harness" or "yoking up." The yogi undoubtedly "gets into harness" in his or her work of controlling the body and mind by the will (Ramacharaka 1960). Similarly, Iyengar (1979, 19) points out that the term *yuj* implies "to direct and concentrate one's attention; to use and apply." It also means *union* or *communion*.

According to the *Yoga Sutras*, an ancient writing, yoga comprises several categories of physiological practices and spiritual exercises, called *angas*, or "limbs." Classical yoga comprises eight limbs whose end is final liberation, *enstasis*:

1. Yama—abstentions
2. Niyama—observances
3. Asanas—posture
4. Pranayama—control of breath
5. Pratyahara—withdrawal of the senses
6. Dharana—concentration
7. Dhyana—meditation
8. Samadhi—a state of superconsciousness, oneness, or unifying concentration

Today, the layperson commonly thinks of asanas as merely physical exercises or postures that often display flexibility and suppleness. However, the asanas are not an end in themselves but a means of facilitating breath control (i.e., pranayama) and subsequently the four remaining angas. Lists and descriptions of asanas are found in many ancient Indian texts, manuals, and manuscripts (Yogendra 1988). According to one ancient text, the *Gheranda Samhita*, "There are eighty-four hundreds of thousands of Asanas described by Shiva. The postures are as many in number as there are numbers of species of living creatures in this universe" (Vasu 1933, 25). In brief, these numerous sources on yoga emphasize the following basic principles that are mystical and transcendental, yet highly logical and rational:

• The body is the temple that houses the Divine Spark.

- The body is an instrument of attainment.
- The yogi masters the body by the practice of asanas.
- The yogi performs asanas to develop complete equilibrium of the body, mind, and spirit.
- The body, mind, and spirit are inseparable.

As an analogy, Iyengar (1979, 24–25) explained yoga as follows:

> To the yogi, his body is the prime instrument of attainment. If his vehicle breaks down, the traveler cannot go far. If the body is broken by ill-health, the aspirant can achieve little. Physical health is important for mental development, as normally the mind functions through the nervous system. When the body is sick or the nervous system is affected, the mind becomes restless or dull and inert and concentration or meditation becomes impossible.

Thus, whether one practices the asanas to improve the mind or attain Samadhi, an additional side benefit will be the development of flexibility.

Relaxation of Stress and Tension

Stress is an inescapable part of life that generally can be described as the "wear and tear." It can be defined as the body's generalized reaction to stimuli (Christiansen and Baum 1991). Any stimuli that an organism perceives as a threat is termed a *stressor*. Stressors occur in varying degrees and different forms. They may be physical, psychological, or psychosocial in nature. All forms of stress affect the individual in ways that are sometimes good and sometimes harmful to health. Normal levels of stress are healthy and desirable. Love and work, for example, involve this beneficial kind of stress. Intense and persistent stress, however, such as continuous anger, fear, frustration, inhibition, or tension, can become bottled up inside an individual and threaten health. This buildup of stress without release of tension leads to problems.

As stated earlier, "the body, mind, and spirit are inseparable." One of the advances of modern medicine is the increasing recognition or rediscovery of the major influence of emotions on physical health. In fact, the knowledge that illness must be considered and treated in relation to the *whole person* forms the basis for *psychosomatic* medicine (from *psyche*, mind, and *soma*, body). Today, many scientists believe that prolonged emotional tensions play a major role in triggering ailments such as high blood pressure, peptic ulcer, headache, and joint and muscular pains (Asterita 1985; Dobson 1983; Larson and Michelman 1973).

Coping is defined as the process through which individuals adjust to the stressful demands of their daily environments (Christiansen and Baum 1991). In the method-of-coping classification (Moos 1974), coping efforts are viewed as either cognitive, behavioral, or avoidant in nature. *Avoidant* strategies attempt to reduce emotional attention through diversion or conscious efforts to circumvent or sidestep the source of stress. For example, when you are upset, angry, or frustrated, you can try to reduce these negative feelings through exercise. Exercise can be implemented as an avoidant strategy to reduce or prevent unwanted stress. The literature contains abundant evidence that therapeutic exercise alleviates stress (de Vries 1975; de Vries et al. 1981; Levarlet-Joye 1979; Morgan and Horstman 1976; Sime 1977). Just as exercise has been found to be immeasurably therapeutic for many people, empirical evidence indicates that individualized flexibility training programs may be similarly beneficial.

Muscular Relaxation

One of the most important benefits of a flexibility program is the potential promotion of relaxation. From a purely physiological perspective, *relaxation* is the cessation of muscular tension. Undesirably high levels of muscular tension in the human organism result in several negative side effects. Excessive muscular tension tends to decrease sensory awareness of the world and raise blood pressure (Larson and Michelman 1973). It also wastes energy; a contracting muscle obviously requires more energy than a relaxed muscle. Furthermore, habitually tense muscles tend to cut off their own circulation. Reduced blood supply results in a lack of oxygen and essential nutrients and causes toxic waste products to accumulate in the cells. This process predisposes one to fatigue, aches, even pain. Common sense and everyday experience show that a relaxed muscle is less susceptible to these and many other ailments.

Our chief concern, however, is flexibility. When a muscle stays partially contracted, an abnormal state of prolonged shortening called *contracture* develops. Contracture and chronic muscle tension not only shorten the muscle, but also make the muscle less supple, less strong, and unable to absorb the shock and stress of various types of movement. Consequently, undue muscular tension can produce excessive muscular tightness. Here, too, common sense indicates that the most appropriate remedy for such a disorder would be to facilitate muscular relaxation and immediately follow with some type of stretching. In support of this position, de Vries and Adams (1972) found exercise to be more effective than medication in decreasing muscular tension.

Self-Discipline

Most of us live undisciplined lives; that is, our responses are often conditioned by mindless habit. However, self-discipline must be cultivated, because sustained effort is required to attain any goal. When the goal is success in an endeavor (e.g., performing a split), effort must be backed up with unflagging persistence that does not recognize failure. The goal must be pursued until it is achieved.

Because the body is controlled by the mind, if the body is disciplined or mastered, then the mind must be disciplined or mastered. Herein lies the fundamental importance of the asanas in yoga. The yogi masters the body by the practice and self-discipline of asanas and thus makes the body a fit vehicle for the spirit. This concept that disciplining the mind disciplines the body also holds true for the athlete, artistic performer, and layperson. If one aspect of life can be disciplined, then anything in one's life can be mastered. A flexibility training program offers an ideal opportunity to seek mastery over oneself. Stretching can give one something to struggle for and against, just as a marathon race does for a runner.

Another benefit of stretching is that it offers a unique opportunity for spiritual growth. A stretching program can provide quiet intervals for thought, meditation, or self-evaluation. During such moments, you can also listen to and monitor your own body—something most of us today seldom do. Thus a stretching program provides the opportunity to get in touch with yourself or with the cosmos. And the beauty of stretching is that it can be done anywhere at any time.

In the world of artistic performance and sports, an individual's successes and failures are visible for all to see, and the measures of success are objectively accurate. One can do little to hide a poor arabesque or a failed split jump. One of the most helpful benefits of a stretching program (or any exercise program) is that it can enable you to understand your own development and abilities. Not everyone can perform a split. Each of us has different abilities and talents—some of which have gone unrecognized. Stretching can teach you lessons about your own human limits and provide opportunities to test yourself physiologically.

Body Fitness, Posture, and Symmetry

The desire to be healthy and attractive is almost universal. The best way to improve bodily measurements and proportions is through a combination of appropriate diet and exercise. To develop body symmetry and good posture, one should engage in gross motor activities rather than specialize in an activity that develops only one area of the body. By incorporating an individualized flexibility program into an overall fitness program, you can improve not only your health and fitness, but also your bodily appearance.

The relationship of flexibility to posture is mainly theoretical and clinical. Crawford and Jull (1993) found that increased kyphosis (flexion in the thoracic region) in older subjects is related to reduced range of arm elevation. Corbin and Noble (1980) and Holland and Davis (1975) suggest that an imbalance in muscular development and a lack of flexibility in certain muscle groups can contribute to poor posture. Rounded shoulders, for example, are thought to be associated with poor flexibility in the pectoral muscles and a lack of muscular endurance in the scapular girdle adductors (i.e., rhomboids and middle trapezius). This condition presumably may be alleviated by stretching the shortened connective tissue and muscles and by strengthening the weakened muscles (Holland and Davis 1975).

Health can be greatly enhanced by daily physical activity. When physical activity is not a regular part of one's life, many ailments and debilitating conditions are more likely to occur such as *asthenia* (loss of strength), *ataxia* (inability to coordinate bodily movements), and *hypokinesis* (diminished ability to move; Larson and Michelman 1973). Conversely, if one makes physical activity a regular part of one's life, many of these conditions can be avoided. Depending on the method and technique of stretching that are employed, individuals can enhance their agility, coordination, flexibility, and muscular strength.

Relief of Low Back Pain

Low back pain (LBP) is one of the most prevalent complaints afflicting people in modern society. Thousands of people seek relief from low back pain by various treatments every year. In fact, most people will probably be affected by low back pain at some point in their lives. Numerous articles and books dealing with the problem appear annually. The question is "What is the relationship between flexibility, or lack of it, and low back pain?" Although the etiology remains controversial, strong evidence supports the need for adequate mobility of the trunk. Farfan (1978), for example, reported that flexibility of the lumbar spine provides a mechanical advantage for function and efficiency. Furthermore, numerous authorities and studies suggest that adequate flexibility or stretching may help reduce the risk or severity of low back pain (Cailliet 1988; Deyo et al. 1990; Khalil et al. 1992; Locke 1983; Rasch and Burke 1989; Russell and Highland 1990). However, doubts regarding the relationship between flexibility and low back pain have been raised in various quarters.

In the opinion of Battié and colleagues (1990, 768), there exists a common public perception "that greater spinal flexibility is associated with improved back health and lesser risk of 'injury.'" To illustrate this contention, they state that improved range of motion may be associated with symptomatic relief in patients with subacute and chronic back problems (Mayer et al. 1985; Mayer et al. 1987; Mellin 1985). However, when reviewing the scientific literature, there is little evidence to support the use of exercises to maintain or increase spinal ROM as a protective measure against back problems (Battié et al. 1987; Battié et al. 1990). Nonetheless, Battié et al. (1990, 771) emphasize that

> lack of such an association does not prove that a program that induces changes will have no effect. . . . However, these data suggest that it is unlikely that increasing flexibility alone in the sagittal and frontal planes will reduce back pain reports.

The argument against programs designed to increase flexibility is based on the fundamental notion that other factors may be associated with the cause or prevention of injury. Furthermore,

additional factors associated with a program may also influence the eventual outcomes. "Flexibility measurements may be influenced by a number of factors such as pain, fear, and motivation, in addition to anatomic or physiologic limitations" (Battié et al. 1990, 772). This notion of a nonanatomic or nonphysiologic limitation of ROM has been raised by a number of researchers (Marras and Wongsam 1986; Pearcy, Portek, and Shepherd 1985; Seno 1968; Stokes et al. 1981). Consequently, changes in flexibility due to injury may be a form of protective behavior to reduce pain or irritation or to reduce moment (force times the perpendicular distance from a fulcrum) and thus the force about the spine.

Another important factor related to low back pain is the velocity of the trunk (i.e., lumbar spine). In a study by Marras and Wongsam (1986), the results indicated significant differences for both angle and velocity measures between patients with low back pain and a normal control group. Their investigation suggested that "trunk velocity be used as a quantitative measure of low back disorder and that it be used as a means to monitor the rehabilitative progress of patients with LBP" (p. 213).

In conclusion, two important issues need to be recognized. First, Battié et al. (1987) emphasize that longitudinal studies assessing premorbid spinal flexibility are needed to clearly define the relationship between spinal flexibility and back problems. Second, Jackson and Brown (1983) point out that clinical assessment of sufficient mobility remains undefined. Consequently, until adequate flexibility can be scientifically defined and the clinical means are developed to measure the achievement of goals (i.e., of ROM), the use of mobility and flexibility exercises to reduce the risk of low back pain will remain theoretical.

Relief of Muscular Cramps

Painful involuntary skeletal muscle contractions are generally called *cramps* (McGee 1990). Ordinary cramps are neural, not muscular, in origin. The ordinary cramp begins when a muscle already in its most shortened position involuntarily contracts (Norris, Gasteiger, and Chatfield 1957; Weiner and Weiner 1980). This may explain the susceptibility of swimmers to calf cramps. That is, good kicking form, with the toes pointed, involves contraction of the shortened gastrocnemius (calf) muscle (Weiner and Weiner 1980). Ordinary cramps cease when the involved muscle is passively stretched (Bertolasi et al. 1993;

Davison 1984; Graham 1965; Weiner and Weiner 1980) or there is an active contraction of its antagonist (Fowler 1973), as in one of the proprioceptive neuromuscular facilitation stretching techniques to be discussed later. Both of these maneuvers have been found to decrease a muscle's electrical activity (de Vries 1966; Helin 1985; Norris, Gasteiger, and Chatfield 1957). The mechanisms proposed to explain the ability of these techniques to relieve cramps are conjectural (McGee 1990). Since stretching has been found to relieve the acute cramp, some individuals propose that stretching exercises will prevent cramps (Daniell 1979; Matvienko and Kartasheva 1990; Sontag and Wanner 1988). One study found that a group of 44 patients was cured of nocturnal cramps after one week of brief calf stretch exercises performed three times per day (Daniell 1979).

Another cause of cramping in some women is dysmenorrhea. *Dysmenorrhea* is defined as excessive or painful menstruation. A number of theories have been propounded to explain its cause. The physiologic theories range from an imbalance in the normal estrogen-progesterone equilibrium to poor posture. Theoretically, the postural deviation involves shortening of fascial and ligamentous connective tissue around the uterus that restricts the extent of the posterior tilt of the pelvis, resulting in the subsequent pain (Billig 1943, 1951; Golub 1987; Holland and Davis 1975; Rasch and Burke 1989). The poor posture theory has led to a number of studies on the effect of exercise on dysmenorrhea.

The findings of several investigators (Billig and Lowendahl 1949; Golub 1987; Golub and Christaldi 1957; Golub, Lang, and Menduke 1958; Golub, Menduke, and Lang 1968) indicate that painful menstruation can be prevented or at least reduced in severity through regular stretching of the pelvic area. Presumably, stretching the fascial bands and ligamentous tissue relieves the compression irritation of the involved nerves and prevents recurrence of the symptoms (Billig 1943, 1951).

Relief of Muscular Soreness

Everyday experience and research appear to indicate that slow stretching exercises can reduce and sometimes eliminate muscular soreness. Two types of pain are associated with muscular exercise: pain during and immediately after exercise, which may persist for several hours, and delayed, localized soreness, which usually does not appear until 24 to 48 hours following exercise (i.e., delayed muscle soreness or DMS). Currently, there is still disagreement regarding the physiological cause or causes of muscular soreness and how stretching supposedly reduces or eliminates it. This topic will be discussed in chapter 9 in greater detail.

Through a series of experiments, de Vries (1961a, 1961b, 1966) found that electromyography (EMG) did not demonstrate reduced soreness after stretching. Rather, EMG demonstrated reduced muscle activity level after stretch, which was correlated with reduced complaint of soreness by subjects in these experiments. The theory to explain this reduction is based on the notion that muscle soreness and spasms are associated with elevated muscle action potentials (MAPs), and so reducing excess muscular tension will reduce soreness (de Vries 1966). It would therefore seem that muscle soreness could be prevented if stretching reduced MAPs. The studies showed that static stretching can significantly decrease electrical activity in the muscle to bring symptomatic relief of muscle soreness. In a study by Thigpen et al. (1985), static stretching was found to bring about a statistically significant reduction of the H/M ratio (this term relates to the level of alpha motoneuron excitability). However, not all research supports the hypothesis that stretching reduces or eliminates delayed muscle soreness. Buroker and Schwane (1989) found that exercise-induced DMS in eccentrically contracting muscles was not reduced either chronically over the prolonged postexercise period by a regimen of intermittent stretching or immediately after the exercise by an acute bout of stretching. Similar findings were observed by McGlynn, Laughlin, and Rowe (1979). Recently, a study by Rodenburg et al. (1994) found that the combination of a warm-up, stretching, and massage reduced some negative effects of eccentric exercise, but the results were inconsistent. Additional research is needed to resolve this issue.

Injury Prevention

The use of stretching exercises to increase flexibility is commonly based on the idea that it may decrease the incidence, intensity, or duration of musculotendinous and joint injury (Arnheim 1971; Aten and Knight 1978; Bryant 1984; Corbin and Noble 1980; Davis, Logan, and McKinney 1965; Garrett et al. 1989; Hilyer et al. 1990; Wiktorssohn-Möller et al. 1983). More than minimal joint extensibility appears to be advantageous in *some* sports and vocations to prevent muscle strain or joint sprain. In other words, there seems to be an *ideal* or *optimal* range of flexibility that will prevent injury when muscles and joints are accidentally overstretched. However, this statement should not be interpreted to mean that *maximum* joint flexibility will prevent injury. In further elaborating this point, the question of whether there is any benefit in stretching a muscle to an extreme ROM must be asked. In addressing this question with regard to athletics, Hubley-Kozey and Stanish (1990) point out that some athletes, such as gymnasts, must be able to reach an extreme ROM without damaging the surrounding tissues. Not all athletes, however, need this extreme ROM. Distance runners, for example, require a smaller ROM. Nevertheless, their range of motion should be adequate to allow them to run without excessive soft tissue resistance.

Insufficient data are currently available to assess the average ROMs required for different athletic activities. Normal ROMs have been determined only for healthy, nonathletic patients. Physicians, therapists, and trainers must rely on their empirical experience and knowledge of a particular sport when suggesting how far an athlete should stretch. Thus, in determining whether there is any benefit in stretching a muscle to an extreme ROM, Hubley-Kozey and Stanish (1990, 22) conclude that "most athletes do not need, and therefore should not attempt to reach, maximum or extreme ranges of motion." Furthermore, available data do not document the minimal amount of flexibility that is necessary to prevent injuries or whether a lack of flexibility predisposes one to injury.

In summarizing the research, Corbin and Noble (1980) state that a wealth of clinical data support the need for flexibility training to prevent muscle and connective tissue injuries. Furthermore, conventional wisdom suggests that shortness of muscle and connective tissue limits joint mobility and may predispose a tight muscle or connective tissue to injury. Thus, although "a wealth of empirical data on the subject is lacking, common sense suggests that adherence to lengthening (stretching) and strengthening programs for athletes, vocational or avocational, would be wise" (p. 59).

Enjoyment and Pleasure

Developing and following a flexibility training program can provide many physical and mental advantages, not the least of which are enjoyment and pleasure. Stretching is refreshing and makes you feel good, often resulting in a tingling and warm sensation. In addition, it is a simple way to both relax and reenergize. Participation in a flexibility training program also provides personal gratification received from doing so; for example, the pleasure of doing something good for yourself and the pride in accomplishing set goals.

Summary

Simply stated, *flexibility* is the range of motion available in a joint or group of joints. Flexibility is usually classified as ballistic, dynamic/functional, or static. Research indicates that flexibility is specific to particular joints or directions of movement. In addition, research has substantiated that patterns of flexibility are specific to sports groups and even within sports groups. Proponents contend that a flexibility training program can result in benefits that can be qualitative or quantitative: relaxation of stress and tension; muscular relaxation; self-discipline; improvement in body fitness, posture, and symmetry; relief of muscular cramps; relief of muscular soreness; and reduced risk of low back injury or pain. In particular, optimal flexibility increases efficiency of movement.

Chapter 2

Osteology and Arthrology

Ultimately, range of movement at a joint is restricted by both bone and joint structure. Consequently, some knowledge of the disciplines of *osteology* (the study of bones) and *arthrology* (the classification of the major joints and the movement potential of each joint) is prudent. It should be noted that conventional stretching procedures can be effective in cases where loss of motion is due to abnormal joint structure.

Just as the railroad or subway track determines the route available to the train, so the shape and contour of the articular surfaces ultimately determine the movement pathways available to bones (Steindler 1977). Obviously, these pathways are also further influenced by cartilage, ligaments, tendons, and other connective tissues that frequently serve as restraining factors. However, in this chapter we will limit our discussion to only the structure of skeletal joints. Connective tissue is the subject of chapter 4.

Classifications of Study

Virtually every bone moves at some joint. (The hyoid bone situated at the base of the tongue is an exception, since it does not articulate with any other bone). *Arthrokinesiology* is the study of the structure, function, and movement of skeletal joints (Neumann 1993). This term is derived from the combination of the word *kinesiology*, which is the science of movement, with the Greek prefix *arthro*, which means joint. *Osteokinematics* is the science that describes the motion of a rotating bone about an axis of rotation that is oriented

perpendicular to the path of the moving bone. In contrast, *arthrokinetics*, or intraarticular kinetics, describes the relative rotary and translatory movements that occur between joint surfaces (Williams et al. 1989). Therefore, it has to do with the movement of one articular surface upon another and is concerned with what happens between joint surfaces during joint movement.

Classification of Joints and Their Influence on Motion

The junction of two or more bones is an *articulation*, commonly known as a *joint*. Joints may be classified in two ways: according to the amount of movement that they allow and according to their structural composition. The simpler form of classification is based on the amount of gross movement that is available at the joint. There are three types of joints according to this classification:

- *Synarthroses*, or immovable joints
- *Amphiarthroses*, or slightly movable joints
- *Diarthroses*, or freely movable joints

Articulating bones of freely movable joints have a variety of shapes. There are six different types of joints according to classification by structural composition.

- *Ball-and-socket joints.* These joints provide the freest movement and the greatest range of motion. Specifically, movement can take place in three directions. In this type of joint, a bone with a more or less rounded head lies in a cuplike cavity or bowl-shaped socket. An example of this joint is the hip (Figure 2.1a).

• *Condyloid or ellipsoid joints.* In this type of joint, movement is permitted in two directions: flexion-extension and abduction-adduction. The surface of the articulation is oval shaped, with one bone received by an elliptical cavity on the other bone. Such an example is the wrist joint between the radius and carpal bones (Figure 2.1b).

• *Hinge joints.* This type of joint allows angular movement in only one plane. Therefore, in this joint, motion is limited to flexion and extension. This movement is similar to a door on a hinge, hence the origin of its name. Examples of hinge joints are the ankle, elbow, and knee (Figure 2.1c).

• *Pivot joints.* These joints permit a rotary movement in one axis. In this type of joint, a ring rotates around a pivot, or a pivotlike process rotates within a ring that is formed of bone and connective tissue. Rotation is the only movement possible. Examples of this kind of joint occur between the first and second cervical vertebrae (atlas and axis, respectively), where head rotation occurs on the neck, and between the radius and ulna, where forearm pronation and supination take place (Figure 2.1d).

• *Plane or gliding joints.* As the name implies, this type of joint permits gliding movements only. The facet joints of the vertebrae in the spine and the intercarpal joints of the hand are good examples. With this type of joint, the articular surfaces are nearly flat, or one may be slightly convex and the other slightly concave (Figure 2.1e).

• *Saddle joints.* This joint resembles a saddle on a horse's back, as its name implies. That is, the surface of each bone is concave in one direction, but is convex in the perpendicular direction. This joint allows movement in two directions, such as flexion-extension and abduction-adduction. The best example of this type of joint is the carpometacarpal joint at the base of the thumb (Figure 2.1f).

Types of Motion

There are six primary types of osteokinetic (voluntary or active) movement that a body segment

can pass through (see Figure 2.2). At this point, you will need to understand the proper terminology used to describe different types of motion.

Flexion

Flexion is a movement that generally decreases an angle. Flexion involves bending and folding movements, or what may be thought of as "withdrawing" movements. Examples are bending the arms at the elbow, bending the head forward as when praying, or bending the knee to press the heel toward the buttocks (see Figure 2.2a).

Extension

Extension refers to lengthening or stretching to a greater length. Therefore, whereas bending movements are flexions, straightening movements are extensions. Consequently, extension movements return a part from the flexed position to its former anatomical, or neutral, position, thus increasing the angle formed between the two segments. When extension continues beyond the anatomical position, it is called *hyperextension* (Figure 2.2b).

Abduction

Abduction refers to the movement of a body segment away from the midline of the body or of the body part to which it is attached (i.e., away from the median plane of the body). Examples of abduction are the moving of the arms or legs straight out to the sides (e.g., a jumping jack; Figure 2.2c).

Adduction

Adduction is the opposite of abduction. It refers to the movement of a body segment toward the midline of the body or of the body part to which it is attached. An example of adduction is bringing the arms back to the sides (Figure 2.2d).

Rotation

Rotation is the pivoting or moving of a body segment around its own axis. An example is holding the head in an upright position and turning it from side to side (Figure 2.2e).

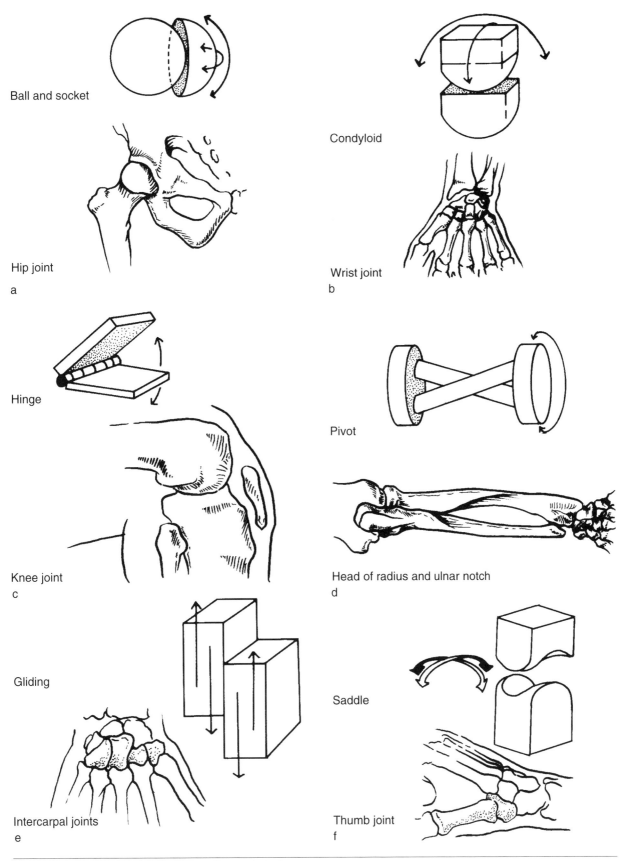

Ball and socket

Hip joint
a

Condyloid

Wrist joint
b

Hinge

Pivot

Knee joint
c

Head of radius and ulnar notch
d

Gliding

Saddle

Intercarpal joints
e

Thumb joint
f

Fig 2.1. Joints may be classified according to their shapes.
Reprinted from Loeper (1985).

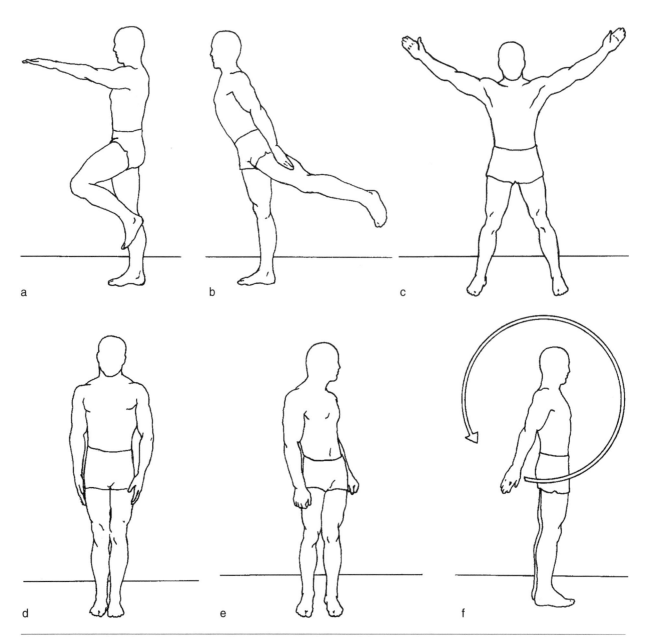

Fig. 2.2. Examples of six primary types of movement. (a) Flexion of the knee. (b) Hyperextension of the hip. (c) Abduction of the arms and legs. (d) Adduction of the arms and legs. (e) Rotation of the head and upper torso. (f) Circumduction of the arm.
Reprinted from Alter (1988).

Circumduction

Circumduction refers to movement that allows the end of the segment to describe or trace a circle. Circumduction is often a combination of flexion, abduction, extension, and adduction movements. An example is circling the arms (Figure 2.2f).

Special Movements

There are several terms to describe certain special types of movements. *Supination* refers to the outward rotation of the forearm. Thus, this movement is associated with turning the palm forward (when standing with arms at the side of the body). In contrast, *pronation* is the inward rotation of the forearm. This movement is used in turning a doorknob or a screwdriver, or when a tennis player follows through with a topspin swing.

Inversion is the turning of the sole of the foot inward, which is what often happens when a person sprains an ankle. In contrast, *eversion* involves the outward rotation of the sole of the foot.

There are other unique movements that occur

at the ankle and foot joints. *Dorsiflexion* involves bending the ankle so that the dorsum (top) of the foot comes closer to the anterior (front) surface of the shin. Conversely, *plantar flexion* involves straightening the ankle, or pointing the foot so that the foot dorsum moves away from the shin.

The last two types of special movement are *protraction* and *retraction* of the shoulder girdle. The former involves a pushing or forward motion of the shoulder, scapula, and clavicle. Protraction is exemplified during the lifting or rising phase of a push-up. In contrast, retraction commonly involves a pulling or backward motion of the shoulder, scapula, and clavicle. Examples of retraction include rowing and pulling back on a bowstring to shoot an arrow.

Bone Growth and Flexibility

Longitudinal growth occurs in bones along with the soft tissues, such as the muscles and tendons. However, during periods of rapid skeletal growth, there can be an increase in muscle-tendon tightness about the joints and a loss of flexibility. Theoretically, this increase in muscle-tendon tightness is thought to be due to the bones growing much faster than the muscles grow and stretch (Kendall and Kendall 1948; Leard 1984; Micheli 1983; Sutro 1947). Since the muscles and their respective connective tissues lag behind in growth, there is greater tension and tightness. This passive tension then stimulates the production of additional sarcomeres (the functional unit of a muscle) and a subsequent decrease in tightness. Consequently, Leard recommends that children perform stretching exercises consistently to maintain flexibility and prevent injuries.

However, a study by Pratt (1989) found no evidence of such deficits in a cross-sectional sample of 84 male students. Rather, Pratt determined that

the Tanner staging (TS) assessment (TS assessment determines sexual maturity using a rating of I [immature] to V [mature] based on assessment of pubic hair growth and pattern) had greater predictive value than age for strength and flexibility. Boys at TS II and TS III tend to be markedly less flexible than boys at TS IV and TS V!

There is also a possibility that the relative growth rate of connective tissue disproportionately exceeds that of bones—a situation that is a likely cause of *hypermobility* (Sutro 1947). That is, in certain stages of development of the skeleton, the rate of bone growth may not keep up with that of the ligamentous and capsular tissues. Thus, an excess of ligament length could lead to joint hypermobility.

Close-Packed Position and Flexibility

The *close-packed position* is defined as the final position in which "the joint surfaces become fully congruent, their area of contact is maximal, and they are tightly compressed having in a sense been 'screwed-home,' while the fibrous capsule and ligaments are maximally spiralized and tense, and no movement is possible" (Williams et al. 1989, 483). Close-packed joint surfaces can be described as having their articulating bones temporarily locked together, as if there were no joint between them. In other positions, when the articulating surfaces are not congruent and some parts of the articular capsule are lax, the joint is said to be *loose-packed*. (See Table 2.1.)

Summary

Arthrokinesiology is the study of the structure, function, and movement of skeletal joints. There

Table 2.1. Close-Packed Versus Loose-Packed Position

Joint	Close-packed position	Loose-packed position
Ankle	Dorsiflexion	Neutral
Knee	Full extension	Semiflexion
Hip	Extension + medial rotation	Semiflexion
Vertebrae	Hyperextension	Neutral
Shoulder	Abduction + lateral rotation	Semiabduction
Wrist	Hyperextension	Semiflexion

are numerous methods of classifying or describing joints and their motions, and basic knowledge of such terminology is essential if one wishes to describe a given movement with accuracy and precision. Ultimately, range of motion at a joint is restricted by both bone and joint structure.

Research has yet to determine if, during periods of rapid skeletal growth, there is an increase in muscle-tendon tightness about the joints and a loss of flexibility due to the bones growing much faster than the muscles grow and stretch.

Chapter 3

Contractile Components of Muscle: Limiting Factors of Flexibility

Skeletal muscle is one of the most highly ordered, structurally specialized cell types. In recent years, it has been increasingly recognized that striated muscle possesses a *cytoskeleton*. Cooke (1985) defines the cytoskeleton of striated muscle as "the system of regulatory components . . . [which] provide the actual physical framework for contraction" (p. 287). With Cooke's definition in mind, a significant part of this chapter will review the major lines of research regarding the myofibrillar cytoskeleton as it pertains to stretching and developing flexibility.

A General Overview of Muscles

Muscles vary in shape and size. The central portion of a whole muscle is called the *belly*. The belly comprises smaller compartments called *fasciculi*. Each fasciculus consists in turn of approximately 100 to 150 individual muscle *fibers* that range from 1 to 40 mm in length and 10 to 100 μm (micrometers) in diameter (1 millimeter equals 0.03937 in.; 1 inch equals about 25.4 mm; 1 micrometer equals 0.000039 in.). Each muscle fiber constitutes a single muscle cell. When viewed under a microscope, individual muscle fibers are seen to have a banded or striated structure. This banding pattern of the muscle fiber reflects the ultrastructural organization of each myofibril. Thus, to understand how muscles contract, relax, and elongate, we must understand the structure of the myofibril.

Composition of Myofibrils and Their Constituents

As viewed from a typical electron micrograph (Figure 3.1) and in the classical illustration (Figure 3.2), each muscle fiber is actually composed of many smaller units called *myofibrils*. Myofibrils range in diameter from 1 to 2 μm. They are grouped in clusters and run the length of the muscle fiber. In turn, each myofibril is comprised of a long, thin strand of serially linked sarcomeres (*sarco* = flesh; *mere* = unit). *Sarcomeres* represent the functional unit of a muscle. Sarcomeres measure approximately 2.3 μm in length and repeat themselves in a specific pattern in each myofibril. At the end of each sarcomere is a dense boundary, termed the Z-line (also known as the Z-band or Z-disk). The term Z-line is derived from the German word *zwischen*, meaning *between*. Thus, the segment between two successive Z-lines represents the functional unit of a myofibril.

Myofibrils are comprised of even smaller structures called *myofilaments*, or *filaments* for short. (We will use the term *filament* throughout the text.) Originally, there were thought to be two

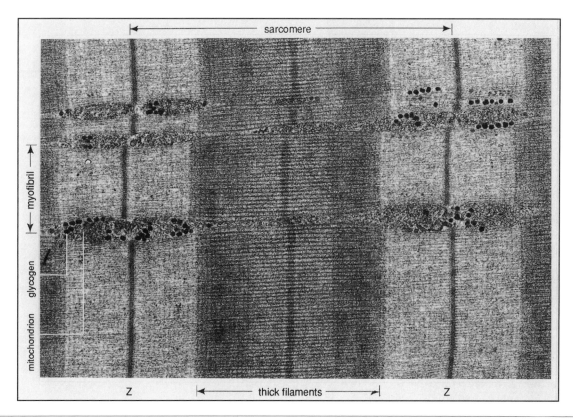

Fig. 3.1. Electron micrograph of a skeletal muscle fiber. The micrograph shows a fiber region containing several distinct myofibrils. Large variation of myofibril width is an illusion of the ultrathin sectioning method: Apparent width is greatest when the section coincides with the diameter of myofibril, less when the section is offset from its center. Reprinted from Pollack (1990).

types of filaments, one thin and one thick, that reside within the sarcomere. Based upon early research, it was determined that a typical myofibril contains about 450 thick filaments in the center of the sarcomere and about 900 thin filaments at each end of the sarcomere. From this data, it was then calculated that a single muscle fiber 10 nm in diameter and 1 cm long contains about 8,000 myofibrils and that each myofibril consists of 4,500 sarcomeres. Consequently, this results in a total of 16 billion thick and 64 billion thin filaments in a single fiber (Vander, Sherman, and Luciano 1975)! According to the sliding filament theory (discussed later), these filaments were thought to be the sole protein elements responsible for causing muscle to *contract* (shorten), *relax*, and *elongate* (stretch). However, during the 1970s and 1980s, a third connecting filament was discovered. The role of the connecting filament will be reviewed later in this chapter.

At the molecular level of analysis, the chemical composition of these three filaments can be determined. The filaments are made of protein, which is formed by a sequence of amino acids

and manufactured within the muscle cell. The synthesis of amino acids is under control of the chromosomes in the muscle cell nucleus. These chromosomes are a spiraled form of deoxyribonucleic acid (DNA), which contains the sequence of genes necessary to tell the muscle how to order the amino acids correctly. In a later section we will review how stretching theoretically modifies gene expression.

Regions of the Sarcomere

In the preceding section it was pointed out that myofibrils are characterized by alternating light and dark areas when observed with an optical microscope (see Figure 3.1). Altogether, there are five well-defined bands or zones within a sarcomere. As was previously mentioned, the Z-line or Z-disk forms the dense line at either end of the sarcomere (i.e., the terminal point of the sarcomere). With high resolution, the Z-line has a zig-

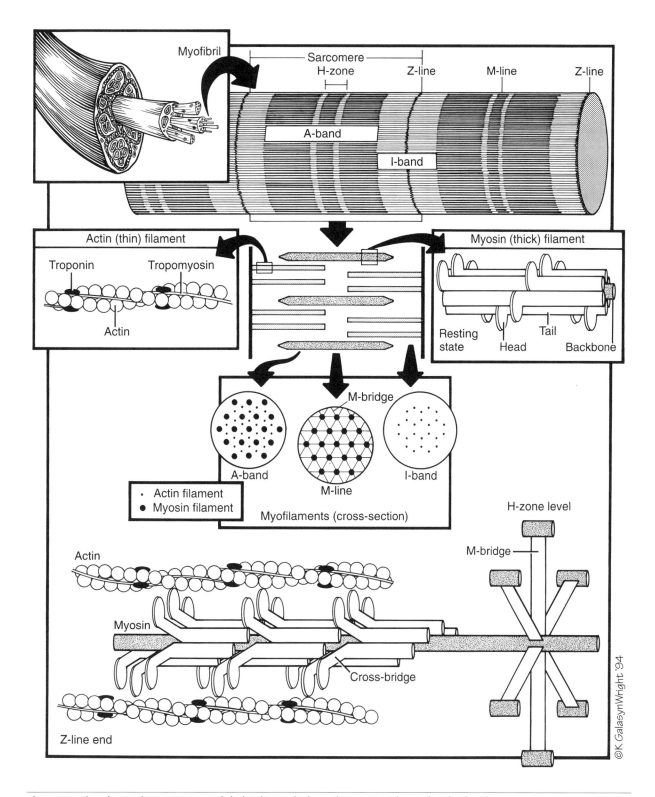

Fig. 3.2. The classical organization of skeletal muscle from the gross to the molecular level.

zag appearance. This appearance is partially because the thin filaments on either side of the Z-line are not collinear. Instead, they are offset by half the filaments' lateral separation. In Figure 3.3, one of the more popular models of the Z-line is illustrated. This two-line configuration has the capacity to accommodate substantial variation in the myofibrillar diameter by either increasing or

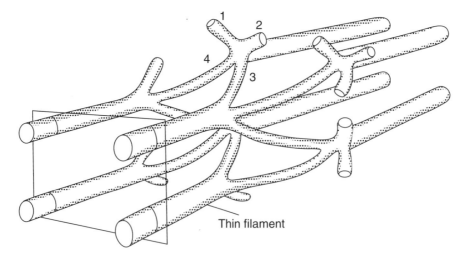

Thin filament

Fig. 3.3. Schematic model of Z-disk, including thin filament origins. Intersecting plane shows square lattice of thin filaments.
Reprinted from Pollack (1990).

decreasing the lateral separation between the filaments. This structural malleability can possibly contribute to muscle's pliability.

Adjacent to the Z-line is the *I-band*, an optically less dense band of the muscle striations. When passed through the muscle's I-band, the velocity of the emerging light is *isotropic* (the same in all directions). Hence, the band's name. The I-band contains actin filaments, titin filaments, and I-bridges. The I-band measures approximately 1.5 μm in length. The dark areas of the sarcomere are called *A-bands*. This region is so called because a light wave passing through the A-band is *anisotropic* (its velocity is not equal in all directions). The A-bands measure approximately 1.0 μm and correspond to the length of the thick filaments (see later section on myosin). The center of each A-band is occupied by a relatively less dense and lighter area, the *H-zone*. The H-zone is found between the tips of the thin filaments. Hence, its size depends on the muscle length, or the extent of overlap of the filaments. Last, there is the *M-line*. This dense, transverse structure is found at the center of the sarcomere, corresponding to several closely spaced, parallel M-bridges.

Ultrastructure of the Thin Filament: Actin

The thin filament is called *actin*. Actin has a diameter of about 5 or 6 nm and a length of about 1 μm. At low resolution, this filament resembles a two-stranded pearl necklace with the strands twisting about one another (see Figure 3.2). The twisting pattern of the two strands is not regular, as once thought; it is semirandom (Egelman, Francis, and Derosier 1982). Actin is not the sole component of the thin filament. In or alongside the filament lie several additional proteins (some with more certainty than others), including nebulin, troponin, and tropomyosin. These proteins serve to regulate the binding of the filaments.

Ultrastructure of the Thick Filament: Myosin

The thick filament is *myosin* (see Figure 3.2). It measures about 10 to 15 nm in diameter and about 1.5 μm in length. Hence, it is thicker and shorter than the actin filament. Myosin filaments are unique in that they possess numerous short lateral projections or rods that extend toward the actin filaments. These projections are collectively referred to as *cross-bridges* and are the sites of binding between the actin and myosin filaments that produce muscle tension. Later in this chapter, we will examine in more detail the function of these projections.

The Myosin Head

Research has found that the HMM also can be cleaved into two subfragments, S-1 and S-2. The S-2 subfragment is the segment of the myosin rod situated between the head and the distal segment of the rod. In contrast, the S-1 subfragment is the segment of the myosin molecule comprising the head. The S-1 subfragment, in turn, is thought to be further made up of *light chains* and *heavy chains*. Each heavy-chain segment lying within the head is divisible into three fractions. The functional significance of this division is not yet clear. In addition to the heavy chain, each head contains two, sometimes three, light chains. Research has confirmed that these light chains play a role in molecular binding and ordering of the heads (Chowrashi, Pemrick, and Pepe 1989).

The Myosin Tail

Through exposure to certain enzymes, the myosin molecule can be cleaved into several fragments or subfragments. When analyzed in greater detail, the myosin molecule is seen to consist of two parts: a tail and a head (see Figure 3.2). The *tail* is often referred to as the rod or rod region of the myosin molecule. This segment of the myosin molecule, consisting of the distal end of the myosin rod, is also known as *light meromyosin* (LMM). The LMM does not have the ability to interdigitate or bind with the actin filament. Connected to the LMM is *heavy meromyosin* (HMM). This component of the myosin molecule comprises the proximal segment of the rod and the head. In contrast to the LMM, the HMM possesses the ability to interdigitate with actin.

Ultrastructure of the Connecting or Gap Filament: Titin

As pointed out earlier, the contemporary two-filament sarcomere model proposed by H.E. Huxley

and Hanson (1954) as well as by A.F. Huxley and Niedergerke (1954) suggested that muscle shortened due to the binding and movement of the actin and myosin filaments. The two sets of discontinuous, inextensible filaments move or slide across each other, varying their degree of overlap while undergoing no change in filament length themselves. However, if one looks at the classic illustration of the organization of a sarcomere (see Figure 3.2), two puzzling questions come to mind: (1) How is it that the myosin filaments appear to float? and (2) What is holding the sarcomere together?

The structure of the sarcomere seems almost illogical. Yet a consistent feature of muscle is the myosin's central position in the sarcomere, midway between the Z-lines. This position is maintained even when the sarcomere is stretched. What is it that keeps the myosin centered? The answer is the presence of a connecting filament, which is now known as *titin* (see Figures 3.4 and 3.5). These connecting filaments are only now becoming more well known. Up until the early 1990s, they had been ignored in most textbooks of physiology, histology, and even anatomy. Yet they are well studied and apparently uncontroversial. According to Maruyama (1986), one reason they were neglected was "the lack of a clear-cut image of the compatibility of the third filament model with the sliding theory of muscle contraction" (p. 83). Hence, at this time, it may be appropriate to digress and review in detail the history of this important filament.

Titin's Structure

Several years after its identification, Wang (1985) began a detailed biochemical analysis of the protein connectin. Wang's research indicated that connectin was composed of two proteins: titin and nebulin. To date, titin is the largest protein identified, with a subunit molecular mass of 2.5

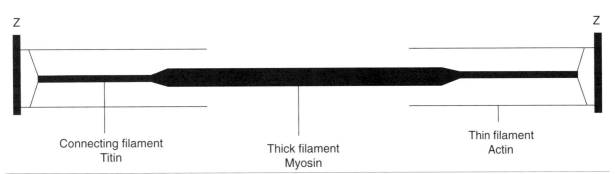

Fig. 3.4.   Schematic diagram illustrating the arrangement of the sarcomere's basic structural elements.
Reprinted from Pollack (1990).

Discovering Titin

Titin has a long history of doubt, neglect, and revival (Maruyama 1986; Pollack 1990; Figure 3.5). The first three-filament model incorporating an elastic filament was proposed by H.E. Huxley and Hanson (1954; Figure 3.5a). They hypothesized the existence of *S-filaments*, described as fine, extensible filaments that linked up the ends of the actin filaments. However, the S-filament was not included in their final two-filament sarcomere model (Page and Huxley 1963). Several years later, A.F. Huxley and Peachey (1961; Figure 3.5d) mentioned in their study the possible presence of "fine filaments" connecting the ends of both the myosin and actin filaments from their observations of highly stretched muscle fibers. In that same year, Carlsen, Knappels, and Buchthal (1961) reported seeing filamentary structures in the "gap space" between overly stretched actin and myosin filaments. In 1962, Sjostrand also observed very thin filaments at the gap region between the myosin and actin filaments when muscle was extremely stretched beyond the overlap of the two sets of filaments. Sjostrand (1962) called these filaments that were thinner than actin filaments "gap filaments" and assumed that they were continuous with the tapered ends of the myosin filaments. This finding was also confirmed by Page and Huxley (1963).

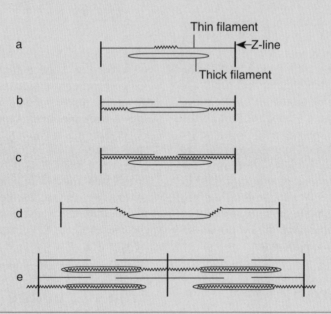

Fig. 3.5. Schematic diagrams of several three-filament sarcomere models. Reprinted from Wang (1985).

In this same period, Auber and Couteaux (1962, 1963; Figure 3.5b) described the myosin filaments of the insect flight muscle to be connected to the Z-lines by means of a second kind of thin filament. Pringle (1967) later designated these "C-filaments." However, at this same time McNeil and Hoyle (1967; Figure 3.5c) discerned from photographs the presence of "superthin" filaments. These were thought to run parallel to the thick and thin filaments and continue from Z-line to Z-line. They were called "T-filaments" to emphasize their thinness. Again, similar findings were published by Walcott and Ridgeway (1967). Then, in 1968, a symposium on muscles was held at which various three-filament models were discussed with no apparent resolution (Wang 1984).

The question of the existence of the third filament lay dormant until the mid-1970s, when a series of highly interesting and revealing papers were published by Locker and Leet (1975, 1976a, 1976b) and by Locker, Daines, and Leet (1976). Their papers detailed the behavior of gap filaments in highly stretched beef muscle. Eventually, these became known as "G-filaments" (Figure 3.5e). Figure 3.6a, b, and c is a series of exquisite photographs clearly displaying the presence of these connecting filaments.

(Continued next page)

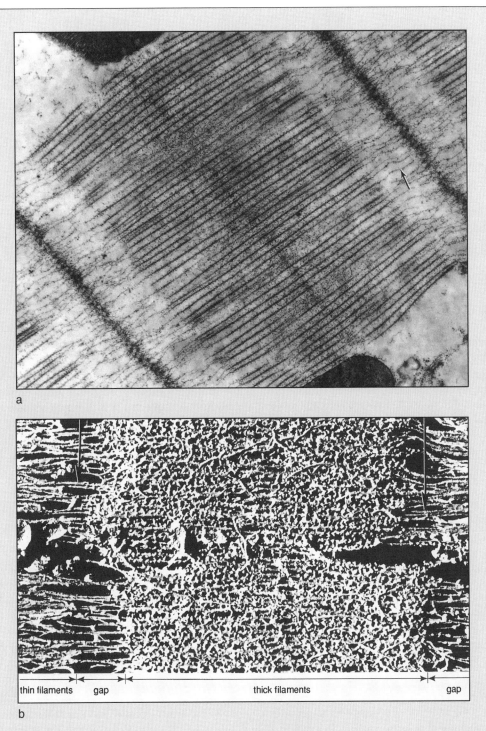

a

b

(continued)

Fig. 3.6. (a) Direct evidence for connecting filaments in flight muscle of honeybee. During fixation, thin filaments were depolymerized and washed away. Connecting filaments remain intact and visible (arrow). Photo by Trombitas and Tigyi-Sebes. (b) Examples of connectin filaments (titin). Overstretched frog muscle, prepared by freeze-fracture, deep-etch method. Thick filaments (center) do not terminate; they give way to thinner "connecting" filaments (arrows), which run out of the field toward the Z-line. Thin-filament tips, seen at edges of figure, do not overlap the thick filaments. Photo by M.E. Cantino and G.H. Pollack.

(Continued next page)

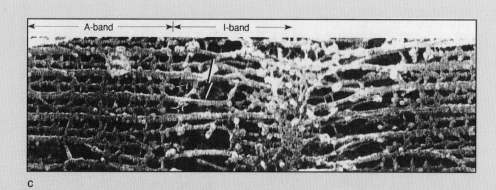

Fig. 3.6. (continued) (c) Freeze-fracture image of honeybee flight muscle in rigor. Thin filaments dislodged from Z-line (arrowheads). Connecting filaments are visible in the I-band (arrow).
Reprinted from Pollack (1990).

In 1976, Maruyama, Natori, and Nonomura began pursuing the question of muscle elasticity. They were able to isolate an elastic protein from myofibrils that was clearly distinguishable from elastin or collagen. Maruyama (1976) proposed to call the intracellular elastic protein *connectin.* One year later, the connectin structure was determined to be responsible for mechanical continuity and tension transmission in striated muscle (Maruyama et al. 1977).

Independently, Wang, Ash, and Singer (1975) attempted to find a smooth-muscle filament protein in striated muscles. Instead, Wang accidentally discovered three high-molecular weight proteins. Wang, McClure, and Tu (1979) tentatively named this protein *titin*, a name derived from Greek referring to a giant deity or anything of great size. Eventually, Maruyama and colleagues (1981) confirmed that Wang's titin was identical to connectin. Thus, after almost 20 years of research, the sarcomere's third filament was identified.

to 3.0 daltons (Maruyama et al. 1984; Kurzban and Wang 1988). Titin constitutes about 10% of myofibril mass (Trinick, Knight, and Whiting 1984). Wang, Ramirez-Mitchell, and Palter 1984.

Research indicates that each titin molecule extends from the Z-line (the end of the sarcomere) to the M-line (the center of the sarcomere) (Furst et al. 1988; Itoh et al. 1988; Wang, Wright, and Ramirez-Mitchell 1985; Whiting, Wardale, and Trinick 1989). In addition, these studies indicate that the A-band portion (the dark areas of a sarcomere) of titin is firmly bound to the thick filament. Hence, when the sarcomere is stretched, the region of the titin molecule found in the A-band behaves as if it were rigidly bound to the thick filaments. In contrast, the region of the titin molecule that links to the Z-lines behaves elastically. It is this elasticity or stretchability that is so critical to our understanding of the nature of flexibility. Herein may lie one of the elusive answers to the mystery of why some muscles possess flexibility and others are more stiff. Needless to say, as our technology improves, we will come to understand more about the complexities of the body as they relate to this topic.

What Makes the Titin Filament So Elastic?

There are several factors that theoretically contribute to titin's tremendous extensibility. First, titin is rich in the amino acid *proline*, which breaks the alpha-helical chains that ordinarily confer rigidity on polypeptides (Pollack 1990). Second, as a consequence, a single titin molecule does not contain any alpha-helical structure. Instead, it consists of *random coils* (Trinick, Knight, and Whiting 1984). Third, a single peptide of 3 million daltons could have a length up to 7.0 μm. However, at rest a sarcomere's length is about 2.4 μm, and at extreme stretch it is 7.0 μm. Based on this data, it has been suggested that titin must be *compactly folded* within a sarcomere (Maruyama 1986). Thus, when stretch is initially applied to muscle, the segment of titin between the end of the myosin filament and the Z-line is the primary contributor to the increased sarcomere length (Trombitas et al. 1993). Once the limit of this titin segment's length is reached, recruitment of additional segments of titin that are "folded" or somehow attached to the myosin filament accounts for an extra increase in length (Wang et al. 1991). However, this structure has its limits.

Regulation of Muscle Extensibility

At this point, several critical questions need to be raised. First, what regulates muscle extensibility? Second, can the factor(s) regulating this muscle extensibility be modified to enhance one's flexibility? Wang et al. (1991) investigated this first issue. Their research found that the length and size of titin appears to be an important factor in determining when sarcomeres will develop resting tension upon stretch and where the sarcomere will yield under stress. For example, muscles that express larger titin *isoforms* (structural variants) tend to initiate tension at a longer sarcomere length and to reach their elastic limit at higher sarcomere lengths. Also, muscles that express the longest titin develop the lowest tension. Their research also concluded that different muscle groups express various types of titin isoforms and thus exhibit various stress-strain curves.

Thus, the data suggested "skeletal muscle cells may control and modulate stiffness and elastic limit coordinately by selective expression of specific titin isoforms" (Wang et al. 1991, 7101). It is interesting that observed anatomical variations in titin isoforms have been reported in muscles from various regions of the body (Akster, Granzier, and Focant 1989; C. Hill and Weber 1986; Horowits 1992; Hu, Kimura, and Maruyama 1986; Wang and Wright 1988).

The pertinent question is: Can training influence the specific titin isoforms? To date, no research has been carried out in this arena. But it would make a fascinating and intriguing study to compare and contrast the titin isoforms in identical muscle groups among performers involved in various disciplines, such as ballet, rhythmic gymnastics, and weightlifting. Then, if differences were found, it would be prudent to identify what type of stretching program could most efficiently and safely be implemented to enhance the optimal titin isoform production. This issue leads to another crucial question: Does the body possess critical periods of titin isoform modification, that is, periods during development when titin is being manufactured and its structure can be modified? It is tempting to speculate that the earlier one starts on a stretching program, the greater the titin isoform modification.

Another significant factor that has been recently investigated is the relationship between titin degradation and various neuromuscular diseases such as Schwartz-Jampel syndrome (Soussi-Yanicostas et al. 1991) and Duchenne muscular dystrophy (DMD). Matsumura and colleagues (1989) are of the opinion that the degradation of titin "even though secondary, is presumed to play an important role in the pathogenesis of myofibrillar degeneration in DMD" (p. 147). Last, another important issue that needs to be investigated is the influence of various medications upon titin isoforms.

Perhaps of greater significance is the question: Does titin isoform modification occur as a result of trauma? If so, how does the body react in the case of a macrotrauma, as in a car accident? Similarly, can isoform modifications develop due to microtraumatic insults, such as long-term poor posture? Of equal importance, clinical research needs to be carried out on the effects of immobilization or reduced movement on titin isoforms.

Function of Titin

Currently, titin is thought to serve two major functions, although this does not mean that other functions do not exist. First, since the elastic elements link each end of the thick filament to the Z-line, the titin filaments are in a position to produce resting tension—a tension that is present when the muscle fiber is at its normal physiological length and that increases as a relaxed fiber is elongated—as well as to provide a force that tends to center the thick filaments within the sarcomere (Horowits 1992). Second, it is speculated that titin plays a role in the morphogenesis of the myofibril (Fulton and Isaacs 1991; Pollack 1990). Models of the sarcomere's assembly have been suggested, but details of the chronology need to be substantiated (Pollack 1990).

Sarcomere Structural Bridges

Not only is the myofibrillar sarcomere held together in the axial direction, it must also be supported in the transverse direction. For example, something must protect a muscle when it is squeezed or sat upon (as are the gluteals). The source of the transverse resistance that maintains the sarcomere's integrity are three bridgelike

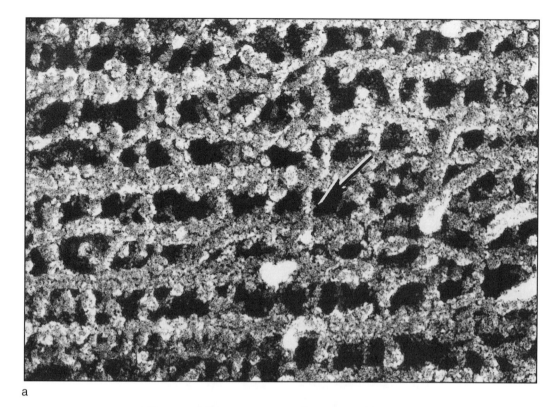

a

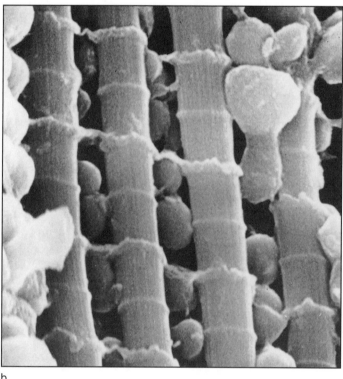

b

Fig. 3.7.   (a) Runglike interconnections between thick filaments. (b) Scanning electron micrograph of honeybee flight muscle. Cylindrically shaped myofibrils run horizontally. Bloblike structures between myofibrils are mitochondria. Lateral interconnections are seen at the level of the Z-line (arrow). Photo by K. Trombitas.
Reprinted from Pollack (1990).

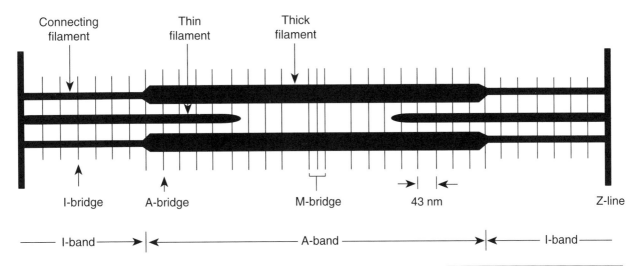

Fig. 3.8. Diagrammatic summary of the sarcomere's principal structures. Reprinted from Pollack (1990).

structures: the M-bridges, A-bridges, and I-bridges (see Figures 3.7, and 3.8).

M-Bridges

In the center of some muscles, the organizing center of the sarcomere contains transverse interconnections between the thick filaments. These runglike structures that interconnect neighboring thick filaments at their midregions are termed *M-bridges*. Their function is to help organize and stabilize the filament lattice (Pollack 1990). However, something in addition to the M-bridges must help to stabilize the filament lattice since some muscles lack M-bridges (Pollack 1990). These structures are the A-bridges and I-bridges.

A-Bridges

For some time, it has been recognized that an additional structure must be present to organize and stabilize the myosin filaments. If not, the filaments would pull apart and suffer serious misalignment. What is the mechanism responsible for maintaining the lattice organization? In 1983, Pollack revealed that the interconnections had been apparent in numerous published electron micrographs, though their significance had not been appreciated at the time. More recent systematic investigations, especially with the high-resolution freeze-fracture method, have revealed the runglike structures with new and unanticipated clarity (Baatsen, Trombitas, and Pollack 1988;

Magid et al. 1984; Pollack 1990; Suzuki and Pollack 1986;). These runglike interconnections between adjacent, parallel thick filaments have been termed *A-bridges* (Suzuki & Pollack 1986).

I-Bridges

Another bridge structure that has been recently identified is the *I-bridge*. The I-bridge is a runglike interconnection that spans the gap between connecting (i.e., titin) and thin (i.e., actin) filaments. These bridges were noted over 20 years ago by Franzini-Armstrong (1970) and then again by Reedy (1971) but did not receive much attention. More recent research has confirmed the structure. It is postulated that the I-bridge is built of troponin. Unfortunately, there is much that we do not know about this structure. In the meantime, it is suggested that the function of these struts is to confer lateral stability and maintain separation of the filaments (Pollack 1990).

The Sarcomere's Principal Structures: A Working Model

A schematized model of the sarcomere's principal structures is seen in Figure 3.8 (Pollack 1990). Today we know that a sarcomere contains at least three longitudinally oriented structures: actin

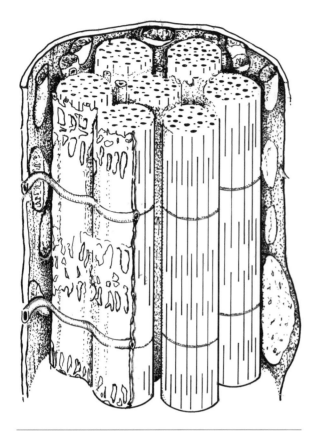

Fig. 3.9. The sarcotubular system.
Reprinted from Fawcett (1986).

(thin filaments), myosin (thick filaments), and titin (connecting filaments). In addition, the sarcomere contains at least two transverse interconnections, not only between thick filaments in the A-band (M- and A-bridges), but between connecting filaments in the I-band (I-bridges). Other possible filaments or structures may also be present, but have yet to be identified.

The Sarcotubular System

The *sarcotubular system* consists of two components (see Figure 3.9). The first part is the *sarcoplasmic reticulum*. It envelops each of the contractile elements of the sarcomeres and is the site of calcium storage. The second component is the *T-system*. The T-system derives its name from the fact that it consists of tubules that run across or transversely into the sarcoplasm (i.e., the cytoplasm and protoplasm of the sarcomere). At the Z-line between sarcomeres, the two portions of the sarcoplasmic reticulum associated with each sarcomere come in close contact with a transverse tubule of the T-system to form a *triad*. The basic

function of the T-system is communication. When the sarcolemma (i.e., the sarcomere's tubular sheath or cell membrane) is excited by an incoming nerve impulse, it undergoes *depolarization*. Simultaneously, the entire T-system also depolarizes, thus communicating an electrical impulse to all sarcomeres in the muscle fiber.

The impulse is then transmitted to a sleevelike system of sacs and tubules of the sarcoplasmic reticulum, where calcium ions are stored. When the T-system depolarizes, this electrical charge is transmitted to the membrane of the sarcoplasmic reticulum, causing it to become more permeable. As a result, calcium ions escape from the sacs of the reticulum.

Theory of Contraction

The function of muscle is to develop or generate tension. This process of tension generation is called *contraction*. The primary function of muscular contraction is to produce movement. Two other essential functions associated with contraction are to maintain posture and to produce body heat. Once a muscular contraction is initiated, a reversible chain of physical and chemical events is set into motion.

Ultrastructural (Physical) Basis of Contraction

The mechanism by which muscles contract, relax, or elongate can be explained by the ultrastructure of the sarcomere. The most well-known theory is the sliding filament theory (see Figure 3.10, a-c). It asserts that the changes in sarcomere length are mediated exclusively by relative sliding of thick and thin filaments. The exact mechanism that regulates the contractile elements, however, is not yet completely understood, and Pollack (1983, 1990), for example, asserted that the theory does not stand on firm ground. "Few of the theory's central predictions are confirmed, and many are badly contradicted by experimental evidence" (Pollack 1990, 35). A more recent hypothesis that has received some attention and interest suggests that periods of sarcomere shortening are punctuated by pauses during which there is little or no length change, conferring a stairlike character on the shortening waveform (Pollack et al. 1977). Of greater interest to us, similar steps are thought to occur during lengthening.

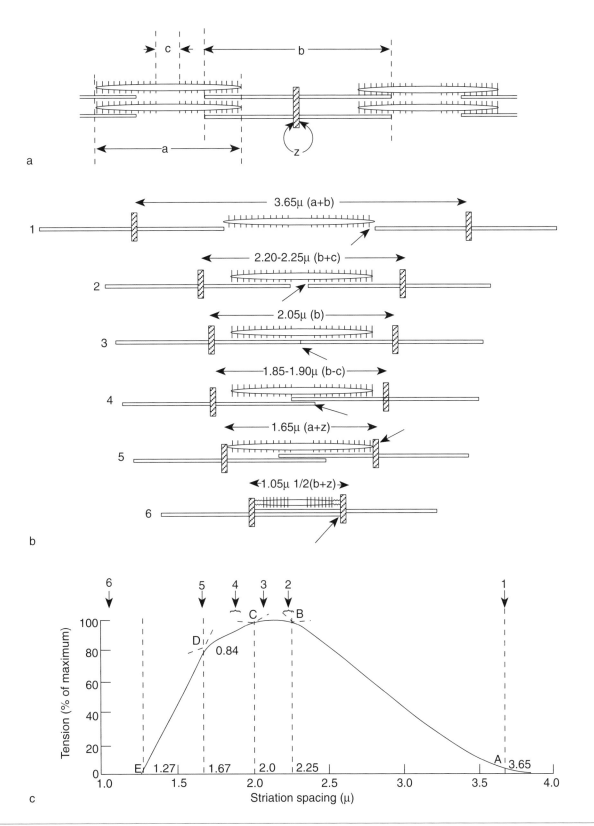

Fig. 3.10. (a) Schematic summary of the variation of tetanus tension with striation spacing. The arrows along the top are placed opposite the striation spacing at which the critical stages of overlap of filaments occur, numbered as in (c). (b) Schematic diagram of filaments, indicating nomenclature for the relevant dimensions. (c) Critical stages in the increase of overlap between thick and thin filaments as a sarcomere shortens.
Reprinted from Gordon, Huxley, and Julian (1966).

When maximally contracted, a sarcomere may shorten from 20% to 50% of its resting length. When passively stretched, it may extend to about 120% of its normal length. Careful microscopic measurements of the length of the A-bands and I-bands from intact muscle in the contracted, relaxed, and elongated states have conclusively proved that the A-bands, and thus the thick filaments, always remain constant in length. Similarly, the distance between the Z-line and the edge of the H-zone also remains constant at all stages of a normal contraction, indicating that the thin actin filaments likewise undergo no change in length. Based on these observations, researchers have concluded that change in muscle length must be due to the sliding of the thick and thin filaments along each other.

Thus, when a muscle contracts, the actin and myosin filaments slide over each other so that each fiber shortens (i.e., the sliding filament theory). For this process to occur, the Z-line of the sarcomere must be drawn in toward the A-band, resulting in the gradual narrowing and eventual elimination of the I-bands and H-zone. The question that is now being debated in the scientific community is whether or not sarcomeres shorten in steps, punctuated by pauses (A.F. Huxley 1984, 1986; Pollack 1986, 1990).

Molecular (Chemical) Basis of Contraction

The immediate source of energy for muscular contraction is the breakdown of the compound adenosine triphosphate (ATP), which is triggered by nerve impulses. When nerve impulses arrive at a skeletal muscle fiber, they spread over its sarcolemma and move inward via its T-tubules. This increases the permeability and triggers the release of *calcium ions* (Ca^{2+}) from the sacs of the sarcoplasmic reticulum in the sarcoplasm. In the resting state, tropomyosin molecules are believed to lie on top of active sites on the actin filaments, preventing binding on the myosin cross-bridges and actin filament. Once Ca^{2+} are released, they bind with the troponin molecules on the actin filament. This is referred to as the "turning on" of active sites on the actin filament. Simultaneously, the uncharged ATP cross-bridge complex is charged, permitting the actin and myosin to form an actomyosin complex. This activates an enzyme component of the myosin filament called myosin ATPase. Myosin ATPase breaks down ATP into ADP and P_i (inorganic phosphate) with the

release of energy. This release of energy allows the cross-bridges to swivel to a new angle and slide over the myosin filament toward the center of the sarcomere. Consequently, the muscle shortens and develops tension. Thus, it is apparent that muscles are completely subservient to nerve impulses for activation. Without a nerve impulse, no muscular tension can be generated.

Theory of Muscular Relaxation

The ability of muscle to relax is essential for optimal movement and health. Hence, the process of muscular relaxation has been studied intensively at both the physical and chemical levels. Like contraction, the exact mechanism of relaxation is not yet fully understood. The physical and chemical basis of relaxation will be analyzed in the following sections.

Ultrastructural (Physical) Basis of Relaxation

Muscular relaxation is completely passive. When muscle fibers no longer receive nerve impulses, they relax. Thus, relaxation is basically a cessation of the production of muscular tension. As the cross-bridges detach and separate at relaxation, the internal elastic force that accumulated within the filaments during contraction is released. Thus, the recoil of the elastic components is what restores the myofibrils to their uncontracted lengths (Gowitzke and Milner 1988). A second possible restoring force could arise from the overlapping thin filaments, which repel one another because of their similar net charge. It is suggested that "such restoring forces may be more than mere luxuries; they reduce the energetic cost of relaxation" (Pollack 1990, 142). In addition, the elasticity of the connective tissues in the tendons, which attach the ends of the muscle to the bone, restores the muscle to its original length.

Molecular (Chemical) Basis of Relaxation

The chemical reactions associated with relaxation are not yet fully understood. Most scientists believe that relaxation is brought about by a reversal of the contraction process. In relaxation, *calcium-troponin* combinations separate, and the calcium ions reenter the sacs of the sarcoplasmic reticulum. Because the troponin is no longer bound to the calcium, it inhibits the actin and myosin from interacting. This inhibition allows for dissociation of actin and myosin and "resliding" of the filaments back to their resting positions. In short, contraction is turned on by the release of calcium and turned off by its withdrawal.

Theory of Muscular Elongation

Muscular fibers are incapable of lengthening or stretching themselves. For lengthening to occur, a force must be received from outside the muscle itself. Among these forces are gravity, momentum (motion), the force of antagonistic muscles on the opposite side of the joint, and the force provided by another person or by some part of one's own body. The latter can be accomplished by a pushing or pulling motion, either manually or through the use of special equipment.

The theoretical limitation of the response to stretch by a muscle cell's contractile component, based on the sliding filament theory, can be determined by microscopic measurements of the length of the sarcomere, the myosin filaments, the actin filaments, and the H-zone. For the purposes of this text, we will look more closely at sarcomere elongation in comparison to resting lengths (see Table 3.1).

Table 3.1. Resting Length of Contractile Components

Sarcomere	2.30 µm
Myosin	1.50 µm
Actin	2.00 µm
H-zone	0.30 µm

When a sarcomere is maximally stretched to the point of rupture, it can reach a length of approximately 3.60 µm. A rupture of the sarcomere, however, is undesirable. Our main concern is to stretch the sarcomere to a length at which there is a slight overlap of the filaments, with at least one cross-bridge maintained between the actin and myosin filaments. This length has been found to be approximately 3.50 µm. Thus, with the sarcomere's resting length 2.30 µm, the contractile component of the sarcomere is capable of increasing 1.20 µm. This represents an incredible increase of over 50% from the resting state. If the sarcomere's resting length is 2.10 µm and all other factors remain constant, the contractile component of the muscle can then increase by 67% of its resting length. This extensibility enables our muscles to move through a wide range of motion. In chapters 4 through 6, we will examine how connective tissues and the nervous system (e.g., muscle spindles) interact with muscle to limit range of motion.

Sliding Filament Theory

According to the original sliding filament theory, the thick and thin filaments merely slide further apart when a sarcomere is stretched. During this change in sarcomere length, neither the thick nor thin filaments change length. There is simply less overlap between them (see Figure 3.10). However, we now know that the mechanism by which the sarcomere elongates is more complex than originally hypothesized. Something, for example, must ultimately prevent sarcomere overextension. This protective mechanism is accomplished by the connecting filament.

Previous structural studies indicate that each titin filament in the sarcomere consists of two segments. The segment between the Z-line and the edge of the A-band has been found to be pliant and extensible. In contrast, the remaining segment that overlaps with the thick filaments has been determined to be stiff and inextensible. Based on this research, several illustrated working models have been developed. In Pollack's model (1990; Figure 3.11), the connecting filament is hypothesized to absorb stretch in two of its elements: tropomyosin and titin. At first, stretch comes easily (Figure 3.11, a and b). During this low level of stretch, the tropomyosin recrystallizes (a phase transition during which a regular, crystalline state is restored from an amorphous state) and confers a little static force to the sarcomere. At this stage, the titin is not extended to the point at which its retractile force is appreciable. Consequently, the sarcomere extends without much difficulty. As the stretch continues, all of the tropomyosin will crystallize. As a result, the tropomyosin strand becomes rigidly inextensible and the sarcomere can no longer be stretched. Thus, it is thought that the tropomyosin maintains the sarcomere within its working length range (Figure 3.11c).

However, even this restrictive system has its limits. With continued elongation, the tropomyosin strand ruptures (Figure 3.11d), and remnants of the torn tropomyosin strand shrivel up against natural foci such as the A-I junction or the Z-lines. However, the tearing of the tropomyosin strand does not spell death for the sarcomere. A backup system stands ready to maintain the sarcomere's integrity during repair: the titin strand (Figure 3.11d).

Shortly after Pollack's 1990 text was published, a new model was developed based on a series of experiments. In the model of Wang et al. (1991), as the sarcomere extends, the extensible segment of titin takes up the early displacement via its elongation. With increasing elongation, the extensible segment becomes longer by recruiting previously inextensible titin when its anchorage to thick filaments starts to slip or when the distal ends of the thick filaments become distorted (Figure 3.12). Eventually, further elongation will result in breakage of the titin strand.

In a sense, titin can be conceptualized as being the scaffold or template of the sarcomere. If it ruptures, then the sarcomere's integrity is compromised. As an analogy, in the Pollack model, the tropomyosin can be compared to a railroad car and the titin to the railroad track. If a railroad car (i.e., tropomyosin) falls off the railroad track, all is not lost. The train needs only to be remounted onto the railroad track. However, if the railroad track is severed, even getting the train back on the rails won't make a difference. Similarly, it is the titin that keeps the sarcomere intact.

In this section, we have dealt almost exclusively with the relationship of stretch and the sarcomere's filaments. However, the reader must keep in mind that the most important component of muscle related to flexibility is the connective tissue that envelops and surrounds the muscle at its various levels of organization (i.e., muscle fiber, bundle, and whole muscle). These tissues are the endomysium, perimysium, and epimysium, explored in chapter 4.

Other Limitations to Range of Motion

There are several factors which may limit a joint's range of motion including improper muscle balance, inadequate muscle control, the age of the muscle, and whether the muscle is immobilized.

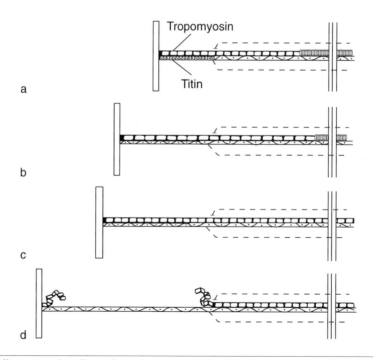

Fig. 3.11. Schematic illustrating the effect of stretch on connecting-filament extension. Once the strand of tropomyosin is fully crystallized (c) further extension can occur only if the strand tears. (Dotted lines indicate thick filaments.) Reprinted from Pollack (1990).

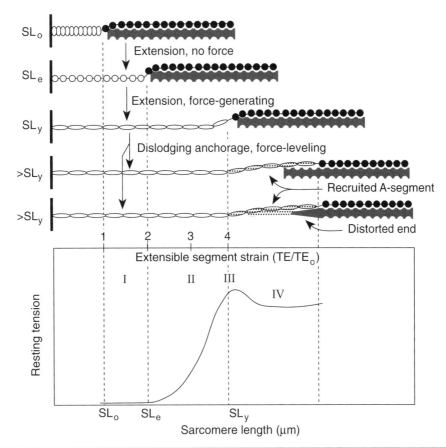

Fig. 3.12. Segmental extension of titin filaments as the structural basis of stress-strain curves of resting muscles. The postulated structural events of the titin filaments that underlie the stress-strain curves are shown. The titin filament that extends from the Z-line to the M-line consists of two mechanically distinct segments: an extensible segment in the I-band (open symbols) and an inextensible segment that is constrained by interaction with thick filaments (solid symbols). At slack sarcomere length (SL_o), titin may be flaccid, and stretching to SL_e causes no net change in contour length and generates no significant force. Beyond SL_e, a linear extension of titin segment generates an exponential increase in tension. At SL_y, the extensible segment becomes longer by recruiting previously inextensible titin when its anchorage to thick filaments starts to slip or when distal ends of thick filaments become distorted, resulting in the leveling of tension. The net contour length of the extensible segment of titin is thought to be longer in a sarcomere expressing a larger titin isoform. As a consequence, SL_e and SL_y increase, and the stress-strain curves of various muscles can be plotted as a function of extensible segmental strain of titin (TE/TE_0).
Reprinted from Wang, McCarter, Wright, Beverly, and Ramirez-Mitchell (1991).

Improper Muscle Balance

Healthy muscles maintain a structural homeostasis. A key to this structural balance is an equal pull by antagonistic, or opposing, muscles located on the opposite side of the joint (see Figure 3.13). An imbalance in these forces can affect range of motion. Muscle imbalance can be due to several factors, including the presence of *hypertonic muscles* (i.e., muscles in a state of contracture or spasm) or weak muscles. Treatment in such cases is to strengthen the weak muscle and stretch the shortened muscle.

Inadequate Muscle Control

Even if a person is endowed with natural flexibility and suppleness, local muscular control may still be inadequate to execute specific flexibility skills. This is because many flexibility skills are composed of additional components. For our purposes, *muscular control* is considered to be the presence of adequate balance, coordination, or control of one's body part(s), or sufficient muscular strength to perform a given skill. As an example, to perform a skill as delicate and elegant as an arabesque (scale) in ballet, one must have

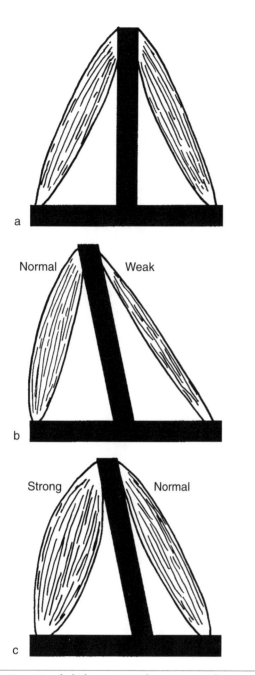

Fig. 3.13. Muscle balance. (a) Balance in muscle gives structural balance. (b) Balance is most often lost because one muscle is weak. (c) Sometimes balance is lost because a muscle is too strong.
Reprinted from Walther (1981).

Effects of Aging on Muscle

The normal aging process brings about an almost imperceptible diminution in normal muscle functions, including muscular strength, endurance, agility, and flexibility. When complicated by the deconditioning of inactivity, disease, and injury, these functions decline rapidly. Physiologically, one of the most conspicuous degenerative changes associated with aging is the progressive *atrophy*, or wasting away, of muscle mass. This loss is due to the reduction in both size and number of the muscle fibers (Grob 1983; E. Gutmann 1977; Hooper 1981; Rockstein and Sussman 1979). According to Wilmore (1991, 236), "This decrease in sarcomere number may contribute to the reduced mobility commonly associated with old age." The age at which these changes in the muscles begin is highly variable. These changes also vary in degree depending on the muscles involved and their degree of use as one grows older. The number of nerve cells in the musculoskeletal system also decreases with age (E. Gutmann 1977).

Last, as muscle fibers atrophy, replacement by fatty and fibrous (collagen) tissue occurs. Collagen, the chief component in connective tissue, has an extremely low compliance. This low compliance implies that small increases in the quantity of collagen in a muscle would increase the stiffness of the tissue considerably. This phenomenon was investigated by Alnaqeeb, Al Zaid, and Goldspink (1984), using the soleus and extensor digitorum longus muscles of rats. Their research confirmed that total collagen content increased continuously with age. Furthermore, the investigation revealed in young muscle a lower rate of passive tension development for every unit increase in length. In contrast, the adult muscle developed passive tension at a higher rate.

> The data for the stiffness of the muscles and those for connective tissue are in accord [with one another] at the ages studied, with the exception of the soleus in the senile animal. With this exception, the passive mechanical behaviour of the muscle appears to be related directly to collagen concentrations. (p. 677)

Collectively, these changes appear to be partly responsible for the age-related loss of flexibility.

Effects of Immobilization

The ability of muscle to adapt in length to an imposed position was demonstrated early by the

the necessary balance. One must also have enough strength to be able to achieve, support, and maintain the desired position. To perform more intricate skills, sufficient coordination, rhythm, or timing may also be necessary. More complex motor skills can be performed only with the proper combination of all the required skill and fitness components.

experiments of Marvey (1887). During the past 20 years, the mechanisms of length adaptation have been studied at the cellular and ultrastructural levels. Research by Goldspink (1968, 1976) and P.E. Williams and Goldspink (1971) has shown that the increase in muscle fiber length during normal growth is associated with a large increase in the number of sarcomeres along the length of the fibers. Because the length of the actin and myosin filaments is constant, the adaptation of adult muscles to a different functional length presumably must involve the production or removal of a certain number of sarcomeres in series in order to maintain the correct sarcomere length in relation to the whole muscle (Goldspink 1976; Tabary et al. 1972).

When adult cat soleus muscle is immobilized in a lengthened position by plaster casts, it adapts to its new length. Tabary et al. (1972) found that this lengthening is accomplished by a production of approximately 20% more sarcomeres in series. P.E. Williams and Goldspink (1973) found that the new sarcomeres are added on the end of the existing myofibrils. In the case of denervation (loss of nerve supply to the muscle) and immobilization in a lengthened state, 25% more sarcomeres in series were produced (Goldspink et al. 1974). Upon removal of the plaster cast, both the normal and denervated muscle rapidly readjusted to their original lengths (Goldspink et al. 1974; Tabary et al. 1972; P.E. Williams and Goldspink 1976). Recently, a study was employed to determine if the extraocular muscle system of three monkeys adapted in the same way as cats' limb muscles (A.B. Scott 1994). The investigation found that the eye muscles lengthened 18%, 25%, and 33% as a result of suturing. The data substantiated previous findings that an addition of sarcomeres was responsible for the increase in muscle length.

On the other hand, when a limb was immobilized with the muscle in its shortened position, the muscle fibers were found to have lost 40% of the sarcomeres in series (Tabary et al. 1972). With denervation and immobilization in its shortened position, a 35% reduction of sarcomeres in series was found (Goldspink et al. 1974). The sarcomere number of these muscles also was found to readjust rapidly on return to their original length (Goldspink et al. 1974; Tabary et al. 1972).

Thus, the results for the normal and denervated muscles immobilized in both the extended and shortened positions indicated that the adjustment of sarcomere number to the functional length of the muscles does not appear to be directly under neuronal control. Rather, it appears to be a myogenic (i.e., originating in the muscle) response to the amount of passive tension to which the muscle is subjected (Goldspink 1976; Goldspink et al. 1974; P.E. Williams and Goldspink 1976).

Associated with the reduction in fiber length and in the number and length of the sarcomeres, researchers found a reduced extensibility (increase in passive resistance) of the muscles immobilized in the shortened position (Goldspink 1976; Goldspink and Williams 1979; Tabary et al. 1972). This loss of flexibility occurred whether or not the muscle was denervated (Goldspink 1976). Along this line, Goldspink and Williams (1979) found that connective tissue was lost at a slower rate than muscle contractile tissue. Hence, the relative amount of connective tissue increased (Goldspink 1976; Goldspink and Williams 1979; Tabary et al. 1972). In addition, P.E. Williams and Goldspink (1984) documented that collagen fibers in immobilized muscle were found to be arranged at an angle more acute to the axis of the muscle fibers than was found in normal muscle. This change would be expected to affect the compliance of muscle.

The decrease in extensibility appears to be a safety mechanism that prevents the muscle from being suddenly overstretched (Goldspink 1976; Goldspink and Williams 1979; Tabary et al. 1972). This mechanism is particularly important in the shortened muscle (i.e., muscle that has lost sarcomeres), because stretching even through the normal range of movement would cause the sarcomeres to be pulled out to the point where the myosin and actin filaments do not interdigitate or overlap, thus causing permanent damage to the muscle (Goldspink 1976; Tabary et al. 1972). In contrast, changes in the elastic properties of the muscle immobilized in the lengthened position do not occur, because the adaptation is in the reverse direction and the chance of the muscle being overstretched is no greater than for a normal muscle (Tabary et al. 1972).

However, the aforementioned decrease in extensibility is not just a protective function. The main effect of changes in sarcomere number and in muscle length is a shift in the muscle's length-tension curve to the left (for shortened immobilized muscle) or to the right (for lengthened immobilized muscle). These length changes serve to adapt the muscle to generate optimal tension levels at its new position and length.

Based upon the foregoing results, P.E. Williams et al. (1988) decided to determine whether lack of stretch or whether lack of contractile activity is responsible for the loss of serial sarcomeres, for the increase in the proportion of collagen, and for the increased muscle stiffness that occurs when muscles are immobilized in a shortened position. Their study found that the connective tissue accumulation that occurs in inactive muscles can be prevented by either passive stretch or by active (i.e., electrical) stimulation.

The logical question that this finding naturally raises is whether or not short periods of stretch are effective in preventing the changes in muscle connective tissue, in fiber length, and in sarcomere number and thus maintain range of joint motion. Research by P.E. Williams (1988) utilizing mice demonstrated that periods of passive stretch of only 15 minutes every other day maintained normal connective tissue proportions. However, it did not prevent the reduction in muscle fiber length, which in itself resulted in considerable loss of range of motion.

The Mechanism of Passive Stretch on Myofibrillogenesis

In the previous section it was documented that immobilization in the lengthened position results in an increase in muscle fiber length. This increase in length is associated with an increase in the number of sarcomeres in series along the myofibrils and hence along the length of the fibers. The specific site of the newly synthesized sarcomeres is near the muscle-tendon junction. In recent years the cellular control mechanism behind muscle fiber elongation and hypertrophy (i.e., myofibrillogenesis) has been investigated.

Research by Dix and Eisenberg (1990, 1991a, 1991b) found the accumulation of slow oxidative myosin mRNA at the end of the muscle in stretched fibers was greater than in control fibers. "These local accumulations of mRNA provide for regional synthesis of contractile proteins, rapid sarcomere assembly, and extension of the myofibrils" (Dix and Eisenberg 1990, 1893). In particular, "a large cytoplasmic space containing polysomes opened up between the myofibrils and the sarcolemmae of the myotendon junction of lengthening fibers and many developing myofibrils were found" (B. Russell, Dix, Haller, and Jacobs-El 1992, 192; see Figure 3.14). In addition, stretched muscles also lengthen by the addition of proliferating myotubes, which may later fuse with existing fibers (Moss and LeBlond 1971; P.E. Williams and Goldspink 1973).

The question that needs to be resolved is: How does stretch increase mRNA production? It is known that cells require hormonelike molecules called growth factors to grow. A review of several proposed "master regulators" is presented by B. Russell, Dix, Haller, and Jacobs-El (1992). However, an additional area that needs to be ex-

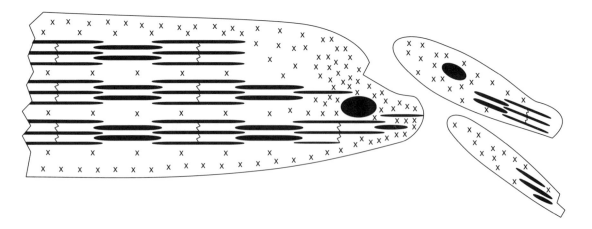

Fig. 3.14.   Distribution of mRNA at the myotendinous junction of stretched skeletal fibers. Myosin mRNA (X) accumulates at the ends of stretched fibers in the increased cytoplasmic space between sarcolemmae and the myofibrils (thin and thick filaments). This mRNA supports local contractile protein synthesis and myofibrillogenesis. Nuclei are often proximal to the ends of these lengthened fibers. Stretched muscles also lengthen by the addition of proliferating myotubes (smaller cells at right), which may later fuse with existing fibers.
Reprinted from Russell, Dix, Haller, and Jacobs-El (1992).

plored is the potential relationship of *streaming potentials* on myofibrillogenesis (discussed in chapter 4). A study by Sutcliffe and Davidson (1990) recently investigated the transduction of mechanical force (i.e., stretching) into gene expression by smooth muscle cells. Additional research is needed in this area.

Proposed Methods of Modulating Gene Expression via Stretching

Muscle cells consist of several structural compartments that are all interrelated and involved in the perception of mechanical signals that takes place during contraction and stretching. These interfacing units are three-dimensional networks whose organization is tissue specific and reflects the unique functions of each tissue. In striated muscle cells these compartments are extracellular, cytoplasmic, and nuclear. Each compartment transmits information across at least one membrane interface that sets the boundary of the particular compartment (Simpson et al. 1994). This integration of mechanical stimulation within and between these three arbitrary compartments has been described as a system of dynamic reciprocity (Bissell, Hall, and Parry 1982). Recently, it has been suggested that mechanical stimulation may affect gene expression.

The proposed pathway begins with mechanical stimulation being transmitted to the extracellular matrix (ECM). The ECM consists primarily of collagen, noncollagenous glycoproteins, and proteoglycans. Then signals from the ECM are transmitted across the sarcolemma (i.e., the membrane surrounding the muscle cell) at specific sites near Z-bands. This interaction appears to be mediated in part by specific receptors identified and termed *integrins* by Tamkun et al. (1986). These receptors link the externally located ECM components with the elements of the cytoskeleton and are important in the transmission of mechanical information (Ingber et al. 1990; Tamkun et al. 1986; Terracio et al. 1989; Vandenburgh 1992). However, the precise mechanism(s) of the transmission of mechanical stimulation are not understood (Goldspink et al. 1992; Simpson et al. 1994). Several cytoskeletal components include vinculin, talin, nonsarcomeric actin, titin, and desmin. These cytoskeletal components are im-

portant because they play an important role in the generation of force and transmission of mechanical tension (Price 1991) and provide positional information to the contractile fibers. In turn, the cytoskeleton attaches to the contractile apparatus and to the nuclear compartment. This interconnection is important in determining the positioning of the nucleus within the cell. Currently, little is known concerning nuclear positioning in striated muscle, although it is thought to be very important in other systems (Simpson et al. 1994). Nuclear positioning as established by the cytoskeleton may be important in establishing the regional domains of protein synthesis that may be essential for myofibrillogenesis and the turnover of myofibrillar components (Blau 1989; B. Russell and Dix 1992). Next, these forces are transmitted to the nuclear membrane complex and, in turn, to the nuclear matrix that contains the genetic material necessary for cellular functions. Recent research on the spatial and positional organization of DNA has invited the speculation that mechanical alteration of the nuclear membrane would in turn cause an alteration of the DNA; these forces thereby may alter gene expression (Simpson et al. 1994). Potentially, altered gene expression may be responsible for enhanced flexibility.

The fundamental issue is to define the underlying mechanism(s) by which muscle and connective tissues modulate their isoforms (i.e., structural variants) in response to mechanical stimulation. Several distinct possibilities, which might operate singly or in combination, include neurological stimulation, transmission of biochemical signals (Kornberg and Juliano 1992), stretch-activated ion channels, or streaming potentials. (The latter is reviewed in chapter 4.)

Because of economic, ethical, moral, and philosophical factors, investigators have used several animal models, including cats, rabbits, many rodents, and chickens, to study length-associated changes in muscles. Researchers have suggested applicability to humans. However, several problems must be addressed when relating animal studies to stretching and to the development of flexibility in humans. First, there has been no documented proof of an increase of sarcomeres in humans via a "traditional" stretching program (i.e., stretching in a recreational or athletic program). Second, the applicability of investigations of immobilization in a lengthened position is dubious at best. The average length of time muscles were under stretch varied from 4 days to 4 weeks. How can this stimulus relate to a person stretching one set of 10 repetitions, each held for 10 seconds? Third, since all of the studies employed traction (passive and static force), what is their practical relationship to the development of active or ballistic flexibility?

Summary

Muscle is a complex structure comprising progressively smaller units that in part determine one's flexibility. The discovery of a third filament, named titin, has shown that the sliding filament theory of the 1950s is incomplete. This filament has been proved to be primarily responsible for the sarcomere's resting tension. Furthermore, research has demonstrated that muscle tissue is very adaptable. The theoretical limit of a sarcomere's elongation while still maintaining at least one cross-bridge between the actin and myosin filaments exceeds 50% of its resting length. Thus, the contractile elements of a muscle are capable of increasing over 50% from resting length, thereby allowing muscles to move through a wide range of motion.

In addition, sarcomere number, fiber length, and sarcomere length have been shown to adjust to the functional length of the whole muscle. Currently, it is speculated that stretching can modulate gene expression and influence muscle extensibility. Additional research is needed to investigate the relationship of various types of stretching programs to identify the regimen that produces the optimal amount of flexibility.

Chapter 4

Connective Tissue: A Limiting Factor of Flexibility

In this chapter we will review the present state of knowledge about the mechanical properties, mechanical ultrastructure, and biochemical constituents of connective tissues and the effects of aging and immobilization on them. Our goal will be to understand how these variables affect and determine the function of connective tissues. This information will enable us to better understand the behavior of connective tissue, which to a major extent determines our degree of flexibility.

Connective tissue contains a wide variety of specialized cells. Different types of cells perform the functions of defense, protection, storage, transportation, binding, connection, and general support and repair. In this chapter we will concentrate on cells that provide binding and support functions.

Collagen

Collagen is the most abundant protein in the mammalian body. It is generally regarded as a primary structural component of living tissue. In higher vertebrates, for example, collagen constitutes one third or more of the total body proteins. Collagen is defined as a protein that contains three chains of amino acids wound in a triple helix. The two major physical properties of collagen fibers are their great tensile *strength* and relative *inextensibility*.

Collagenous fibers appear virtually colorless or off-white. They are arranged in bundles and, except under tension, run a characteristically wavy course. Collagen fibers are capable of only a slight degree of extensibility. They are, however, very resistant to tensile stress. Therefore, they are the main constituents of structures such as ligaments and tendons that are subjected to a pulling force.

A large number of different types of collagen are known. Currently, at least five classes have been identified, each of which has subclasses (Jungueira, Carneiro, and Long 1989). Each type of collagen is identified by a roman numeral, which merely reflects the order in which the collagen types were discovered. Type I collagen is the most common form and is important to our interest in range of motion. Type I collagen is located in skin, bone, ligament, and tendon. Genetic mutations that affect the structure or processing of the chains of Type I collagen are often expressed as generalized connective tissue disorders.

Ultrastructure of Collagen

The structural organization of collagen is analogous to that of muscle (see Table 4.1 and Figure 4.1). However, the classification system is not widely agreed upon due to a lack of consistent terminology used in the field (Kastelic, Galeski, and Baer 1978; Strocchi et al. 1985). When viewed

Table 4.1. A Comparison of Muscle and Collagen
Structures

Muscle	Collagen
Muscle	Tendon
Muscle bundle (fasciculus)	Fascicle
Muscle fiber	Fibril
Myofibril	Subfibril
Myofilament	Microfibril
Sarcomere	Collagen molecule
(functional unit)	(functional unit)
Actin	$Alpha_1$ chains (2)
Myosin	$Alpha_2$ chains (1)
Titin	
Cross-bridges	Cross-links

Note. From *Science of Stretching* (p. 24) by M.J. Alter,
1988, Champaign, IL: Human Kinetics. Copyright 1988
by M.J. Alter. Reprinted by permission.
Reprinted from Alter (1988).

under a microscope, individual collagen fibers are
seen to have a banded or striated structure. The
characteristic pattern of cross-striations of collagen reflects its ultrastructural organization.
Knowledge of this pattern is fundamental to un-

derstanding the mechanism of collagen's two
major physical properties: its great tensile
strength and relative inextensibility.

The collagen of a tendon is arranged in wavy
bundles called *fascicles* (see Figure 4.1). A fascicle
varies from 50 to 300 μm in diameter. The fascicle is composed of bundles of *fibrils*, each of
which is approximately 50 to 500 nm in diameter. The fibrils are in turn composed of bundles
of collagen *subfibrils*, each of which is approximately 10 to 20 nm in diameter. Each subfibril is
composed of bundles of collagen *microfibrils* or
filaments, each of which is approximately 3.5 nm
in diameter. The sizes of the filaments in a given
tissue vary with age and other factors.

According to Inoue and Leblond (1986), the
least known of the fibrous components of connective tissue is the collagen microfibril. The microfibril was given its present name by Low
(1961a, 1961b, 1962). Various and conflicting descriptions have been made of this structure. In
an attempt to clarify these uncertainties, Inoue
and Leblond (1986) examined microfibrils of the
connective tissue of a mouse at high resolution
in the electron microscope. Their study revealed
that microfibrils are composed of two parts: the
tubule proper and a surface band. The *tubule* is
characterized in cross section by an approxi-

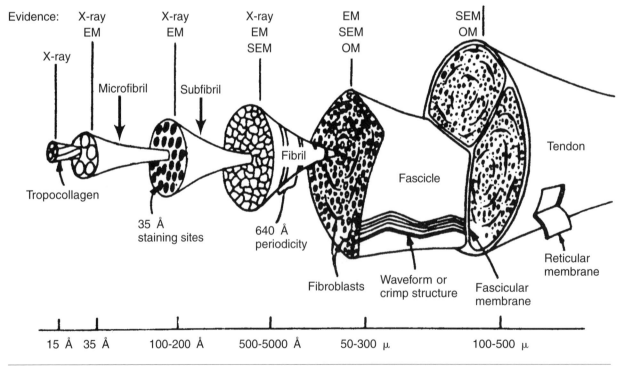

Fig. 4.1. Collagen hierarchy.
Reprinted from Kastelic, Galeski, and Baer (1978).

mately pentagonal wall and an electron-lucent lumen containing a bead, referred to as a *spherule*. The *surface band* is a ribbonlike structure wrapped around the tubule. The band has dense borders called *tracks* with *spikes* attached at intervals (Figure 4.2). Additional research is recommended to confirm whether this structure is also present in human microfibrils and to determine its relationship to range of motion.

The collagen microfibril is composed of regularly spaced, overlapping collagen molecules (Figure 4.3b). These units are analogous to the sarcomeres of muscle cells. The collagen molecules are in turn made of coiled helices of amino acids. The collagen molecules are very small; they measure about 300 nm in length and 1.5 nm in diameter (Figure 4.3c). They lie in parallel alignment with a staggered overlap of almost one fourth their length. This overlapping is what creates the prominent cross-bands or striations. Col-

lagen fibrils have a cross-band periodicity of from 60 to 70 nm depending on their source and degree of hydration. Actual measurements indicate that a gap or hole of about 41 nm occurs between the end of one collagen molecule and the beginning of the next in the same line.

Upon extreme magnification, the collagen molecule is seen as three polypeptide chains that are coiled in a unique type of rigid helical structure. Of the three intertwining amino acid chains in human collagen, two (the $alpha_1$ *chains*) are identical and one (the $alpha_2$ *chain*) is distinct in its sequence of amino acids. The three chains are thought to be held together by hydrogen bonds that form cross-links (Figure 4.3d).

In addition to the presence of a cross-banding periodicity or striation pattern, connective tissues possess wavelike undulations of the collagen fibers. This undulating phenomenon is known as *crimp* (Portenfield and De Rosa 1991). The crimp

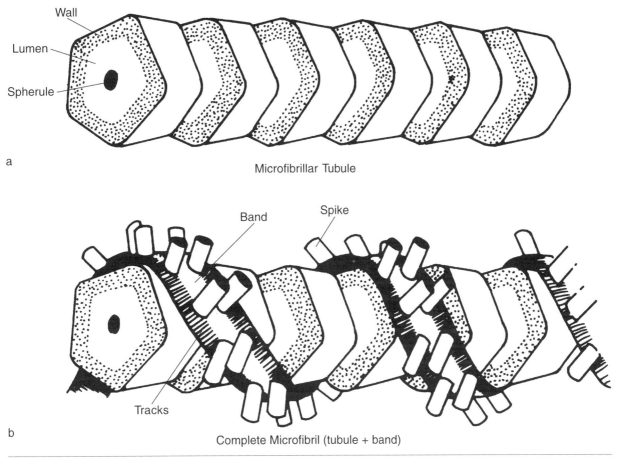

Fig. 4.2. Model of the tubular portion of a typical microfibril. It is composed of pentagonal segments associated in a column (a). Segments are all the same size, but larger and smaller spaces alternate between them. (b) Model of a typical microfibril. At the surface of the tubular portion, represented as in (a), the surface band is associated with protruding spikes. The band is depicted as a helix but may be differently organized. In any case, it is in close association with the surface of the segments. Approximate magnification × 2,700,000.

Reprinted from Inoue and Leblond (1986).

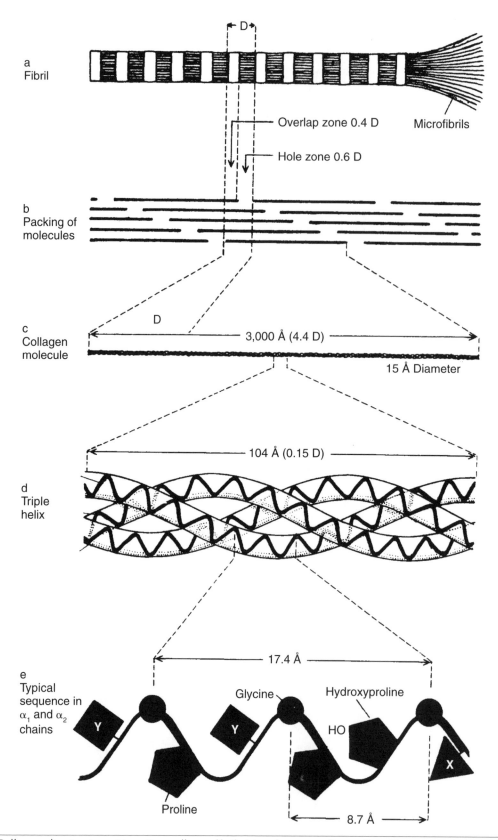

Fig. 4.3. Collagen ultrastructure. Many tiny collagen fibrils (a) make up a collagen fiber. The cross-striations in the fibril result from the overlapping of collagen molecules (b). The collagen molecule itself (c) is composed of three polypeptide chains that are organized into a ropelike triple helix (d). The amino acid sequence of these polypeptide chains is unique in having glycine as every third amino acid (e). The X position following glycine is frequently proline and the Y position preceding glycine is frequently hydroxyproline. Drawing by B. Tagawa.

Reprinted from Prockop and Guzman (1977).

organization of collagen is one of the major factors behind the viscoelastic response of connective tissue. Collagen is composed of crimped fibrils that are aggregated into fibers. The mechanical properties of collagen fibrils are such that each fibril can be considered a mechanical spring and each fiber an assemblage of springs. Whenever a fiber is pulled, its crimp straightens, and its length increases. Like a mechanical spring, the energy supplied to stretch the fiber is stored in the fiber, and it is the release of this energy that returns the fiber to its unstretched configuration when the applied load is removed (Ozkaya and Nordin 1991). Fibril crimp has been attributed to collagen-ground substance interactions, properties of the molecular structure, and cross-linking effects, but the exact cause is not known (Gathercole and Keller 1968).

Collagenous Tissue Cross-Links

A major factor that adds tensile strength to collagenous structures is the presence of both *intramolecular cross-links* between the alpha$_1$ and alpha$_2$ chains of the collagen molecule and of *intermolecular cross-links* between collagen subfibrils, filaments, and other fibers. In a sense, cross-links act to weld the building blocks (i.e., the molecules) into a strong, ropelike unit. Generally, the shorter the length between one cross-link and the next or the larger the number of cross-links in a given distance, the higher the elasticity (R.M. Alexander 1975, 1988).

Researchers speculate that the number of cross-links relates to a collagen turnover; that is, collagen is continuously and simultaneously being produced and broken down. If collagen production exceeds collagen breakdown, more cross-links are established and the structure is more resistant to stretching. Conversely, if the collagen breakdown exceeds collagen production, then the opposite holds true. Some research has suggested that exercise or mobilization can decrease the number of cross-links by increasing the collagen turnover rate (W.M. Bryant 1977; Shephard 1982). Recent findings have also suggested that exercise or mobilization may play a determining factor in preventing cross-linking.

The Biochemical Composition of Collagen

The collagen molecule is a complex helical structure whose mechanical properties are due to both its biochemical composition and the physical arrangement of its individual molecules. Although collagen is composed of many complex molecules called *amino acids*, three stand out. They are the amino acids *glycine*, which constitutes one third of the total, and *proline* and *hydroxyproline*, each of which constitutes one-fourth or more (see Figure 4.3e). The presence of proline and hydroxyproline keeps the ropelike packing arrangement of collagen stable and resistant to stretching. Thus, the higher the concentration of these amino acids, the higher the stretch resistance of the molecules will be. Because the nitrogen of the proline is fixed in a ring structure, its presence prevents easy rotation of the regions in which it is located (Grant, Prockop, and Darwin 1972; Gross 1961). To help visualize this idea, think of these additional amino acids as being comparable to eggs added to a meat loaf or tin combined with copper to make bronze. In all these cases, the result is increased rigidity and stability of the end product.

The Influence of Ground Substances on Collagen

A major factor affecting the mechanical behavior of collagen is the presence of *ground substances*. Ground substances are widely distributed throughout connective tissue and supporting tissues. At many sites, they are known as *cement substances*. They form the nonfibrous element of the matrix in which cells and other components are embedded. This viscous, gel-like element is composed of *glycosaminoglycans* (GAGs), plasma proteins, a variety of small proteins, and water.

Water makes up 60% to 70% of the total connective tissue content. GAG, which has an enormous water-binding capacity, is considered partially responsible for this high level of water content. According to Viidik, Danielsen, and Oxlund (1982), the importance of the hyaluronate molecule in this regard cannot be overestimated because it takes up a hydrodynamic volume of 1,000 times the space occupied by the chain itself in an unhydrated state.

Hyaluronic acid and its attached or entrapped water is the principal fibrous connective tissue lubricant. Specifically, hyaluronic acid with water is thought to serve as a lubricant between the collagen fibers and fibrils. The lubricant appears to maintain a critical distance between the fibers and fibrils, thereby permitting free gliding of the fibers and fibrils past each other and perhaps preventing excessive cross-linking (Figure 4.4).

> # *Glycosaminoglycan (GAG)*
>
> A glycosaminoglycan (GAG) is a polysaccharide composed of repeating disaccharide (two-sugar) units. The four major GAGs found in connective tissue are hyaluronic acid, chondroitin-4-sulfate, chondroitin-6-sulfate, and dermatan sulfate. Generally, GAGs are bound to a protein and collectively referred to as *proteoglycan*. In connective tissue, proteoglycans combine with water to form a proteoglycan aggregate. A proteoglycan, by definition, consists of a protein or a polypeptide to which one or more GAG chains are covalently attached. Each disaccharide group in the GAG chain often has two negatively charged groups. Their high fixed negative charge attracts counter ions, and the osmotic imbalance caused by a local high concentration of ions draws water from the surrounding areas. Proteoglycans thus keep the matrix hydrated and function physically as creators of a water-filled compartment. Proteoglycans are deformable and not rigid because the GAG chains are freely mobile and can be forced together. This proximity produces a rise in internal charge density that counterbalances compressive forces.

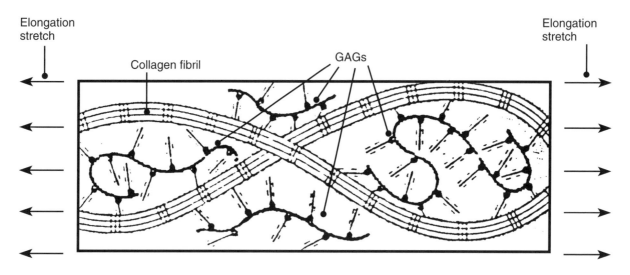

Fig. 4.4. The action of GAGs. Stretch is applied to collagen fibrils, but the GAGs keep the fibrils separated and aligned. Reprinted from Meyers, Armstrong, and Mow (1984).

Electromechanical and Physiological Properties

Solid crystalline materials demonstrate an electromechanical phenomenon when deformed. This phenomenon is referred to as the *piezoelectric effect* (Athenstaedt 1970; Shamos and Lavine 1967). A similar effect is also present in biological tissues. One example is the molecular structure of the native collagen fibril. The knitted tropocollagen molecules that make up the fibril are electrically dipolar rods that have a permanent electric moment in the direction of the longitudinal tropocollagen axis (Athenstaedt 1970). When a connective tissue such as cartilage is compressed, a mechanical-to-electrical transduction occurs, resulting in measurable electrical potentials (Grodzinsky 1983). In recent years, the piezoelectric mechanism has received wide attention, especially in terms of its possible function in growth and remodeling of connective tissues as well as in the healing of bone fractures.

In biologic tissues, the piezoelectric effect is commonly referred to as *electrokinetics* or *streaming potentials*. In addition to streaming potentials and currents, deformation of biologic tissues can produce hydrostatic pressure gradients, fluid flow, and cell deformation in the matrix. Currently, the mechanism(s) that account for these responses are unknown, although several theories have been proposed. However, it is now apparent that an electrokinetic or streaming-potential mechanism is the primary source of this transduction response (Grodzinsky 1987). An excellent overview of the relationship between electromechanical and physiochemical properties of connective tissue can be found in the work of Grodzinsky (1983). At the present time, two important questions are being investigated: (1) What is the mechanism that makes it operate? and (2) What is the transduction phenomenon at the cellular level?

Mechanical Properties

It is interesting to speculate one step further that the streaming potentials represent the mechanism by which the mechanical forces of stretching are transduced into various types of gene expression and therefore into protein synthesis (e.g., developing specific isoforms of titin and other tissues). In this regard, a study by Sutcliffe and Davidson (1990) demonstrated that transduction of mechanical force into elastin gene expression by smooth muscle cells during stretching may contribute to their specific adaptations.

To date, most research has concentrated on articular cartilage under compression. Nonetheless,

important information can be extrapolated from such studies on two grounds. First, articular cartilage is in the family of connective tissue. Second, elongation occurs simultaneously as a result of compression. It has long been known that electrostatic forces are among the intermolecular interactions that can significantly affect rheological behavior of biological tissues (Grodzinsky, Lipshitz, and Glimcher 1978). In particular, the extracellular matrix has the important function of resisting tensile, compressive, and shear mechanical stresses. As was previously discussed, electrostatic repulsion forces between GAG fixed-charge groups tend to stiffen the matrix, thereby increasing its ability to withstand deformation and loading (Grodzinsky 1983, 1987; Muir 1983; Figure 4.5). Thus, proteoglycans act like "molecular springs" (Muir 1983).

This swelling pressure of certain tissues (e.g. intervertebral disks or cartilage) is crucial to the tissue's ability to withstand compressive loads. J. Urban et al. (1979) investigated the swelling

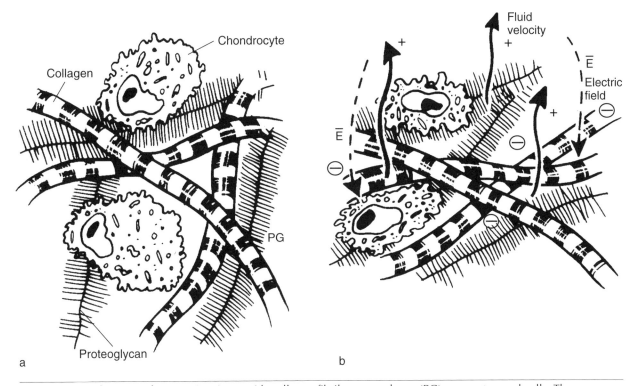

Fig. 4.5. (a) Schematic of connective tissue with collagen fibrils, proteoglycan (PG) aggregates, and cells. The extracellular matrix contains negative fixed charge, and the interstitial fluid therefore contains enough extra (+) counterions to satisfy electroneutrality. (b) Dynamic compression of the tissue will produce deformation, pressure gradients, fluid flow, and streaming potentials (and currents) within the extracellular matrix in the environment of the cells; compression-induced changes in fixed charge density will alter the concentration of all mobile ionic species within the extracellular matrix according to Donnan and electroneutrality laws.
Reprinted from Grodzinsky (1987).

pressure of proteoglycan solutions. They found the swelling was independent of proteoglycan molecular size and aggregation state. Furthermore, they found that the final hydration of intact tissues is determined not only by fixed charge density, but by various other factors, including the arrangement of collagen fibrils, intra- and intermolecular cross-linkages, and proteoglycan-collagen interactions. Additional research is needed to investigate the effect of tensile forces applied under varying conditions (e.g., ballistic and static) on muscle fascia, ligaments, and tendons as it relates to the phenomenon of electrokinetic transport fields, forces, and flows.

Effect of Static Versus Dynamic Loading

Research dealing with articular cartilage in vivo has demonstrated that static immobilization, reduced loading, or static compression of a joint results in regions of increased fixed charge density, an increased concentration of positive counterions, and an increased osmotic pressure. Such factors have been found to inhibit proteoglycan synthesis and processing (Gray et al. 1988; Schneiderman, Kevet, and Maroudas 1986; J.P.G. Urban and Bayliss 1989) and to impair cartilage nutrition. In contrast, dynamic or oscillatory compression results in increased hydrostatic pressure, increased fluid flow, increased streaming potentials, and altered cell shape that may stimulate biosynthesis (A. Hall, Urban, and Gehl 1991; Y.-J. Kim et al. 1994; Sah et al. 1992). Therefore, cyclic loading and unloading is good for maintaining cartilage health. However, during impacts or excessive loading, there is an increase in fluid flow, strain, and strain rate. High levels of strain or strain rate may cause matrix disruption, tissue swelling, and accentuate diffusion within cartilage (Sah et al. 1991), resulting in permanent cartilage damage.

Based on the preceding information, it may seem plausible to extrapolate from these findings that certain types of stretching techniques (e.g., ballistic) or specific stretches (e.g., hurdler's stretch, inverted hurdler's stretch, or bridges) are potentially harmful. However, these studies utilized high-amplitude, 24-hour cyclic compression in 2-hour-on/2-hour-off intervals. The important question is: Does this information have practical implications and relevance for those people who incorporate into an exercise program "traditional" stretches that maintain a stretch for 5 to 10 seconds up to 1 minute? Additional research must be initiated to ascertain the consequences of loading for such brief periods of time before

definitive statements can be made regarding supposed advantageous or detrimental effects.

Effects of Aging on Collagen

As collagen ages, specific physical and biochemical changes take place. Ultimately, these changes reflect a reduction of the minimal extensibility that existed earlier and an increased rigidity. For instance, aging increases the diameter of the collagen fibers in various tissues. Also, with the passage of time, the fibrils become more crystalline. This increase in crystallinity or orientation strengthens the intermolecular bonds and increases resistance to further deformation. Furthermore, aging is believed to be associated with an increased number of intra- and intermolecular cross-links. These additional cross-links apparently restrict the ability of collagen molecules to slip past each other. Dehydration also occurs with the aging process. The amount of water (i.e., hydration) associated with connective tissues such as tendon declines with age. Although the degree of dehydration reported varies from source to source, tendon water content, approximately 80% to 85% in babies, has been found to decrease to 70% in adults (Elliott 1965; Figure 4.6).

The Ultrastructural Basis and Physiological Limit of Collagen Elongation

Unlike a sarcomere, a collagen fiber is comparatively inextensible. The collagen fiber is so inelastic that a weight 10,000 times greater than its own will not stretch it (Verzar 1963). Research indicates that microscopic fibers can be stretched to a maximum of about 10% more than their original length before they break. However, at the molecular level, the collagen fibrils undergo an extension of about 3% (Ramachandran 1967). Under a microscope, when collagen is elongated it displays progressive alteration in intrafibril periodicity and lateral dimensions. One early study (Cowan, McGavin, and North 1955) found that stretching increased the repeated axial interval from 0.286 to 0.310 nm or more.

Such an extension is believed to occur initially through a straightening of the fibers followed by a gradual slip of one fiber relative to the next. Ultimately, this movement results in an increase in crystallinity or orientation that strengthens the intermolecular bond and increases resistance to further elongation. This process can be compared

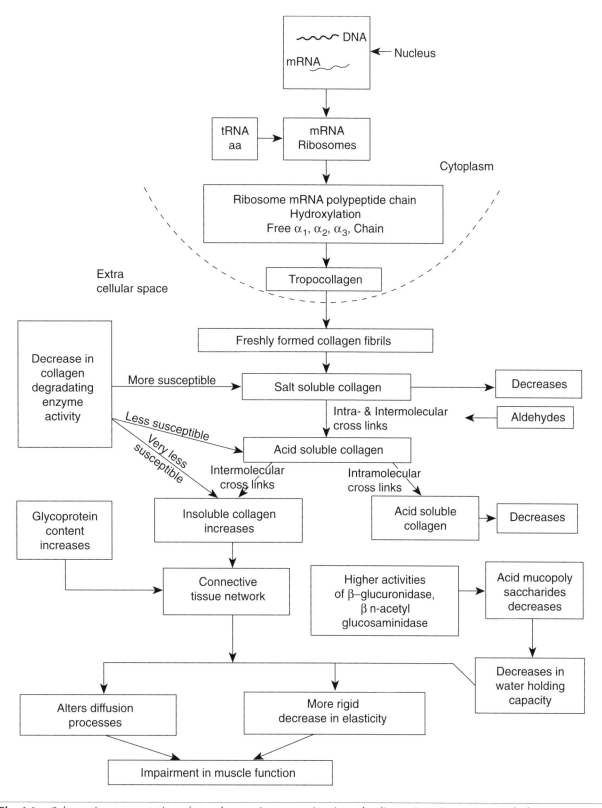

Fig. 4.6. Schematic representation of age changes in connective tissue leading to impairment in muscle function. Reprinted from Mohan and Radha (1981).

to spinning wool: With an increase in crystallinity there is an increase of the intermeshing of the adjacent molecules. Consequently, there is an increased regularity in packing and enhanced interchain forces which permits increased resistance to deforming forces. Thus, simply stated, collagenous fibers allow elongation until the slack of their wavy bundles is taken up. However, if stretch continues, a point will be reached where all intermolecular forces are exceeded and the tissue parts (Laban 1962; L. Weiss and Greep 1983).

Elastic Tissue

Elastic tissue is a primary structural component of living tissue and is found in various quantities throughout the body. Electron photomicrographs have shown that there is a large amount of elastic tissue in the sarcolemma of a muscle fiber (the connective tissue that surrounds the sarcomere). Thus, elastic tissue plays a major role in determining the possible range of extensibility of muscle cells. In certain locations, rather large amounts of almost pure elastic fibers can be found, particularly in the ligaments of the vertebral column. Consequently, to a major extent, elastic tissue determines the possible ranges of motion.

Elastic fibers perform a variety of functions, including disseminating stresses that originate at isolated points, enhancing coordination of the rhythmic motions of the body parts, conserving energy by maintaining tone during relaxation of muscular elements, providing a defense against excessive forces, and assisting organs in returning to their undeformed configuration once all forces have been removed (Jenkins and Little 1974).

The Composition of Elastic Fibers

Unfortunately, elastic fibers have not been studied as extensively as collagen fibers and therefore are less understood. This situation is primarily due to technical difficulties encountered in solubilizing them (Modis 1991). Another compounding factor is that elastic and collagen fibers are usually very closely associated anatomically, morphologically, biochemically, and physiologically. In fact, elastic fibers may have collagen fibers interwoven with their principal components and are usually dominated by them.

Elastic fibers are optically homogenous. Hence, they are highly refractile and almost isotropic. Under an electron microscope, each fiber appears to consist of a fused mass of fibrils twisted in ropelike fashion. Unlike collagenous fibers, elastic fibers display a complete lack of periodic structure (i.e., banding or striation).

Elastic Tissue Cross-Links

Elastic fibers are thought to be composed of a network of randomly coiled chains, which are probably joined by covalent (atoms that share electrons) cross-links. However, the noncovalent interchain forces are considered weak, and the cross-links themselves are believed to be widely spaced (L. Weiss and Greep 1983). Consequently, elastic cross-links do not weld the molecules into a strong, ropelike unit similar to collagen. The significance of this difference will be discussed later.

Elastin

When the term elastic tissue or elastic fiber is utilized, it has a structural connotation. In contrast, elastin refers to the biochemical character of elastic fibers. Elastin is a complex structure with a mechanical property of elasticity due both to its biochemical composition and to the physical arrangement of its individual molecules. Like collagen, elastin is also composed of amino acids. Unlike collagen, however, elastin is composed mostly of nonpolar hydrophobic amino acids, and it has little hydroxyproline and no hydroxylysine. Also, elastin is unique in that it contains *desmosine* and *isodesmosine*, which function as covalent cross-links in and between the polypeptide chains. Similar to collagen, about one third of the residues of elastin are *glycine* and about 11% are *proline*.

Effects of Aging on Elastic Fibers

Elastic fibers display specific physical and biochemical changes as a result of aging. They lose their resiliency and undergo various other alterations, including fragmentation, fraying, calcification and other mineralizations, and an increased number of cross-linkages. Biochemically, there is an increase in amino acids containing polar groups as well; for example, the content of desmosine, isodesmosine, and lysinonorleucine all increase as elastin ages. Other changes are an increase in the proportion of chondroitin sulfate B and keratosulfate. Altogether, these alterations appear to be responsible for age-related loss of resiliency and increased rigidity (Bick 1961; Gosline 1976; Schubert and Hammerman 1968; Yu and Blumenthal 1967).

Ultrastructural Basis and the Physiological Limit of Elastin Elongation

Elastic fibers yield easily to stretching. However, when released they return to virtually their former length. Only when elastic fibers are stretched to about 150% of their original length do they reach their breaking point; a force of only 20 to 30 kg/cm^2 is necessary to bring this about (Bloom and Fawcett 1986).

Several models have been developed to explain the elastic force associated with elastin. One theory is the two-phase model of elastin proposed by Partridge (1966) and later adopted by Weis-Fogh and Anderson (1970a, 1970b). According to this model, elastin exists as distinct particles attached to one another by cross-linkages with water in spaces between the particles. The globules are initially spherical in shape. During stretching, the globules are drawn out and form the ellipsoid shape of an American or rugby football. This change of shape is opposed by the surface tension. When the stretch is released, surface tension makes the globules become spherical again and so drives the elastic recoil. However, this model has been challenged by Hoeve and Flory (1974) based on thermodynamic considerations.

A second explanation for the elastic force is that the elastin is thought to be composed of a network of randomly coiled chains joined by covalent cross-links. These cross-links impose a restriction on the relative movement of the elastic fibers, so that when the tissue is stretched the individual chains are constrained and cannot slip past one another (Franzblau and Faru 1981). However, the covalent interchain forces are weak, and the cross-links widely spaced. As a result, minimal unidirectional force can produce extensive elongation of chains before the cross-links begin to restrict movement. Thus, similar to the collagenous fibers, elastic fibers allow extensibility until the slack and spacing between the chains are taken up (Figure 4.7).

A third model has been proposed by Urry (1984). This model also relies on an entropy-driven mechanism to provide the elastomeric force. However, it relies on a different molecular

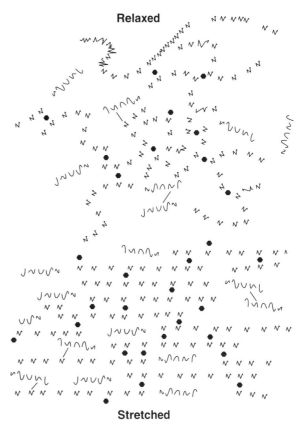

Relaxed

Stretched

Fig. 4.7. Diagrammatic representation of cross-linked elastin in relaxed and stretched states. The potential cross-linking domains, some of which are probably in an alpha-helical conformation, are in bold. For clarity of presentation only some of the tetrafunctional desmosine (•) or bifunctional (/) cross-links are shown. The hydrophobic domains in the relaxed state are probably largely random coils, although limited portions may exist in a β-spiral conformation. In the stretched state, the imposed force brings the chains into relative alignment and limits their conformational freedom.
Reprinted from Rosenbloom, Abrams, and Mecham (1993).

conformation, which has been summarized by Rosenbloom, Abrams, and Mecham (1993):

> The entropic elasticity derives from the β-spiral structure, with essentially fixed end-to-end chain lengths. The peptide segments suspended between the β-turns are free to undergo large-amplitude, low-frequency rocking motions called librations. Upon stretching, there is a decrease in amplitude of the librations that results in a large decrease in the entropy of the segment, and this provides the driving elastomeric force for return to the relaxed state. (p. 1217)

Further studies are required to prove whether one of these models is uniquely valid or whether the structure of elastin incorporates some features of each of them. It is also possible that at a later date all of these models may be found to be inadequate or completely incorrect.

The Relationship Between Collagen and Elastic Fibers

As mentioned above, elastic fibers are almost always found in close association with collagenous tissues. Furthermore, the performance of this combined tissue is a result of blending and integrating the distinctly different mechanical properties of these two tissues. First, the elastic fibers themselves are typically responsible for what may be called reverse elasticity (the ability of a stretched material to return to its original resting state). Second, the collagen meshwork provides the rigid constraints that limit the deformations of the elastic elements and that are largely responsible for the ultimate properties (tensile strength and relative inextensibility) of those composite structures. Logically, where collagenous fibers dominate, rigidity, stability, tensile strength, and a restricted range of movement will prevail (Eldren 1968; Gosline 1976).

Structures Composed of Connective Tissue

The human body contains numerous structures composed of connective tissue. The three structures that are of greatest concern to us include tendons, ligaments, and fascia. In the sections that follow, individual tissues will be analyzed and discussed.

Tendons

Muscles are attached to bones by tough cords called *tendons*. The primary function of a tendon is to transmit tension from the muscle to bones, thereby producing motion. Tendons are extremely important in determining one's quality of movement. Verzar (1964, 255) vividly described this concept:

> The importance of inextensibility, from a physiological point of view, is that the smallest mus-

cular contraction can be transmitted without loss to the articulations. If tendons, i.e., collagen fibers, were only slightly extensible, the finest movements, such as those of the fingers of a violinist or pianist, or the exact movements of the eye, would be impossible.

The chief constituents of tendons are thick, closely packed, parallel collagenous bundles that vary in length and thickness. They show a distinct longitudinal striation and in many places fuse with one another. The fibrils making up the tendon are virtually all oriented in one direction, that is, toward the long axis, which is also the direction of normal physiological stress. The tendon is thus especially adapted to resist movement in one direction. Therefore, the greater the proportion of collagen to elastic fibers, the greater the number of fibers that are oriented in the direction of stress, and the greater the cross-sectional area or width of the tendon, the stronger the tendon.

The connective tissue wrappings of tendon have a similar arrangement to those of a muscle fiber and have analogous names. However, as was pointed out previously, this terminology has not been universally employed. The following terms have been adopted by the International Anatomical Nomenclature Committee (1983). The *endotendineum* surrounds the tendon bundle. At the next layer, the *peritendineum* surrounds the tendon fascicle. Last, there is the *epitendineum*, which surrounds the entire tendon. These wrappings are also made of loosely woven collagen fibers.

In tendon, a stress of about 4% is regarded as especially significant and corresponds to the elasticity limit (length of reversibility), and therefore to elasticity (Crisp 1972). At this point, the tendon's surface waviness disappears, and if the stretch continues, injury may result.

When stretch tension is applied to tendon, the amount of deformation that follows a pattern is called a load-deformation curve. At low levels of tension, the wavy structure of the tendon's collagen bundles straightens, allowing rapid, slight deformation (the "toe" region of the curve). Beyond this threshold, further stretch results in deformation that is linearly related to the amount of tension (the linear phase of the curve). Within this range of loads, the tendon will return to its original length when unloaded. At loads greater than this range, permanent length changes will occur, accompanied by microtrauma to the tendon's structural integrity (the "yield" point of the curve).

Ligaments

Ligaments bind bone to bone. Consequently, unlike tendons, they attach (insert) to bones at both ends. Their function is primarily to support a joint (the place where two or more bones meet) by holding the bones in place. There is abundant research information about the types of neural sensory receptors located in ligaments (Brand, 1986; Rowinski, 1985) that function as sensors for the nervous system. Thus, "they may have played a larger role in normal joint function than has been realized and may make a correspondingly large contribution to the pathological consequences of injuries" (C.G. Armstrong, O'Connor, and Gardner 1992, 276).

Ligaments are similar to tendons, except that the elements are less regularly arranged. Like tendons, they are composed mainly of bundles of collagenous fibers placed parallel to, or closely interlaced with, one another. Ligaments are found in different shapes, such as cords, bands, or sheets. However, they lack the glistening whiteness of tendon because there is a greater mixture of elastic and fine collagenous fibers woven among the parallel bundles. Consequently, they are pliant and flexible so as to allow freedom of movement but strong, tough, and inextensible so as not to yield readily to applied forces.

A biochemical analysis reveals that ligament contains mostly collagenous tissue. The exceptions to this rule are the ligamentum flavum and ligamentum nuchae, which connect the laminae of adjacent vertebrae in the lower spine and neck, respectively. These ligaments are made up almost entirely of elastic fibers and are quite elastic in their behavior. Another reason for differences among some ligaments and tendon in their viscoelastic properties is the percentage of GAGs (glycosaminoglycan). Research by Woo, Gomez, and Akeson (1985) found that only 1% to 1.5% of tendon is made up of GAGs. Similarly, collateral ligament also consisted of 1% to 1.5% GAGs. In contrast, the cruciate ligaments totaled 2.5% to 3.0% GAG concentration. It would make an interesting study to find out whether there are quantitative differences in the GAG content between the ligaments of gymnasts, dancers, or contortionists and those of the "normal" population. The question here is: Does a higher percentage of GAGs increase the extensibility of ligaments?

A study by Johns and Wright (1962) determined that tendons provide only about 10% of the total resistance to movement. In contrast, they found that the ligaments and joint capsule contribute about 47% of the total resistance to movement. Consequently, the latter tissues are extremely significant in determining the ultimate range of movement of a joint. As a general rule, stretching exercises employed by laypeople should not be directed toward elongating the joint capsule and ligaments that are of normal length, because stretching these structures may destabilize the joint and increase the likelihood of injury. However, stretching of the ligaments and joint capsule should not be absolutely prohibited. The application of a chiropractic adjustment or general manipulation under the care of a trained and certified practitioner (e.g., chiropractor, osteopath, or physical therapist) has been demonstrated in many cases to be effective in correcting subluxations, increasing range of motion, reducing pain, and improving performance in many patients. In fact, stretching a joint capsule is absolutely essential if it has become shortened and is limiting ROM (as in adhesive capsulitis at the shoulder).

Fascia

The word *fascia*, taken from Latin, means a band or bandage. Technically, fascia is a term used in gross anatomy to designate all fibrous connective structures not otherwise specifically named. Similar to other previously mentioned tissues, fascia varies in thickness and density according to functional demands and is usually in the form of membranous sheets.

The fascia can be broken down into three general divisions or types. The *superficial fascia* lies directly below the dermis (i.e., skin). It is composed of two layers. The outer layer is called the *panniculus adiposus*. It usually contains an accumulation of fat that varies in amount among individuals and regions of the body. The *inner layer*, by contrast, is a thin membrane that ordinarily has no fat. In many parts of the body the superficial fascia glides freely over the deep fascia, producing the characteristic movability of skin (Clemente 1985). The *deep fascia* is directly beneath the superficial fascia. This fascia is usually tougher, tighter, and more compact than the superficial fascia. It covers and is fused with the muscles, bones, nerves, blood vessels, and organs of the body. In addition, it compartmentalizes the body by separating such things as muscles and the internal visceral organs. The *subserous fascia* is innermost around body cavities. It forms the fibrous layer of the serous membranes that cover and support the viscera. Examples include the pleura around the lungs, the pericardium around the heart, and the peritoneum around the abdominal cavity and organs.

The deep fascia that envelops and binds down the muscle into separate groups is named according to where it is found. The sheaths of connective tissue that encase the entire muscle are called the *epimysium*. Next, the *perimysium* encases the bundles of muscle fibers known as fasciculi and interconnect them to the epimysium (Borg and Caulfield 1980). Not only does the perimysium bind muscle fibers into bundles, it also binds each muscle fiber within a bundle to its immediate neighbor (Rowe 1981). Within the perimysium, as many as 150 individual fibers may be found. Surrounding each muscle fiber is the *endomysium*, which also interconnects to the perimysium (Borg and Caulfield 1980). Last is the *sarcolemma*, the connective tissue that covers the functional unit of the muscle, the sarcomere (Figure 4.8).

Function of Fascia

According to Rowe (1981), there are at least three probable functions of intramuscular connective tissue. First, it provides a framework binding the muscle together and ensuring the proper alignment of muscle fibers, blood vessels, nerves, and

so on. Second, it enables forces, either actively developed by the muscle or passively imposed on the muscle, to be transmitted by the whole tissue safely and effectively. Last, it also probably provides the necessary lubricated surfaces between muscle fibers and muscle fiber bundles that enable the muscle to change its shape.

Connective tissue makes up as much as 30% of muscle mass. Furthermore, it is this tissue that allows muscle to change length. During passive motion, the sum of the muscle's fascia accounts for 41% of the total resistance to movement (Johns and Wright 1962). Hence, the fascia represents the second most important factor limiting the range of motion (Table 4.2). A stretching program should be directed primarily toward elongating

Table 4.2. Comparison of the Relative Contribution of Soft Tissue Structures to Joint Resistance

Structure	Resistance
Joint capsule	47%
Muscle (fascia)	41%
Tendon	10%
Skin	2%

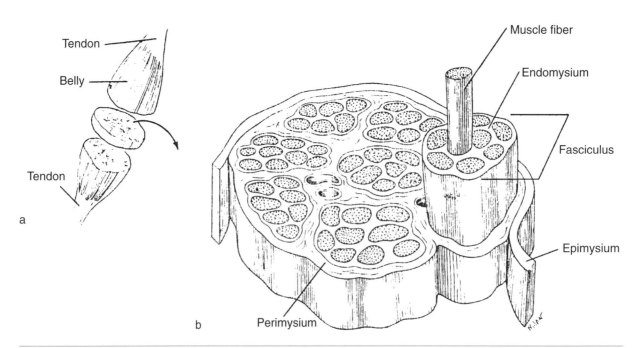

Fig. 4.8. Connective tissue of a muscle. (a) Entire muscle, with the belly sectioned. (b) Enlargement of a cross section of the belly.

From *Human Anatomy and Physiology, 3rd edition* (p. 215), by A.P. Spence and E.B. Mason, 1987, Menlo Park, CA: Benjamin/ Cummings Publishing Company. Copyright 1987 by Benjamin/Cummings Publishing Company. Reprinted by permission.

the fascia. Generally, stretching should not be targeted to the ligaments because stretching these structures may result in destabilization of the joint.

Unfortunately, the functional relationships between fascia and the forces and pressures generated by underlying muscular contractions are poorly understood (Garfin et al. 1981). Few research projects have studied the biomechanical effects of fascia on muscle or explored the effect that removal of the fascia has on the underlying muscle and osseofascial compartment (Manheim and Lavett 1989). However, one research study clearly demonstrated the importance of the fascial tissues. Garfin et al. (1981) found that using a surgical fascial release to apply a small slit in the epimysium of a dog's hindlimbs resulted in an approximately 15% reduction in forces produced and a 50% decrease in the intracompartmental pressure developed during muscle contraction.

Myofascial Restrictions and the Anatomy of Fascia

All too often, various health practitioners view the body from a myopic point of view as determined by their scope of practice, philosophy, mastered techniques, or time limitations. Traditionally, chiropractors are concerned with a subluxation of the vertebrae, osteopaths with an osteopathic lesion, medical doctors with pain or symptom relief, acupuncturists with treating a trigger point, and so on. But what happens if the problem is with the fascia and not with the joints, muscles, or nerves? Fascia has the capacity to adapt to various conditions. Furthermore, it must be recognized that fasciae are continuous (fasciae can be traced from one area of the body to another) and they are contiguous (they all touch). To better understand myofascial interaction, imagine that the body is like a giant balloon that is filled with smaller balloons that are attached to it inside. These smaller balloons represent the body's various organs and muscles. If just one part of the balloon is distorted by tightness or restriction, then all parts of the balloon must be distorted to compensate. Several different models can be employed to represent this concept (Kuchera and Kuchera 1992).

Diagnosis of Myofascial Restrictions

These fascial interconnections can be demonstrated on two levels: visual and tactile. First, visualize a skeleton with a tight plastic overlay representing the muscles and fascia. As the overlays are stretched, they change to white along the lines of stress. Second, fascial connections can be sensed by palpation. Have a partner lie on a table. Place your fingers gently on his or her scalp, close your eyes, and concentrate on any movement being transferred to the scalp. Have the partner move his or her head, and feel the subsequent movement transmitted to the scalp. Next, have the partner shrug his or her shoulders, and once again feel the movement being transmitted to the scalp. Gradually, work down the body, having the hips, knees, ankles, and even toes flex and extend. Even at the most distal parts of the extremities, well-trained people will be able to detect the most subtle movements.

Last, imagine your car was hit in the rear bumper by another car at a moderate speed. Extensive damage may occur to the rear of the car (the rear bumper and fenders), but body damage may also be found throughout the vehicle including the front of the hood. Thus, the body shop would need to replace the damaged fender and repair the additional body damage throughout the car. Patients may not be treated as well as a car in a body shop—the "rear fender" is fixed, but the subtle damage to the rest of the body is ignored. With a car, this oversight may reduce its efficiency and decrease its life expectancy. With a human being, it may also result in a decrease in quality of life.

Treatment Strategies for Compromised Fascia

When the body is subjected to insult, fascial restrictions may occur in all directions: parallel, perpendicular, and oblique to the muscle fibers. To relieve such restrictions, biomechanical forces of tension, compression, shearing, bending, stress, and strain can be applied to the tissue (Mottice et al. 1986). These forces can be applied using a variety of techniques (e.g., general massage, rolfing, mobilization, manipulation, stretching). It is claimed that many of these techniques do not alter or modify the powerful fascial restrictions that occur in a high percentage of patients (Barnes 1991). However, in recent years the *myofascial release technique* (MRT) has been added to the arsenal of the field of manual medicine. MRT can target connective tissues or muscles. Several books and chapters of books have been written on this subject, from which this discussion was culled (Barnes 1991; Cantu and Grodin

1992; Manheim and Lavett 1989; Souza 1994; Ward 1985, 1993). However, as yet there have been no peer-reviewed research articles demonstrating the effectiveness of this technique.

A grossly overgeneralized version of this technique follows. The patient is evaluated by "reading the tissues" for areas of symmetry-asymmetry and looseness-tightness. Then, a force is applied in the appropriate direction and held until the soft tissues are felt to relax. This "softening" or "letting go" is called a *release*. The process is then repeated until the targeted tissues are fully elongated. A variety of force application techniques can be employed using MRT. In one method, termed *transverse muscle play*, a shearing force is applied by both palms of the therapist. The hands do not slide over the skin. Rather, the fascial layers slide on one another. Another method is referred to as *stripping*. Here, using a broad contact over the area of tightness, a firm pressure is applied as the patient actively moves through a full range. A variation of this technique is to perform a stripping massage while the muscle is under stretch with no active movement by the patient. *Strumming* is a deep-release technique that is usually performed with the fingers held in rigid extension, or the hand may be cupped in a clawlike position. Pressure is then applied to the restricted site using deep pressure

across and perpendicular to the muscle fibers. For a more detailed discussion, the reader is referred to the works of Cantu and Grodin (1992) and Manheim and Lavett (1989).

Effects of Immobilization on Connective Tissue

As a result of abnormal physical and chemical states, fascia may thicken, shorten, calcify, or erode, often causing pain (Mottice et al. 1986). In particular, when joints are immobilized for any length of time, the connective tissue elements of the capsules, ligaments, tendons, muscles, and fascia lose their extensibility. In addition, immobilization is associated with a concomitant change in chemical structure: 40% decrease in hyaluronic acid, 30% decrease in chondroitin-4- and chondroitin-6-sulfate, and 4.4% loss of water (Akeson, Amiel, and LaViolette 1967; Akeson et al. 1977; Akeson, Amiel, and Woo 1980; Woo et al. 1975). If we assume that distances between fibers are reduced when GAG and water volumes decrease, then this loss of GAG and water will result in a reduction of the critical fiber distance between collagen fibers. Consequently, the connective tis-

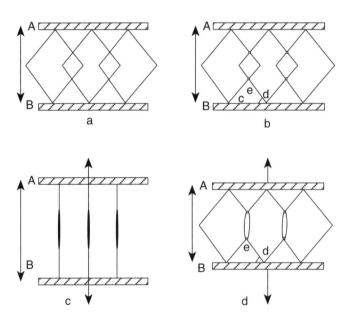

Fig. 4.9. The idealized weave pattern of collagen fibers. It can be demonstrated that fixed contact at strategic sites (e.g., points d and e) can severely restrict the extension of this collagen weave. (a) Collagen fiber arrangement; (b) collagen fiber cross-links; (c) normal stretch; and (d) restricted stretch due to cross-link.
Reprinted from Akeson, Amiel, and Woo (1980).

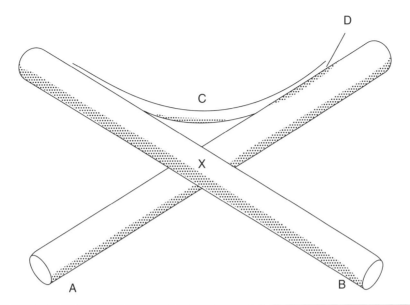

Fig. 4.10. An idealized model demonstrating the collagen cross-links' interaction at the molecular level. A and B represent the preexisting fibers; C represents the newly synthesized fibril; D represents the cross-links created as the fibril becomes incorporated into the fiber; and X represents the nodal point at which adjacent fibers normally move freely past one another.
Reprinted from Akeson, Amiel, and Woo (1980).

sue fibers will come into contact with each other and eventually stick, thereby encouraging the formation of abnormal cross-linking. The result is the loss of extensibility and an increase in tissue stiffness (Figures 4.9 and 4.10; Akeson, Amiel, and Woo 1980; McDonough 1981).

In addressing the significance of immobilization and mobilization, Donatelli and Owens-Burkhart (1982, 72) succinctly point out:

> If movement is the major stimulus for biological activity, then the amount, the duration, the frequency, the rate, and the time of initiation of the movement are all important in producing the desired therapeutic effects on connective tissue structures. These factors must be determined before we can comprehend the optimal benefits of mobilization.

Metabolic and Nutritional Influences on Connective Tissue

Normal tissue growth and wound healing represent a highly dynamic, integrated series of cellular, physiologic, and biochemical events that oc-

cur exclusively in whole organisms. Two factors that have significant implications in terms of optimal function, growth, and wound healing are metabolic and nutritional influences (e.g., vitamins A, E, and C and the minerals calcium, copper, iron, magnesium, and manganese). It has been recognized that a number of dietary deficiencies, excesses, and imbalances influence the metabolism and maturation of connective tissue proteins (Figure 4.11 and Table 4.3). Furthermore, research has demonstrated that inherited genetic disorders influence enzyme activity and, in turn, influence the metabolic pathways involved in the synthesis of connective tissue (Table 4.4). Since several enzymes participate in tissue formation, defects in any of the several steps of modification could become manifest. In turn, these connective tissue defects may ultimately influence tissue elasticity, stiffness, range of motion, and wound healing.

The interested reader is referred to two works. The first, by Tinker and Rucker (1985), offers the most detailed analysis on the subject of the proposed mechanisms by which diet changes can modify connective tissue metabolism. The second article, by Mead (1994), provides an interesting examination of how research suggests that diet may improve one's suppleness. Unfortunately, the article does not provide any references.

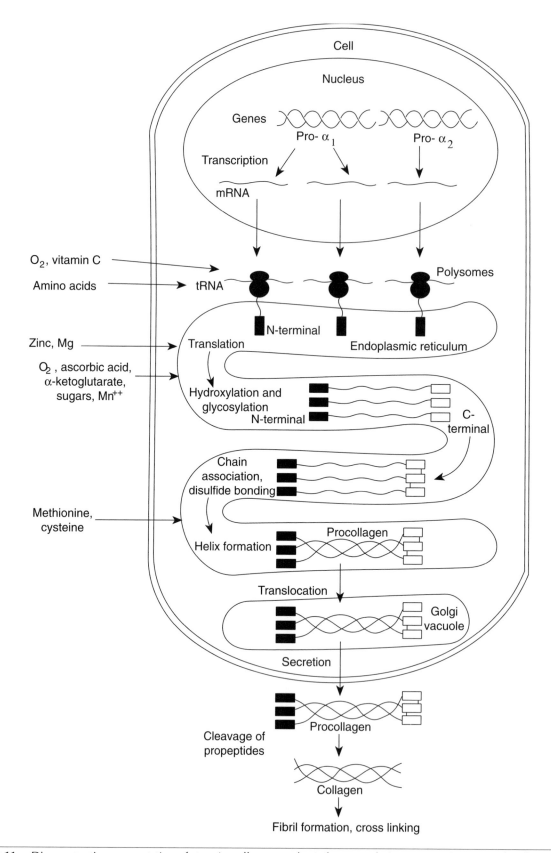

Fig. 4.11. Diagrammatic representation of steps in collagen synthesis from translation to secretion. Note the cleavage of the registration peptide (the rectangles at the ends of the molecule) that occurs in the extracellular space before final polymerization. Important nutrients at certain steps are noted on the left.
Reprinted from Hunt and Winkle (1979).

Table 4.3. Roles of Selected Nutrients in Maintenance of Connective Tissue

Nutrient	Functions important for connective tissue maintenance	Metabolic defects arising from deficiency
Copper	Collagen and elastic cross-linking, perhaps in sulfation or glycosylation of proteoglycans	Skin friability, aneurysms, bone fragility, and loss of coat color and structural integrity
Manganese	Cofactor for glycosyl transferases	Decreased proteoglycan accumulation, chondrodystrophy, and perosis in growing chicks
Zinc	Cell differentiation and histone assembly and structure	Poor wound healing, poor growth, and skeletal and cranial anomalies in young animals
Ascorbic acid	Cofactor in prolyl and lysyl hydroxylation, perhaps a cofactor in certain glycosylation reactions	Poor wound healing, decreased collagen synthesis, impaired bone development, and loss of basement membrane integrity
Pyridoxine	Elastin and collagen cross-linking (?)	Poor growth, abnormal protein synthesis and amino acid metabolism, and homocystinuria
Thiamine	Collagen synthesis (?)	Poor wound healing and decreased NADP production, neurological defects
Vitamin A	Differentiation of epithelium and putative role in proteoglycan synthesis	Poor wound healing and keratinization of epithelial tissue
Vitamin E	Collagen cross-linking (?)	Altered wound healing
Vitamin D	Bone collagen synthesis and osteoblast differentiation	With deficiency, poor bone growth and development; with an excess, decreased collagen synthesis
Vitamin K	Cofactor in carboxylations of glutamyl residues in osteocalcin	Altered bone mineralization

Table 4.4. Inherited and Experimentally Induced Disorders That Interfere With Collagen Biosynthesis and Degradation

Experimentally induced by	Pathway of collagen biosynthesis	Hereditary disorder
	Regulation of synthesis	Osteogenesis imperfecta
	↓	Ehlers-Danlos, Type IV
	Synthesis of pro α chains	
Proline analogs	Signal peptidase	Ehlers-Danlos, Type VI
α.α' dipyridyl	Prolyl and lysyl hydroxylases	(lysyl hydroxylase deficiency)
Ascorbic acid deficiency	Glycosyl transferases	Osteogenesis imperfecta
	Disulfide bond formation	
	↓	
	Procollagen	
Antimicrotubular agents,	Intracellular translocation	Ehlers-Danlos, Type IV
e.g., colchicine	and secretion	
	↓	
	Extracellular procollagen	
	Procollagen protease	Ehlers-Danlos, Type VII
		Dermatosparaxis
		(in cattle and sheep)
	↓	
	Collagen	
	Molecular packing	Spondyloepiphyseal dysplasia
		Ehlers-Danlos, Type I, in humans; dominant EDS in cats, mink, and dogs
	↓	
	Collagen fibril	
β-aminopropionitrile	Lysyl oxidase, Cu^{2+}	Cutis laxa, X-linked
(Osteolathyrism)	Cross-link formation	Aneurysm-prone mice
Copper deficiency		Menkes' kinky hair syndrome
D-Penicillamine		Homocystinuria
		Alcaptonuria
		Aging process
	↓	
	Collagen fiber	
	Collagenase	Epidermolysis bullosa
	↓	
	Collagen breakdown	

Reprinted from Bornstein and Byers (1980).

Summary

Connective tissue plays a significant role in determining one's range of movement. This tissue is influenced by a variety of factors, such as aging, immobilization, insults to the body, metabolic disorders, and nutritional deficiencies or excesses. Total resistance to movement has been determined to be 10% from tendon, 47% from ligament, and 41% from fascia. Because connective tissues are one of the most influential components in limiting range of motion, they must be optimally stretched.

Chapter 5

Mechanical and Dynamic Properties of Soft Tissues

For years, numerous research labs throughout the world have directed their efforts toward identifying the mechanical properties of muscle and connective tissue. *Biophysics* is the science that deals with the study of biological structures and processes with reference to principles and phenomena of physics. A knowledge of biophysics can help one to distinguish between fact and fallacy, cause and effect, the possible and impossible. Understanding the biophysics of muscle and connective tissue under various types of stress is therefore essential for determining the optimal means of increasing range of motion.

Unfortunately, the discipline of biophysics is complicated (Figure 5.1). The principles of physics do not always readily lend themselves in their application to biological tissues, which often behave in nonlinear ways. When dealing with such tissues it is necessary to take into simultaneous consideration their mechanical, electrical, and biochemical responses, particularly at the microlevel (G.C. Lee 1980). In addition, when dealing with living human beings one must take into consideration nonbiophysical factors such as feelings (e.g., pain and pleasure) and emotions (e.g., fear and joy). Nonetheless, there is much to be gained by learning how soft tissues respond to stresses such as postural distortion or trauma and, most significant, by learning how to correct and maintain them through an understanding of this discipline.

Terminology

Before we begin our examination of biophysics, you should understand some of its basic terminology and concepts. At times you will find several different terms used for essentially the same thing (distensibility, extensibility, or stretchability) and some words with definitions not commonly known or accepted (e.g., elasticity, sprain, or strain). The most precise and accurate terminology possible was adopted for use in this book.

Types of Force and Deformations

Whenever a tissue or material is subjected to a *force* (i.e., a pull or a push), a change in the shape or size of the material can occur. This response is, of course, dependent upon several variables: the type of material, the amount of force, the duration of the force, and the temperature of the material, to name a few.

These changes are called *deformations*, and the types of forces and the resulting deformations experienced by biological tissues and other materials fall into three major categories (Figure 5.2). A material subjected to a *compressive* force, for instance, shortens in length, and this decrease in length is its deformation. Such a deformation is called *compression*. An example of compression

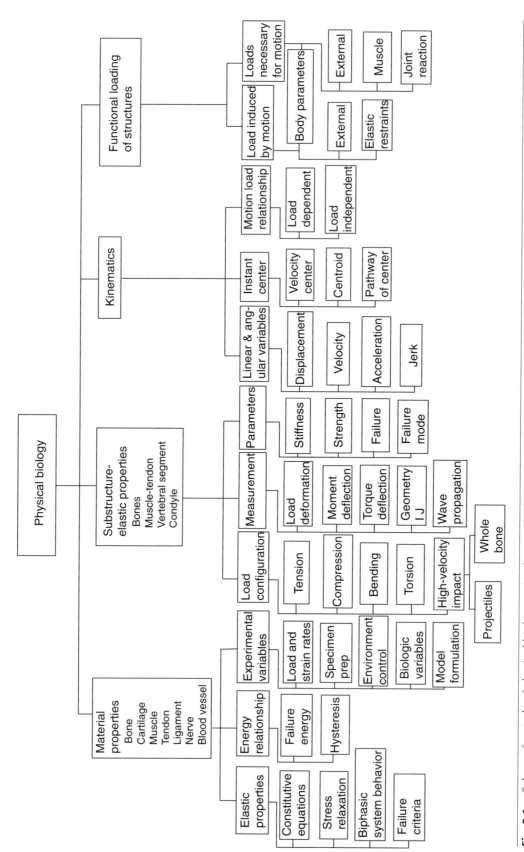

Fig. 5.1. Schema for study of physical biology as it relates to the locomotor system. Reprinted from Frankel and Burnstein (1974).

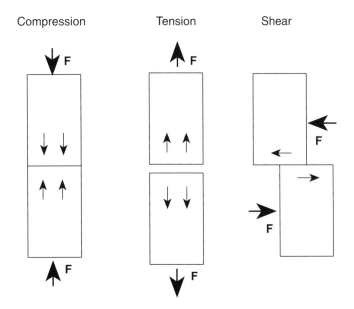

Fig. 5.2. Schematic representation of the three basic types of stress: compression, tension, and shear.

is weight bearing on the cartilage of a joint surface. In contrast, when a *tensile* or *horizontal* force is applied to a material, its length is increased. Such a lengthening is called an *axial* or *tension* deformation. In layperson's terms, *stretching* refers to the process of elongation and *stretch* refers to the elongation itself. Another type of deformation, called *shear*, results from shear forces that, when applied to an object, tend to cause one layer of the object to slide over another layer.

Elasticity

The property that enables a tissue to return to its original shape or size when a force is removed is called *elasticity*. Elasticity is measured as the amount of counterforce within the material itself. Since elastic stretch represents springlike behavior, it is often symbolized pictorially by a zigzag line representing a spring. It is sometimes called the *Hookean element* (Figure 5.3).

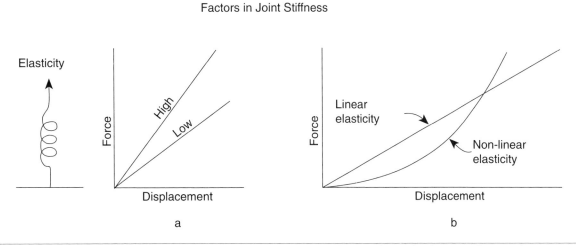

Fig. 5.3. Elastic stiffness as exemplified by an ideal spring showing a linear relationship between force and displacement. (a) A stiffer spring exhibits a higher degree of stiffness (steeper slope). (b) Linear and nonlinear elasticity of the common type in which stiffness (slope) increases with displacement.
Reprinted from Wright and Johns (1960).

Stress

When a force acts on a body or material, resisting forces within the body react. These resisting forces are called *stresses*. A stress is an internal resistance to an external force. Stress is measured by the force applied per unit area that produces or tends to produce deformation in a body, that is, the applied force divided by the cross-sectional area of the material that resists the force. Examples of stress units are lb/ft^2, N/m^2, and $dynes/cm^2$. Thus,

$$\text{Stress} = \frac{\text{Force}}{\text{Area of surface on which force acts}} = \frac{F}{A}$$

There are three principal kinds of stresses. These are compressive, tensile, and shear. A *compressive* stress is the force in the matter which resists its being pushed together. It results from two forces that are directed towards each other along the same straight line. *Tensile* stress represents a force in a material that resists the pulling apart or separating of the material. It is produced when two forces are directed away from each other along the same straight line. In contrast, a *shear* stress is the force in a material that opposes or resists two forces directed parallel to each other but not along the same line.

Strain

Strain is the change in length or amount of deformation occurring as a result of the applied force. Strain is defined as the ratio of length after stress is applied to original length. Because it is a ratio of lengths, strain has no dimensions or units. Thus, strain is a pure number or a percentage of original length. Thus,

$$\text{Longitudinal strain} = \frac{\text{Change in length}}{\text{Initial length}} = \frac{L}{l}$$

The amount of strain produced by a stress is determined basically by the electrochemical forces between the material's atoms. The stronger these forces are, the greater the stress will have to be before producing a given amount of strain. Mathews, Stacy, and Hoover (1964) have clearly described this concept. The molecules of a material are held together by attractive forces. When there is no external force applied, the length of a material is determined by a balance of attractive and repulsive forces between molecules. When a material is lengthened, the molecules spread far-

ther apart; the attractive forces then grow stronger while the repulsive forces grow weak. "Therefore, there is a force generated within the molecules of the material itself which tends to pull the ends of the sample back toward the unstressed condition. This is the elastic force" (p. 69).

Stiffness

Stiffness is a term that means different things to different people or in different disciplines. Common words that are synonymous to stiffness are soreness, tension, and tightness. In everyday usage, stiffness can imply anything from a difficulty in moving a joint to a low level of discomfort at the end of the range of movement (Gifford 1987). To the manipulative therapist, stiffness is generally taken to mean a painless abnormal restriction of movement (Maitland 1979). To the exercise physiologist, stiffness can also be used to describe postexercise soreness felt in muscles that is exacerbated when the affected tissues are stretched or contracted. (The topic of delayed muscle soreness will be discussed in chapter 9.) To the psychiatrist and psychologist, stiffness may reflect a psychosomatic disorder.

In biophysics stiffness is defined as the ratio of stress to strain, or of force to deformation. As force increases, deformation also increases, but the amount of deformation from any given force depends on the tissue. Stiffness can be plotted on a stress-strain, or load-deformation, curve and is indicated by the slope of the stress-strain relationship. A tissue with a steep load-deformation plot (such as bone) is said to have a high stiffness. It will exhibit relatively less deformation for a given amount of force. In contrast, a tissue with a more gradual slope for a given amount of force (such as cartilage) is said to have less stiffness. It will exhibit relatively more deformation.

Hooke's Law and the Modulus of Elasticity

The numerical relationship between stress and strain was first discovered by Robert Hooke. *Hooke's law* states that there is a constant or proportional arithmetical relationship between force and elongation. One unit of force will produce one unit of elongation, two units of force will produce two units of elongation, and so forth. Within the context of Hooke's law, body tissues may be *perfectly elastic*. There are two requirements that need to be fulfilled for a material to be perfectly elastic. First, the elastic element must have full recovery and regain its exact original dimensions from the deformation. Second, an instantaneous force application or removal must be accompanied by the appropriate change in dimension without delay.

The equation constant in Hooke's law is the material's *modulus of elasticity*. This modulus value varies for different tissues. With materials of a higher modulus, there is a greater degree of stiffness. Therefore, a stiffer material will require a greater stress for a certain strain or a greater load for a given deformation than will a more flexible tissue. The modulus of elasticity is the ratio of the unit stress to the unit of deformation or strain, where Y is the proportional constant. Thus, the modulus of elasticity equals the stress required to produce one unit of strain.

$$Y = \frac{\text{Longitudinal stress}}{\text{Longitudinal strain}} = \frac{F/A}{L/l} = \frac{Fl}{AL}$$

Because the strain is a dimensionless ratio, the units of Y are identical with those of stress, namely, force/length^2. Thus, Y may be expressed in lb/in^2, N/m^2, or dynes/cm^2. The value of Y differs for different materials and does not depend on the material's dimensions. The value for a cross-linked polymer (i.e., a material that has molecules built up from large numbers of more or less similar units) depends on the spacing of the cross-links. The shorter the length of molecule between one cross-link and the next, the higher the modulus of elasticity and thus the harder the material is to stretch (R.M. Alexander 1975, 1988).

Elastic Limit

In materials that are not perfectly elastic, the arithmetical relationship between force and elongation reaches a value known as the *elastic limit*. The elastic limit is the smallest value of stress required to produce permanent strain in the body. Below the elastic limit, materials return to their original length when the deforming force is removed. However, the result of applying a force beyond the elastic limit is that the stressed material will not return to its original length when the force is removed. The difference between the original length and the new length is called the amount of *permanent set* or *sprain*. This unrecoverable or permanent elongation is also called *plastic stretch*. When stress is applied beyond the elastic limit, deformation and force are no longer linearly proportional. The material elongates much

further for each unit of force above the elastic limit than it did below it.

When stress slightly beyond the elastic limit is applied, a deformation occurs without additional stress. This transition is called the *yield point*. As increased forces are applied beyond this point, the curve tends to flatten. As further stress or force is applied, gradual tissue failure occurs. Eventually, the maximal force that can be tolerated by the tissue is reached. The maximum stress recorded—that is, the unit stress that occurs just at or below rupture—is called the *ultimate strength* of the material.

These concepts are extremely significant for athletes and laypeople alike. If one wishes to reduce the probability or degree of tissue damage from overstretching, the appropriate course of action is to strengthen those parts of the body that are most likely to receive insults. This practice is commonly seen in athletics where resistance training (e.g., free weights or machines) is incorporated to strengthen the musculature and appropriate tissues (e.g., ligaments and tendons). By so doing, the tissues adapt to a higher level of stress as a result of the overload, and their ultimate strengths are increased.

Factors Influencing Stiffness

Stiffness not only varies between tissues, it also changes with other factors, such as age, immobilization, and repetition of stress. Under all three of these conditions, stiffness decreases and the resistance of tissues to applied force is therefore reduced, leading to increased risk of injury.

Plasticity

Plasticity is the property of a material to permanently deform when it is loaded beyond its elastic range. Consequently, there is no tendency for elastic recoil or recovery. Past the yield point, a tissue's plastic response involves considerable amounts of deformation with very small increases in force. There are probably no perfectly plastic materials (Figure 5.4). However, modeling clay is an example of a plastic material that exhibits extremely plastic behavior.

Plasticity is crucial in terms of both the cause and treatment of various injuries. It is recognized that long-term, repetitive microtrauma can result in deformed (i.e., plastic) tissues that exhibit reduced stability, leading to reduced efficiency and quality of life. A classic example is long-term improper posture when sitting in a chair. Over

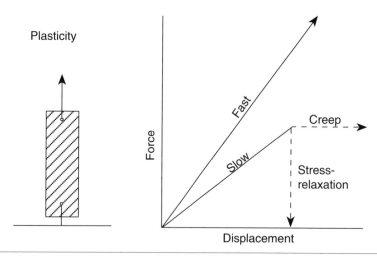

Plasticity

Fig. 5.4. Plastic or viscoelastic stiffness. The elastic stiffness of a plastic substance is typically greater with faster stretch (steeper slope). Maintenance of a constant force results in continued elongation (creep). If stretched and maintained at constant length, the force required wanes (stress-relaxation).
Reprinted from Wright and Johns (1960).

time, the body adapts to the stresses by increased deformation of the back tissues and shortening of anterior trunk tissues, leading to reduced range of motion and the development of discomfort and pain.

Conversely, the application of stretching exercises, traction, and other remodeling procedures plays an important part in improving performance or in rehabilitation. For improving performance, most knowledgeable athletes are aware that proper stretching (i.e., plasticity training) results in increased flexibility. That is, the tissues adapt to the stretching forces with increased flexibility. For many disciplines this adaptation is essential to success or failure. In rehabilitation, the achievement of plasticity is essential. Therapeutic stretching procedures are used to create a

beneficial deformation back to a more efficient position (Garde 1988).

Viscosity

Viscosity is the property of materials to resist loads that produce shear and flow. Unlike elasticity and plasticity, it is truly time dependent. A dashpot, a plunger or piston immersed in a viscous fluid, classically illustrates viscosity. The behavior of a dashpot is closely mimicked by a syringe filled with fluid. The faster one tries to move the plunger, the higher the pressure within the fluid (Figure 5.5).

Viscosity is a concept that is especially important as it relates to sports. Athletes are commonly told to warm up. One reason is to reduce their

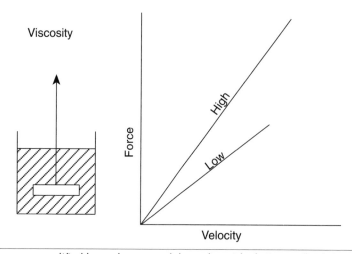

Viscosity

Fig. 5.5. Viscous stiffness as exemplified by a plate moved through an ideal viscous fluid showing a linear relationship between force and velocity. Increased viscosity results in higher viscous stiffness (steeper slope).
Reprinted from Wright and Johns (1960).

tissue viscosity. By warming up, the bodily tissues and fluids become warmed. This reduces viscosity, and consequently extensibility is enhanced. As an analogy, think of a syringe filled with warm honey and another with cold honey. Which fluid do you think will flow faster?

Viscoelasticity

Most biological materials are neither perfectly elastic nor perfectly plastic. They exhibit a combination of properties, referred to as viscoelastic behavior. When subjected to low loads, they exhibit elastic behavior. At higher loads, they exhibit plastic response. In addition, when loads are applied over time, the tissue exhibits viscous deformation.

Hysteresis

Hysteresis is a phenomenon associated with energy loss exhibited by viscoelastic materials when they are subjected to loading and unloading

cycles (Figure 5.6). As explained by Frost (1967), when an elastic tissue is loaded and unloaded, the stress-strain curve is identical during the loading and unloading phases. In contrast, with viscoelastic material, the curves for the two phases are *not* identical. If the loading ceases prior to tissue failure and an unloading test is performed, the descending curve for the decreasing stress will not precisely coincide with the ascending curve, despite the absence of permanent deformation at the end. The area between the loading and unloading curves represents energy lost (converted into heat).

As with plasticity, hysteresis is important in therapeutic techniques such as traction and other remodeling procedures. Hence, two points made by Garde (1988) deserve mention. First, hysteresis is the desired effect of those procedures that produce a beneficial deformation back to a more efficient position. If the tissues remained resilient after their initial and negative deformation, there would be no change in condition. Consequently, a beneficial deformation back to a more efficient position could not take place. Second, it must be

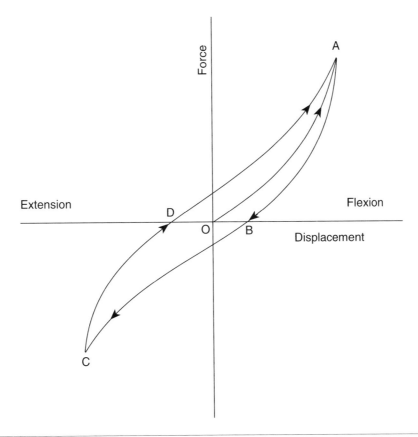

Fig. 5.6. Diagram of the stiffness of joints, with extension to the left, flexion to the right, and force (torque) vertically. Joint rotation begins at the midposition (O) and proceeds to full flexion (A). It is then extended (A, B, C) and flexed (C, D, A). It is apparent that the elastic stiffness (slope) is nonlinear and that there is hysteresis.
Reprinted from Wright and Johns (1960).

remembered, however, that hysteresis is also part of the pathological deforming cycle due to macrotrauma or repetitive microtrauma.

Soft Tissues

Tissues may be divided into two categories: hard and soft. The former includes bone for the most part, as well as teeth, nails, and hair. Soft tissues include tendons, ligaments, muscles, skin, and most of the other tissues (Mathews, Stacy, and Hoover 1964). Soft tissues are divided into two groups: contractile and noncontractile.

Properties of Soft Tissues

Soft tissues vary in physical and mechanical characteristics (Figure 5.7). Both contractile and noncontractile tissues are extensible and elastic, but contractile tissues are also contractible. *Contractility* is the ability of a muscle to shorten and develop tension along its length. *Distensibility* (commonly known as *extensibility* or *stretchability*) is the ability of muscle tissue to stretch in response to an externally applied force. The weaker the forces generated within the muscle, the greater will be the amount of stretch.

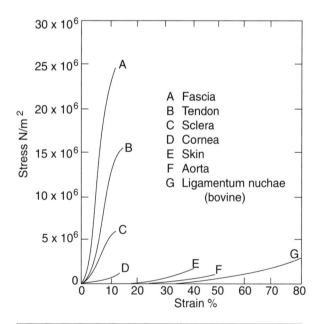

Fig. 5.7. Stress-strain curves for various connective tissues.
Reprinted from Soden and Kershaw (1974).

The Relationship of the Mechanical Properties of Soft Tissues to Stretching

The greater the stiffness of a soft tissue, the greater the force must be that can produce an elongation. A tissue of low stiffness cannot resist a stretching force as well as a tissue that is very stiff, and it will need a lesser force than the stiffer tissue does to produce the same degree of deformation. Therefore, soft tissues with greater stiffness are less susceptible to injuries such as sprains (which involve tears of ligamentous tissue) and strains (which involve tears of contractile tissue or muscle).

Soft tissues are not perfectly elastic. Beyond their elastic limit, they cannot return to their original length once the stretching force is removed. The difference between the original length and the new length is called the amount of *permanent set* (plastic stretch or deformation) and correlates to minor tissue damage. Thus, when one suffers a minor sprain or strain, the soft tissues do not return to their original length after the excessive stress is removed, leading to permanent laxity and joint instability.

A natural question then arises: For flexibility to be developed, should one stretch up to the elastic limit or slightly beyond it? Most authorities recommend stretching to the point of "discomfort" or "tension," but not pain. What, then, is the difference between discomfort and pain? The meaning of these terms in medicine (and other disciplines) can be interpreted in various ways, depending on who does the interpreting (de Jong 1980). In 1979, the International Association for the Study of Pain (IASP) was organized to develop an internationally acceptable definition of pain and a classification system of pain syndromes. Eventually, pain and 18 other common terms were defined (de Jong 1980; Merskey 1979). Three terms are most relevant to this discussion:

Pain: "An unpleasant sensory and emotional experience associated with actual or potential tissue damage or described in terms of such damage"

Pain threshold: "The least stimulus intensity at which a subject perceives pain"

Pain tolerance level: "The greatest stimulus intensity causing pain that a subject is prepared to tolerate"

Based on the preceding definitions, most authorities state that the stretch should be at least to the pain threshold point. However, because these three concepts are based upon subjective factors, there is no way that coaches or trainers can determine this level for a person under their charge. Remember, there is no such thing as an average person; each person is unique in his or her own sensory and emotional experience, and this experience continually changes.

Another point deserves special consideration and caution. That is, for those individuals who are undergoing rehabilitation and have healing tissues, the point before pain is reached may be sufficient to rupture these already weakened tissues. Hence, extreme caution must be employed when applying tension to previously damaged tissues.

This discussion raises another question: Is the point of discomfort below, at, or beyond the elastic limit? Although the literature is not conclusive on this subject, research indicates that the type of force, the duration of the force, and the temperature of the tissue during and after stretching will determine whether the elongation is recoverable or permanent.

The Length-Tension and Stress-Strain Relationship

The length of a soft tissue depends on the relation of the internal force developed by the tissue to the external force exerted by the resistance or load. If the internal force exceeds the external force, the tissue shortens. Conversely, if the external force exceeds the internal force, the tissue lengthens.

Stress-Relaxation and Creep During Passive Tension

Living tissues are characterized by the presence of time-dependent mechanical properties. These properties include creep and stress-relaxation. When a resting muscle is suddenly stretched and held at a constant length, after a period of time there is a slow loss of tension. This behavior is called *stress-relaxation* (Figure 5.8a). In contrast, the lengthening that occurs when a constant force or load is applied is called *creep* (Figure 5.8b).

We are most interested about how these time-dependent mechanical properties operate on

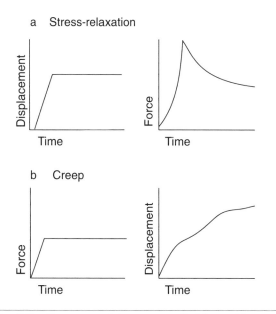

Fig. 5.8. Responses of tissues to applied force. (a) Stress-relaxation results when there is a reduction in force that occurs when a tissue is held at a constant length. (b) Creep is the lengthening that occurs over a period of time when a constant force is applied.
Reprinted from Alter (1988).

muscle cells and connective tissues. Among the pertinent questions that need to be addressed in future research are:

- How is tensile force transmitted through the sarcomere and through the structures of the various connective tissues?
- What is the effect of tensile force on a sarcomere's sarcolemma, sarcoplasm, and cytoskeleton (i.e., the supporting framework of minute filaments and tubules within every cell)?
- Where and through what structures in the sarcomere do the creep and stress-relaxation phenomena operate?
- What is the relationship (if any) of creep and stress-relaxation in sarcomeres to pressure gradients, fluid flow, and streaming potentials of the structures of the various connective tissues?

The Molecular Mechanism of Connective Tissue's Elasticity Response

Connective tissues are composite materials linked to form long, flexible chains. Two essential variables that influence the stiffness (or elasticity) for connective tissues are the spacing of their cross-links and the temperature. For example, imagine a long, flexible molecule composed of a number of segments. The letter n will represent this number. Each segment has a given length, represented by the letter a. It is also given that each segment in itself is stiff, but the joints between the segments are flexible. We will also assume that the molecules of the segments are not restrained in any way, but are free to move.

All molecules move in a random fashion to some extent or another. However, as temperature decreases, molecules become less free to move. When the temperature of absolute zero (i.e., –273° C) is reached, all movement ceases. Due to the random molecular movement, at a particular given instant, the distance from one end of a segment to another may have any value from 0 (if the ends are in contact) to na (if the molecule is stretched out straight). However, the maximum length position is unlikely. It can be shown that the most probable length for the molecule is its midlength $n^{1/2}a$.

In a "normal" state, molecular chains in a network will continue to move, and the junctions at which they end will move together and apart. The distance between the ends of a particular chain will vary, but the average distance in a sample containing many chains will always be $n^{1/2}a$. (This value is actually a root mean square value, not a simple mean.)

Now, let's look at Figure 5.9a. Assume an external tensile force is applied to the connective tissue. The network will be deformed (Figure 5.9b), and the chains will align in the direction of stretch. Consequently, the chains aligned in the direction of the tensile force (for example, AB) now have average lengths greater than $n^{1/2}a$. In contrast, those chains aligned across the direction of stretching (BC) have average lengths less than $n^{1/2}a$. What has happened is that the arrangement is no longer random. Then, when the distorting force is removed, the chains move back into random configurations. As a result, the connective tissue returns to its original shape; it recoils elastically.

As described by R.M. Alexander (1988),

a theory developed from these ideas predicts the force required for equilibrium of the deformed network, and hence the modulus of elasticity. The shear modulus G and Young's modulus E are given by the equation:

$$G = NkT = E/3$$

where N is the number of chains per unit volume of material, k is a physical constant (Blotzmann's constant) and T is the absolute temperature. *Notice the importance of the number of chains. If more cross-links are inserted, dividing the molecules into a larger number of shorter chains, the material becomes stiffer. Also, the modulus is proportional to the absolute temperature because the energy associated with the writhing of the molecules increases with temperature. Similarly, the pressure exerted at constant volume by a gas increases with temperature, because the kinetic energy of the molecules increases with temperature.* (p. 14, emphasis added)

Research Findings Regarding Stretching of Connective Tissue

With a basic knowledge of the biophysics of connective tissues and muscles, we are now ready

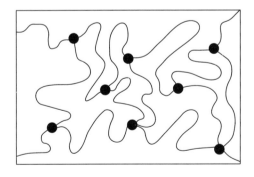

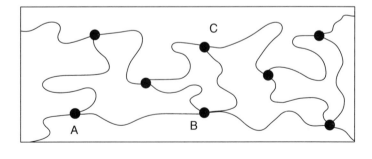

a   b

Fig. 5.9. A diagram of a rubbery polymer (a) unstrained and (b) stretched horizontally. The sinuous lines represent polymer molecules and the dots represent cross-links.
Reprinted from Alexander (1988).

to examine the research findings. When a tensile force is applied to connective tissue or muscle, the original length increases and its cross section (i.e., width) decreases. Are there different types of forces, or conditions under which a force can be applied, that will create an optimal change in connective tissue? Sapega et al. (1981) addressed these questions clearly and succinctly:

When tensile forces are continuously applied to an organized connective tissue model (tendon), the time required to stretch the tissue a specific amount varies inversely with the forces used (C.G. Warren, Lehmann, and Koblanski 1971, 1976). Therefore, a low-force stretching method requires more time to produce the same amount of elongation as a higher-force method. However, the proportion of tissue lengthening that remains after tensile stress is removed is greater for the low-force, long-duration method (C.G. Warren et al. 1971, 1976; Laban 1962). Higher-force, short-duration stretching favors recoverable, elastic tissue deformation, whereas low-force, long-duration stretching enhances permanent, plastic deformation (C.G. Warren et al. 1971, 1976; Laban 1962). This principle does not necessarily rule out combining higher forces with a prolonged duration of stretch, but in the clinical setting, high-force application has a greater risk of causing pain and possibly tissue rupture. In addition, laboratory studies have shown that when connective tissue structures are permanently elongated, some degree of mechanical weakening takes place, even though outright rupture has not occurred (C.G. Warren et al. 1971, 1976; Rigby, Hirai, Spikes, and Eyring 1959). The amount of weakening depends on the way the tissue is stretched as well as how much it is stretched. Of particular interest is that for the same amount of tissue elongation, a high-force stretching method produces more structural weakening than a slower, low-force method (C.G. Warren et al. 1971, 1976).

Temperature has a significant influence on the mechanical behavior of connective tissue under tensile stress. As tissue temperature rises, stiffness decreases and extensibility increases (Laban 1962; Rigby 1964). Raising the temperature of tendon samples above 103°F increases the amount of permanent elongation that results from a given amount of initial stretching (Laban 1962; Lehmann, Masock, Warren, and Koblanski 1970). At about 104°F a thermal transition in the microstructure of collagen occurs which significantly enhances the viscous stress relaxation of collagenous tissue, allowing greater plastic deformation when it is stretched (Mason and Rigby 1963; Rigby 1964; Rigby et al. 1959). The mechanism behind this thermal transition is still uncertain, but it is thought that intermolecular bonding becomes partially destabilized enhancing the viscous flow properties of the collagenous tissue (Rigby 1964; Rigby et al. 1959).

When connective tissue is stretched at an elevated temperature, the conditions under which the tissue is allowed to cool can significantly affect the amount of elongation that remains after the tensile stress is removed. After the heated tissue has been stretched, maintaining tensile force during tissue cooling has been shown to significantly increase the relative proportion of plastic deformation compared with unloading the tissue while its temperature is still elevated (Lehmann et al. 1970). Cooling the tissue before releasing the tension apparently allows the collagenous microstructure to restabilize more toward its new stretched length (Lehmann et al. 1970).

When stretching connective tissue at temperatures within the usual therapeutic range (102–110°F), the amount of structural weakening produced by a given amount of tissue elongation varies inversely with the temperature (C.G. Warren et al. 1971, 1976). This is apparently related to the progressive increase in the viscous flow properties of the collagen as it is heated. It is possible that thermal destabilization of intermolecular bonding allows elongation to occur with less structural damage.

The factors influencing the viscoelastic behavior of connective tissue can be summarized by stating that elastic or recoverable deformation is most favored by high-force, short-duration stretching at normal or colder tissue temperature, whereas plastic or permanent lengthening is most favored by lower-force, longer-duration stretching at elevated temperatures, but allowing the tissue to cool before releasing the tension. In addition, the structural weakening produced by permanent tissue deformation is minimized when prolonged, low-force application is combined with high therapeutic temperatures, and it is maximal when higher forces and lower temperatures are used. (pp. 59–61)

Tables 5.1, 5.2, and 5.3 summarize these factors.

Research by others (Becker 1979; Glazer 1980; Jackman 1963; Kottke, Pauley, and Ptak 1966; Light et al. 1984) has also demonstrated that stretching at low to moderate tension levels is effective. However, other than the clinical successes of Sapega et al. (1981), no additional studies have been reported that combine tissue temperature manipulation and therapeutic stretching.

Table 5.1. Summary of Factors That Influence the Proportion of Plastic and Elastic Stretch

Influential factors	Elastic stretch	Plastic stretch
Amount of applied force	High force	Low force
Duration of applied force	Short time	Long time
Tissue temperature	Low temperature	High temperature

Reprinted from Sapega, Quedenfeld, Moyer, and Butler (1981).

Table 5.2. Summary of Factors that Influence the Viscoelastic Behavior of Connective Tissue

Elastic deformation	Viscous (plastic) deformation
High-force short-duration stretching	Low-force long-duration stretching
Normal or colder tissue temperatures	Elevated temperatures with cooling before release of tension

Reprinted from Sapega, Quedenfeld, Moyer, and Butler (1981).

Table 5.3. Summary of Factors That Influence Amount of Tissue Weakening Produced by Deformation

Minimal structural weakening	Maximal structural weakening
Lower forces	Higher forces
Higher temperatures	Lower temperatures

Note. Adapted from "Biophysical Factors in Range-of-Motion Exercise" by A.A. Sapega, T.C. Quedenfeld, R.A. Moyer, and R.A. Butler, 1981, *The Physician and Sportsmedicine*, 9(12), pp. 59-60. Copyright 1981 by McGraw-Hill. Adapted by permission.

Reprinted from Sapega, Quedenfeld, Moyer, and Butler (1981).

Summary of Research

One of the most interesting aspects of research is that it raises more questions than it answers, for we are still in the dark about many aspects of flexibility and stretching. We remain uncertain, for instance, about the exact mechanism by which tissues actually develop elasticity. We still do not fully understand what structural or chemical changes occur in tissues as a result of stretching. It is far too early to promise any panacea for those who desire to increase their flexibility in a short period of time. The exciting possibility of applying new and powerful techniques may lie in the future, but such techniques will need to be investigated vigorously at the clinical as well as the experimental level. In the meantime, there are no shortcuts for diligent and hard practice.

Muscle

We know a great deal about the various mechanical properties of muscle, as they have been among the favorite topics of researchers for decades. There are several reasons why we should study the mechanical properties of muscle. One is so that we may comprehend the mechanical responses of a whole muscle; another is to help us understand the mechanical properties of the contractile components themselves (Zierler 1974). Yet for our needs here, the most important reason for studying the mechanical properties of muscle is so that we may understand and determine the factors that limit flexibility and the best means of increasing flexibility.

Muscle Connective Tissues

Muscle is composed of three independent mechanical components or elements, which may be classified as either *elastic* or *viscous*. These mechanical components are important because they resist deformation, and therefore play a major role in determining one's flexibility. Elastic components exert a restoring force in response to a change in length. Viscous components exert a force in response to the rate (velocity) and duration of a change in length. The three mechanical components are

1. the parallel elastic component (PEC),
2. the series elastic component (SEC), and
3. the contractile component (CC).

The Parallel Elastic Component (PEC)

The component responsible for passive or resting tension in muscle is the *parallel elastic component* (PEC). The PEC is so named because it lies parallel to the contractile mechanism (see Figure 5.10). If a muscle is removed from a body, it will naturally shorten by about 10% of its original, intact (in situ) length (Garamvölgyi 1971). This shortening is independent of (passive) contraction. The length of the isolated, uncontracted muscle is called its *equilibrium length*; this shortening means that muscles are under tension at their intact length. The in situ length of an uncontracted or unstretched muscle is called its *resting length*, symbolized as Rl or L_o.

Resting muscle is elastic and resists lengthening. At lengths less than equilibrium length ($0.90L_o$) there is no resting tension and the PEC is slack. However, when an unstimulated muscle is stretched, it develops tension in a nonlinear fashion. That is, little tension is developed with initial stretch, and increasingly more tension is developed as stretch continues. The same effect can be seen when a knitted stocking is stretched (Carlson and Wilkie 1974). But of what is the PEC composed, and what structures are responsible for a muscle's resting tension?

Originally, the PEC was thought to consist primarily of the sarcolemma, sarcoplasm, and elastic fibers of the epimysium, perimysium, and endomysium. Later, H.E. Huxley and Hanson (1954) proposed the S-filament, which was thought to link up the ends of the actin filaments on either side. However, one year later, S-filaments were dropped without explanation from the muscle model of H.E. Huxley (1957). Another explanation for the passive resting tension was an *electrostatic force*. For example, it is a fact that the volume of muscle fibers remains constant even when muscle is stretched. The cross-sectional area (i.e., width) of a muscle, however, must decrease as well as the side spacing between the actin and myosin filaments as they move closer to each other. However, if a mutual electrostatic repulsive force exists between the filaments, work must be done to move them closer together. That is, some force must exist that maintains the filaments in a regular array. Consequently, the force necessary to move the filaments closer against the electrostatic repulsion would appear as the resting tension or the "parallel" resistance to stretch (Davson 1970; H.E. Huxley 1967). Although the electrostatic force may contribute to resting tension at high degrees of stretch, research has shown that it cannot be a dominant source.

As was discussed in chapter 3, unequivocal evidence has finally demonstrated that titin is the major source of muscle elasticity. This proof has been accomplished by destroying the titin filament while recording the muscle's degree of tension under stress. In the first study of this type, titin was preferentially destroyed by radiation (Horowits et al. 1986). The result was a reduction in resting tension. One year later, Horowits and Podolsky (1987b) published additional data from another study that supported the hypothesis that

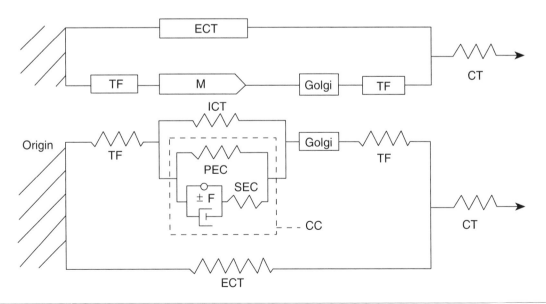

Fig. 5.10. Composite diagram of viscoelastic components of muscle fiber and surrounding connective tissue, with Golgi tendon organ in series. TF, tendon fascicles; ECT, extra connective tissue; M, muscle fibers; Golgi, tendon organ; PEC, parallel elastic component; CC, contractile component; SEC, series elastic component; ICT, intramuscular connective tissue; CT, common tendon.
Reprinted from Long (1974).

the elastic titin filaments produce most of the resting tension in muscle. In another study (Yoshioka et al. 1986), titin was preferentially destroyed via controlled proteolysis (i.e., the use of digestive enzymes). Once again, there was a reduction of resting tension. Similarly, in a more recent study (Funatsu, Higuchi, and Ishiwata 1990), it was also reported that there was a decrease in the resting tension with the degradation of titin via its enzymatic digestion (by plasma gesolin).

What then happens as the sarcomere is stretched and released? As was discussed in chapter 3, during stretch, neither the thin filament (actin) nor the thick filament (myosin) changes length. Instead, the filaments merely slide past one another—the well-known sliding filament theory. During the application of stretch, the sarcomere resists the deforming force by its resting tension. At first, the resting tension is modest. After a considerable stretch the resting tension rises steeply and resists any further extension (elastic stiffness). It is the titin that is responsible for this behavior. Upon release, the stretched titin filaments retract. Hence, titin can store potential energy.

If titin contributes to resting tension, what about nebulin? Research has suggested that nebulin constitutes a set of inextensible filaments attached at one end to the Z-line and that nebulin filaments are in parallel, not in series, with titin filaments (Wang and Wright 1988). Hence, nebulin could potentially represent a fourth filament in the sarcomere. Insofar as the proposed nebulin filament is concerned, research has confirmed that it is not a factor in the resting tension. When nebulin is degraded, there is no decrease in resting tension (Funatsu, Higuchi, and Ishiwata 1990; Wang and Wright 1988). Therefore, nebulin does not produce the elasticity.

The Series Elastic Component (SEC)

When a muscle is stretched, the contractile component (i.e., the actin and myosin filaments and their cross-bridges), PEC, and SEC all contribute to the development of tension. The *series elastic component* (SEC) is so named because the elastic components occur directly in line with the contractile components (see Figure 5.10). The SEC has the important function of smoothing out rapid changes in muscle tension. One of the chief anatomic parts making up the SEC is thought to consist of tendon. However, Pollack (1990) has postulated that the Z-line may also constitute a modest source of the sarcomere's series elasticity. This function is accomplished by the thin filaments pulling on the Z-line. For example, when a force on the thin filaments is transmitted to the Z-line, the lateral separation between the filaments is reduced (Figure 5.11). Yet, in order to accommodate a decrease in interfilament spacing, the fold angle in the Z-line structure simply becomes accentuated and more acute (Figure 5.12). Consequently, the Z-line effectively thickens, creating a kind of "elasticity."

The Contractile Component (CC)

The muscle's ability to increase tension is called the *contractile component* (CC). The CC of muscle may be regarded as a tension generator. It consists

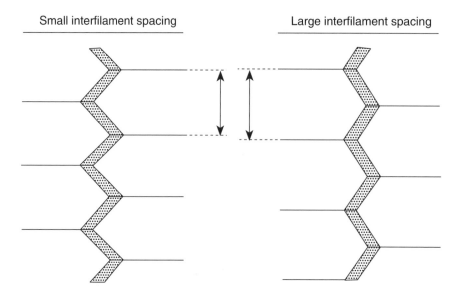

| Small interfilament spacing | Large interfilament spacing |

Fig. 5.11. Effect of change of interfilament spacing on Z-line structure. The Z-line accommodates such changes through variation of the angle between contiguous elements.
Reprinted from Pollack (1990).

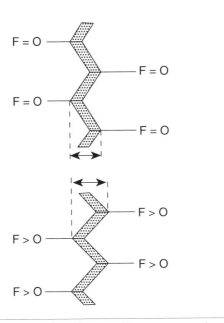

Fig. 5.12. Force on thin filaments (F) accentuates zigzag pattern of Z-line structure, resulting in changes of effective "width" of the Z-line. Such accordionlike changes may give rise to series elasticity.
Reprinted from Pollack (1990).

of the filaments and their cross-bridges. If tension is proportional to the number of chemical links established between the two filaments, then the greater the overlap between the filaments, the more binding sites can interact and the greater the tension that can be developed. Maximal contractile tension is assumed to be developed when sarcomere lengths are such that maximal single overlap of actin and myosin filaments exists. At greater muscle length, the number of cross-links diminishes as filament overlap decreases, resulting in reduced tension. As the stretch continues, the tension developed becomes smaller until, finally, the tension developed during the stretch is no greater than that in a passive muscle. This fact can be explained by the fact that at such lengths, actin and myosin filaments no longer interdigitate. Thus, they can develop little or no tension.

Total Tension of Active Muscle During Stretch

In general, the maximum total active tension is found at about 1.2 to 1.3 times the muscle's original or rest length. At greater lengths, total active tension diminishes until the muscle is at about 1.5 times the muscle's rest length, at which point active tension generation is zero. At lengths beyond $1.3L_o$, the number of cross-links diminishes as overlap decreases, resulting in reduced ten-

sions. Furthermore, although the PEC is increasing in its passive tension output, this total does not match the corresponding decline in active tension of the contractile components. Consequently, total tension decreases. At extremes of muscle length, passive tension generated by the SEC increases substantially, compensating for the decline in active tension, resulting in an increase in total tension (Figure 5.13). Other explanations for the mechanism underlying the extra tension during slow lengthening to contraction include heterogeneity of sarcomere lengths, an elastic structure other than the cross-bridges recruited or formed during activation, and axial shifts of cross-bridges (Yagi and Matsubara 1984).

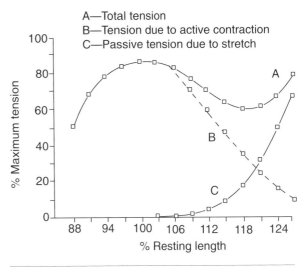

Fig. 5.13. Length-tension diagram of the total and passive tension. Length-tension diagram for passive stretch of an unstimulated muscle is shown in lower curve C. Curve A, showing total isometric tension when the muscle was stimulated at various lengths from maximal stretch through moderate shortening, represents the summation of active contraction (B) plus tension due to passive stretch (C). Active tension due solely to muscular contraction is obtained by subtracting passive tension, C, from total tension, A, and is represented by curve B. Normal resting length is 100%.
Reprinted from Schottelius and Senay (1956).

Muscle Stretches Applied During Contraction at Long Muscle Lengths

When tissues are stretched, they develop tension. This tension is known as the *stretch response*, which is independent of the central nervous system (CNS) and is a mechanical property of the tissues stretched. On the other hand, the *stretch reflex* is a response mediated by the CNS that causes the stretched muscle to contract in response to stretch stimulus (Gowitzke and Milner 1988).

One of the major arguments against the use of ballistic stretching (i.e., bobbing or bouncing) is that it initiates a stretch reflex. However, if one were to begin such stretching beyond the length of $1.5L_o$, the stretch reflex should not result in any increase of tension in the CC because the filaments are no longer capable at such lengths of interdigitating and developing tension. This reasoning would be true if all sarcomeres in the muscle fiber were stretched to the same extent. However, not all sarcomeres stretch to the same extent. That is, when a muscle is stretched, the stretch is not uniform along its entire length. Sarcomeres near tendons stretch to a much lesser extent than sarcomeres in the middle of a muscle. Hence, sarcomeres at the end of the muscle may still have considerable filament overlap, while those filaments in the middle sarcomeres are stretched beyond the point of overlap (Davson 1970). Therefore, the sarcomeres near tendons can still develop reflex tension and influence the degree of extension. Furthermore, it seems reasonable to argue that the resistance to continued stretching arises either from the reattachment of cross-bridges previously broken, or from the attachment of additional cross-bridges to sites on the actin filament that are not available initially, but that become accessible as a result of the movement (Flintney and Hirst 1978). Thus, activation of the stretch reflex, even when the muscle fiber is beyond $1.5L_o$, will probably result in some additional tension being produced by the CC.

Vascular Tissue

Numerous structures of the body are exposed to a wide range of forces during movement, and during stretching in particular. Among the most obvious structures subjected to forces are the connective tissues (e.g., tendons, ligaments, and fascia) and the muscles. But there are two other broad categories of structures that must not be overlooked. They are the gross structures of the vascular system and nervous system. In the following sections, the effect of stretch applied to these structures will be analyzed.

Anatomy of the Vascular System

Upon leaving the heart, the blood enters the vascular system. The vascular system is composed of numerous types of blood vessels, which transport the blood throughout the body. In addition, they permit the exchange of nutrients, metabolic end products, hormones, and other substances between the blood and the interstitial fluid. Eventually, the blood returns to the heart. There are three major kinds of blood vessels: arteries, veins, and capillaries.

An *artery* is a vessel that carries blood away from the heart. All arteries (except the pulmonary artery and its branches) carry oxygenated blood. When an arterial vessel has a diameter of less than 0.5 mm, it is referred to as an *arteriole*. Arteries can be classified as *elastic* or *muscular* according to the prevalent tissue component in their walls. Examples of elastic arteries are such large vessels as the aorta, common carotid, subclavian, and common iliac. The great majority of arteries belong to the muscular category. Through arteries' constriction and dilation, blood flow can be regulated (Figure 5.14).

A *vein*, on the other hand, is a vessel that carries blood toward the heart. All of the veins (except the pulmonary vein) contain deoxygenated blood. Small veins are called *venules*. The main difference between the veins and the arteries is the comparative weakness of the vein wall's middle coat. Its much smaller content of muscle and elastic fibers is related to the much lower venous blood pressure. In addition, veins have valves, unlike arteries.

Capillaries are microscopic blood vessels that connect arterioles with venules. Their walls are composed of a single layer of endothelial cells. The average diameter of capillaries is small, varying from 7 to 9 μm. Their length usually varies from 0.25 mm to 1 mm, the latter length being characteristic of muscle tissue. Capillaries serve a variety of functions: transporting the blood with all its necessary components and permitting them to be exchanged with the surrounding tissues, maintaining normal blood pressure and circulation, and serving as a blood reservoir.

Applications of Stretch to Blood Vessels

When blood vessels are loaded (stretched by blood flow or the effects of stretch on blood vessels), they display typical viscoelastic properties in response to the constantly changing stress that accompanies each cardiac cycle. The effect of skeletal muscle sarcomere length on total capillary length was investigated by Ellis and colleagues (1990) in the extensor digitorum longus of the rat. Normalized data

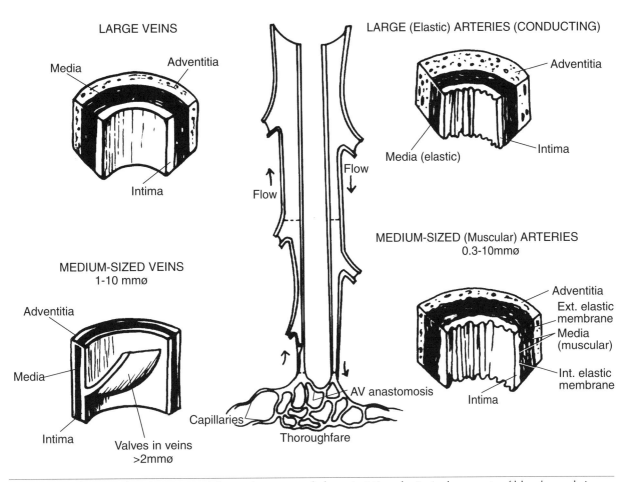

LARGE VEINS

Media
Adventitia
Intima

LARGE (Elastic) ARTERIES (CONDUCTING)

Adventitia
Media (elastic)
Intima

Flow
Flow

MEDIUM-SIZED VEINS
1-10 mmø

Adventitia
Media
Intima
Valves in veins
>2mmø

MEDIUM-SIZED (Muscular) ARTERIES
0.3-10mmø

Adventitia
Ext. elastic membrane
Media (muscular)
Int. elastic membrane
Intima

AV anastomosis
Capillaries
Thoroughfare

Fig. 5.14. Schematic drawing summarizing major structural characteristics of principal segments of blood vessels in mammals.
Reprinted from Rhodin (1988).

from six capillaries "indicated that four [vessels] stretched to the same degree as the muscle, one stretched more and another less" (p. 63). It was suggested that the variations in capillary distensibility may be due to variations in vessel diameter, wall thickness, and degree of tethering to adjacent muscle cells. Thus, the study essentially substantiated the hypothesis that capillaries are generally in a tortuous (winding) configuration, and muscle extension will merely cause them to straighten with no change in vessel length. Once capillaries have been pulled into a straight configuration, further muscle extension will result in capillary stretching and a linear increase of individual vessel length from L_o.

Research has shown that artery length changes very little in vivo (i.e., in the living body). Dobrin (1983), citing Lawton (1957) and Patel and Fry (1964), reported a 1% increase in length of the thoracic aorta and a 1% decrease in length of the abdominal aorta during each cardiac cycle. The ascending aorta and pulmonary arteries change 5% to 11% in length, but this effect results from

gross motion of the heart (Patel, Greenfield, and Fry 1963). Although artery length changes negligibly over a wide range of pressures, it may change with alterations in body position. Browse, Young, and Thomas (1979) radiographically determined the changes in arterial length and diameter as well as the patterns of blood flow in the femoral and brachial arteries of 10 males. Beginning with the leg straight (i.e., a knee joint angle of 180°), the knee was then fully flexed. The average amount of flexion was 100° (from a straight leg to one bent to 80°), and this movement caused a mean shortening of 4.5 cm in the femoral artery, 20% of the initial mean length, while the vessel's diameter was maintained. The only noticeable change was the appearance of crinkling of the internal surface of the vessel when the artery was fully bent. Measurements on a human brachial artery showed that at the elbow, this vessel shortened by 2.3 cm—16.3 cm at 180° (arm straight) to 14 cm at 105° (elbow flexed), that is, 3 mm/10° of joint movement—with no measurable change in vessel diameter.

In part, the mechanical characteristics of blood vessels are attributed to the properties of the connective tissues in the wall, specifically to those of elastin and collagen. With development and maturation, the collagen-to-elastin ratio of arteries increases, and therefore their stiffness also increases. Vessel stiffness under distention may be plotted as a function of several parameters and depends on whether the vessels are constricted or relaxed. The interested reader is referred to the work of Dobrin (1983), which deals with these complexities in greater detail.

Influence of Stretch on Muscle Oxygen Consumption and Regional Blood Flow

It is known that during exercise the body is capable of dramatically increasing the amount of blood transported through the cardiovascular system. But what is the effect on blood flow, oxygen consumption, and oxygen extraction when a stretched muscle is relaxed; contracting isometrically in an elongated state; contracting eccentrically; or under compression either before, during, or after stretching? With improved technologies, several of these questions have been investigated.

Over 100 years ago, Gaskell (1877) showed that dogs' muscular blood flow decreased during contraction of calf muscles, a finding that has been confirmed in many later works. In general, blood flow is reduced in proportion to the force of contraction. But, what happens to the blood flow of a muscle and its oxygen consumption during and after stretch? These questions were investigated by Stainsby, Fales, and Lilienthal (1956). They found that when the gastrocnemius-plantaris muscle group of the dog was stretched, the rate of oxygen consumption fell on the average to half of the resting rate and remained at this low level until tension was released. When the tension was released, the oxygen consumption returned to the previous resting rate with little payment of the oxygen debt created during stretch. Several explanations were proposed to explain this phenomenon.

Several years later, Gray and Staub (1967) observed that less reduction of blood flow occurred during passive stretching than during the same degree of active tension. They suggested the decreased blood flow due to stretch was due to local pinching of vessels. Following this study

Hirche, Raff, and Grün (1970), working on muscles dilated with papaverine (a vasodilator drug), found the increase in resistance to blood flow was the same, whether produced by passive or active muscle tension. Later, research by Wisnes and Kirkebø (1976) determined that active contraction or stretching of the calf muscles of rats mechanically impeded muscular blood flow, most pronouncedly in the central inner zone at high tensions. That is, the blood flow in the inner, central zones of the muscle groups was reduced far more than flow in the outer, peripheral zones. As a result, Wisnes and Kirkebø (1976) suggest that "since blood flow may vary regionally within a single muscle, measurements of total organ flow should not be regarded uncritically to represent a similar flow in every locality of the organ" (p. 265). A later study by Kirkebø and Wisnes (1982) explained the disproportionate reduction of blood flow in the central zones as due to differences in regional tissue pressure. In addition, they suggested that "the heterogeneous pattern of muscle fiber directions and relative displacement of various elements during work, may induce shear forces causing focal vessel obstructions that are different during contraction and stretch" (p. 114).

Later, several teams of former Soviet researchers continued to investigate various phenomena that pertain to the blood flow and stretch. The first investigation by Matchanov, Levtov, and Orlov (1983) reported that a longitudinal stretch of cat gastrocnemius muscles by 10% to 30% of initial length increased the passive strength and regularly decreased the blood flow. The decreased blood flow was dependent on the value of the passive tension and not on the degree of deformation. Postelongation hyperemia (increased blood flow) developed after stretching. A subsequent study by Matchanov, Shustova, Shuvaeva, Vasil'eva, and Levtov (1983) found that longitudinal stretch of cat gastrocnemius muscle to between 111% and 117% of its initial length was followed by increases in passive strength and in mechanical displays of the 15-s isometric tetani. In addition, blood flow in the muscle vessels decreased at rest during the longitudinal stretching, whereas oxygen (O_2) extraction from the blood increased, but oxygen consumption did not change. In a third investigation, Shustova, Maltsev, Levkovich, and Levtov (1985) once again applied stretch to the gastrocnemius of cats. Longitudinal stretch of the muscle by 1 to 2 cm decelerated the capillary blood flow up to its complete rest. After 1 min of stretch, the blood flow velocity increased by 0.30±0.06 mm/s in 148 capillaries, decreased by 0.22±0.07 mm/s in 35 capillaries, and remained the same in 5 capillaries. Responses of individual capillaries seemed to be unrelated to the initial flow velocity at their location within the vessel network. Next, the team of Shustova, Matchanov, and Levtov (1985) investigated the effect of the compression of cat gastrocnemius muscle vessels on the muscle blood supply during stretching. A 10% to 20% longitudinal stretch of the muscle reduced the blood flow from 5.0 to 3.0 ml/min. However, the decrease of the blood flow in stretching and the postelongation hyperemia could not be reproduced by external compression of the muscle equal to the balancing pressure at a given extent of stretching. Furthermore, they concluded that the effect of longitudinal muscle stretch on its vessels is not limited to their compression by the intramuscular pressure. In the last published report, Levtov and colleagues (1985) found that mean blood velocity increased in capillaries during postelongation hyperemia. However, the velocity was slower in distal capillaries. The blood flow velocity in the capillaries was determined to depend on the ratio of the total resistance of incoming and outgoing vessels to the resistance of the capillary.

Peripheral Nerves

Normally both active and passive joint movements can be freely carried out over a wide range. During such movements, nerves are subjected to various stresses and strains that usually are tolerated without pain or any functional impairment. However, under certain conditions, nerve injuries do occur. Traumatic and stretch injuries to peripheral nerves represent considerable clinical problems to allied health practitioners and to those involved with treating athletes and performing artists. A knowledge of those features that relate to nerve compression and stretch is important on several levels. For the athlete, dancer, coach, and trainer, it is important to know the limiting factors that can influence performance or predispose one to injury. To the medical community, nerve compression and stretch represent practical clinical problems in terms of treatment and rehabilitation. For instance, peripheral nerves may be subjected to stretching during suturing of severed nerve trunks under tension by surgeons. Similarly, physical therapists must be cognizant of nerve vulnerability during mechanical traction procedures. Health care practitioners who employ adjustment and manipulative techniques need to be vigilant to avoid causing or compounding preexisting nerve damage by the application of excessive force.

Nerve Structure and Sheaths

For over 100 years, numerous researchers have investigated the structure of peripheral nerves (a nerve lying outside of the central nervous system). With improved microscopic techniques and technologies, a greater understanding of the nature of peripheral nerves has become possible. In the peripheral nervous system the nerve fibers are grouped in bundles to form the nerves.

Nerves have three separate connective tissue sheaths: the epineurium, the perineurium, and the endoneurium (Figure 5.15). The obvious functions of the connective tissue sheaths are to provide structural support to the peripheral nerve and to contribute to the elasticity that allows a nerve to be stretched during body movement. In addition, research has shown that some of the sheaths serve as a blood-nerve barrier that protects the nerve fiber from various noxious agents, limits the penetration of macromolecules, and may also control the passage of ions. Last, the

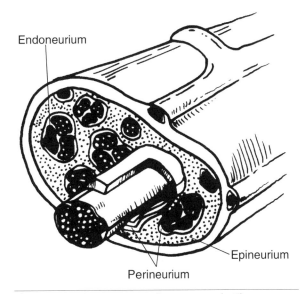

Fig. 5.15. Microanatomy of a nerve trunk. The axons are collected in fascicles surrounded by a perineurium. A small number of fascicles often constitute a well-defined fascicular group.
Reprinted from Lundborg (1993).

sheaths serve to separate and compartmentalize the nerve fibers.

The Epineurium

The *epineurium* is the nerve's external fibrous coat of dense connective tissue. This outermost sheath encloses the entire nerve and lies between fiber bundles. It contains connective tissue fibers, blood vessels, and some small nerve fibers that innervate the vessels. The components of the epineurium, the most prominent of which are collagen fibrils, are mainly oriented longitudinally. Elastic fibers are also present.

The Perineurium

The *perineurium* lies deep within the epineurium and separately encloses each bundle (fascicle) of nerve fibers. Therefore, each bundle is surrounded by the perineurium, which consists of 3 to 10 concentric layers of cells. The number of layers depends on the size of the nerve fascicle being ensheathed and its proximity to the central nervous system. The cells in these layers are joined at their edges by tight junctions, an arrangement that makes the perineurium a barrier to the passage of most macromolecules. The collagen fibrils are thinner than those of the epineurium and contain only a few scattered elastic fibers.

The Endoneurium

The *endoneurium* represents the deepest of the nerve sheaths and encloses each individual nerve fiber. The endoneurium consists of a thin layer of collagen fibrils that are mainly oriented longitudinally. These fibrils are generally similar in diameter to those of the perineurium.

Application of Stretch to Nerves

Numerous studies on the behavior of peripheral nerves subjected to stretching (i.e., tensile load) date from the later half of the 19th century. Despite this long history, little is known about the biomechanical properties of peripheral nerves or about the limits of stretching that the nerve may undergo before structural damage occurs. Research has shown that chronically injured nerves may have altered mechanical properties, for example, increased stiffness (Beel, Groswald, and Luttges 1984). However, the available data regarding tensile properties and the critical limits of stretching is limited and often conflicting (Beel,

Stodieck, and Luttges 1986; Denny-Brown and Doherty 1945; Haftek 1970; Highet and Sanders 1943; Hoen and Brackett 1970; Rydevik, Lundborg, and Skalak 1989; Sunderland 1991; Sunderland and Bradley 1961). In the following sections, we will review the research regarding stretching forces as related to the biomechanics of nerves, the blood flow to the nerves, and the effect on neural transmission.

Comparison between the reported experiments is often impossible due to a lack of biomechanical standardization (Wall et al. 1992). Among some of the variables relating to the nerve to be tested are in situ versus in vitro experimentation, the type of animal, the specific nerve, the age of the nerve, the preparation of the nerve, and the test itself.

In general, when a nerve is subjected to a gradually increasing tensile load, there is a linear relationship between load and elongation until a certain point is reached beyond which the nerve ceases to behave as an elastic structure (Sunderland 1978, 1991). The principal component imparting elasticity to the nerve trunk and giving it tensile strength is the perineurium. The elastic range is between 6% and 20% of resting length. If stretching continues beyond the elastic limit, deformation and force are no longer linearly proportional. As greater forces are applied, the curve tends to flatten until the maximum stress or ultimate strength level—the point at or before rupture—is reached.

Existing data regarding the amount of stretching that leads to structural changes are limited, with values from 11% to 100% elongation. These structural changes are highly dependent on the magnitude and character of the deforming force, as well as on the length of time during which they operate.

Stress-Strain Properties of Peripheral Nerve Trunk

Sunderland and Bradley (1961) performed a series of experiments on the stress-strain phenomena in stretched human peripheral nerves that are subjected to progressively increasing loads up to the point of mechanical failure. Human specimens of the median (*n* = 24), ulnar (24), medial popliteal (13), and lateral popliteal (15) nerves were obtained from the autopsy room within 12 hours of death and tested immediately. All specimens were from adult individuals from 30 to 50 years old. The tests provided the following data about the range of maximum load irrespective of size:

Median	7.3 to 22.3 kg
Ulnar	6.5 to 15.5 kg
Medial popliteal	20.6 to 33.6 kg
Lateral popliteal	11.8 to 21.4 kg

Maximum Tensile Strength of the Nerve Trunk

Nerves are not homogeneous structures and do not behave as perfect cylinders. The range of maximum tensile stress (kg/mm^2) was calculated on the cross-sectional area of the nerve trunk:

Median	1.0 to 3.1 kg/mm^2
Ulnar	1.0 to 2.2 kg/mm^2
Medial popliteal	0.5 to 1.8 kg/mm^2
Lateral popliteal	0.8 to 1.9 kg/mm^2

Maximal Elongation of the Nerve Trunk

Provided that a nerve was not strained beyond its elastic limit, the nerve specimen regained its original length. Further testing showed that it also retained its elastic properties when the load was removed. However, when the elastic limit was exceeded, the specimen did not regain its original length but acquired a permanent set or deformation. Tests showed a linear (elastic) relationship between load and elongation over a range of elongation, which may be summarized as follows:

Median	6% to 20%
Ulnar	8% to 21%
Medial popliteal	7% to 21%
Lateral popliteal	9% to 22%

Percentage of Elongation at Mechanical Failure

While there were substantial individual variations among the nerves, it was clear that the greatest elongation at the elastic limit was about 20%. Complete mechanical failure occurred at maximal elongations of approximately 30%. The elongation at mechanical failure, as a percentage of resting length, were:

Median	7% to 30%
Ulnar	9% to 26%
Medial popliteal	8% to 32%
Lateral popliteal	10% to 32%

Implications of Nerve Stretch for Health Care Practitioners

Rydevik and colleagues (1990) made several important observations that have implications for health and medical practitioners. First, they observed that when the nerve failed mechanically, it appeared to be grossly intact, although there were multiple ruptures of the perineurial sheaths. "It is thus not reliable to assess the structural integrity of a nerve trunk through visual examination" (p. 699). Furthermore, the perineurial sheath ruptures did not occur at one given point in the specimen, but were spread over some distance. Hence, this observation "indicates that stretch injuries to a peripheral nerve may not be localized and may occur along the length of the nerve" (pp. 699–700; Figure 5.16).

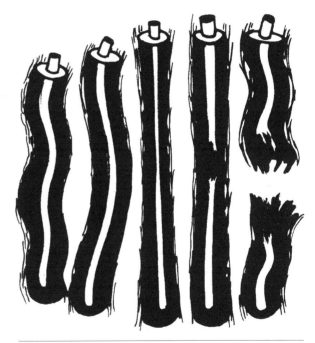

Fig. 5.16. The behavior of the fascicle and contained nerve fibers of a nerve trunk stretched to the point of mechanical failure.
Reprinted from Sunderland (1978).

Intraneural Microvascular Flow

An important consequence of stretching a nerve is the effect on the intraneural microvascular blood flow (Figure 5.17). When a nerve is stretched, its cross-sectional area is gradually reduced. This change introduces compression that results in further deformation of the nerve fiber as well as impairment of its blood supply. The

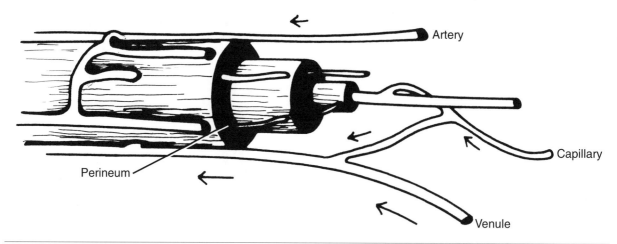

Fig. 5.17. Diagrammatic representation of the intrafascicular microvascular architecture as revealed by vital microscopic studies in perineurium, arteriole, venule, capillary. Note the capillary loops, sometimes arranged in planes perpendicular to the longitudinal axis of the nerve. Arrows denote direction of blood flow.
Reprinted from Lundborg and Branemark (1968).

importance of a sufficient blood supply for the function of the nerve is well known and discussed in many textbooks. Therefore, stretching that interferes with the intraneural microvascular flow can be expected to impair nerve function. Experimental studies by Lundborg (1975), Lundborg and Rydevik (1973), and Ogata and Naito (1986) found that intraneural microvascular flow was impaired beyond an 8% elongation of the nerve. Complete intraneural ischemia (a decrease in blood supply) occurred at a 15% elongation. After stretches to these lengths, circulation recovers following relaxation.

Effect of Stretch on Nerve Transmission

Another significant consequence of stretch on nerves is the failure of electrical conduction. Failure to conduct is reported to begin at stretch extents ranging from 6% to 100%, depending on the animal tested. Recently, a study by Wall et al. (1992) suggested that mechanical deformation, not ischemia, is responsible for early conduction loss.

Protective Structures of Nerve Trunks

How is it possible that the peripheral nerves of the legs allow a person to stand upright, flex forward from the trunk with the knees fully ex-

tended, and rest the palms of the hands flat on the floor? During such movements the tissues involved with the stretch must elongate sometimes as much as 5 cm. The answer is that most peripheral nerves have three features that protect them from physical deformation: (1) slackness, (2) the course of the nerves in relation to the joints, and (3) elasticity.

Slackness of the Nerve Trunk and Nerve Fibers

A nerve trunk runs an undulating course in its bed. So, too, the fiber bundles (fasciculi) run an undulating course within the epineurium sheaths, and each nerve fiber runs an undulating course inside the fasciculi. When there is little or no tension on these nerves, they shorten in an accordionlike arrangement (J.W. Smith 1966). As a result, the length of a nerve trunk and its contained nerve fibers traveling between any two fixed points on the limb is considerably greater than the linear distance between those points (Figure 5.18).

During initial stretching the undulations are taken out of the nerve. With continued stretching the undulations are eliminated in the fasciculi and finally in the individual nerve fibers. Therefore, it is only at this last point that all the slack is taken up and the nerve fibers are subjected to tension. If stretching is allowed to continue, conduction in the nerve fibers is progressively impaired and then fails completely, until finally the nerve fibers fracture inside the fasci-

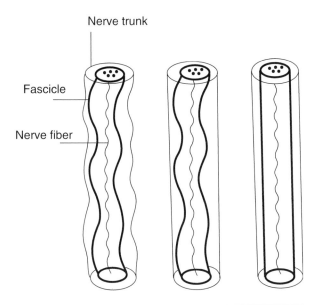

Fig. 5.18. Diagram illustrating the undulations in nerves, fasciculi, and nerve fibers, which protect nerve fibers when nerves are stretched during a full range of limb movements.
Reprinted from Sunderland (1991).

culi. The perineurium is the last component to fail structurally.

The importance of this slack system cannot be overstated. As explained by Sunderland (1991, 66), "The slack provided in the system in this way absorbs and neutralizes traction forces generated during limb movements so that the contained nerve fibers are at all times protected from being overstretched."

Course of the Nerve in Relation to Joints

A second important feature that protects nerves and facilitates range of movement is the course or path of the nerve in relation to the joints. With two notable exceptions, nerves typically cross the flexor aspect of joints (the "inside" of the joint when flexed). Because the range of joint flexion is much greater than that of extension, a nerve crossing the flexor aspect of a joint remains relaxed during flexion and is only slightly stretched during extension. In contrast, a nerve crossing the extensor aspect of a joint is relaxed during extension but is put under considerable tension during flexion. In other words, there is a greater "safety margin" and more "nerve play" with flexion than extension. It is clear that nerves crossing the extensor aspect of a joint are at a disadvantage in regard to exposure to forces generated during limb movements. The advantage of crossing the flexor aspect of a joint explains why most nerves do so.

The only notable exceptions are the ulnar nerve, which crosses the extensor aspect of the elbow joint, and the sciatic nerve where it crosses the extensor aspect of the hip joint. As a result, these two nerves are repeatedly subjected to undue tension during full flexion. Since movements involving forward trunk flexion with the knees extended are common to many sports and activities, this fact is particularly relevant to individuals involved in stretching.

Sunderland (1991) points out that where the sciatic nerve crosses the extensor aspect of the hip joint, the epineurial tissue represents as much as 88% of the cross-sectional area of the nerve. He speculates that this structure is probably a special protective feature, for much time is spent squatting or sitting on the sciatic nerves with the thighs flexed, putting stretch on that nerve.

Elasticity of the Nerve Trunks

The third feature that protects a nerve from deformation is its elasticity. Elasticity is a material's resistance to distortion—that property which enables it to return to its original shape or size. As was previously pointed out, when a nerve is subjected to a gradually increasing tensile load, there is a linear relationship between load and elongation until a certain point is reached beyond which the nerve ceases to behave as an elastic structure. The principal component responsible for elasticity in the nerve trunk and for giving it tensile strength is the perineurium. Various test data have been published regarding the stress-strain values for different peripheral nerves. Research indicates that in peripheral nerves the elastic range is between 6% and 20%.

Factors Reducing the Elasticity and Mobility of Nerves

Peripheral nerves display the attributes of strength, elasticity, and mobility. However, over a course of time these characteristics can be modified. Among several of the factors that can alter the mechanical characteristics of nerve fibers are

- adhesions and scar tissue,
- changes in the ratio of collagenous tissue to elastic tissue of the nerve,
- deformities,
- trauma, and
- sutures.

Can Training Modify Peripheral Nerves?

To date, no known studies have been attempted to determine how different types of traditional stretching regimens or protocols influence peripheral nerve strength, elasticity, and mobility. Thus, it is not known if, or how, stretching (as employed in athletics, dance, yoga, or physical therapy) affects peripheral nerve elasticity and mobility. Research is needed to explore these issues.

Factors Affecting the Mechanical Properties of Connective Tissues and Muscles

The behavior of connective tissues (collagenous or elastic) and of muscle under stress are influenced by a number of related factors, including the following:

- The alignment or orientation of the fibers
- The influence of different interweaving patterns of fibers within specific tissues
- The influence of different interweaving patterns of collagen molecules within each fibril
- The presence of interfibrillar substances
- The number of fibers and fibrils
- The cross-sectional area of the fibers
- The proportion of collagen and elastin
- The chemical composition of the tissues
- The degree of hydration
- The degree of relaxation of the contractile components
- The tissue temperature before and during the applied force
- The tissue temperature before releasing the applying force
- The amount of applied force (load)
- The duration of the applied force (time)
- The type of applied force (ballistic vs. static)

The Need for Additional Research

Research is a never-ending process. In the area of soft tissue mechanics, there is an array of is-

sues that needs to be addressed. These are two such relevant issues, pointed out by G.C. Lee (1980, 30–33):

1. Soft tissue contains largely fluids. Movement of this fluid compartment within the tissue therefore plays an important role in the tissue's response to deforming forces. In addition, the deformational responses of the tissue are dependent on the mechanical, electrical, and biochemical characteristics of the tissue's cellular and molecular constituents. These factors are believed to be responsible for the loading path and rate-dependent nature of the biomechanical response of soft tissues. However, additional quantitative research in this area needs to be performed.

2. Most soft tissue responses are more or less controlled and coordinated by the nervous system. The passive mechanical properties of elastic fibers and biological membranes have been studied separately by many investigators. The interactive nature of the muscles with the passive soft tissue components needs to be clearly established.

Summary

All tissues (connective, muscular, nervous, and vascular) undergo predictable changes when force is applied. If excessive tensile force is experienced, all tissues will eventually rupture. The amount of damage will be determined by such factors as the degree of force, the speed with which the force is applied, and the length of time that the force is applied.

Research has demonstrated that elastic or recoverable elongation is optimized by high-force, short-duration stretching at normal or colder than normal tissue temperatures. Plastic or permanent lengthening is more likely to be produced by low-force, long-duration stretching at elevated temperatures, followed by tissue cooling before releasing the tension. In addition, minimal structural weakening is associated with low-force stretching combined with high therapeutic temperatures, whereas maximal structural weakening is associated with higher forces and lower temperatures.

Therefore, the ideal stretching program to optimize increase in tissue length without damage should increase tissue temperature prior to stretching (by exercise or therapeutic modalities that increase body core temperature), apply low-intensity force, maintain stretching force for a prolonged period of time, and cool the tissue to normal temperature before releasing the stretching force.

Blood vessels and peripheral nerves are capable of elongation. Applications of stretch to blood vessels results in decreased blood flow. Ex-cessive stretching of nerves impairs function and eventually results in mechanical failure. Three features protect peripheral nerves from physical deformation via elongation: the nerve's slackness, path, and elasticity.

Chapter 6

The Neurophysiology of Flexibility: Neural Anatomy and Neural Physiology

The nervous system constitutes one of the main communication systems for the body. Consequently, it plays a significant role in determining the quality and quantity of movement available to the body. The nervous system comprises the central nervous system (the brain and spinal cord) and the peripheral nervous system (the cranial and peripheral nerves). A simplified model of the functional elements of the nervous system is illustrated in Figure 6.1.

Structural Foundation: Cellular Neuroanatomy

The structural and functional unit of the nervous system is the *neuron* (nerve cell). Knowledge of how the neuron functions is basic to understanding the nervous system. Neurons, like all of the body's cells, are structurally designed in ways

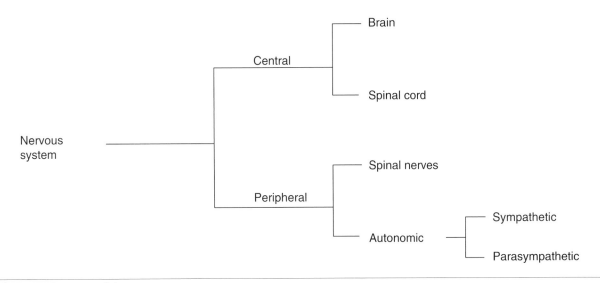

Fig. 6.1. Structure of the nervous system.

that are appropriate for their primary function, which is receiving and transmitting electric impulses. For a nervous system response to occur, three things are necessary. First, there must be a means of detecting a stimulus, or a change in the environment (e.g., stretching). Structures called *receptors* perform this function. Second, the stimulus, after it is received, must be transmitted. This function is accomplished by the nervous system's conductors—the neurons. Finally, responding organs must carry out the appropriate responses to the stimulus. This function is accomplished by the *effectors* (such as muscles and glands).

The Neuron

In the structural make-up of a neuron, there are four distinct morphological regions: the cell body (*soma*), one or more *dendrites*, a single *axon*, and the *presynaptic terminal* (see Figure 6.2). The cell body, or soma, contains a nucleus and protoplasm. Protoplasm is all the living substance within a cell surrounding the nucleus. The nucleus is responsible for controlling the various processes of the cell.

The dendrite is one type of nerve fiber extending from the cell body. Dendrites branch extensively, similar to tiny trees. In fact, the term *dendrite* comes from the Greek word *dendron*, meaning tree. Its function is to receive and convey impulses toward the cell body and is therefore known as the *afferent process*.

The long part of a neuron leading away from the cell body is the axon. Most axons conduct impulses away from the cell body. They can, however, transmit impulses in either direction. In addition, the axon usually gives off branches that are referred to as *collaterals*. The ending point of an axon involved in a synapse is known as the presynaptic terminal. This structure is the contact point that provides the means for the neuron to transfer its signal to the target cell. Covering large axons is a fatty insulating sheath called *myelin*. In the peripheral nerves myelin is produced by the *Schwann cells*. Gaps between the adjacent Schwann cells are referred to as *nodes of Ranvier*. At these points, charged ions can cross the axon membrane, allowing electrical signals to be regenerated. Axons make up what is known as the *efferent system*.

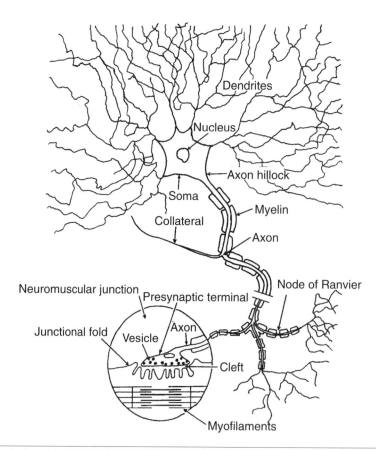

Fig. 6.2. The four morphological regions of a typical neuron: dendrites, soma, axon, and presynaptic terminals.
Reprinted from Enoka (1988).

Nerves

Bundles of neuron fibers are called *nerves*. These bundles are bound together by connective tissue sheaths (the epineurium, perineurium, and endoneurium). Nearly all nerves are mixed nerves (i.e., they contain both afferent and efferent fibers). *Afferent* fibers conduct impulses toward the central nervous system (CNS). They are classified by size and conductivity into Groups I–IV. In humans, no function of the body can be performed independently of some type of control by the CNS. Even a simple response to a stimulus involves at least the spinal cord. In contrast, *efferent* fibers conduct impulses away from the CNS and toward the effectors.

Nerve Electrical Potential

The function of a nerve is to transmit signals in the form of nerve impulses from one part of the body to another. This transmission of impulses is an electrochemical process. In the following sections, two types of electrical potentials related to nerve function will be discussed: the resting potential and action potential.

Resting Potential

Neurons are *polarized*. That is, they have an unequal number of different types of ions outside and inside the membrane. An *ion* is an atom that has gained or lost one or more of its electrons, thereby acquiring a positive or negative charge. These ions move through a fluid in response to an electric field, or a concentration gradient (the difference in ion concentration between two fluid areas).

When a neuron is at rest, there are more sodium ions (Na^+) on the outside of the membrane than there are on the inside, and more potassium ions (K^+) on the inside of the membrane than there are on the outside. Sodium ions, however, can be transported outward through the membrane by an active transport mechanism called the *sodium pump*. A continuous expenditure of energy is necessary to maintain the resting membrane potential (the potential difference across a nonconducting neuron's membrane) in this way. Potassium ions can pass through the membrane by passive transport. Therefore, some of them diffuse out of

the cell. They are returned to the cell by the Na^+-K^+ pump, in exchange for Na^+, which is pumped out.

The difference in ionic concentration across the neuron membrane is basic to the establishment of a potential difference across the cell membrane, a *membrane potential*. In resting cells, the inside is negatively charged relative to the interstitial fluid. Therefore, the neuron can be considered analogous to a battery, with its negative terminal on the inside. The membrane potential difference at rest is approximately 0.1 V.

Action Potential Generation

When an axon is stimulated, changes in this potential occur. A stimulus alters the permeability of the neural membrane. With stimulation, the membrane becomes more permeable to sodium ions (Na^+). As a result, sodium ions diffuse quickly into the nerve fiber. This inward movement of the sodium ions causes a reversal of the membrane's resting potential. That is, the outside of the nerve fiber becomes negative in relation to the inside. Consequently, the nerve's polarity is reversed. The nerve fiber *depolarizes* (polarity inside becomes less negative or closer to zero). When depolarization reaches a critical voltage level, an *action potential* is generated. Thus action potential and depolarization are related, but are not synonymous. Depolarization is the flow of ions that initiates the action potential. At the peak of depolarization, entry of sodium ions into the cell slows down, and the membrane becomes impermeable to sodium.

At this time, another cell membrane permeability change occurs. After a brief interval, the membrane becomes highly permeable to potassium (K^+). The potassium is able to diffuse out with great ease because of the high concentration on the inside (and because of the reduced electrical attraction of the less negative neuron potential). Consequently, the potassium ions begin to leave the cell, carrying the positive charges with them. The outflow of the potassium ions restores the original negative charge of the interior of the membrane. Thus, the membrane voltage difference returns to normal. This process, called *repolarization*, brings the action potential to an end (Figure 6.3).

In order for the membrane to return to its original resting potential, the sodium ions must be returned to the outside and the potassium ions must be returned to the inside of the membrane. The sodium-potassium pump is the active trans-

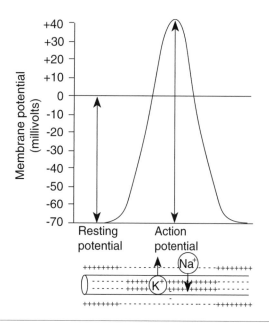

Fig. 6.3. The action potential. Ionic movements across the nerve fiber membrane (below) coincide with changes in electric potential (above). As sodium ions (Na$^+$) rush into the axon, the membrane potential becomes positive. Movement of potassium ions (K$^+$) to the outside of the fiber follows. At the point of the action potential, the potential across the membrane is reversed about +40 mV.
Reprinted from Alter (1988).

port mechanism that returns the ions to their original locations. Thus, the original potential of the membrane is restored.

The All-or-None Law

If the stimulus (e.g., stretch) is strong enough to initiate a nerve impulse in the axon, it causes a full-strength action potential to be generated. This observation is known as the *all-or-none law*, which can be compared to the process of shooting a gun. As soon as a pull on the trigger is strong enough to drop the firing pin, the gun fires. This critical value is called the *threshold*. A harder pull on the trigger will not change the velocity of the bullet, because it is the powder charge in the bullet, and not the pull on the trigger, that causes the response (Sage 1971). Therefore, either a stimulus is strong enough to stimulate the fiber or it is not. Stronger stimulations do not result in larger action potentials.

CNS Feedback About Intensity of Stretching

How, then, does the nerve differentiate between various intensities of stretching? The nerve has

two means by which it can transmit information about stretching of different intensities. First, it can transmit stretching sensation simultaneously over varying numbers of nerve fibers. Therefore, a greater intensity of stretching sensation can bring more sensory nerve fibers into action. This process is called *recruitment*. Consequently, intensity of stretch can be increased by increasing the recruitment of receptor organs and sensory neurons. For example, a weak stretching stimulus activates only those stretch receptors with the lowest thresholds. However, as intensity is increased, a greater number of less-excitable stretch receptors are also activated, thereby involving more sensory units.

Second, the nerve can transmit different numbers of impulses per unit of time over the same fiber. Thus, changes in intensity of stretch may be reflected in different frequencies of firing (i.e., rate of discharge) of nerve impulses in single fibers: The more intense the stretch stimuli, the greater the frequency of the stretch impulse. This process is called *rate of frequency coding*.

In summary, the stronger the stretching stimulus, the greater the number of active sensory neurons, and the greater the impulse frequency in each. Consequently, the bombardment of motoneurons in the spinal cord and the cortical centers of the brain will be more intense, leading to increased reflex motor activity and a stronger sensation.

Sensory Receptor Adaptation

If a stimulus is applied to a sensory receptor and maintained at a steady strength, the receptor usually responds with an initially high rate of discharge. The generator potential is at first proportional to the stimulus intensity. With time, however, the generator potential declines gradually during the steady stimulation. As a result, the rate of discharge slows. This phenomenon is known as *adaptation*. If, however, the stimulus is even momentarily stopped and then reapplied, an initial burst of impulse activity will reoccur, and the process will be repeated.

Stretch receptors can be categorized as either fast or slow adapting. *Fast-adapting* units show a more rapidly decreasing rate of discharge with maintained stretch (because the generator potential declines more rapidly in the fast-adapting units). Conversely, the *slow-adapting* units display a continued rate of discharge with sustained stimulation. Slow-adapting units display long-maintained generator potentials. The terms *pha-*

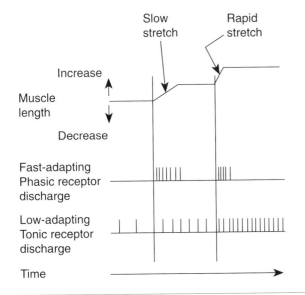

Fig. 6.4. Phasic and tonic receptor discharges. Fast-adapting or phasic receptors are characterized by a more rapidly decreasing rate of discharge with maintained stretch. Hence, their frequency of discharge is proportional to the rate of change. In contrast, slow-adapting or tonic receptors display a continued rate of discharge with sustained stimulation.
Reprinted from Alter (1988).

sic and *tonic* are interchangeably used for fast- and slow-adapting receptors, respectively (Figure 6.4).

Research has demonstrated that fast-adapting receptors, such as the pacinian corpuscles (which are skin and joint receptors), behave like mechanical high-pass filters. These filters are thought to be composed of both viscous and elastic components. When a force is delivered to the viscous components over a sufficiently rapid time course, it is transmitted directly to the central core of the receptor, where the nerve ending is loaded. The time course of this dynamic component parallels that of the early receptor potential of the intact corpuscle. However, this dynamic component declines rapidly regardless of the duration of the applied stimulus. Only force stored in the stretched elastic components is then transmitted with a marked reduction to the central core. As a result, no steady generator potential results.

In contrast, slow-adapting receptors, such as muscle spindles (which are muscle length receptors), have no mechanical high-pass filter at the nerve endings. Consequently, steady generator potentials are produced by steady stretch. The degree of adaptation that does occur from the initial high-frequency discharge to the following steady state (the newly adapted state of discharge) is thought to be due to the presence of

viscous components in series within the spindle itself (Mountcastle 1974).

Sensory Receptors Related to Stretching

Three major receptors have implications for stretching and maintaining optimal ROM. These receptors are the muscle spindles, Golgi tendon organs (GTOs), and articular (joint) mechanoreceptors. In the following sections, their structure, function, and relationship to stretching will be reviewed.

Muscle Spindles

The primary stretch receptors in muscle are the muscle spindles. Muscle spindles have been the most widely studied proprioceptors. (Proprioceptors are receptors located in muscles, tendons, and the vestibule of the ear whose reflex is connected with locomotion or posture.) They are located in various numbers in most skeletal muscles of the body. Muscle spindles are particularly numerous in the small, delicate muscles of the hand and eye. Because the muscle fibers are encased within the fusiform (spindle-shaped) capsule (the connective tissue sheath that envelops the receptor), they are referred to as *intrafusal* fibers. In contrast, the *extrafusal* fibers are the regular contractile units of the muscle. The spindles attach at both ends to the extrafusal fibers and are therefore parallel to those fibers. So, when the whole muscle is stretched, the spindle is stretched too.

Spindle Intrafusal Muscle Fibers

There are two major types of intrafusal fibers: the nuclear bag fibers and the nuclear chain fiber. The former contain an abundance of sarcoplasm and cell nuclei in a dilated, swollen, baglike structure. This noncontractile structure is located in the center, or equatorial, region of the intrafusal fiber. Hence its name, *nuclear bag intrafusal fiber*. At the distal, or polar, ends of the nuclear bag fiber are striated contractile filaments, near the spindles attached to the extrafusal fibers. In recent years, it has been verified that there are actually two subtypes of nuclear bag fiber. They have been termed bag_1 and bag_2 (Gladden 1986; Figure 6.5).

The second type of intrafusal muscle fiber is the *nuclear chain intrafusal fiber*, which is thinner and shorter than the nuclear bag fiber. Further-

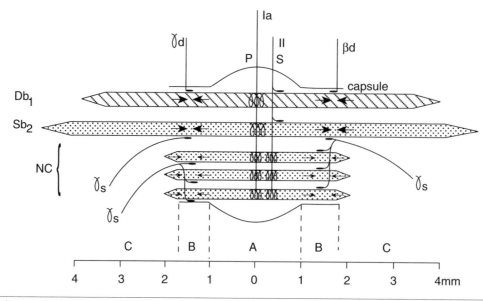

Fig. 6.5. Relation of primary sensory ending (P) and secondary sensory ending (S), supplied by Group Ia and II axons, respectively, to the three types of intrafusal fibers, bag$_1$ (b$_1$), bag$_2$ (b$_2$) and nuclear chain fibers (NC), and to their motor endings.
Reprinted from Gladden (1986).

more, it contains only a single row of nuclei, which are spread out in a chainlike structure through the noncontractile equatorial region. Like the nuclear bag fibers, the polar ends of the nuclear chain fiber are also composed of striated contractile filaments. Their ends often connect to the nuclear bag fibers, which in turn attach to the endomysium of extrafusal fibers.

Spindle Sensory Nerves

There are two types of sensory (afferent) endings in each spindle. These are the *primary*, or annulospiral, endings and the *secondary*, or flower-spray, endings. The primary endings terminate as a spiral wrap around the central region of a nuclear bag fiber and as a side branch to a nuclear chain fiber. Afferent axons of primary endings belong to the large Group I fibers. To distinguish these sensory nerves from others in the Group I size category, large spindle afferents are known as Group Ia.

Primary endings have a very low threshold to stretch and are thus easily excited. Their response includes both a phasic (dynamic) and a tonic response. A phasic response measures the rate or velocity of the stretch by changing the neuron impulse frequency during the stretch. Specifically, the frequency of discharge increases rapidly with the initial stretch. Then, when the stretching reaches its new length, the frequency of discharge drops to a constant level appropriate to the new tonic length. Hence, a tonic response measures

the length of a muscle. In other words, the primary endings measure length plus velocity of stretch.

Secondary endings form branched or flower-spray-shaped endings. Consequently, in older terminology they were referred to as *flower-spray endings*. They are restricted almost entirely to the juxta-equatorial segment (near the equator) of the nuclear chain fibers. However, there is some disagreement among authorities regarding the limitation of secondary endings to the chain intrafusal fibers (Gowitzke and Milner 1988). Axons of the secondary endings belong to the smaller Group II afferent fibers. In contrast to the primary endings, secondary endings measure tonic muscle length alone.

These motoneurons cause contraction of the muscle filaments in the polar ends of the intrafusal muscle fibers. When these ends shorten, passive stretch occurs at the center equatorial region, where the sensory neuron receptors are located. Thus, activation of gamma motoneurons by the CNS can increase the amount of stretch perceived by the sensory endings (Banker 1980).

Spindle Motor Nerves

The motor nerves that innervate each intrafusal muscle fiber at its polar regions are the *gamma efferent fibers*, which make up the *fusimotor system*. The two types of gamma axons are classified on the basis of their effects on the sensitivity of the primary and secondary sensory nerve endings. Stimulation of what is called the *static gamma* axon can increase the length sensitivity of a primary ending with little or no effect on its velocity sensitivity. In contrast, *dynamic gamma* axons can markedly enhance the velocity sensitivity of a primary ending with little or no alteration in its length sensitivity.

The function of the *gamma system* is to control spindle sensitivity to stretch. This process of sensitization of the spindle through the gamma efferents is known as *gamma bias* (Norback and Demarest 1981). Activation of gamma motoneurons (by higher-brain motor centers) results in contraction or shortening of the intrafusal muscle fibers at their polar regions. When intrafusal fibers contract, the equatorial bag region is stretched, just as if the main muscle had been extended in length. This central deformation pulls the coils on the annulospiral part of the primary endings and increases the rate of firing of the Group Ia and II afferents.

The second function of gamma motoneurons is to maintain spindle sensitivity during shortening contractions of the whole muscle. When muscles shorten, the parallel spindle is also passively shortened. This passive approximation of the spindle's two ends removes the tension on its primary endings (*spindle unloading*) as well as its secondary endings, and this unloading thereby deprives the brain of information from the spindle about the muscle length changes, as well as eliminating stretch reflex input to the spinal cord. To prevent this spindle unloading, gamma motoneurons are activated to adjust the spindle sensitivity.

> Through the gamma efferent stimulation, the slack in the muscle spindle (a consequence of the shortened muscle) is taken up by the pull exerted on the bag by the intrafusal muscle fibers. This acts to maintain spindle firing, which, through excitatory influences conveyed via Ia fibers to the alpha motoneurons, acts to reflexly maintain the muscle contraction. (Norback and Demarest 1981, 190)

The Process of Muscle Spindle Excitation

As a general rule, the process of excitation of a muscle spindle may be outlined as follows: First, a minimal stretching stimulus is applied to a muscle spindle. Second, a change in the permeability of the sensory neuron ending develops, resulting in the production of a generator current (a transfer of charge across the nerve terminal membrane). In turn, this current flow produces a depolarization, called the generator potential. With a slightly greater degree of stretch, a generator potential of greater amplitude is evoked in the muscle spindle endings. When depolarization reaches threshold, a conducted action potential results. If the stretch is even stronger, it can lead to a "train" or series of conducted nerve impulses. The steps in muscle spindle excitation are summarized in the chart at the bottom of this page.

Golgi Tendon Organs (GTOs)

Golgi tendon organs (GTOs) are contraction-sensitive mechanoreceptors of mammalian skeletal muscles innervated by large-diameter fast-conducting Group Ib afferent nerve fibers (Jami 1992). GTOs were first identified and described by Golgi in 1903. Initially, Golgi called these structures *musculotendinous end-organs*. Later, the name *Golgi tendon organ* was adopted. Due to technical difficulties, GTOs have not been studied as much as muscle spindles. Nonetheless, their importance in regard to stretching and the development of flexibility cannot be overemphasized. In the following sections, factors such as the location, structure, function, and misconceptions regarding the GTOs will be discussed.

Location and Structure

GTOs are located almost exclusively at the *aponeuroses*, or muscle-tendon junctions, and not within tendons (Figure 6.6). In the material of Pang (quoted in Barker 1974), which is the largest sample ever studied, 92.4% of 1,337 receptors from different portions of cat muscles were located at musculotendinous junctions, versus only 7.6% within the tendon proper. The functional properties of these purely tendinous receptors are not known (Jami 1992).

In nonmammalian species, the GTOs are unencapsulated receptors located along the length of the tendon fascicles (collagen fiber bundles). Conversely, GTOs of mammals are encapsulated and, as previously mentioned, are located at the musculotendinous or musculo-

(1)	(2)	(3)	(4)	(5)
Stimulus	→Local Change in Permeability	→Generator Current	→Local Depolarization	→Conducted Action Potential
(stretch)		(charge transfer)	(generator potential)	

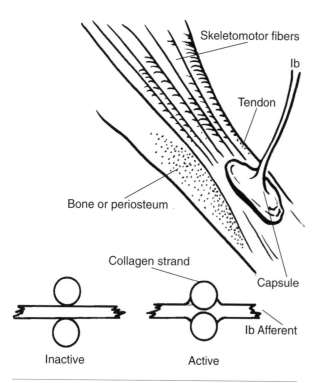

Fig. 6.6. The Golgi tendon organ. The encapsulated Ib afferent encircles the tendons of several skeletomotor fibers. Contraction of the skeletomotor fibers causes the collagen strands (tendon) to squeeze and thus activate the Ib afferent.

Reprinted from Enoka (1988).

apo-neurotic junctions. The significance of these differences is twofold. First, encapsulated organs are believed to be more sensitive to a given amount of stimuli and are more precise in localizing and relaying information to the CNS. Second, the location of the GTOs enables these receptors to be extremely sensitive to any degree of change in tension in the individual muscle fibers to which they are attached (J.C. Moore 1984).

Because GTOs lie directly in line with the transmission of force from muscle to the insertion on bone, they are said to be in series with the muscle. This arrangement is in direct contrast to the muscle spindles, which are located parallel to the muscle fibers. The significance of the GTOs' location will be discussed later in greater detail. The number of muscle fibers attached in series with a GTO varied, with a range of 3 to 50 in the sample of Pang. Each GTO is usually innervated by a single fast-conducting Group Ib afferent nerve fiber (Jami 1992).

GTO Function

Currently, the multidimensional function of GTOs is only partially understood. However, in-

vestigators are realizing that this receptor is more complex than was originally thought (J.C. Moore 1984). Of major significance, GTOs are now known to monitor all degrees of muscle tension. However, GTOs are most sensitive to tension forces generated by muscle contraction (i.e., active tension as opposed to passive stretch tension; see Figure 6.6b). Another speculated function of the GTOs is contribution to conscious sensations. This belief is based on the fact that input from the GTOs reaches the cerebral cortex, the portion of the brain that interprets the sensory activity of the body (Roland and Ladegaard-Pedersen 1977).

It has also been suggested that the GTOs appear to function in reducing muscle fatigue (Barr 1979; Kandel and Swartz 1981; Lundberg 1975; J.C. Moore 1984). As tension builds up in a group of muscle fibers, the GTOs and their Group Ib afferent sends an increasing number of signals to the CNS. These sensory nerves terminate in the spinal cord, on small interneurons, which then inhibit the motoneuron cell bodies that are activating the contracting muscle. This process is known as *autogenic inhibition*, since the muscle's contraction is being inhibited by its own receptors. The resulting reduction in muscle force decreases activation of the GTOs and the amount of inhibitory feedback being received by the CNS from these muscles. This momentary inhibition in feedback enables more tension to develop in these muscles.

Further studies are needed to fully understand the cooperation of information from GTOs and other muscle, skin, and joint receptors in feedback control of muscle contraction and in conscious proprioception (Jami 1992).

Misconceptions about GTOs

Over the years, numerous misconceptions regarding GTOs have developed and persisted. One example deals with the relationship between GTOs and measuring stretching forces. GTOs have often been called "stretch receptors." Unfortunately, this term implies that passive tension accompanying muscle stretch might also represent an adequate stimulus for the GTOs. While it is true that GTOs can be activated by passive tension, their threshold for this kind of stimulus is very high. Therefore, extremely intense stretch is necessary to activate GTOs (Houk, Singer, and Goldman 1971). Also, GTO discharge rarely persists during maintained muscle stretch.

Another misconception regarding GTOs is their lack of sensitivity to active (contractile) tension. Research has demonstrated that GTOs display a very low threshold and an appreciable *dynamic sensitivity* when tested with their adequate stimulus. Thus, GTOs are capable of signaling very small and rapid changes in contractile forces (Houk and Henneman 1967; Houk, Singer, and Goldman 1971; Jami 1992).

The function of GTOs was once postulated in the research literature to be autogenic inhibition, that is, inhibition of agonists and synergists and facilitation of antagonists. It is now known that this is just one of many functions of the GTOs, which are assisted by at least two other known receptors in this task: low-threshold joint capsule receptors and low-threshold cutaneous receptors (J.C. Moore 1984). The purpose of this autogenic inhibition was related to "protective functions." If, for example, when forces of muscle contraction together with forces resulting from external factors reach a point that musculotendinous damage could ensue, then the GTOs act to "shut off" the agonist contraction and stimulate the antagonist muscle. Consequently, this process helps prevent injury in the associated muscles, tendons, ligaments, and joints.

However, this system is not a fail-safe mechanism. It is known that the effects of the GTOs can be counterbalanced by additional signals from higher centers. The process of minimizing the influence of GTOs is referred to as *disinhibition* of the agonist motoneurons. The relevance of disinhibition as it applies to athletics has been raised by Brooks and Fahey (1987):

> Indeed, practicing disinhibition appears to be part of athletic training, the purpose of which is to push performance to the limits of tissue capacity. In the sport of wrist wrestling, ruptured muscles or tendons and broken bones occasionally occur. In highly motivated individuals and disinhibited individuals the combination of active muscle contraction plus tension exerted by the opponent can exceed the strength of tissues. (p. 194)

Articular Mechanoreceptors (Joint Receptors)

All the synovial joints of the body (including the apophyseal joints of the vertebral column) are provided with four varieties of receptor nerve endings. These joint receptors sense mechanical forces on joints, such as stretch pressure and distension. Hence, they are called *articular mechanoreceptors*. These receptors may be classified as Types I–IV (Table 6.1). This classification is based on the respective morphological and behavioral characteristics of the nerve endings. In the following sections, the four types of articular mechanoreceptors will be reviewed. This material was culled from Wyke (1967, 1972, 1979, 1985).

Type I Joint Receptors

Type I mechanoreceptors consist of clusters of thinly encapsulated globular corpuscles. They are located mainly in the external (i.e., superficial) layers of the fibrous joint capsule. Each cluster consists of up to eight corpuscles. Furthermore, each member of a cluster is supplied from a single Group II myelinated fiber (6–9 μm in diameter). Type I mechanoreceptors are found with an increased density in the proximal (e.g., hip) joints than in more distal (e.g., ankle) joints.

Physiologically, the Type I corpuscles behave as low-threshold, slow-adapting receptors. Consequently, they respond to very small mechanical stresses and they continue to fire nerve impulses throughout the duration of mechanical stimulus. For example, a force of approximately 3 g is sufficient to stimulate them. Furthermore, a proportion of these lowest-threshold receptors are always active in every position of the joint, even when it is immobile. Their rate of resting discharge usually has a frequency of some 10 to 20 Hz (impulses per second).

Type I mechanoreceptors are reported to have several functions, including signaling the direction, amplitude, and velocity of joint movements produced actively or passively; regulating joint pressure changes; contributing significantly to postural and kinesthetic sensation; facilitating the CNS in regulating postural muscle tone and muscle tone during joint movement; and producing an inhibitory effect on the flow of nociceptive (pain-sensing) afferent activity from the Type IV articular receptor system. Type I receptors may be categorized as static or dynamic mechanoreceptors.

Type II Joint Receptors

The *Type II receptor* is represented by larger, thickly encapsulated, conical corpuscles. They are located in the fibrous joint capsule, but in its deeper layers and in articular fat pads. Each cluster usually consists of two to four corpuscles. In addition, each member of the cluster is innervated by a branch of Group II myelinated articular nerve fibers (9–12 μm in diameter). Type II mechanoreceptors are also located in greater density in the more distal joints (e.g., the ankles) than in the more proximal joints (e.g., the hip).

Table 6.1. Characteristics of Articular Receptor System

Type	Morphology	Location	Parent Nerve Fibers	Behavioral Characteristics
I	Thinly encapsulated globular corpuscles (100 μm × 40 μm), in tridimensional clusters of 3–8 corpuscles	Fibrous capsules of joints (in superficial layers)	Small myelinated (6–9 μm)	Static and dynamic mechanoreceptors: low-threshold, slowly adapting
II	Thickly encapsulated conical corpuscles (280 μm × 120 μm), individual or in clusters of 2–4 corpuscles	Fibrous capsules of joints (in deeper subsynovial layers). Articular fat pads	Medium myelinated (9–12 μm)	Dynamic mechanoreceptors: low-threshold, rapidly adapting
III	Thinly encapsulated fusiform corpuscles (600 μm × 100 μm), individual or in clusters of 2–3 corpuscles	Applied to surfaces of joint ligaments (collateral and intrinsic)	Large myelinated (13–17 μm)	Dynamic mechanoreceptors: high-threshold, slowly adapting
IV	(a) Tridimensional plexuses of unmyelinated nerve fibers (b) Free unmyelinated nerve endings	Fibrous capsules of joints. Articular fat pads. Adventitial sheaths of articular blood vessels Joint ligaments (collateral and intrinsic)	Very small myelinated (2–5 μm) and unmyelinated (<2 μm)	Nociceptive receptors: very high-threshold, nonadapting. Chemosensitive (to abnormal tissue metabolites) nociceptive receptors

Reprinted from Wyke (1985).

Physiologically, like the Type I receptors, Type II receptors have a low threshold. But, in contrast, they behave as rapidly adapting mechanoreceptors and do not fire at rest. Hence, they are totally inactive in immobile joints. Type II receptors have no static discharge because their firing is velocity dependent. Consequently, they are known as acceleration or dynamic mechanoreceptors. When stimulated, each cluster will emit a brief, high-frequency burst of impulses for less than 1 s, and very often less than 0.5 s. Their primary function is to measure quick changes in movement, such as acceleration and deceleration.

Type III Joint Receptors

Type III mechanoreceptors are thinly encapsulated corpuscles confined to the intrinsic (within the joint capsule) and extrinsic (outside the joint capsule) ligaments of most joints. They are not found in the ligaments of the vertebral column. Type III receptors are the largest of the articular corpuscles and are like the Golgi tendon organs in behaving as high-threshold, slowly adapting mechanoreceptors. They are serviced by a large Group I myelinated afferent axon that may be up to 17 μm in diameter.

Physiologically, joint ligament mechanoreceptors have a high threshold and become active to-

ward the extremes of joint movement. Therefore, Type III receptors are completely inactive in immobile joints and respond only when high tensions are generated in joint ligaments. When stimulated, Type III receptors emit a discharge frequency that is a continuous function of the magnitude of that tension. Because these receptors are slow adapting, the discharge will decrease only very slowly (i.e., over many seconds) if the extreme joint displacement or joint traction is maintained.

Type III mechanoreceptors appear to have two basic functions, although others are possible. First, their primary function is to monitor the direction of movement. Second, they may produce profound reflex inhibition of activity in some of the muscles operating over the joint. Thus, they may act with a reflex effect to produce a braking mechanism against overstress of the joint.

Type IV Joint Receptors

Unlike the mechanoreceptors, *Type IV nerve endings* are unencapsulated. They are subdivided into two types. Type IVa endings are represented by latticelike plexuses that are found in joint fat pads and throughout the entire thickness of the joint capsule. However, they are entirely absent from synovial tissue, intraarticular menisci, and articular cartilage. The Type IVb receptors are free nerve endings with a bare nerve and no associated specialized structures. They are sparse and are confined largely to the intrinsic and extrinsic ligaments. These terminations are derived from the smallest (Group III) afferent fibers in the articular nerves. Those Group III nerve fibers that are thinly myelinated range between 2 and 5 μm in diameter.

Both Types IVa and IVb constitute the pain receptor system of the articular tissues. They are often referred to as nociceptors. Needless to say, these receptors are of major importance to those health care practitioners (i.e., medical doctors, osteopaths, chiropractors, physical therapists) who endeavor to relieve their patients of pain. Under normal conditions, these receptors are entirely inactive. However, they become active when the articular tissues containing this type of nerve ending are subjected to marked mechanical deformation or chemical irritation. Examples of chemical irritants are agents such as bradykinin, prostaglandin-E, lactic acid, potassium ions, polypeptides, and histamines. These substances appear in conditions of ischemia (lack of blood) and hypoxia (lack of oxygen) and are also constituents of inflammatory exudates. Of significance for individuals who are potential surgical candidates to relieve certain types of pain, Wyke (1972, 97) emphatically states:

> Type IV category of receptors is entirely absent from the synovial lining of every joint that has been examined, and is also lacking from the menisci present in the knee and temporomandibular joints, and from the intervertebral disks. There is no mechanism, then, whereby articular pain can arise directly from the synovial tissue or menisci in any joint, and surgical removal of synovial tissue or joint menisci likewise does not involve removal of pain-sensitive articular tissues per se.

Thus, this type of surgery will not stop the pain.

Reflexes and Other Spinal Neural Circuits

A reflex is a neuron circuit consisting of a sensory neuron, an internuncial or communicating neuron, and a motoneuron with its effector. When an appropriate stimulus is applied to the receptor ending, an impulse is initiated, which passes along the afferent process to the spinal cord where it synapses with a connecting neuron. Finally, a motoneuron is excited, and the nerve impulse is conducted down the efferent fiber to a muscle or gland cell. In other words, a reflex is a response to a stimulus.

The Myotatic or Stretch Reflex

According to the classical description of the stretch reflex, whenever a muscle is stretched, the stretch reflex mechanism is initiated (Figure 6.7). Stretching a muscle lengthens both the extrafusal muscle fibers and the muscle spindles (i.e., the intrafusal fibers). The consequent deformation within the muscle spindles activates the primary and secondary endings, which results in action potentials in their Group Ia and II sensory neurons. These neurons travel to the spinal cord, where they terminate on the cell bodies of alpha (large) motoneurons. If the sensory afferents produce enough depolarization in the motoneuron, it will fire action potentials. Its axon, which travels to the skeletal muscle, will transmit an impulse resulting in a reflex contraction.

The stretch reflex response can be divided into two components: *phasic* and *tonic*. The phasic response is an initial burst of action potentials that results in a rapid rise of muscle tension, proportional to the velocity of the stretch. The tonic response is a later phase of slow (low-frequency) firing lasting for the entire duration of the stretch, which is proportional to the amount of stretch.

The classic example of the phasic type of stretch reflex is the *knee jerk* or *patellar reflex*. For example, when the patellar tendon (located below the knee) is given a light tap, the muscle spindles located in parallel with the muscle fibers in the quadriceps (front thigh muscles) are stretched, creating a deformation in its muscle spindles. As a result, the firing of the Group Ia muscle spindle afferents is increased. (The primary ending is excited more than is the secondary ending because the former is the more extensible central region of the spindle intrafusal muscle fiber, while the latter is located on the less extensible juxta-equatorial area.) The message is then sent to the spinal cord (via the dorsal root) and to the brain. Completing the reflex arc, the spinal cord sends an efferent nerve impulse to the quadriceps muscles and causes them to briefly contract, thus shortening the muscle and taking the tension off the muscle spindles (Figure 6.8).

Another type of stretch reflex is the static, or tonic, stretch reflex. In this type of reflex, the

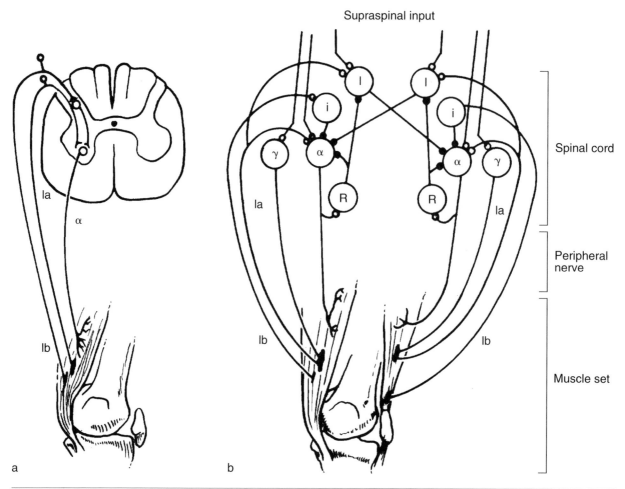

Fig. 6.7. Spinal connections between sensory receptors located in muscle and alpha motoneurons. The Ia axon conveys afferent information from the muscle spindle to the central nervous system. The Ib axon represents a similar connection but from the tendon organ. (a) Homonymous relationships—muscle spindles and tendon organs located in a muscle connect with the alpha motoneurons that activate the same muscle. Afferent and efferent axons that serve muscles located on the right side of the body enter and exit the spinal cord on the right side, and vice versa. (b) The same connections for an agonist-antagonist muscle set (e.g., the hamstrings and quadriceps for the right leg), but this time emphasizing the complexity of the interneuronal connections. Open synapses (○) represent excitatory connections; filled synapses (●) indicate inhibitory effects. (α) = alpha motoneuron, (γ) = gamma motoneuron, i = interneuron, I = Ia inhibitory interneuron, Ia = muscle-spindle afferent, Ib = tendon-organ afferent, R = Renshaw cell. Reprinted from Enoka (1988).

stimulus is a maintained stretch, and the response is a corresponding maintained muscle contraction. The response to maintained stretch results in part from the effect of the Group II afferents. A common example of a tonic response may be found in the postural reaction to stretch, exemplified by the contracting of the gastrocnemius (calf) muscle to correct an excess forward shifting of one's center of gravity while standing.

Reciprocal Innervation

Muscles usually operate in pairs, so that when one set of muscles, the *agonists*, are contracting,

the opposing muscles, the *antagonists*, are relaxing. This organization of coordinated and opposing agonist and antagonist muscles is called *reciprocal innervation*. For example, when the arm is flexed at the elbow, by contraction of the biceps brachii, the triceps brachii muscle, which normally extends the arm at the elbow, must relax. If not, the two muscles would be pulling against each other and no movement would occur (see Figure 6.8).

In summary, when the motoneurons to one muscle receive excitatory impulses leading to muscle contraction, the motoneurons to the opposite muscle receive neural signals that make it

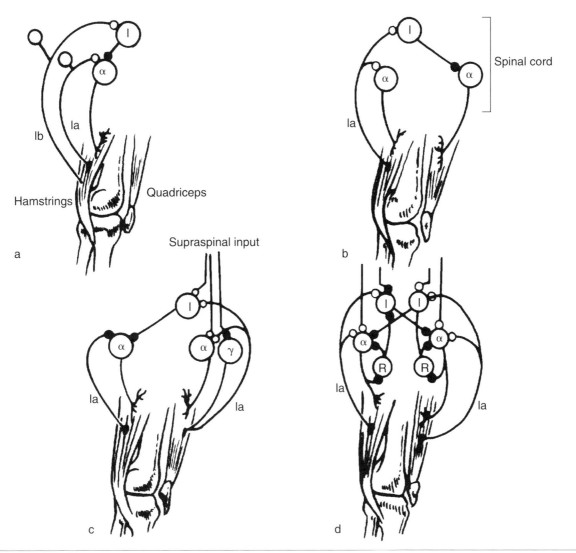

Fig. 6.8.   Selected central connections (• = inhibitory, ○ = excitatory) of the muscle spindle (Ia) and tendon organ (Ib) efferents to the schematized quadriceps and hamstrings muscle groups. (a) Effects of homonymous alpha (α) motoneurons. (b) Transmission of the reciprocal-inhibition reflex through the Ia inhibitory interneuron (I). (c) Supraspinal input to the quadriceps muscle group activating the reciprocal-inhibition circuit to the hamstrings. (d) Recurrent inhibition of the alpha motoneuron, and the Ia inhibitory interneuron through the Renshaw (R) cell. I = Ia inhibitory interneuron, i = interneuron, R = Renshaw cell, (α) = alpha motoneuron, (γ) = gamma motoneuron.
Reprinted from Enoka (1988).

less likely that they will fire and produce muscle contraction (*inhibition*). The antagonist is therefore inhibited at nearly the same instant that the agonist contracts. Reflex inhibition is controlled by a small inhibitory neuron (located in the spinal cord) to the motoneurons innervating the antagonistic muscle of the reciprocal pair. Conversely, if the antagonist muscle were similarly stretched, the agonist muscle would show reciprocal inhibition by the same process. Without this reciprocal innervation, coordinated muscular activity would be impossible.

Advances in Reflex Knowledge

In the previous sections, two types of spinal reflex actions were described in classical ways that have direct implications when utilizing various stretching techniques. They were the myotatic, or stretch, reflex and reciprocal inhibition. (Strictly speaking, reciprocal inhibition is not a reflex.) However, in most physiology textbooks the concepts were grossly generalized. Almost 30 years ago, Buller (1968) raised the point that much of the loose thinking that takes place regarding reflex activity stems from the use of oversimplified diagrams. Anatomical complexity renders the production of meaningful diagrams difficult. Further compounding the problem, the diagrams became accepted as anatomical facts. Elaborating on this concept, Buller writes:

> To make but a few of the possible additions, the incoming afferent will give off collaterals which ascend in the posterior columns. Further collaterals will synapse with interneurons which pass to synapse with the motoneurone of antagonistic muscle groups. The single incoming afferent will synapse not with a single large anterior horn cell but with each motoneuron of the motoneuron pool. The motor axon of the large anterior horn cell is likely to give off a Renshaw recurrent collateral—and so one could go on. The point to be stressed is that it is the very complexity of the interconnections within the spinal cord which are at the root of its behaviour. No truer phrase has been written than that stating that the simple spinal reflex arc just does not exist! (p. 209)

This similar view was stated by none other than Sherrington, the father of neurophysiology (1906):

> A simple reflex is probably a purely abstract conception because all parts of the nervous system are connected together and no part of it is probably ever capable of reaction without affecting and being affected by various other parts, and it is a system certainly never absolutely at rest. (p. 7)

But what then is the significance of the preceding reflex information in terms of stretching and understanding the nature of flexibility? According to Enoka (1988), because our knowledge and understanding of the nature and role of reflexes is insufficient, it is folly to carry these ideas too far in attempting to discuss the use of reflex concepts to develop flexibility protocols. Nonetheless, in chapter 13 we will review several reflex concepts utilized in rationalizing a flexibility protocol.

Coactivation/Cocontraction

Coactivation or *cocontraction* can be defined as contraction of two opposing muscles with "a high-level activity in the agonist muscles simultaneously with low-level activity in the antagonistic muscle of the same joint" (Solomonow and D'Ambrosia 1991, 396). Ironically, Sherrington as long ago as 1909 pointed out that antagonist

muscles may be in contraction concurrently. He attributed it to *double reciprocal innervation*. Several years later, Tilney and Pike (1925, 333) concluded that "muscular coordination depends primarily on the synchronous cocontractive relation in the antagonistic muscle groups." Eventually, Levine and Kabat (1952) summarized their observation by stating that, in a human's normal voluntary movement, there was insufficient evidence of the assumption that reciprocal innervation plays the dominant role in the coordination of the contraction of antagonist muscles. Furthermore, "cocontraction seems to be the rule rather than the exception" (p. 118). In more recent years, the central and peripheral control of agonist-antagonist coactivation has been established for various types of joint movement (DeLuca 1985; Kudina 1980; Rao 1965).

Having established the fact that cocontraction exists, the question arises as to its purpose. Unfortunately, there is surprisingly little data available on cocontraction. In particular, movement conditions under which we use cocontraction have been largely unexplained (Enoka 1988). However, in reviewing the existing literature Solomonow and D'Ambrosia (1991) identified two distinct purposes. First, it produces smooth, highly regulated, and accurate joint motion. Without such regulation, high-performance capacity in performing daily tasks as well as sports activities would be impossible. Second, cocontraction preserves joint stability, having the mechanical effect of making a joint stiffer. Consequently, movement becomes more difficult (Enoka 1988). Hence, muscles can provide a substantial and important basis for the stability of the joint via cocontraction.

Autogenic Inhibition (Inverse Myotatic Reflex)

Up to a point, the harder a muscle is stretched, the stronger is the resistance to the movement. The increase in resistance is explained by the myotatic stretch reflex. But, after a certain limit is reached the resistance suddenly yields, collapsing like the blade of a pocket knife snapping shut. Consequently, this phenomenon is often referred to as the *clasp-knife response*. The physiologic name for it is the *lengthening reaction*. This phenomenon was originally thought to be the responsibility of the GTOs, but that view has been disproved. It is now believed to be the result of afferent input from Group II nerve fibers coming from the muscle spindles and perhaps from thinly myelinated fibers subserving pain sensation from the joints (Moore, 1984). However, additional research is needed to substantiate this view.

Plasticity of the Spinal Cord Neural Circuits

The mechanisms of memory, or long-term adaptive change, in the CNS have long been of interest. According to Wolpaw and Carp (1990),

> The spinal cord in general, and spinal reflexes in particular, were widely viewed as fixed and inflexible, responding in a stereotyped manner to inputs from periphery or from supraspinal areas. This common perception is not correct. Spinal cord neurons and synapses, like those of cerebral cortex and other supraspinal structures, change in the course of development and in response to trauma. (p. 138)

More recently, it has been recognized that neuronal activity can produce persistent changes in the CNS. These *plastic changes*, which could be as striking as the sprouting of new synaptic connections or as subtle as modification in specific membrane ionic conductances, are thought to be responsible for subsequent changes in CNS activity that are expressed as altered behavior (Wolpaw and Lee 1989). In order to investigate this phenomenon, several experimental tasks need to be undertaken. First, it is mandatory to define the neuronal and synaptic substrates, or memory traces, of learned changes in behavior. Second, it is essential to know where these substrates are located. Third, it is necessary to describe the characteristic memory trace—the change in the CNS that is responsible for a particular change in behavior. In other words, it will be important to describe learning, the process that creates the trace.

Method of Plasticity Research and Findings

Since the early 1980s, researchers have examined the capability of nonhuman primates to alter the magnitude (size) of the *spinal stretch reflex* (SSR) as a systematic study of the anatomical and physiological substrates governing memory. The SSR, also called the *tendon jerk* or *M1*, is the initial response to sudden muscle stretch. The SSR is the simplest behavior of which the vertebrate CNS is capable (Matthews 1972). The Hoffman reflex (H-reflex) is comparable to the SSR, except that it is elicited by direct electrical stimulation of the Ia afferent fibers rather than by mechanical stretch, so that the muscle spindle is removed from the reflex arc. We can then more easily control the magnitude of the reflex stimulus to investigate the SSR and H-reflex phenomena.

In a series of experiments, the biceps brachii and triceps surae muscles in monkeys were operantly conditioned through the use of an implanted EMG-electrode biofeedback device and juice reward. Monkeys were exposed to a conditioning task that required prolonged change in neuronal activity influencing the SSR pathway and that was thus likely to produce a memory trace located in this pathway (Wolpaw 1983; Wolpaw, Braitman, and Seegal 1983). Over a span of 250 days, it was found that the monkeys could increase (uptrain) or decrease (downtrain) the magnitude of the SSR and H-reflex. It was determined that the monkeys could even be trained to reverse the changed response, thereby demonstrating an adaptive plasticity (Figures 6.9). Perhaps the most important finding was that, even following total spinal cord transection above the lumbosacral site of the SSR pathway (which would eliminate the influence of the brain), the animals previously subjected to the operant conditioning still displayed their trained reflex. This study substantiated the hypothesis that altered reflex activity eventually modifies the spinal cord (Wolpaw, Lee, and Carp 1991).

Site of the Plastic Changes

Currently, three possible locations of the spinal cord memory traces responsible for change in SSR size have been hypothesized (Figure 6.10). The most likely site is the Ia afferent terminal on the motoneuron (Figure 6.10a). Literature readily acknowledges that transmission through the Ia synapse is inhibited by presynaptic inputs from several supraspinal sites (Baldissera, Hultborn, and Illert 1981; R.E. Burke and Rudomin 1978). Furthermore, recent studies suggest that short-term changes in presynaptic inhibitions are important in motor behavior (Capaday and Stein 1987a, 1987b). Thus, chronic alterations or long-term change in this inhibition might modify the Ia terminal. Wolpaw and Carp (1990) have suggested that presynaptic inhibition may affect depolarization-induced calcium entry and transmit-

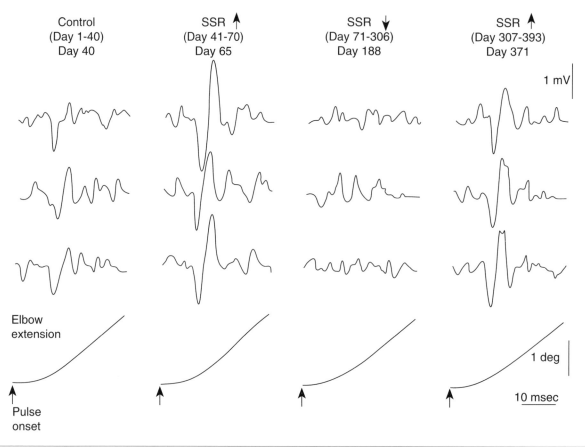

Fig. 6.9. Series of individual trials of raw EMG from a monkey under the control mode (left side), after initial SSR (up) exposure, after SSR (down) exposure, and, finally, after SSR (up) reexposure (right side). Each series is made up of consecutive trials. Pulse onset is indicated by the arrows, and the average course of pulse-induced extension is shown by the bottom trace. Background EMG, represented here by the 10 msec immediately following pulse onset, and pulse-induced extension are stable across the four series. In contrast, SSR amplitude increases well above control with minimal SSR (up) exposure, decreases well below control with subsequent SSR (down) exposure, and increases again with SSR (up) reexposure.
Reprinted from Wolpaw (1983).

ter release, and thereby alter the size of the excitatory postsynaptic potential (EPSP) produced in the motoneuron when the Ia sensory afferent is stimulated.

A second possible source could be a memory trace produced by prolonged change in the motoneuron that alters its response to any input. For example, motoneuron membrane properties that control resting potential and input resistance, such as ion permeability, could be altered. Needless to say, a modification in a motoneuron membrane's properties would have widespread effects on motoneuron function and would help determine the response of the motoneuron to any input (Figure 6.10b). However, Wolpaw and Carp (1990) and Wolpaw, Lee, and Carp (1991) are of the opinion that generalized membrane modifications present a less likely and more complex explanation for the reflex change.

A third explanation is a very localized postsynaptic modification. This process could perhaps be manifest as a change of receptor sensitivity or dendritic architecture. However, pathways capable of producing such a selective modification are not known at present (Figure 6.10c).

Implications of Neural Plasticity

The confirmation that the spinal cord can be altered (i.e., plasticity of the spinal cord) presents several highly significant implications. These implications deal with understanding the mechanism by which neurological insults potentially affect the body, the means to most optimally rehabilitate the injured part, and the factors related to motor learning and to developing flexibility in particular.

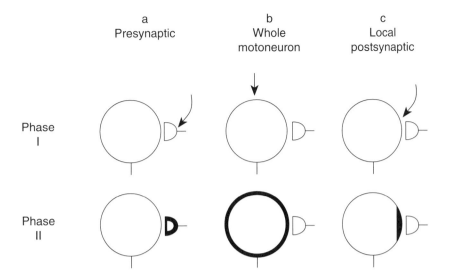

Fig. 6.10. Possible locations of the spinal cord memory traces responsible for change in SSR, or H-reflex, amplitude. In each case, phase I change in descending influence on a site in the SSR pathway (indicated by the arrow) eventually produces phase II change (that is, the memory trace at the site). (a) The most likely site is the Ia afferent terminal on the motoneuron. A memory trace here could be produced by prolonged change in presynaptic inhibition. (b) The memory trace could be a generalized change in the motoneuron that alters its response to any input. However, such a modification would have widespread effects on motoneuron function. (c) The trace could be a very localized modification in the postsynaptic membrane, such as a change in receptor sensitivity or dendritic architecture. Reprinted from Wolpaw and Carp (1990).

Clinical Perspectives on Neural Plasticity

From a clinical perspective, the question of interest becomes whether human SSRs can be experimentally conditioned and, if so, whether hyperactive SSRs (found in spastic muscles) might be successfully downtrained or hypoactive SSRs (in flaccid muscles) uptrained with less effort and in a more timely manner than demonstrated with nonhuman primates. According to Wolf and Segal (1990), the data of several researchers suggests that the human nervous system can be conditioned by monitoring and feedback of the SSR (Evatt, Wolf, and Segal 1989; Neilsen and Lance 1978).

Relationship of Neural Plasticity to the Development of Flexibility

Specifically, for individuals concerned with increasing their flexibility (i.e., range of motion), research regarding plasticity of the spinal cord may possibly substantiate the reason why static stretching has been so effective when utilized by practitioners of yoga. That is, perhaps, static stretching held for a given period of time may modify the stretch reflex excitability and thereby reduce the muscle's resistance to stretch. If a controlled test could be designed, it would make a fascinating study to determine which technique of stretching (i.e., ballistic vs. static) most facilitates beneficial plastic changes of the spinal cord.

Relationship of Neural Plasticity to Motor Learning

Changes in the SSR appear to occur throughout one's life. In children, gradual changes in the SSR occur with acquisition of fundamental motor skills (Myklebust, Gottlieb, and Agarwal 1986). Reviewing the literature, Wolpaw, Lee, and Carp (1991) suggest that comparable changes seem to take place later in life during learning of skills such as ballet (Goode and Van Hoven 1982; Nielsen, Crone, and Hultborn 1993) and aerobic versus anaerobic activities (Rochcongar, Dassonville, and Le Bars 1979). Thus, "slow activity-driven changes in the spinal cord and elsewhere in the CNS may account for much learning, and serve to explain why acquisition of many skills depends on prolonged practice" (Wolpaw, Lee, and Carp 1991, 344). This observation has major implications in such fields as athletics, the performing arts, ergonomics, medicine, chiropractic, and physical therapy, to mention just a few.

In the arena of sports medicine, the discovery of plasticity of the spinal cord has additional implications. For example, abnormal gait patterns following an injury may be a cause of foot, knee, hip, and back pain (Day and Wildermuth 1988;

Subotnick 1979). Furthermore, these changes could result in plastic changes in the spinal cord that could further complicate and delay full recovery. In this regard, research has found that up to 33% of the patients suffering acute sprains will have residual symptoms long after their rehabilitation programs have terminated (Bosien, Staples, and Russell 1955; Evans, Harcastle, and Frenyo 1984; Itay et al. 1982). It has been speculated that the subsequent functional instability may be due to lost and unrecovered joint, limb, and body proprioception (Freeman, Dean, and Hanham 1965). Perhaps, in part, this loss may be a consequence of plastic changes to the spinal cord.

Effects of Stretching Techniques on Neural Plasticity

Given that insults to the body can result in plastic changes to the spinal cord, the question that needs to be investigated is, What clinical techniques, either alone or in combination, can most efficiently, effectively, and rapidly correct the physical alteration to the spinal cord: a chiropractic adjustment or osteopathic manipulation, various stretching techniques (e.g., muscle energy, proprioceptive neuromuscular facilitation [PNF], static, ballistic), mobilization, traction, or employment of physical modalities? Similarly, it must be asked whether or not the use of medications that are commonly employed as an adjunct to therapy actually facilitate or impede this process.

Relationship of Neural Plasticity to Athletics and Sport Rehabilitation

In sports there is an old adage that it takes at least twice as long to correct something that was incorrectly learned. Thus, when an incorrect technique is learned, mastered, and ingrained, the neuromuscular pathways become "grooved," and subsequent neural plastic changes may take place. During the relearning phase, the undesired motor pattern must be "unlearned." This will necessitate not only unlearning the "grooving" of the neuromuscular pathways, but also proper modification of the plastic changes that took place during the initial learning.

Neurological and Other Factors of Flexibility Training

Gains in muscle strength are believed to result from two principal factors. Whereas muscle hy-pertrophy (i.e., an increase in size) occurs in the later stages of training (Enoka 1988; Komi 1986; McDonagh and Davies 1984; Sale 1986), strength gains achieved during the first weeks of training reflect an increased ability to activate motoneurons and therefore appear to be neural in origin (Figure 6.11). Abundant evidence demonstrates neural changes that occur soon after strength training begins. Voluntary strength increases rapidly before muscles exhibit hypertrophy (Ikai and Fukunaga 1970; D.A. Jones and Rutherford 1987; Liberson and Asa 1959; Moritani and de Vries 1979; Rose, Radzyminski, and Beatty 1957; Tesch, Hjort, and Balldin 1983) and before increases in electrically evoked tension occur (Davies and Young 1983; McDonagh, Hayward, and Davies 1983). These early strength increases are accompanied by increased integrated EMG (Komi 1986; Sale 1986) and increased reflex gains (Milner-Brown, Stein, and Lee 1975; Sale et al. 1982, Sale, MacDougall, Upton, and McComas 1983; Sale, Upton, McComas, and MacDougall 1983; Upton and Radford 1975).

Extrapolating from strength training to flexibility training, the pertinent question that is raised is, What is responsible for the initial increase of flexibility during the first weeks of training versus many months of training? Also, does the type of training (ballistic, static, PNF, etc.) influence the nature of these changes? Research has demonstrated that certain reflexes are modified in dancers as compared to the untrained (Goode and Van Hoven 1982; Koceja, Burke, and Kamen 1991; Nielsen, Crone, and Hultborn 1993). However, nonneural factors may also be involved. Koceja, Burke, and Kamen (1991) suggest that the difference between the two groups in their previous studies is their relative tissue compliance. They argue that long-term training can result in a change in the composition of the connecting tendon and that these changes might result in less loading on the muscle spindle apparatus given equal tendon-tap force. Byrd (1973) was cited as demonstrating that endurance training produced less tension per unit of cross-sectional area in the tail tendons of rat. This evidence suggested a greater fraction of soluble collagen. Last, Viidik (1973) was cited as having demonstrated that stretched tendon exhibits a tendency to remain in a stretched state. Consequently, any subsequent loading on the tendon will result in less force being transmitted to the muscle.

In returning to our question, only one study was located that investigated this area. Stevens et al. (1974) tested 232 physical education students, identifying the 15 subjects most supple and the 15 stiffest in the hamstring muscle group. They found a

Factors in Muscle Strength Gain

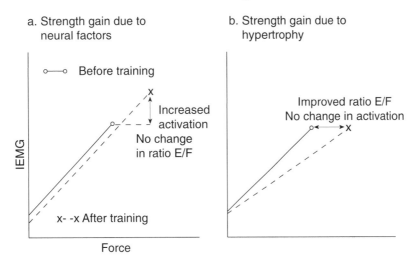

a. Strength gain due to neural factors

b. Strength gain due to hypertrophy

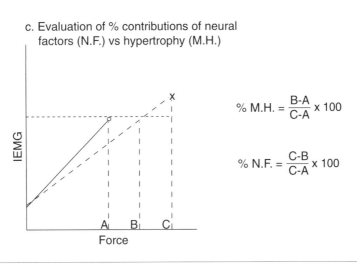

c. Evaluation of % contributions of neural factors (N.F.) vs hypertrophy (M.H.)

$$\% \text{ M.H.} = \frac{B-A}{C-A} \times 100$$

$$\% \text{ N.F.} = \frac{C-B}{C-A} \times 100$$

Fig. 6.11. Schema for the evaluation of the percentage of contributions of neural factors and hypertrophy to the gain of strength through progressive resistance exercise.
Reprinted from Moritani and de Vries (1979).

stronger EMG activation in the stretch patterns of the hamstrings and of the other muscles and an earlier onset (the last 40° of the stretch movement) and a longer duration of stretch reflex muscle activity in the stiff subjects than in the compliant, lithe subjects. In contrast, the lithe people of this sample showed stretch reflex activation in the last 20° of the stretch movement. This data "encouraged the hypothesis of a stronger sensitivity of the muscle spindles (fusimotor bias) as well as a stronger excitability of the circuit downstream from the spindles or an enhanced gamma activity among stiff subjects" (p. 496).

In a follow up study, Stevens et al. (1977) applied a vibration (to elicit the tonic vibration reflex) to the tendon of the biceps femoris for 2 min, followed by stretch. The mean integrated EMG

activity did not significantly differ in both groups. However,

> it was only in the stiff subjects that repeated stretch movements provoked a decreasing gradient of the maximum angle and the point at which the stretching activity started (i.e., the stretch reflex started later as a function of the repeated stretch movements). (p. 508)

In the opinion of the researchers, these findings "may suggest the hypothesis that viscoelastic components of a stiff muscle changes by stretching while the neurological component remains constant" (p. 509). In contrast, these tendencies were not found in the lithe subjects.

However, two recent studies challenge the previous reports. Vujnovich and Dawson (1994) demonstrated a significant effect of passive muscle stretch on decreasing the activity of neurons within the L5-S1 spinal segment by both static and ballistic stretch, which correlates with increased flexibility. Halbertsma and Göeken (1994) investigated the concept that stretching exercises lengthened the hamstrings by changing the elasticity of the muscles. The results showed that a slight but significant increase in the extensibility of the hamstrings was accompanied by a significant increase of the stretching (moment) force tolerated by the passive hamstring muscles. However, the elasticity remained the same. It was concluded that "stretching exercises do not make short hamstrings any longer or less stiff, but only influence the stretch tolerance" (p. 976).

The question that needs to be further investigated is, Are neural influences more or less important than other factors in flexibility training? The application of therapeutic stretch has been demonstrated to increase ROM. Two simple explanations for increased ROM include the mechanical elongation of muscle and of intervening connective tissue and the reduction of the levels of neuronal excitability. Additional research is needed to quantify how therapeutic stretching modifies the viscoelastic component of soft tissues and neural response among different populations—the healthy and those with disorders—and to establish the most efficient technique to achieve the desired outcome.

Speculations for the Future

The nervous system plays a major role in determining our quality and quantity of movement.

During this century and especially in recent years, there have been major advances in understanding the nervous system. With newer technological advances we will possibly learn more about the nervous system in the next 10 years than in the previous 100 years. Perhaps this increased knowledge will enable individuals involved with developing and maintaining optimal flexibility and range of motion to develop and implement new, effective approaches based on research findings to improve one's quality of life as well as the body's efficiency.

Summary

The structural and functional unit of the nervous system is the neuron. Two significant mechanoreceptors are the muscle spindles and Golgi tendon organs (GTOs). The primary stretch receptors in muscle are the muscle spindles. In contrast, the GTOs are primary contraction-sensitive mechanoreceptors. Joint receptors that sense mechanical forces on joints, such as stretch pressure and distention, are called articular mechanoreceptors. These nerve endings may be classified as Types I–IV based on morphological and behavioral criteria.

The nervous system operates through a complex set of interactions called reflexes, a few of which are the stretch reflex, reciprocal inhibition, and the inverse myotatic reflex. In addition, coactivation or cocontraction has been established during various types of joint movement. Currently, research has demonstrated that neuronal activity can produce persistent changes in the CNS, referred to as plastic changes. These changes have implications for rehabilitation, motor learning, and developing flexibility in particular.

Chapter 7

Hypermobility of the Joint

Hypermobility, or joint laxity, has long been recognized as a curiosity and source of entertainment. The earliest known clinical description of this trait is attributed to Hippocrates. He drew attention to a race of individuals called Scythians. According to Hippocrates, the Scythians' elbows were so lax they could not effectively draw their bows to shoot arrows! The old German diagnosis of *konstitutionelle Bindegewebenschwache* (connective tissue weakness) carried our awareness of this condition into the early 20th century, after which it received only scant attention in standard textbooks (Rose 1985). In the 1880s, a series of articles on contortionists appeared in several leading British medical journals ("The American Contortionist" 1882; "A Contortionist" 1882; Owen 1882; "Voluntary Power" 1882). One book that briefly dealt with the subject was *Anomalies and Curiosities of Medicine* by Gould and Pyle (1896, 473–475). Later, Finkelstein (1916) and Key (1927) presented the first detailed reports on joint hypermobility. Several years later, Wiles (1935) used radiography to perform a detailed analysis of the lumbar vertebrae of two extremely flexible professional acrobats.

During the 1950s and 1960s, the recognition developed of the importance of generalized joint laxity in the pathogenesis of joint dislocation (Bowker and Thompson 1964; Carter and Sweetnam 1958, 1960; Carter and Wilkinson 1964; Massie and Howarth 1951). However, it was not until the work of Kirk, Ansell, and Bywaters (1967) that the terms *hypermobility syndrome* and *hypermobility* were finally described in the medical literature. The former was defined as the situation in which joint laxity is associated with musculoskeletal complaints. In contrast, *generalized hypermobility* is said to be present when the joints are unduly lax and the range of motion is in excess of the accepted norm in most of the joints.

Terminology

Over the course of time, numerous papers have been published with reference to an excessive range of motion in joints. Among the lay public, this characteristic has been commonly referred to as being "double jointed." In the allied health arena the condition of excessive range of motion has been variously described as *ligamentous laxity* (Grana and Moretz 1978), *loose jointed* (Lichtor 1972), *joint hypertonia* (Finkelstein 1916; Jahss 1919), *joint looseness* (Marshall et al. 1980), *joint laxity* (Balaftsalis 1982–1983; Barrack et al. 1983; Bird 1979; Bird et al. 1980; Brodie, Bird, and Wright 1982; Cheng, Chan, and Hui 1991) and *hypermobility* (Ansell 1972; Child 1986; Grahame and Jenkins 1972; Gustavsen 1985; Key 1927; Kirk, Ansell, and Bywaters 1967; Klemp and Learmonth 1984; Klemp, Stevens, and Isaacs 1984; Rose 1985). An entire text has been devoted to this topic, and it adopted the term *hypermobility*. The reason for its adoption was as follows:

> It has been argued that the word "hypermobility" is inaccurate in its medical context and that it should be replaced by "hyperlaxity" or "hyperextensibility." However, for the sake of clarity we have adhered to the terminology used in previous publications and have employed

these terms interchangeably. (Beighton, Grahame, and Bird 1989, xi)

In this text we will use the terms *hypermobility* and *joint laxity* interchangeably.

Assessment of Joint Hypermobility

Over the years, many different systems of measuring hypermobility, or joint laxity, have been devised. They range from simple clinical tests (Carter and Wilkinson 1964), a modified system (Beighton, Solomon, and Soskolne 1973), and a global index (Bird, Brodie, and Wright 1979) to more sophisticated methods using radiologic assessment (Bird et al. 1980; Harris and Joseph 1949), photographic techniques (Troup, Hood, and Chapman 1968), a pendulum machine (Barnett 1971), and a fixed torque measuring device (Silman, Haskard, and Day 1986).

The first scoring system that established the criteria for hypermobility was devised by Carter and Wilkinson (1964) and assessed the following joint movements:

- Passive opposition of the thumb to the flexor aspect of the forearm
- Passive extension of the fingers so that they lie parallel with the extensor aspect (backside) of the forearm
- The ability to hyperextend the elbows more than 10°
- The ability to hyperextend the knees more than 10°
- An excessive range of passive dorsiflexion of the ankle and eversion of the foot

They defined generalized joint laxity as being present when three of the five movement tests were positive and were found when both upper and lower limbs were involved.

A more complex assessment was suggested by Kirk, Ansell, and Bywaters (1967). However, this testing procedure proved to be too time-consuming for routine use. Several years later, Beighton and Horan (1969) revised the 1967 test to measure joint laxity in people with Ehlers-Danlos syndrome (EDS), an inherited connective tissue disorder. Because passive extension of the fingers was too severe, it was replaced by passive extension of just the little finger beyond 90° with the

forearm flat on a table. In addition, the range of ankle movement was replaced by forward flexion of the trunk with the hands flat on the floor and with the knees fully extended (i.e., legs kept straight). Individuals were then given a score between 0 and 5.

Grahame and Jenkins (1972) modified the latter system to include passive dorsiflexion of the ankle to beyond 15° past the right angle. This modification was made because many of the subjects under study were ballet dancers. Therefore, six movements were evaluated in this test. Beighton, Solomon, and Soskolne (1973) slightly amended the test. Their generally accepted method utilized a rapid and easily applied screening test. In this test, a score from 0 to 9 is allocated, with the highest score denoting maximum joint laxity. However, there is disagreement as to the number of points necessary to be classified as possessing a generalized hypermobility. According to Child (1986), a score of 4 or more out of 9 possible points indicates generalized hypermobility of the joints. In contrast, Beighton, Grahame, and Bird (1989) state that the majority of clinicians require a minimum score in adults of between 4 and 6 out of 9 before making the diagnosis. Yet Rose (1985) states that it is generally accepted that a score of 6 or more allows definite classification of the syndrome. These are the movement tests used in this 9-point scoring system:

- Passive dorsiflexion and hyperextension of the fifth metacarpophalangeal (MCP) joint (i.e., the little finger) beyond 90° (1 point for each hand, 2 points for both)
- Passive apposition of the thumb to the flexor aspect of the forearm (1 point for each thumb, 2 points for both)
- Hyperextension of the elbow beyond 10° (1 point for each elbow, 2 points for both)
- Hyperextension of the knee beyond 10° (1 point for each knee, 2 points for both)
- Forward flexion of the trunk with the knees fully extended so that the palms of the hands rest flat on the floor (1 point)

In addition to the preceding assessment tools that examine multiple joints, there are several other methods of measuring joint laxity using a single joint. A hyperextensometer method was developed that used passive extension of the MCP joint of the little finger and a goniometer (a device for measuring joint motion) to measure the range of motion. Because this procedure is relatively imprecise, Grahame and Jenkins (1972) employed a predetermined force of 0.91 kg (2 lb) to standardize the testing. Later, Jobbins, Bird, and Wright (1979) constructed a device that measured torque (joint movement force). It was found that a torque of 2.6 kg/cm was of most use in the detection of hyperlaxity in a Caucasian population.

A final method to determine joint hypermobility is the *global index* (Brodie, Bird, and Wright 1982). This procedure score is based on the method proposed by the American Academy of Orthopaedic Surgeons (1965). It is derived by using goniometry to assess the range of movement at almost all joints in the body and summating the measured arcs of movement. Then the result is divided by 100.

Determining Factors of Hypermobility

The prevalence of hypermobility in the general population has been found to be 4% to 7% (Carter and Wilkinson 1964; Jesse, Owen, and Sagar 1980; D. Scott, Bird, and Wright 1979; Sutro 1947). In contrast, Klemp, Stevens, and Isaacs (1984) found a 9.5% rate among 377 ballet dancers. What factors contribute to joint laxity and how can it be altered? Range of motion is multifaceted in nature and is discussed throughout this text. Generally, it is affected by such things as skin tension, muscle tone, muscle fiber length (sarcomere number), various connective tissues (e.g., fascia, ligament, and tendon), and joint structure. Joint laxity can also be affected by such things as training, hormonal variations, temperature, gender, and genetic predisposition.

Ethnic and Racial Differences

If either generalized hypermobility or hypermobility syndrome is hereditary, the question then arises about ethnic and racial variations (Ansell 1972; Beighton 1971; Bird 1979; Child 1986; Wood 1971). Wood (1971) found no difference between subjects of Caucasian and African origin in Buffalo, New York. However, most research has demonstrated that true ethnic differences exist. People of Asian Indian origin have been shown to have more hyperextension of the

thumb than those of African origin, who in turn have greater hyperextension than those of European descent (Harris and Joseph 1949; Wordsworth et al. 1987). Similar results have been obtained by comparing the finger joints of different racial groups in Southern Africa (Schweitzer 1970) and among Iraqis (Al-Rawi, Al-Aszawi, and Al-Chalabi 1985). In a study by Pountain (1992), it was determined that the flexibility scores in 16- to 25-year-old residents of Oman were considerably lower than those reported in the 20- to 24-year-old Iraqi students previously cited. Finally, studies by Cheng, Chan, and Hui (1991) found that Chinese children were more lax than the Africans measured by Beighton, Solomon, and Soskolne (1973).

Genetic and Biochemical Defects That Influence Joint Hypermobility

Joint hypermobility may have many causes. Three important factors include the anatomical structures of the joints that normally restrict movements, the contribution of muscular tone to restricting joint movement, and the role of the extracellular matrix components in the mechanical properties of joint connective tissues (Beighton, Grahame, and Bird 1989). Having discussed these factors in previous chapters, we will assume that the third factor is most important and will therefore limit our discussion here to hypermobility that is due primarily to an alteration in collagen.

Connective tissue cells synthesize collagen according to instructions carried in the genes of their DNA. Any abnormality of this protein synthesis can result in weakened and therefore distensible connective tissue. Beighton, Grahame, and Bird (1983, 29-30) have proposed the following hypothetical deviations of metabolism that may explain the phenomenon of hypermobility. They include

1. The synthesis of specific messenger-RNA [a nucleic acid which carries genetic coded information] for collagen may be abnormal, leading to variation in amino acid content;
2. Errors may occur at the level of [genetic] transcription, leading to variation in amino acid content;
3. Variation may occur in the natural [hormonal] "fine tuning" mechanism by which

the amino acid content varies slightly from site to site in the same individual;

4. A defect may occur in the cleavage process that connects procollagen to [form] collagen;

5. Variation may occur in the ionic interactions which tend to align and strengthen collagen fibres;

6. There may be a defect in [interfiber] cross-linking;

7. Although collagen is relatively inert, variation in the rate of metabolism of collagen may lead to quantitative rather than qualitative variation in some individuals.

Consequences of Hypermobility

Although generalized hypermobility may be of benefit to dancers, musicians, some athletes (Beighton, Grahame, and Bird 1989; Larsson et al. 1993), and those employed in the circus as clowns or contortionists, there are also potential negative consequences. Some of these negative consequences associated with generalized hypermobility are impaired proprioceptive acuity (Mallik et al. 1994), increased risk of joint trauma (such as sprains), recurrent dislocation, effusions, and premature osteoarthrosis (Beighton, Grahame, and Bird 1989; Grahame 1971). The degree of the negative consequences depends on several factors, such as the degree of hypermobility, the physical condition of the individual, and the individual's vocation and avocation, to mention just a few (Beighton, Grahame, and Bird 1989; Larsson et al. 1993; Stanitski 1995).

General Management of Hypermobility

General treatment for someone with hypermobility syndrome (remember this means one who has joint laxity and musculoskeletal complaints) depends on a number of variables. Among them are the degree or grade of hypermobility, the presence of any other medical conditions (e.g., EDS, rheumatoid arthritis, Marfan syndrome, injury such as dislocation), the degree and quality of pain, and the individual's vocation and avocation. The course of treatment

will be ultimately based on a trained health care practitioner's professional knowledge and experience in his or her respective field.

Conservative Management of Hypermobility

The most conservative treatment is used for individuals with the lowest grade of hypermobility syndrome. The premanagement stage entails gathering information about the patient's history and the clinical evaluation. The management of such cases commences with reassurance as to the absence of serious disease (Biro, Gewanter, and Baum 1983; Kirk, Ansell, and Bywaters 1967). Next, the patient should be counseled about the nature of the condition and how to live with it (Rose 1985). Included at this stage are exploring the most aggravating and relieving factors with the patient and helping to modify the pattern of daily living accordingly (Child 1986). This modification may entail avoidance of strenuous sports, a change in occupation, or modification of the manner of performance of a particular job (Beighton, Grahame, and Bird 1989). Whenever practical, education about adequate joint protection should be facilitated (Child 1986; Rose 1985). Along these lines, practitioners should encourage moderate exercise to keep body weight low and muscular and ligamentous support maximal (Child 1986) and should provide correct postural training (Rose 1985). A recommended sport is swimming, since it involves less joint stress than weight-bearing activities like jogging (Child 1986; Kirk, Ansell, and Bywaters 1967). Another conservative treatment to further enhance joint protection is the utilization of braces, support splints, and surgical corsets (Beighton, Grahame, and Bird 1989; Rose 1985).

More aggressive treatment by health practitioners may include the direct incorporation of manual physical therapy techniques or modalities. These techniques may include massage, gentle mobilization (Beighton, Grahame, and Bird 1989), or gentle manipulation (Child 1986). However, Beighton, Grahame, and Bird (1989, 20) emphasize: "A word of caution is needed as regards the use of forceful manipulation in hypermobile patients, as joint subluxation may result from over-enthusiasm!"

For many patients, symptomatic pain relief may be achieved from hydrotherapy, in which exercises are performed under the supervision of a physical therapist in a pool heated to 35° C. (Beighton, Grahame, and Bird 1989). The application of other modalities in the presence of pain—including acupuncture, transcutaneous electrical nerve stimulation (TENS), and other types of electrical stimulation—may also be of use.

Moderate Management

The topical, oral, or intravenous application of various types of medications is another alternative treatment available to some allied health practitioners. (Chiropractors and massage therapists cannot dispense medication or inject patients.) The goal of this technique is usually to help relieve mild musculoskeletal pain, reduce inflammation, or facilitate the healing process. Among the more common medicinal aids are NSAIDs (nonsteroidal anti-inflammatory drugs, such as aspirin), analgesics (pain-relieving compounds, such as acetaminophen), and corticosteroids (hormones naturally produced by the adrenal gland) (Beighton, Grahame, and Bird 1989; Child 1986; Rose 1985). Almekinders (1993, 141) reminds us that "many questions regarding the exact effects and roles of NSAIDs remain unanswered" and that "choice of NSAIDs, timing and dosage schedules also remain unclear." The potentially negative consequences of the use of drugs or medications should be obvious to practitioners and are being increasingly recognized by an informed public. Needless to say, the possible risk of side-effects should be carefully weighed against the potential benefits to the patient. Therefore, practitioners should be judicious in the utilization of medications and discontinue their use as soon as feasible.

Radical Management

In severe cases, radical management, including major invasive techniques such as surgery, may be necessary. Radical treatment is usually employed as a last resort after conservative and moderate treatments have failed. Among conditions that might require surgery are soft tissue lesions (such as sprains), persistent synovitis (inflammation of the tissue layer lining the interior of the joint capsule), recurrent dislocation, spinal instability, and advanced cases of both rheumatoid arthritis and osteoarthritis (Beighton, Grahame, and Bird 1989).

Inherited Syndromes

A number of genetic syndromes are associated with joint laxity. Perhaps the most well known is Ehlers-Danlos syndrome (EDS). EDS is an inherited connective tissue disorder characterized by articular hypermobility, dermal (skin) extension, and cutaneous scarring. There is considerable variation in the extent to which individuals may be affected by this condition.

Familial undifferentiated hypermobility syndromes are conditions associated with excessive range of motion. These syndromes are a heterogeneous group of disorders in which generalized joint laxity is the primary clinical manifestation (Beighton, Grahame, and Bird 1989). Some of the earliest accounts of familial hypermobility were described by Finkelstein (1916), Key (1927), and Sturkie (1941). Carter and Sweetnam (1958, 1960) and Carter and Wilkinson (1964) further showed a close association between familial joint laxity and the incidence of dislocations in close relatives. Later, Beighton and Horan (1970) described two families in which joint laxity was transmitted as an autosomal (i.e., genetic) dominant trait.

In addition to EDS and the familial undifferentiated hypermobility syndromes, joint laxity is present in a number of other inherited disorders. Among them are Marfan syndrome, osteogenesis imperfecta (OI), Larsen syndrome, and several inherited skeletal dysplasias (malformations) in which dwarfism is the major feature. The interested reader is referred to the concise and well-illustrated work of Beighton, Grahame, and Bird (1989).

Research Perspectives in Heritable Disorders of Connective Tissue

The term *heritable disorders of connective tissue* became embedded in the medical literature with the publication in 1956 of a book of the same name written by Victor McKusick. Since that time, over 200 distinct disorders have been identified. Research has also enhanced our understanding of connective tissues.

It is recognized that many of these disorders not only influence range of motion, but also have a major impact on the patients' well-being and on financial costs for patients and for society. Thus, based on a workshop on heritable disorders of connective tissue at the National Institutes of Health (1990, April), the following areas were identified as research priorities:

1. To identify and characterize genetic mutations in all disease phenotypes
2. To determine structure-function relationships of normal connective tissue matrix molecules
3. To describe developmental regulations of matrix formation
4. To perform multidisciplinary analysis of disease mechanisms
5. To design clinical studies of natural history and clinical trials in the treatment of genetic diseases
6. To establish disease registries
7. To provide periodic workshops and to include disease studies in major symposia on matrix biology
8. To identify and study existing animal models of genetic diseases and to create animal models by transgenic technologies to identify phenotypes produced by mutations in specific genes
9. To apply genetic linkage strategies to heritable disorders of connective tissue
10. To pursue the molecular basis of common disease analogues of specific heritable disorders of connective tissue

During the past 10 years in particular, major advances have been made in identifying the molecular components of the extracellular matrix, in isolating and characterizing the genes that encode these proteins, in identifying and characterizing the biosynthetic pathways of most matrix proteins, in defining interactions among these proteins, and in characterizing mutations in genes that produce a limited variety of these disorders (Byers, Pyeritz, and Uitto 1992). Perhaps in the near future we will have a more complete understanding of those factors that affect connective tissue and that ultimately determine one's range of motion.

Contortionism

Contortionism can be defined as the art of manipulating the body parts in feats of extreme suppleness and skill. The art originated in ancient times and was present in virtually all ancient civiliza-

tions. The early purpose of contortionism was as a source of entertainment. Contortionists are usually classified by those in the profession as "legs," who can perform unusual acts of flexibility about the hips; "front benders," who bend forward from the waist; "back benders," who actually bend their trunk backward; and "dislocationists," who can dislocate major articulations of their body, including the neck (Figures 7.1–7.5). An "elastic person" is a skin-stretching exhibitionist whose skin can be stretched several inches and, on release, immediately returns to its former position (Figure 7.6). Such individuals have Ehlers-Danlos syndrome.

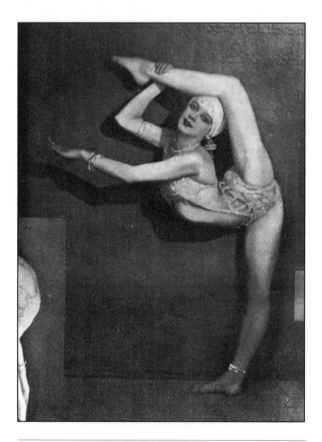

Fig. 7.1. "Legs" Valentine Sayton performing an arabesque. Burns Kattenburg Collection/Harvard Theatre Collection. Reprinted with permission.

One age-old question is whether contortionists are born or are the product of nurturing. Some contortionists are graced with inherent articular laxity. These performers require very little in the way of training or warm-up. In a sense, "they chose their parents wisely." According to Beighton, Grahame, and Bird (1989), a number of well-known circus performing families are affected by an autosomal dominant trait that

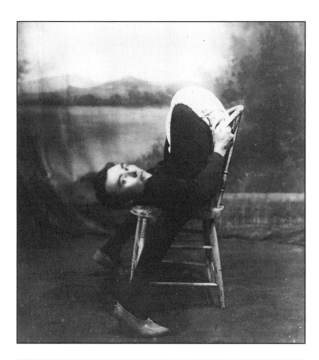

Fig. 7.2. "Front bender" E.C. Biggerstaff, straddle legs. Burns Kattenburg Collection/Harvard Theatre Collection. Reprinted with permission.

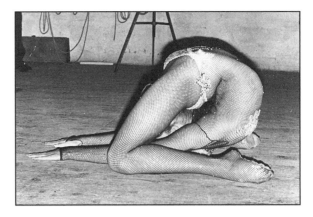

Fig. 7.4. "Back bender" Diane Bennett, chest bridge/ pigeone. Burns Kattenburg Collection/Harvard Theatre Collection. Reprinted with permission.

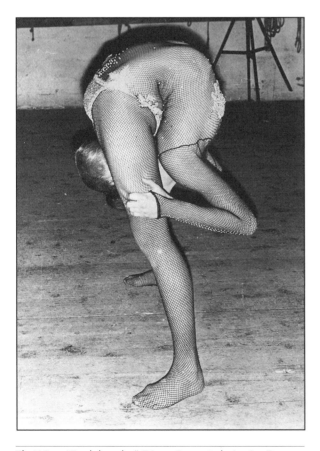

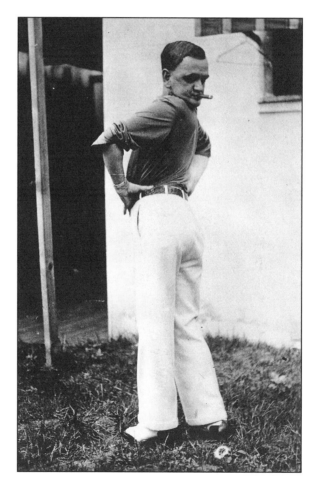

Fig 7.5 "Dislocationist" Martin Laurello. Burns Kattenburg Collection/Harvard Theatre Collection. Reprinted with permission.

Fig 7.3. "Back bender" Diane Bennett, hair pin. Burns Kattenburg Collection/Harvard Theatre Collection. Reprinted with permission.

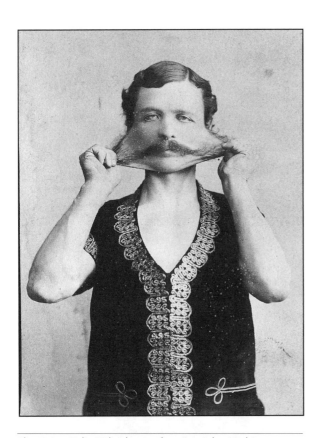

Fig. 7.6. Felix Whorley performing "elastic skin wonders." Burns Kattenburg Collection/Harvard Theatre Collection. Reprinted with permission.

explains their natural suppleness. In contrast, many contortionists have to develop their skills by years of rigorous training. Unfortunately, these contortionists must practice several hours each day and require a long warm-up period before a performance. Furthermore, even a few days of inactivity will result in a marked stiffening of the joints.

Summary

The presence of joint hypermobility has been recognized since antiquity. Numerous systems have been developed to quantify joint hypermobility. Furthermore, there has been extensive research related to its predisposing factors. Various types of medical management can be employed in caring for those individuals with hypermobility syndrome. Treatment will be determined by the extent of the symptoms.

Contortionism can be defined as the art of manipulating the body parts in feats of suppleness and skill. It is an ancient and widespread practice.

Chapter 8

Relaxation

A multitude of articles and books have been written on the topic of relaxation. What is relaxation and why is it so important in facilitating the development of flexibility? We must first define the term *relaxation* before addressing these and other crucial questions.

Defining Relaxation

Relaxation may be defined in several ways. In the discipline of motor learning, it is "the ability to control muscle activity such that muscles not specifically required for a task are quiet, and those which are required are fired at the minimal level needed to achieve the desired results" (Coville 1979, 178). Accordingly, relaxation "can be considered as a motor skill in itself because the ability to reduce muscle firing is as important to motor control as is generation of firing" (Coville 1979, 177). Consequently, relaxation may be regarded as a factor that determines optimal performance.

In skilled performance, movement is characterized by an appearance of ease, smoothness of movement, coordination, grace, self-control, and total freedom. It may also be characterized by beauty, harmony, precision, and virtuosity. Thus, in motor learning the term *relaxation* applies to the absence of anxiety, inhibition, tension, or extraneous motion.

Relaxation is economical energy consumption and resistance to fatigue. It involves a minimal expenditure of energy consistent with the desired ends (Basmajian 1975). When more muscle fibers than necessary are activated, an inefficient energy expenditure results (Coville 1979). To compensate for the shortfall of oxygen and energy in such an instance, the cardiovascular system is taxed that much more. This unnecessary expenditure of energy may actually interfere with the execution of the task at hand and, more significantly, may help to bring on fatigue more quickly (Coville 1979).

Relaxation can help reduce the risk of injury. If one is relaxed, there is an economical expenditure of energy and thus resistance to fatigue. Furthermore, when one is less fatigued, one is less prone to injury, because awkward movements and psychological tension in general should increase the frequency of accidents (Rathbone 1971).

Although muscular relaxation is important for all of these reasons, our concern is with flexibility (i.e., range of motion) and stretching. How does relaxation affect flexibility, and why should a muscle usually be relaxed prior to stretching? Theoretically, stretching should begin when a muscle is in a completely relaxed state. That is, there should be a minimal amount of tension developed by the contractile components. As a result of this reduced internal tension, the individual should then be able to most effectively and efficiently work on stretching out the connective tissue, which truly limits extensibility. Remember, each muscle cell is capable of at least a 50% increase in length, accomplished by the longitudinal sliding of the actin and myosin filaments that leaves at least one cross-bridge maintained. Usually, this phase of muscle lengthening (the stretching phase) is performed slowly or at a constant rate, thus reducing the likelihood of activating the stretch reflex and ultimately the muscular contractile components. However, in an investigation of proprioceptive neuromuscular inhibitory techniques (PNF), M.A. Moore (1979) found that complete relaxation was not a requisite for effective stretching. This topic will be investigated in chapter 13.

Measuring Relaxation

Relaxation can be measured by a variety of technologies, including galvanic skin responses, electroencephalography (EEG), and electromyography (EMG). Their application depends on which physiological response is to be analyzed. Among the physiological responses that can be evaluated are oxygen consumption, respiratory rate, heart rate, blood pressure, skin temperature, muscle tension, and alpha brain waves. EMG is probably the most relevant method for those individuals concerned with measuring muscle tension via a muscle's action potential. In contrast, sleep laboratories would be more concerned with brain wave patterns recorded during sleep.

Methodologies of Facilitating Muscular Relaxation

According to Hertling and Jones (1990), types of relaxation training and related techniques are difficult to classify because they employ a combination of strategies and techniques. Among the strategies and techniques are

- the somatic, or physical, approach, which uses special breathing and movement, special stretching techniques, massage and acupressure, or adjustment and manipulation;
- physiological therapeutic modalities, which use cold, heat, needles or lasers, or traction;
- cognitive, mental, and mind-controlling techniques;
- sophisticated technology, such as biofeedback; and
- drugs or medications.

To determine the most cost-effective and efficient plan of action, one should consider the safety of the plan, any special assistance or instruction necessary, the need for special equipment and ergogenic aids (i.e., anything that enhances performance), the amount of time required, and the financial cost. Ideally, a specific strategy or technique should be implemented only after thoughtful consideration of these issues.

Somatic Approach

Somatic or physical strategies fall into two major categories: *passive distraction* and *active distraction.* The former strategies include progressive relaxation, massage, and certain respiratory techniques. The latter strategies include techniques such as Alexander, Feldenkrais, and tai chi. The interested reader is referred to the summaries of Hertling and Jones (1990).

Breathing Techniques

For thousands of years it has been known that various breathing techniques facilitate relaxation. A classic example is found in hatha-yoga. Today, many relaxation techniques employ specific breathing patterns in conjunction with specific physical and mental strategies. In the area of sports medicine, the close relationship between respiration and the motor system has been recognized and investigated. This relationship has been termed *synkinesis,* which occurs when a certain type of movement is linked either with inspiration or with expiration (Lewit 1991, 27). For example, researchers have investigated the relationship of breathing cycles and the Valsalva phenomenon (an expiratory effort against a closed glottis that results in an impeded blood flow to the heart and a fall in arterial pressure) in weightlifting. Yet another area of interest has been the relationship between the respiratory pattern and the movements in specific athletic activities such as bicycling (Bechbache and Duffin 1977), gymnastics (Mironov 1969a, 1969b), rowing (Clark, Hagerman, and Gelfand 1983; Maclennan et al. 1994; Mahler et al. 1991, Steinacker, Both, and Whipp 1993), running (Pechinski 1966), swimming (Holmer and Gullstrand 1980; Keskinen and Komi 1991), and walking (A.R. Hill et al. 1988). However, to date, there has been no attempt to integrate the anecdotal, empirical, and experimental literature of breathing as it relates to stretching, flexibility, and performance.

How Can Proper Breathing Facilitate Stretching?
Theoretically, coupling the correct breathing pattern with specific movements can facilitate movement itself. This effect can be explained on three levels: neurophysiological, mechanical, and experiential, or subjective. We will analyze these three explanations in their relationship to forward flexion of the vertebral column.

First, during forward flexion of the trunk, the musculature of the lower back is put under passive tension. The greater this tension, the more difficulty in flexing the upper torso toward the thighs. The objective at this point must be to initiate any measure that can minimize the tension of these muscles. This relaxation can be achieved by a gentle expiratory effort. Research has documented that a deep inspiration with the chest expanded and the abdominal muscles drawn in is accompanied by active contraction of the erector spinae muscles (muscles of the lower back) (Campbell 1970; Roaf 1977, 49). However, contraction of the erector spinae is undesirable: Contraction of these muscles will further increase resistance to forward flexion and will initiate extension of the lower torso, which is a motion counter to the desired trunk flexion. Hence, it is self-defeating to deeply inhale during forward

flexion. Instead, the appropriate course would be to slowly exhale in order to facilitate a relaxation of the erector spinae. (Research by Campbell has also shown that in some instances a maximum expiration can result in activity of the sacrospinalis muscles of the lower back.)

Second, to facilitate stretching one can incorporate gravity and appropriate breathing. During inspiration the lungs become inflated, much like a balloon or life preserver used on a boat. Thus, inhalation creates a "lifting" or "rising" effect (Figure 8.1). However, during trunk flexion the objective is to descend and to lower the upper torso, not to raise it. If the lungs are inflated during forward flexion, their lifting effect counters the desired direction of movement.

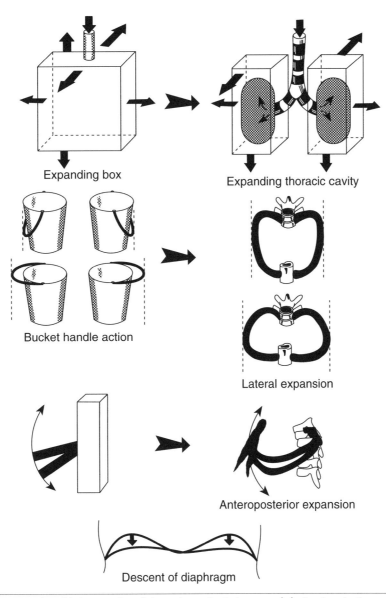

Expanding box

Expanding thoracic cavity

Bucket handle action

Lateral expansion

Anteroposterior expansion

Descent of diaphragm

Fig. 8.1. The different ways in which capacity of thoracic cavity is increased during inspiration. Reprinted from Snell (1992).

When the lungs are deflated, there is an absence of this lifting force. As a result, nothing counters the effect of gravity acting on the upper torso to facilitate its lowering to the thighs. Hence, it is advantageous to exhale during stretches involving forward flexion of the upper torso toward the lower limbs (e.g., the modified hurdler's stretch) and to inhale when raising the torso.

During forward flexion most of the spinal flexion occurs by the time the trunk is inclined 45° forward. The remainder of the forward flexion occurs via forward rotation (anterior tilt) of the pelvis. The pelvis rotates around the fulcrum of the hip joints, like a seesaw or teeterboard. X-ray studies by Mitchell and Pruzzo (1971) documented that the sacral apex (inferior tip) moves posteriorly during exhalation, so that the oppo-

site, top end moves forward. Hence, exhalation facilitates pelvic tilt and trunk flexion (Figure 8.2).

Research has demonstrated that in the upright posture the diaphragm has an inspiratory action on the lower rib cage, whereas in the supine posture the diaphragm has an expiratory action on the lower rib cage (De Troyer and Loring 1986). With trunk flexion the diaphragm is gradually elevated. In part, this action is facilitated by gravity, simulating the action of exhalation.

Third, as the diaphragm rises in the chest with exhalation, it pushes up against the heart and slows down the heart rate. Therefore, by breathing slowly, with the exhalation longer than the inhalation, heart rate and blood pressure decrease. Furthermore, with exhalation there will

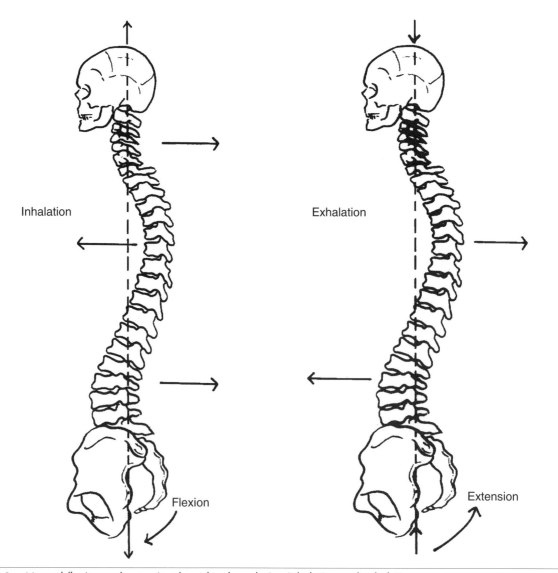

Fig. 8.2.   Normal flexion and extension that take place during inhalation and exhalation. Reprinted from Faucret (1980).

be decreased stress and tension on the ribs, intercostal muscles, abdominal wall, and related musculature and fascia (see Figure 8.1). This decrease in muscle tension will be transmitted by the appropriate muscle spindles and other proprioceptors. Consequently, there will be the subjective perception of less stress and greater relaxation. In contrast, inhalation is associated with increases in the heart rate, blood pressure, and stress on various structures of the body.

Coordinating Breathing and Eye Positioning With Mobilization.   It is widely held that muscular activity is facilitated during inspiration and inhibited during expiration, but this statement is an oversimplification (Lewit 1991). In actuality, there are several important exceptions to the rule with regard to exhalation. For example, Lewit (1991) points out that there is a close connection among looking up, inspiration, and straightening of the body, and among looking down, expiration, and stooping. However, this rule applies only to the cervical and lumbar spine (which are decisive in view of their great mobility) and not to the thoracic spine. In contrast, in the thoracic spine, the following relationship applies.

> Here it is maximum inspiration that facilitates flexion and maximum expiration that facilitates extension, i.e., the thoracic erector spinae, and this to such an extent that deep inspiration is probably the most effective method of mobilizing the thoracic spine into flexion, with maximum expiration most effective for extension. (Lewit 1991, 26)

Furthermore, Lewit (1991), citing the work of Gaymans (1980), points out that there is an alternating facilitation and inhibition of individual segments of the spinal column during side-bending.

> It can be regularly shown that during side-bending resistance increases in the cervical as well as in the thoracic spine in the even segments (occiput-atlas, C2, etc., and again in T2, T4, etc.) during inspiration; during expiration we obtain a mobilizing effect in these segments. Conversely, resistance increases in the odd segments (C1, C3, T3, T5, etc.) during expiration, while we obtain mobilization during inspiration. There is a "neutral" zone between C7 and T1. An important feature of the atlas-occiput segment is that here inspiration increases resistance not only against side-bending but in all directions, while expiration facilitates mobility. This effect is most marked at the craniocervical junction and decreases in a caudal direction; in particular the mobilizing effect of inspiration (in the odd segments) diminishes in the lower thoracic region. (Lewit 1991, 26)

What, then, does the research show regarding the coordination of eye position and breathing to enhance range of movement? Below, we will review two published investigations. The first one was a creative study designed by Fellabaum (1993) that investigated the effect of eye position on flexibility during lumbar flexion. Thirty subjects were tested using a set of specially prepared eyeglasses. The lenses of each pair were painted, with exception of a clear circle about 0.5 cm in diameter placed in the midline vertical plane at "12 o'clock" (up) on one pair and "6 o'clock" (down) on another pair. Half of the subjects started with the downward-viewing glasses, and the other half started with the upward-viewing glasses. The flexibility of subjects was then measured in centimeters from the tip of the subject's fist to the floor on the fourth attempt at forward flexion. "The findings suggested that eye positioning in the vertical plane does significantly affect forward flexion, with downward gaze enhancing forward flexion" (Fellabaum 1993, 15).

In a second study, Sachse and Berger (1989) investigated the efficacy of cervical mobilization induced by eye movement and fixed to a respiratory phase. As illustrated in Figure 8.3a-d, there is restricted rotation of the C2-3 segment to the right. The therapist's left hand stabilizes the vertebral arch of the C3 vertebra by palpation. The fingertips of the therapist's right hand are placed on the subject's chin with the head rotated to the right, thus inducing a very slight resistance at the relevant segment. Then,

> holding the head in an unchanged, rotated position, the patient looks upward and breathes in as slowly as he can. A symmetrical contraction of the neck extensors can be perceived during slight extension of the head [Figure 8.3e]. After deep inspiration the patient looks down, breathes out, and is completely relaxed [Figure 8.3d]. At the end of the second or third expiration cycle, resistance in the particular segment decreases. The therapist may now extend the rotation of the head to achieve the same degree of slight resistance in the segment as before. After about five breathing cycles, rotation will be normalized. (Sachse and Berger 1989, 155)

The efficacy of linking eye movements, breathing, and body movement can be demonstrated using cervicomotograms. In some subjects, rota-

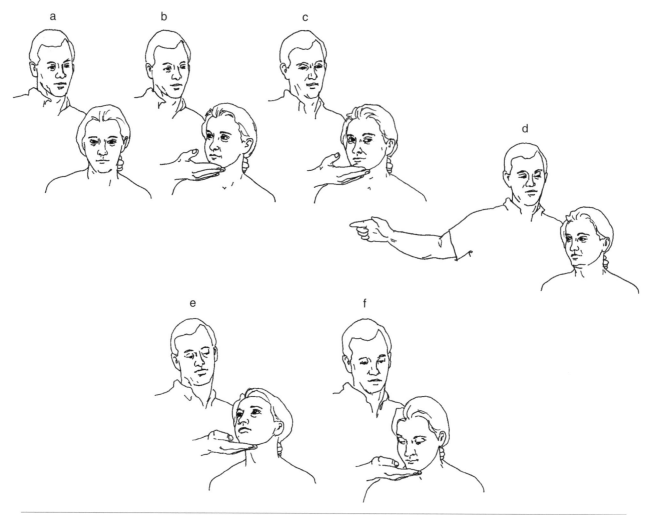

Fig. 8.3. Mobilization of restricted rotation to the right at the C2-3 level by vertical eye movements in correlation with inhalation and exhalation.
Reprinted from Sachse and Berger (1989).

tion increased steadily during the breathing cycles (turning the head to the right makes the curve go up; see Figure 8.4). In others, there was an oscillatory increase and decrease of the rotational angle of the head. The increase can be linked to expiration as expected. However, in some cases increases of the rotational angle took place in the inspiration-extension phase as shown in Figure 8.5a. In one patient tested, the rotational pattern in segment C1-2 was always similar to that of segment C2-3 (Figure 8.5, a and b). In addition, in some people lateral flexion could be seen to correlate with rhythm of flexion and extension (Figure 8.6).

Facilitating Inhalations and Exhalations During Manual Therapy. These findings have practical implications for practitioners of mobilization and

manipulative techniques, such as chiropractors, osteopaths, and physical therapists. The importance of reducing arousal and tension is paramount for those practitioners in particular who utilize thrusting techniques, because the more the patient is aroused, tense, or resistive, the greater the force that must be applied to overcome such resistance. With greater external force there is the increased risk of trauma produced by the manual technique. The perfect technique is that which offers the body the least amount of energy needed to achieve the desired objectives (Gold 1987). Manual techniques require a unique interaction between the patient and doctor or therapist. This interaction can only take place when there is total relaxation and acceptance on the part of the patient. It is no wonder that the thrust is usually timed to coincide with the exhalation and subse-

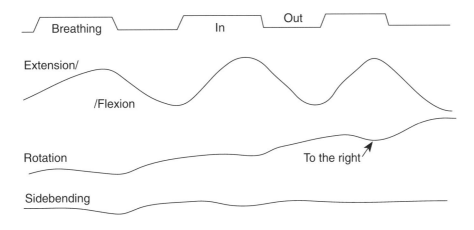

Pat.: G.H.
Active segment cervical 2/3, rotation to right

Fig. 8.4. Cervicomotogram of breathing cycles in a healthy subject, as illustrated by Figure 8.3, c and d: steadily increasing rotation to the right.
Reprinted from Sachse and Berger (1989).

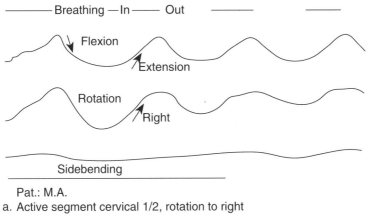

Pat.: M.A.
a. Active segment cervical 1/2, rotation to right

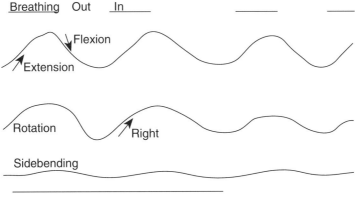

Pat.: M. A.
b. Active segment cervical 2/3, rotation to right

Fig. 8.5. Cervicomotogram of breathing cycles in spinal segments C1-2 and C2-3 in a healthy subject, as illustrated by Figure 8.3, c and d: oscillating rotational synkinesis similar in both segments.
Reprinted from Sachse and Berger (1989).

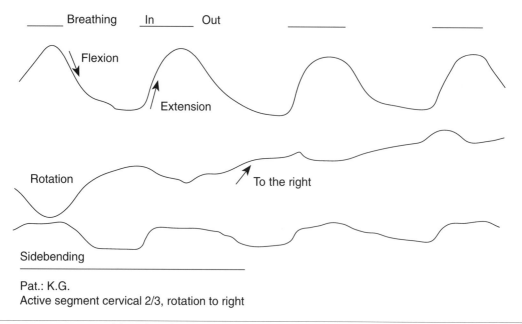

Fig. 8.6. Cervicomotogram of three breathing cycles in a healthy subject, as illustrated in Figure 8.3, c and d: synkinesis of lateral flexion.
Reprinted from Sachse and Berger (1989).

quent "release" of the patient. This timing is especially important when working on the spine, since exhalations decrease *pneumatic* resistance and tend to relax the long extensors as well as flexors of the body (Hellig 1969; Janse, Houser, and Wells 1947, 365). To achieve this end (i.e., facilitating relaxation) appropriate breathing and related strategies should be employed.

Stretching

Stretching can be used to facilitate relaxation. The theoretical basis for this idea is founded primarily on spinal reflex physiology. The two strategies employed to induce muscle relaxation are the static stretch and proprioceptive neuromuscular facilitation.

Static Stretch. *Static stretching* involves stretching the muscle to the point at which further movement is limited by its own tension. At this point, the stretch is held and maintained for an extended period of time, during which relaxation and reduction of tension take place. This relaxation phenomenon has three possible explanations: First, the muscle's stretch receptors (i.e., muscle spindles) become desensitized and subsequently *adapt* to stretch. Hence, the stretch reflex is reduced. Second, if the passive tension from the stretch is great enough, GTO and joint receptors (see chapter 6) will be activated, thus initiating the *autogenic inhibition reflex*. In turn, this reflex

will inhibit the motoneuron of the muscle under stretch. Consequently, the muscle's tension will decrease, thereby facilitating relaxation. Research by Thigpen (1984) has demonstrated that short bouts of static stretching reduce electrical activity within the muscle. Similarly, Etnyre and Abraham (1984) found that static stretching produced a slight depression of the motor pool excitability throughout stretching of the human soleus muscle. The third and last explanation is based on the fact that muscle and connective tissue possess time-dependent mechanical properties. That is, when a constant force is applied, *creep*, or a progressive change in length, occurs along with *stress-relaxation*, a progressive reduction in tension.

Proprioceptive Neuromuscular Facilitation. *Proprioceptive neuromuscular facilitation* (PNF) is a strategy that can induce relaxation of a muscle. Its operation is based in part on the physiology of the muscle spindles and GTOs. Using the *hold-relax* technique, a limb or muscle is stretched to the point where further motion in the desired direction is prevented by the tension in the antagonistic muscle (i.e., the muscle being stretched). At this point, a maximal isometric contraction for 5 to 10 s is gradually exerted by the muscle being stretched. Theoretically, this contraction will cause the GTOs to fire, consequently initiating the autogenic inhibition and relaxing the stretched muscle.

Another modified PNF technique is believed to employ the strategy of reciprocal innervation (see chapter 6). Once again, an antagonistic muscle is stretched to the point where further motion is prevented by the tension in the muscle. However, at this point either an isometric or isotonic contraction of the agonist (i.e., the muscle opposite the antagonist) can be employed. By so doing, the tension in the antagonistic muscle should be reduced via reciprocal innervation.

Massage

Massage is probably the oldest of all remedies since it is used instinctively not only by humans, but by lower animals as well. Most cultures, both ancient and modern, have employed massage as a health aid. We will use the term *massage* to imply the scientific and systematic manipulation of body tissues for the purpose of affecting the nervous and muscular systems and general circulation (Knapp 1990). According to Hertling and Jones (1990), there seems to have been a general decrease in the use of massage lately for several reasons: It is time-consuming and sometimes strenuous and demands skill on the part of the person giving the treatment; increased knowledge and sophistication of equipment and technology has made basic massage too simple to use; and its use has been experiential rather than scientific.

The effects of massage may be classified into two general categories: *reflex effects* and *mechanical effects*. By reflex action, the sensory nerves in the skin act to produce sensations of pleasure or relaxation, which cause the muscles to relax and blood vessels to dilate (Dubrovskii 1990; Longworth 1982). Another reflex effect is sedative, reducing mental tension (Yates 1990). Research has demonstrated that motoneuron excitability can be reduced by massage of the triceps surae (calf muscles; Morelli, Seaborne, and Sullivan 1989). To achieve these results, the massage should be given in a monotonously repetitive manner (Knapp 1990).

The mechanical effects consist of stimulating circulation of venous blood and flow of lymph through or from an area; stimulating metabolism in an area, thus increasing removal of waste or fatigue products; and stretching adhesions between muscle fibers. Furthermore, several studies have found massage to be an effective means of increasing range of motion (Crosman, Chateauvert, and Weisberg 1984; Nordschow and Bierman 1962). In the latter study, the effect of Swedish massage was a statistically significant improvement in muscle relaxation in normal subjects (as measured by trunk flexion). In contrast, a study by Wiktorsson-Möller and colleagues (1983) found that stretching resulted in a significantly increased range of motion in all muscle groups tested, whereas only one muscle group was influenced by massage, warming up, or a combination of the two.

There are three basic types of massage hand movements. *Stroking*, or *effleurage*, may be superficial or deep. The movements must be slow, rhythmic, and gentle. The major objective of this technique is to improve the movement of venous blood and lymph flow. *Compression*, or *petrissage*, includes kneading, squeezing, and friction. This method is used to limit or eliminate adhesions. Finally, *percussion*, or *tapotement*, employs hacking, clapping, or beating and is used to produce stimulation.

Massage is contraindicated with the slightest suspicion of local malignancy (cancer), sepsis (infection) or thrombosis (blood clot). Nor should massage be used in the presence of skin irritations or in inflammatory disease of the joints. In addition, Corbett (1972) is of the opinion that under certain conditions massage used by itself may be very harmful psychologically. The rationale here is that "tense muscles are often the symptom of anxiety or depression and, while stroking away the evil humours is temporarily effective, the long-term effect is often to make the patients dependent on it or even addicted to it" (p. 137). In conclusion, massage is an effective tool when utilized properly.

Manipulation and Chiropractic Adjustment

In general, manipulation can be defined as a form of manual medicine in which passive movement is designed to restore ROM and decrease joint pain. (This term will be extensively reviewed in chapter 14). The use of manipulation dates back to antiquity. Numerous theories have been proposed to explain the relief from pain and decreased muscle tension following manipulation or chiropractic adjustment. Shambaugh (1987) found an average 25% reduction in muscle activity and muscle tension as a result of a chiropractic adjustment. Pain reduction via manipulation has been documented by several studies (Kokjohn et al. 1992; Terrett and Vernon 1984). In addition, research demonstrated that under very controlled and artificial conditions, manipulation performed on an experimental group of young males resulted in a small but statistically significant elevation in levels of plasma beta-endorphin (an opioidlike substance found in the brain and other tissues that produces, among other things, analgesia, or pain relief; Vernon et al. 1986). In contrast, Sanders and colleagues (1990) found a significant reduction in pain via manipulation but with no significant accompanying change in the plasma beta-endorphin concentration. An earlier investigation by Christian and co-workers (1988) also failed to identify any differences in endorphin levels following spinal manipulative therapy.

Currently, the mechanisms by which manipulation decreases muscle tension and pain to potentially assist those attempting to increase ROM is unknown. What is known is that with many patients manipulation has been demonstrated to be effective in improving muscular relaxation, which is an important component in stretching. In chapter 14, the direct implications of using manipulation as a means to enhance ROM will be reviewed.

Physiological Therapeutic Modalities

In the following sections, a variety of methods to facilitate or induce relaxation will be discussed, ranging from the simple to the complex and from the safe to the potentially dangerous. Regardless of the technique employed, increased knowledge will make the treatment more effective, efficient, and safe.

Heat

Probably one of the oldest and most common methods to achieve relief of pain and muscular tension is the use of heat. However, for our concerns, heat is important because it can facilitate relaxation either as an analgesic or as a sedative. The exact mechanisms and effects of heat in these two areas, however, are poorly understood.

Two natural questions arise: First, what method of heating is to be employed? Second, in what dosage should it be used? The advice of a physician, therapist, or athletic trainer will help answer these questions because they are a matter of clinical judgment.

Superficial Heat.   One of the most common methods of applying heat is the application of hot water, including the use of special bottles or wet packs. Agitated water baths, which stir heated water in a whirlpool or Jacuzzi-type de-

vice, may also be used. Because the temperature usually ranges from 40 to 43° C (104 to 110° F), caution must be used not to burn oneself, induce mild fever, or fall asleep while in the bath or tub. In most instances, however, a simple hot bath or shower should more than adequately fulfill one's needs. Research has demonstrated that hot water immersion does temporarily enhance range of motion (Sechrist and Stull 1969).

Electric heating pads offer another simple method of applying heat to a given area. The advantages of a heating pad are its different levels of intensity and its steadily maintained temperature. Because the temperature is maintained, however, one is more likely to be burned if not careful. Wrapping an electric heating pad around a wet hot pack must be avoided to prevent the danger of electric shock.

Deep Heat or Diathermy.   Another method to induce muscle relaxation and facilitate stretching is diathermy. For our purposes, *diathermy* is defined as deep heating (Jaskoviak and Schafer 1986; Lehmann and de Lateur 1990). Generally, three types of diathermic modalities are used for therapeutic purposes.

Shortwave diathermy works on the principle that energy is transferred into deep tissue layers by a high-frequency current. Such currents employ energy generated by means of electromagnetic radiation having frequencies greater than a million Hz (cycles per second). Another high-frequency current is *microwave*, which is also generated by means of electromagnetic radiation. Microwaves have a shorter wave length than shortwaves. The third type of diathermy is *ultrasound*. Ultrasound utilizes a high-frequency sound wave capable of penetrating into the deeper tissue layers. Here, too, high-frequency currents in the neighborhood of a million Hz are used to produce mechanical vibration of deep tissues. Research by Wessling, DeVane, and Hylton (1987) demonstrated that ultrasound combined with static stretch in the triceps surae (calf muscles) of human subjects significantly increased range of motion more than did static stretching alone.

No matter what form of diathermy is used, its immediate effect is purely physical: a rise in temperature in the heated tissue. The degree and extent of the treatment effect will vary in relation to the source of heating, its intensity, and the length of application (Lehmann and de Lateur 1990). Such heating can act as either a sedative or an irritant on sensory and motor nerves. The sedative action explains the relief given by diathermy, which is thought to somewhat lessen nerve sensitivity. Among other effects associated with diathermy are increased blood flow, an initial increase in tissue metabolism, a decrease in muscle spindle sensitivity to stretch, muscular relaxation, and tissue that yields more readily to stretch (Jaskoviak and Schafer 1986; Lehmann and de Lateur 1982).

Common sense indicates that diathermy is not a toy. Each modality must be prescribed by a physician, physical therapist, or athletic trainer who selects it for a precise purpose. Diathermy should be used intelligently, effectively, and safely only by a qualified and trained person.

Cold or Cryotherapy

Cryotherapy is the therapeutic use of cold. In recent years, it has become increasingly popular (Nielsen 1981; Travell and Simmons 1983). A complete text, *Cryotherapy in Sport Injury Management*, has been written on this subject by Knight (1995). The major advantages of cryotherapy are similar to heat in that it acts as an anesthetic and can effectively promote muscular relaxation. Cryotherapy should be used only when the therapeutic goal is to tear connective tissue (such as breaking adhesions) rather than to stretch it, when no other range of motion therapy can be attempted due to pain, or when muscle spasticity significantly interferes with the proper range of motion therapy (Sapega et al. 1981). Additional advantages of cold include decreasing swelling or effusion, decreasing inflammation, and increasing subsequent blood flow.

How does cold affect the nerves? F.A. Harris (1978, 105) provides the following explanation:

> The relaxing effect of deep cold may be based on the same phenomenon as relaxation obtained through slow stretch, with the difference that slow stretch physiologically desensitizes the stretch receptors, thereby lowering the background level of stretch afferent input, while deep cold (penetrating the muscle mass) produces "cold block" of the receptor excitatory process or of the afferent fibers themselves. The latter is a state resembling blockage of impulse conduction which can be achieved by applying a local anesthetic to the nerve fibers. Just as muscle can be reduced to a state of complete flaccidity by interrupting all dorsal root fibers carrying stretch afferent input to it, muscle tone can be diminished by cold block of conduction in the stretch afferent, which temporarily prevents impulse conduction while leaving the fibers themselves intact.

A study by Prentice (1982) found the use of cold followed by static stretching superior to heat combined with stretching in reducing delayed muscle pain. The use of cold spray for the relief of muscle spasm and pain to temporarily increase muscle length by mobilization has been documented (Harvey et al. 1983). Cold used to relieve pain is thought to send impulses to the spinal cord that compete with pain-producing impulses conveyed by much slower fibers. Thus, it has been argued that cold does not produce anesthesia, but rather counterirritation.

Since cryotherapy is relatively simple, an individual may treat oneself at home under a physician's, therapist's, or trainer's directions. One should be aware of the danger of freezing tissue, which can result in frostbite, but this phenomenon occurs only if ice is left directly and continuously on the body part. When ice is applied to a surface, the area goes through various stages of sensations: Initially there is a feeling of cold; subsequently there is a sensation of burning, stinging, or intense aching; and finally there is a partial loss of sensation and numbness.

Meridian Trigger Points

For thousands of years, forms of stimulation to specific sites on the skin have been utilized. Perhaps the most well-known and publicized technique is the Chinese system of acupuncture. Acupuncture is the science and art of passing thin needles through the skin to certain specific points (commonly referred to as meridians) for treating certain painful conditions, relieving various dysfunctions, and producing regional anesthesia (Jaskoviak and Schafer 1986). In the past 30 years, comprehensive studies of acupuncture have taken place and numerous theories have been proposed to explain its mode of operation. Currently, its exact mechanism of operation is still unknown. However, it has been suggested that meridian therapy with needles most likely works by "blocking pain signals in or to the brain by projecting inhibitory impulses to the thalamus and/or cerebral cortex and ultimately to the cord, and finally, by blocking noxious stimuli through the pathophysiological reflex and thus producing muscular relaxation" (Jaskoviak and Schafer 1986, 90). Meridian stimulation need not always be produced by needles. It is known to also work by using finger or thumb pressure (Shiatsu), a specially designed blunt instrument (teishin or a T-bar-like device used in massage therapy), and electrical stimulation modalities. Chiropractic management of trigger points was extensively studied by Nimmo (1958), who developed a technique termed *receptor tonus*. This technique is defined as a method of locating and dissipating neurofascial and tendinous points in the body, which are generative points of noxious nerve circuits that disrupt function and/or produce pain, referred or otherwise.

The most recent addition to the health care armamentarium is the laser. The word *laser* is an acronym for light amplification by stimulated emission of radiation. Since their development in the 1960s, there has been an ever-growing body of data supporting the effectiveness of lasers in a large number of fields. Various types of lasers have been demonstrated to enhance relaxation, reduce pain, and facilitate the healing of open lesions. "It works, but exactly how is one of the modern medical mysteries which is in the process of being systematically and scientifically unraveled" (Ohshiro 1991, 18).

Traction

Another mechanical technique to facilitate relaxation is traction. *Traction* uses a manual or mechanical distraction (separating) force on specific targets of the body. Traction is commonly employed to stretch tissues and separate joints. In addition, traction can facilitate relaxation and decrease pain due to muscle guarding—a muscle contracting to stabilize a joint—and spasm.

Cognitive Approaches

The cognitive approach utilizes mental or mind-controlling techniques. However, it should be recognized that many techniques employ a combination of both the cognitive and somatic approaches. Cognitive strategies include such procedures as meditation, sensory awareness techniques, autogenic training, and sentic cycles. A brief review of a number of these techniques is found in Hertling and Jones (1990). Below, two popular cognitive approaches will be discussed.

Progressive Deep Muscle Relaxation Training

Progressive deep muscle relaxation (PDMR) was developed by Edmund Jacobson (1929). Progressive relaxation seeks to relax the voluntary skeletal muscles by conscious control. The technique is practiced in a quiet setting and with a passive attitude. A muscle is contracted hard and then suddenly relaxed. As a result, the individual becomes aware of the contrast between the feeling of tension and the feeling of relaxation. Then the individual relaxes one muscle group at a time in a systematic order from foot to head or head to foot. Gradually, the entire body is relaxed progressively. With careful and dedicated practice, one can be taught to recognize the most minute contractions and learn to avoid them, thus achieving the deepest degree of relaxation possible (Jacobson 1938).

Later, PDMR was modified by Wolpe (1958) and by Bernstein and Borkovec (1973). The term *relaxation training* (RT) is commonly used interchangeably for PDMR. In some cases, relaxation training may represent an effective and viable adjunctive treatment for those individuals with psychophysiological ailments (Michelson 1987). In particular, PDMR may serve as an adjunct to standard pharmacological and psychiatric therapeutics (Fried 1987, 90). However, there has been some controversy regarding the specific action of relaxation training procedures for producing physiological effects (Borkovec and Sides 1979; King 1980; Lehrer and Woolfolk 1984). According to Michelson (1987), methodological issues account, in large part, for many of the equivocal findings. For thousands of years, various forms of PDMR have been employed by students of yoga.

The Relaxation Response

Almost 40 years after Jacobson's pioneering work, another development in the field of relaxation occurred. The *relaxation response* was discovered and publicized by Dr. Herbert Benson (1980) of the Harvard Medical School. Based on techniques that have been practiced for thousands of years by numerous cultures and cults, Benson identifies four basic components necessary to bring forth the relaxation response:

1. A *quiet environment*. Quiet will allow one to "turn off" both internal stimuli and external distractions and can be likened to a mental and emotional decompression chamber.
2. A *mental device*, or an object to dwell on. This should be a constant stimulus. It may involve word repetition (e.g., *relax* or *stretch*), gazing at an object (e.g., mentally reaching for one's toes); or concentrating on a particular feeling (e.g., imaging the muscles "oozing out" or feeling the connective tissue untwining).
3. A *passive attitude*. In the opinion of Benson,

this attitude "appears to be the most essential factor in eliciting the relaxation response" (p. 111) and is accomplished by emptying all thoughts and distractions from one's mind.

4. A *comfortable position*. The purpose of a comfortable posture is to eliminate any "undue muscular tension" (p. 161) and allow one to remain in the same position for an extended period of time.

Contraindications of Cognitive Approaches

Until rather recently, it was assumed that the clinical use of the relaxation response was a totally harmless therapeutic intervention. However, Everly (1989) points out that "recent data have argued contrary to that position." Therefore, those practitioners who incorporate various techniques to facilitate a relaxation response in conjunction with a stretching regimen need to be aware of potential undesirable side effects. Based on the research of Luthe (1969), Stroebel (1979), Emmons (1978), and Everly (1989), Everly and colleagues (1987) identified five major areas of concern in the elicitation of the relaxation response:

1. *Loss of reality contact.* This problem includes such manifestations as dissociative states, hallucinations, delusions, and perhaps paresthesia (abnormal skin sensations).

2. *Drug reactions.* The relaxation response may actually intensify the effects of some medications or other chemical substances that the patient may be taking. Particular caution should be implemented with patients taking insulin, sedatives or hypnotics, or cardiovascular medications.

3. *Panic states.* These psychological reactions are characterized by high levels of anxiety concerning the loss of control and by insecurity.

4. *Premature freeing of repressed ideation.* It is not uncommon for deeply repressed thoughts and emotions to be released in response to a deeply relaxed state. This response could create negative consequences if such reactions are unexpected or are too intense.

5. *Excessive trophotropic states.* In some instances, relaxation techniques may induce an excessively lowered state of psychophysiological functioning. Among the potential side effects are a temporary hypotensive state as a result of lowered blood pressure, a temporary hypoglycemic state (i.e., low blood sugar), and fatigue.

Biofeedback

Biofeedback is another technology that can be employed to promote relaxation and can serve as an adjunct to therapeutic exercise. Biofeedback is described by Basmajian (1981) as a technique that uses electronic equipment to reveal instantaneously to patients and therapists certain internal physiologic events by means of meters, banks of lights, and various auditing devices. Through this feedback, humans can be taught to manipulate voluntarily those otherwise unsensed events by concentrating on either increasing or decreasing the electronic signals that indicate the level of physiologic activity (Basmajian 1981). Several studies have demonstrated that through appropriate biofeedback techniques it is possible to control even individual motor units (Basmajian 1963, 1967, 1972; Basmajian, Baeza, and Fabrigar 1965; Simard and Basmajian 1967). Recently, Levin and Wolf (1987) demonstrated that biofeedback could be used to downtrain (reduce the amplitude of) the triceps surae spinal stretch reflex (SSR) of stroke patients who displayed increased tone in ankle extensor muscles. In brief, the proponents of biofeedback believe that by recognizing a biological function, you can gain control of that function.

In the arena of athletics and other athletic disciplines (e.g., dance and the martial arts), biofeedback has been suggested as a means that can supposedly facilitate stretching and the development of flexibility. In an early study, Wilson and Bird (1981) found a significant improvement in hip flexion was produced in male gymnasts in both the biofeedback and relaxation groups, with the biofeedback group improving more quickly across trials. For the female gymnasts a significant improvement in hip flexion was noted for the control group, the relaxation group, and the relaxation plus biofeedback group. In a later investigation by Cummings, Wilson, and Bird (1984), it was determined that relaxation or biofeedback training had beneficial effects upon flexibility development of sprinters only in the retention period. Due to the paucity of research, additional studies are still needed to determine the effectiveness of biofeedback as a means to facilitate the development of flexibility.

Medications

Medications offer another potential avenue to reduce tension and facilitate relaxation. We are constantly inundated by an avalanche of advertisements from the pharmacological industry proselytizing and instilling the belief that many problems can be eliminated simply by the use of a specific medication. These supposed "magic bullets" also are a two-edged sword with numerous potential risks. It behooves today's health-conscious public and medical practitioners to employ greater discretion in the dispensing and application of popular, over-the-counter medications. Failure to do so conveys a dangerous message and exacerbates a major drug problem facing the world.

Analgesics and Counterirritant Balms and Liniments

Analgesics and counterirritants are among the most extensively used aids for the treatment of athletic or everyday muscular aches and sores due to overexertion. The most common ingredients are oil of wintergreen (methyl salicylate), peppermint (menthol), red pepper, and camphor. When applied to the skin, they create a mild irritant that counters or masks the sense of pain. Besides creating a slight degree of local anesthesia, they also cause the muscle fibers surrounding the blood vessels to relax and consequently cause the blood vessels to dilate. In turn, the increased circulation helps promote the absorption of inflammatory products and brings more blood and nutrients to the applied area.

Muscle-Relaxant Drugs

Muscle relaxants fall into two categories: *nonprescription*, or over-the-counter, and *prescription* drugs. The precise mechanism of many of these drugs is not fully understood. In many drugs, the therapeutic action may be related to analgesic or sedative properties. Those drugs are understood either to block nerve impulses to skeletal muscles at the neuromuscular junction or to act as general CNS depressants. In many instances, these drugs are indicated as an adjunct to rest, physical therapy, and other measures for the relief of discomfort associated with acutely painful musculoskeletal conditions. There are a number of potentially negative side effects associated with some of these drugs, including depression, allergies, dizziness, headaches, irritability, lightheadedness, nausea, cardiorespiratory depression, coma, and death. In addition, pregnant women or nursing mothers should be especially aware of potential risks. As a rule, prescription drugs should be taken only as a last resort and must be used carefully, following all recommended directions. Medication should be taken in as limited doses as necessary and discontinued as soon as possible.

Summary

Theoretically, relaxation, or the absence of muscular tension, should exist before stretching is begun. Reduced internal tension can aid in effectively and efficiently stretching out muscle and connective tissues, which substantially limit extensibility. Muscular relaxation can be induced or facilitated by the somatic, or physical, approach; physiological therapeutic modalities; cognitive, mental, and mind-controlling techniques; sophisticated instrumentation, such as biofeedback; and the use of drugs and medications. Consideration must be given to the decision of which is the safest, most effective, and most efficient means to achieve the desired goal.

Chapter 9

Muscular Soreness: Etiology and Consequences

Exercise and stretching may result in varying degrees of discomfort, soreness, stiffness, or pain of two general kinds: that which occurs during and immediately after the exercise or stretching and which may persist for several hours and that which usually does not appear until 24 to 48 hours later. First we will examine these two general kinds of pain. Then we will briefly examine the inflammation and remodeling response to injuries.

There are five basic hypotheses that attempt to explain the nature of muscular soreness:

1. The damaged or torn muscle hypothesis
2. The damaged connective tissue hypothesis
3. The hypothesis of metabolic accumulation or osmotic pressure and swelling
4. The lactic acid hypothesis
5. The hypothesis of localized spasm of motor units

Although these possible causes will be reviewed separately, this does not mean that they cannot occur together or that there are no other possible causes for muscular soreness.

The Damaged or Torn Muscle Hypothesis

Hough (1902) first suggested that muscular soreness had its origin in some sort of rupture within the muscle itself, in other words, that it was a direct result of muscle injury from microscopic tearing of muscle fibers. However, de Vries (1961a, 1961b, 1962, 1966) was originally of the opinion that such injury probably occurs much less frequently than is thought by athletes, coaches, and laypeople. He argued that this hypothesis is not a plausible explanation for muscle soreness because "it is somewhat illogical to postulate that a tissue has been structurally damaged by the very function for which it is specifically differentiated" (de Vries 1966, 119). Nonetheless, de Vries reminds us that some types of activity are more likely to result in sore muscles than others, including the following:

- Vigorous contractions while the muscle is in a shortened position.
- Muscle contractions involving jerky or uncoordinated movements. In this case, some fibers in the muscle may be temporarily overloaded when a full load is placed on the muscle before a sufficient number of motor units have been recruited.
- Activity involving repetition of the same movement over a long period of time.
- Bouncing movements, because at the end of a ballistic motion, the movement is stopped by the muscle and its connective tissues, bringing about reflex contractions at the same time the muscle is being forcefully elongated.

However, since the writings of de Vries there have been substantial improvements in technology to substantiate this hypothesis as one of the most probable causes of delayed muscle soreness

(DMS). In particular, during the past 25 years numerous photographs have been taken which clearly show damage to the internal structure of the sarcomere following exercise (Figure 9.1). These published photographs (R.B. Armstrong, Ogilvie, and Schwane 1983; Fridén 1984a, 1984b; Fridén and Lieber 1992; Fridén, Seger, and Ekblom 1988; Fridén, Seger, Sjöström, and Ekblom 1983; Kuipers et al. 1983; Newham, McPhail, Mills, and Edwards 1983; Newham, Mills, Quigley, and Edwards 1982, 1983; Waterman-Storer 1991) clearly show mechanical disruptions of the Z-lines, referred to as *Z-disk streaming*. Their findings indicated that during overloading the Z-lines constitute a potential weak link in the myofibrillar contractile chain (Figure 9.2, a and b).

The damaged or torn muscle hypothesis also comprises such events as damage to the sarcoplasmic reticulum (Byrd 1992; McCutcheon, Byrd, and Hodgson 1992; Newham, Mills, Quigley, and Edwards 1983; Nimmo and Snow 1982) and to

the T-tubule system (Stauber 1989). See chapter 3 for discussion of these structures. Both of these disruptions also interfere with normal calcium metabolism in muscle cells.

Another avenue to verify the damaged or torn muscle theory has been the use of biochemical testing. Abraham (1977, 1979) investigated the relationship between DMS and urinary excretion of myoglobin. Myoglobin is thought to be released from the muscle into the vascular system during muscle injury and thus is indicative of muscle fiber trauma. Abraham's findings were inconclusive. The enzyme creatine kinase (CK) is another potential indicator of muscle damage. Research (Byrnes et al. 1985) has demonstrated that an increased concentration of CK is found after exercise, thus potentially substantiating the theory. However, while CK may be related to soreness, it cannot actually cause DMS because there is a mismatch between the time-courses of the muscle damage, the pain, and the peak enzyme efflux, which is delayed relative to the pain

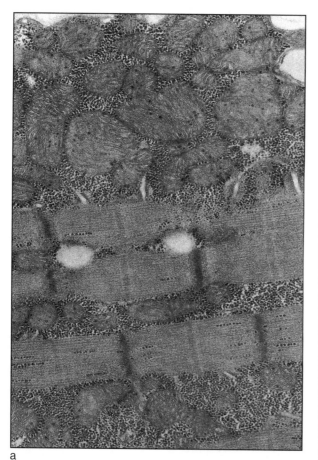

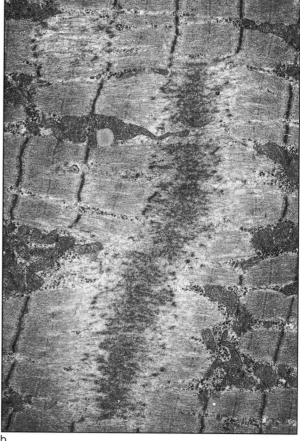

a   b

Fig. 9.1. (a) An electron micrograph showing normal arrangement of the actin and myosin filaments and Z-disk configuration in the muscle of a runner before a marathon. (b) A muscle sample taken immediately after a marathon race shows a damaged sarcomere.
Reprinted from Wilmore and Costill (1994).

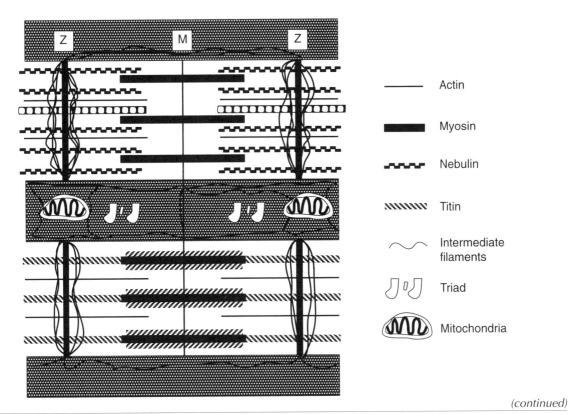

(continued)

Fig. 9.2. (a) A highly schematized representation of the proposed arrangement of cytoskeletal elements in and around the sarcomere. Both sarcomeres show the arrangement of intermediate filaments, composed mainly of the protein desmin, linking neighboring myofibrils both transversely and longitudinally at the Z-line and encircling the Z-line with a doublet structure. The upper sarcomere shows the arrangement of nebulin, running parallel to actin within the I-band. The lower sarcomere depicts titin's proposed location, stretching the full length of the half sarcomere and attaching to myosin within the A-band.

(Cleak and Eston 1992; D.A. Jones, Newham, Obletter, and Giamberardino 1987). That is, peak CK concentrations occurred as the soreness was resolving (Newham 1988).

The Damaged Connective Tissue Hypothesis

In addition to damage to muscle contractile tissue, there is also potential damage to the connective tissues associated with the muscle. Selective damage to the series elastic component (SEC; composed of the epimysium, perimysium, endomysium, fascia, and tendons) is also widely supported. Research by Abraham (1977, 1979) supports the theory that DMS is most closely linked to irritation of the muscle's connective tissue. His investigations revealed a significant positive correlation between urinary excretion of hydroxyproline (OHP) and subjective incidence of

muscle soreness. OHP is a marker of a breakdown product of connective tissue and is an indicator of collagen metabolism. Tullson and Armstrong (1968, 1981) also provide additional support for the relationship between muscle soreness and connective tissue irritation or damage. This theory is based on the finding that the connective tissues are damaged to a greater extent following eccentric contraction due to a greater passive tension on them (Sutton 1984).

The Hypothesis of Metabolic Accumulation or Osmotic Pressure and Swelling

Other explanations for delayed muscle soreness emphasize the accumulation of muscle metabolic by-products, including lactic acid (a by-product of anaerobic metabolism), extracellular potas-

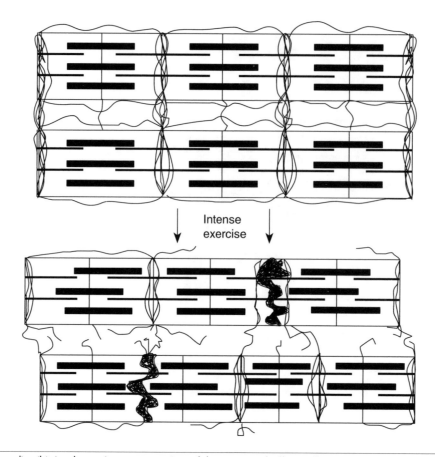

Intense
exercise

Fig. 9.2. (continued) (b) A schematic representation of the proposed effects of intense exercise on the exosarcomeric intermediate-filament system. (above) Before exercise, intermediate filaments run between contiguous myofibrils, linking them at the Z-lines and M-lines, keeping axial register. (below) Following intense exercise, many intermyofibrillar connections are broken, and the Z-lines lose their transverse register. Some Z-lines completely dissipate, their doublet intermediate-filament structure splits, and they give rise to new sarcomeres. Often myosin loses its centralized location within the sarcomere.
Reprinted from Waterman-Storer (1991).

sium, and an excess of other metabolites that causes an increased osmotic pressure inside and outside muscle fibers, leading to retained excess water that causes edema and pressure on sensory nerves (Asmussen 1956; Bobbert, Hollander, and Huijing 1986; Brendstrup 1962; Committee on the Medical Aspects of Sports 1975; Karpovich and Sinning 1971). Yet another theory of soreness is that the swelling of the muscle causes it to become shorter, thicker, and more resistant to stretching (Howell et al. 1985; D.A. Jones, Newham, and Clarkson 1987). This swelling gives rise to a sensation of stiffness when the muscle is stretched during the contraction of the antagonistic muscles (Morehouse and Miller 1971).

Stauber (1989) has suggested that the discomfort and swelling associated with DMS resembles a mini–compartment syndrome and that the ex-

tracellular space may be a major contributing factor. Studies by Fridén, Sfakianos, and Hargens (1986); Fridén, Sfakianos, Hargens, and Akeson (1988); and Wallensten and Eklund (1983) found that tissue fluid pressure was elevated in muscles exercised eccentrically (in which the muscle elongates as it contracts). Howell et al. (1985, 1718) have proposed an analogy comparing the muscle with a water balloon stuffed inside a nylon stocking. "The presence of the balloon would prevent the nylon stocking from being stretched to its full length. Similarly, water of edema within the three-dimensional matrix of the endomysium, perimysium, and epimysium would limit their extension." It is the increased volume of fluid that produces passive tension effects throughout the stocking. Associated with this tension are feelings of pain, swelling, and stiffness. Howell et al. (1985, 1718) have suggested that slow extension occurring beyond the initial stiffness barrier may "represent squeezing of water out of the perimuscular connective tissue matrix into interfascial planes."

However, there are several problems with these explanations. Muscle soreness is usually greater after exercise consisting of eccentric work (in which muscle elongates as it contracts) as opposed to concentric work (in which muscle shortens as it contracts). Research has consistently found that eccentric contractions are less demanding in their energy requirements or oxygen consumption than concentric contractions (R.B. Armstrong 1984; R.B. Armstrong, Warren, and Warren 1991; Bigland-Ritchie and Woods 1976; Davies and Barnes 1972; Dick and Cavanagh 1987; Knuttgen, Patton, and Vogel 1982; Newham, Mills, Quigley, and Edwards 1983). In addition, several studies (Asmussen 1953; Seliger, Dolejs, and Karas 1980) have substantiated a higher electromyographic (EMG) activity for concentric work of a given resistance load than for eccentric contractions. Last, regarding the idea that increased intramuscular pressure is the cause of pain, D.A. Jones, Newham, Obletter, and Giamberardino (1987) are of the opinion that it is unlikely. Their evidence refuting this viewpoint is that during isometric contractions the intramuscular pressure can rise to several hundred mmHg (A.V. Hill 1948). However, this pressure is not perceived as painful in the same way as muscle tenderness is. Furthermore, even in already tender muscle, isometric contractions do not aggravate the pain. Nonetheless, stretching and cool-down after exercise is strongly encouraged to allow the muscles time to promote the removal of accumulated waste products.

The Lactic Acid Hypothesis

One of the oldest and most popular explanations of immediate and delayed muscle soreness is the accumulation of waste products, especially lactic acid. Lactic acid is a by-product of metabolism and can only form in the absence of oxygen. Therefore, lactic acid accumulates when there is an insufficient blood supply to the muscles. Consequently, lactic acid must not be a factor in pain following passive exercise and most static stretching programs.

The Hypothesis of Localized Spasm of Motor Units

As postulated in numerous works by de Vries (1961a, 1961b, 1962, 1966), the delayed localized soreness that occurs after unaccustomed exercise is caused by tonic, localized spasm of motor units whose number varies with the severity of pain:

1. Exercise beyond a minimal level causes some degree of ischemia (i.e., temporary lack of blood supply) in active muscle.
2. Ischemia causes muscle pain. This pain probably occurs by means of the transfer of P-substance (some particular pain substance) across the muscle cell membrane into the tissue fluid, from which location it gains access to pain endings.
3. The resulting pain consequently brings about a protective, reflexive, tonic muscle contraction.
4. The tonic contraction then brings about localized areas of ischemia in the muscle tissue, and a vicious cycle begins, which results in a local, tonic muscle spasm.

Using specially developed EMG equipment, muscular pain has been demonstrated quantitatively by de Vries. That is, using EMG, he found a positive relationship between the severity of exercise-induced pain and the level of muscular electrical activity. More importantly, de Vries found that static stretching furnished symptomatic relief and also caused a significant decrease in the electrical activity of the hurting muscles. Thus, de Vries contends that we may assume some degree of control over the prevention and relief of soreness.

However, when Abraham (1977) attempted to duplicate the EMG experiment of de Vries, he was unable to find significant EMG changes as a result of induced muscle soreness. Similarly, Talag (1973), Torgan (1985), and Newham, Mills, Quigley, and Edwards (1983) were unable to substantiate the findings of de Vries. This discrepancy was probably related to the choice of recording electrodes (de Vries 1986; Francis 1983). However, research by Bobbert, Hollander, and Huijing (1986) has also been unable to find evidence in support of de Vries. Furthermore, recent data raise doubts about the presence of increased EMG activity in relaxed sore muscles (Lund et al. 1991).

This negative opinion is also held by Francis (1983) and Jones, Newham, Obletter, and Giamberardino (1987). Additional research is needed to resolve these discrepancies.

Predisposing Factors of Delayed Muscle Soreness

The etiology of DMS is unknown. However, numerous factors have been proposed. Among them are eccentric contractions, state of training, and insufficient warm-up.

Eccentric Contractions

One explanation of the cause of DMS might relate to the nature of the tension that develops in the tissues during elongation or stretching. When a muscle contracts *concentrically*, the muscle fibers shorten actively and *positive* work is performed. As the muscle continually shortens, its tension output decreases. To maintain tension production, a greater number of fibers are compelled to take part in the contraction, so the pull exerted by each individual muscle fiber on its connective tissue is reduced. The workload is thus shared by a greater mass of muscle cells, and each is spared excessive stress and tension so that the tissues escape injury.

During elongation of a muscle, individual muscle fibers are capable of contracting. This lengthening contraction is called an *eccentric* contraction and produces *negative* work. As in concentric contractions, eccentric contractions produce active tension that is transmitted via connective tissues. The degree of muscle excitation is known to be related to the number and discharge frequency of active motor units. An active motor unit consists of one motoneuron and the muscle cells supplied by its axon branches. A review of the literature by Dean (1988, 233) found that EMG activity has been "reported to be reduced in eccentric muscle contraction compared with concentric muscle contraction at comparable force and speed of contraction. This finding suggests that fewer motor units may be recruited in an eccentric contraction compared with a concentric contraction." However, the potential recruitment pattern on EMG patterns during negative work has not been well established (Aura and Komi 1986).

The reason for the decreasing number of active motor units is that connective tissue passive tension, which increases with length, compensates for the decline in active tension, resulting in increased elastic tension. In addition, Faulkner, Brooks, and Opiteck (1993) suggest that lengthening contraction also reflects an increased strain on individual cross-bridges. "The tension per active unit will consequently be greater in negative work than in positive, and so the chances of strain or damage to parts [i.e., connective tissue and contractile components] of the muscles" (Asmussen 1956, 113). Initially, it was suggested that the structural disturbances may also be secondary, resulting from an activation of lysosomal enzymes, bringing about a concomitant inflammation (Fridén, Sjöström, and Ekblom 1981). However, the assumption that the inflammatory process is secondary to myofibrillar damage has not been supported by other research (R.B. Armstrong, Ogilvie, and Schwane 1983; Fridén, Sjöström, and Ekblom 1983).

State of Training

A popular theory is that the degree of muscular pain, soreness, or stiffness corresponds to the state of training of the tissues involved. That is, people with unexercised and tight muscles usually show a markedly higher reaction when subjected to a variety of physical stresses. Consequently, fibers and connective tissues are more susceptible to strain and rupture. Thus, it can be claimed that "stiffness is a disease of the unfit" (J.C.P. Williams and Sperryn 1976, 301).

In recent years, a number of studies of the attempt to reduce or eliminate DMS by training have been performed. Cleak and Eston (1992) identified several studies that documented the alleviation of the soreness response, along with reduced morphological changes, enhanced performance, and decreased CK concentration in the blood (Byrnes and Clarkson 1986; Byrnes et al. 1985; Clarkson et al. 1987; Clarkson and Tremblay 1988; Fridén, Seger, Sjöström, and Ekblom 1983; D.A. Jones and Newham 1985; Knuttgen 1986; Komi and Buskirk 1972; Miller, Wilcox, and Schwenkel 1988; Schwane and Armstrong 1983; Schwane, Williams, and Sloan 1987). The protective effects of training are suggested to last from up to 6 weeks (Byrnes et al. 1985) to up to 10 weeks (D.A. Jones and Newham 1985). Studies show that the required length of training may vary from many weeks (Fridén, Seger, Sjöström, and Ekblom 1983; Komi and Buskirk 1972) down to a single intense exercise bout (R.B. Armstrong, Ogilvie, and Schwane 1983; Byrnes et al. 1985; Clarkson et al. 1987; Clarkson and Tremblay 1988; Ebbeling and Clarkson 1989).

Insufficient Warm-Up

Yet another explanation of the cause of DMS is the long-held opinion popular among coaches and athletes that muscle soreness results from failing to warm up before exercising or stretching. According to Mellerowicz and Hansen (1971), poor blood circulation and cold muscles and tendons have a greater tendency to result in strains and ruptures than do properly warmed-up ones. Currently, there is very little experimental evidence with human subjects to support this theory, probably because no researcher cares to set up an experiment in which the subjects may be injured (de Vries 1966). Nonetheless, everything that is known of muscle physiology tends to support the need for warm-up as a prudent protective measure. Warming up is discussed at greater length in chapter 10.

Trauma and Overload Injury to the Musculature and Connective Tissues

All tissues have mechanical limits beyond which intrinsic damage can occur. The cause of the insult to the body can vary, but its consequences can be significant in terms of joint dysfunction. In general, musculoskeletal *trauma* falls into two major categories: chronic, or overload, injuries and acute, or sudden, tear and blow injuries. An *overload* injury occurs when a muscle is forced to perform work of an unaccustomed intensity or duration. The resulting histological picture within the muscle tissue resembles that of a necrotic inflammation, with disruption and swelling of muscle fibers and infiltration of the extracellular space by inflammatory cells such as white blood cells (Round, Jones, and Cambridge 1987). In contrast, a *tear* or *blow* injury is a result of strong mechanical forces acting briefly on muscle tissues, disrupting blood vessels and muscle fibers. When a tissue is stretched beyond certain limits, the injury is known as a *sprain* for ligamentous and capsular tissues, or a *strain* for muscle and tendon tissue. Sprains and strains may vary in

degree from mild to severe. In mild cases, there may be only a little hemorrhage with disruption of a few fibers and a mild inflammatory reaction. In contrast, in severe instances, there can be considerable intramuscular hemorrhage, with partial or complete tear of the muscle and its connective tissue. In either case, the response to injury follows an orderly and well-defined but overlapping sequence of events: injury, inflammation, repair, and remodeling. In the following sections, the inflammatory responses and consequences will be reviewed.

The Inflammatory Response

The initial biologic response to virtually all injuries is inflammation. *Inflammation* is a vascular and cellular response that serves to promote the recovery of damaged tissues. The extent of tissue damage depends on the amount of force applied to the fibers involved. In turn, the degree of inflammation is proportional to the amount or degree of damage. The inflammatory reaction is a dynamic and continuous succession of well-coordinated events. These events are complicated but predictable. The gross features associated with inflammation were described some 2000 years ago by five cardinal signs. These signs are *rubor* (redness), *tumor* (swelling), *calor* (heat), *dolar* (pain), and *functio laesa* (altered or loss of function). The most severe sequence ultimately can result in a self-perpetuating pain cycle. According to Rubin and Farber (1994, 34), inflammation can be thought to proceed as follows:

- *Initiation* of the mechanisms responsible for the localization and clearance of foreign substances and injured tissues is stimulated by the recognition that injury to tissues has occurred.
- *Amplification* of the inflammatory response, in which both soluble mediators and cellular inflammatory systems are activated, follows recognition of injury.
- *Termination* of the inflammatory response, after generation of inflammatory agents and elimination of the foreign agent, is accomplished by specific inhibitors of the mediators.

The initial stages of inflammation are characterized by vascular changes. Immediately following injury, a temporary constriction of the local vasculature occurs lasting 5 to 10 minutes. The vasoconstriction is followed by active vasodilation of all local small vessels and by increased blood flow.

Tissue damage triggers several mechanisms that result in an increase in the tissue concentration of endogenous (produced within an organism) biologically active substances, including vasodilators. Among the more potent vasodilators are histamine, kinins, and particularly prostaglandin-E and prostacyclin. Initially, histamine was considered to be the primary mediator of the inflammatory vascular response. This substance is released from mast cells, granulocytes, and platelets. It produces local vasodilation and increases the small vessel permeability. However, histamine acts for short periods (less than 30 minutes) because local sources are depleted rapidly. At the same time, 5-hydroxytryptamine (5-HT), which has a local action similar to that of histamine, is released from the platelets. The increased blood vessel permeability facilitates the removal of cellular debris and injured tissue fragments, an essential part of the injury-healing stage. It also allows the passage of plasma proteins into the affected tissues. The plasma proteins may become an important asset to the defense of the tissues. In addition, the blood may also contain a number of antimicrobial substances and nutrients vital to the repair of damaged cells. Next, the kinins, a series of biologically active peptides, and the prostaglandins (principally PGE1 and PGE2) are released by torn vessels. They facilitate the liberation of bradykinin (BKN). The prostaglandins seem to be the final mediators of acute inflammation, including the reversible, small vessel permeability (Madden and Arem 1986).

It is during this time that tissues exhibit the symptoms of warmth, redness, swelling, pain, and loss of function. The increased blood flow to the region causes the warmth and redness. Swelling is a result of the outpouring of fluid into the tissue. Pain may be produced by various noxious stimuli, including chemical, mechanical, and thermal agents. Accordingly, the body has four major classes of pain receptors: *chemoreceptors*, which respond to chemical stimuli; *mechanoreceptors*, which respond to mechanical stimuli; *thermoreceptors*, which respond to changes in temperature; and *polymodal receptors*, which respond to several or all types of stimuli.

Postinflammation Repair and Remodeling

The next major pathological phases after inflammation are the *repair* and *remodeling* phases. Repair is associated with proliferation of capillaries and fibroblasts (cells that synthesize collagen fibers). Hence, this repair phase is known as *fibroplasia*. The exact mechanisms by which the fibroblasts begin synthesizing scar tissue, primarily collagen and protein polysaccharides, are still debated. During this time the new collagen fibers are randomly oriented and highly soluble; thus, the union established is fragile. During the remodeling and maturation phase, collagen synthesis continues along with a reorientation of the collagen fibrils in the direction of loading and the formation of normal cross-links between fibrils. Thus, microscopically, the weave or architecture of the collagen fibers changes to a more organized pattern. If the damage is relatively severe, there may be considerable scarring. The extent to which a scar remodels varies among individuals and also within the same individual depending on age at the time of injury. Ultimately, the strength and plastic characteristics of scar tissue depend on the formation and density of intermolecular covalent bonds and on the orientation and weave of the individual collagen fibers.

Although scarring represents the lesser evil compared with having an open or unhealed injury, it also presents potential problems, which are most evident when scarring is extensive, as with a severe strain or rupture. Muscle regains strength slowly, and the rate for tendon injuries is even slower due to poorer blood supply. In spite of strength gains, some injuries rarely, if ever, regain their full strength. Strength is not the only important physical parameter affected by scars. Normal elasticity, so important in tissue function, is lost by scar tissue, which often converts an elastic, pliable tissue to an inelastic, brittle mass. As Arnheim (1989) points out, scarring can produce more serious consequences for some people, especially athletes (who often return to practice and competition before healing), because strains have a tendency to recur due to the already brittle nature of scar tissue. The higher the incidence of strains at a particular muscle site, the greater the amount of scar tissue that is present and the greater the potential for recurrent injuries. Worse yet, the fear of another "pull" may become for some individuals an almost neurotic obsession more handicapping than the injury itself.

Medical Management of Acute Soft Tissue Injuries

The three phases of medical management coincide with the three phases of micropathological change. Oakes (1981) and Van der Meulin (1982) have classified the pathological process into three phases, which are similar to one another apart from minor differences in terminology (see Table 9.1).

Treatment During the Acute Inflammatory Phase

This phase may last up to 72 hours depending on the severity of the injury. The primary objective at this phase is to minimize the hemorrhaging and swelling. Accordingly, the principles of management of acute soft tissue injuries have been embodied in the well-known acronym *RICE*.

R = Rest of the injured soft tissues

I = Ice application for 20 to 30 minutes at hourly intervals for 4 hours postinjury

C = Compression and bandaging, which is continuously applied for at least 48 hours

E = Elevation to enhance venous return (see Figures 9.3 and 9.4)

During this stage, Oakes (1981) emphasizes two important don'ts. First, don't apply heat for at least 48 to 72 hours. This is because heat increases bleeding and thus increases edema formation. Therefore, muscle stimulators, ultrasound, and similar modalities should not be used in the acute phase. Second, don't drink alcohol since it is a potent vasodilator. In addition to these cautions, Oakes (1981) and Kellett (1986) warn that the use of exogenous steroids may delay collagen repair and should be avoided.

Treatment During the Repair Phase

The repair phase may last from 48 hours up to 6 weeks. In the opinion of Oakes (1981), this phase is the most difficult to manage because it requires a balance between setting optimal conditions for collagenous, injured muscle, and ligamentous

repair and satisfying the needs of athletes, coaches, and management for a rapid return to competition. In particular, it is necessary to encourage and facilitate injury repair through local mobility while at the same time maintaining cardiovascular fitness through body movement. Special care must be employed to make sure that the athlete does not return prematurely to competition. Otherwise, the participant may retear the muscle or ligament, and a vicious cycle is repeated.

Treatment During the Remodeling Phase

This phase may last from 3 weeks to a year or more. It is during this phase that collagen is remodeled to increase functional capabilities so that it can withstand the stresses imposed on it. The distinction between repair and remodeling is largely that the *quantity* of collagen is increased during the repair phase and that an improvement in the *quality* (orientation and tensile strength) of collagen takes place in the remodeling phase. Such a clear-cut distinction is, however, quite artificial, as there is a merging of the two phases to a large degree.

Effects of Mechanical Stress on Elasticity and Strength of Collagen in Scar Tissue

Can applying a tensile force affect the remodeling of damaged (scar) tissue so as to enhance the optimal regaining of elasticity and strength? The answer is *yes:* Stress and motion have been demonstrated to stimulate a more functional alignment of collagen fibers, to maximize healing by the development of the correct type of connective tissue, and to minimize the development of

Table 9.1. Phases of Soft Tissue Injury

	Oakes (1981)	Van der Meulin (1982)
Phase 1	Acute inflammatory phase	Reaction phase
Phase 2	Repair phase	Regeneration phase
Phase 3	Remodeling phase	Remodeling phase

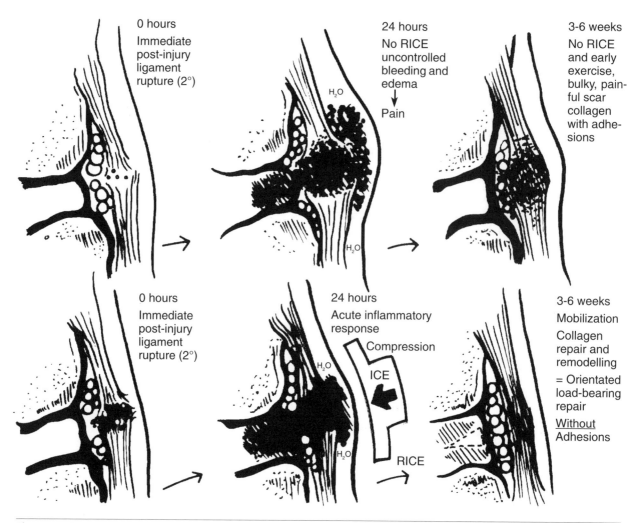

Fig. 9.3. Diagrammatic representation of ligament injury without RICE and antiprostaglandin or early mobilization and with RICE, antiprostaglandin, and early mobilization.
Reprinted from Oakes (1981).

scar tissue adhesions (Cummings and Tillman 1992). Current theory suggests that exercise or therapeutic stress can decrease the number of collagen cross-links by increasing the collagen turnover rate (Shephard 1982). Recall from chapter 4 that the strength of collagen (and so of scar tissue) appears to be in part the result of the intramolecular cross-linking between the $alpha_1$ and $alpha_2$ chains of the collagen molecule and of the intermolecular cross-linking between the collagen fibrils, filaments, and fibers. Bryant (1977) speculates that modifications of adhesions and scars are probably related to the development or dissolution of cross-links between collagen units. This process is called *collagen turnover*, continuous and simultaneous collagen production and breakdown. If the rate of breakdown exceeds production, the scar becomes softer and less bulky. If, on the other hand, the rate of production exceeds breakdown, the opposite effect oc-

curs. (The collagen in debilitating adhesions and scars is thought to be shorter and more compactly organized.) Thus, if exercise can in fact decrease the number of collagen cross-links by increasing the collagen turnover rate, stretching could possibly determine the ultimate degree of extensibility, elasticity, and strength of the remodeled tissues.

According to Cummings and Tillman (1992, 47), "time must be given for connective tissue to remodel in proportion with the increased demands of the new situation." The effect of stress on strength of new scar tissue is a function of the intensity and duration of stress applied. If excessive stress is applied to newly formed and weak tissue, the scar is pulled apart and weakened.

In particular, stretching scar tissue can be dangerous because it might tear not only the remodeling connective tissue, but also the vascular bed, resulting in more bleeding. Consequently, inflam-

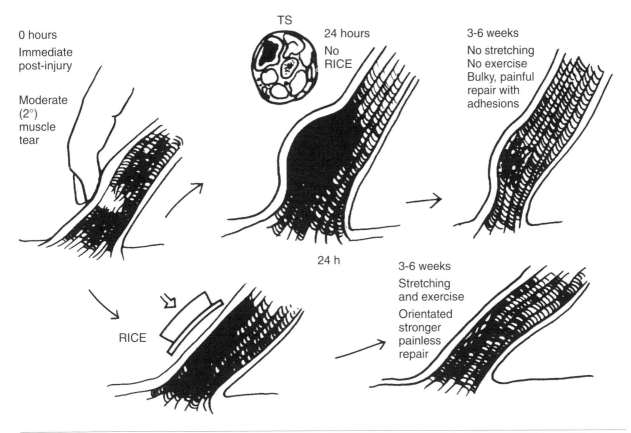

Fig. 9.4. Diagrammatic representation of muscle pathology following a tear, with and without RICE and stretching. Reprinted from Oakes (1981).

mation will increase, and rehabilitation will be prolonged. Furthermore, inflammation may result in pain and muscle spasms, thus limiting range of motion (Burkhardt 1982). It must be remembered at such times that the new collagen has not yet matured with increased quantity, cross-linkages, and fiber diameter and is thus susceptible to new injury (Booth and Gould 1975; Ciullo and Zarins 1983). Thus, Tillman and Cummings (1992, 29) caution:

> For the therapist who is physically stressing scar to bring about remodeling, it is important to visualize the highly cellular, fragile structure of new scar. Use of stress to "stretch" scar tissue at this stage will cause elongation of the scar by one of only two mechanisms: disruption of cell membranes and cell death, in response to high or sudden loads, or cell migration, in response to gentle and prolonged loads.

Summary

Two types of muscle soreness sometimes develop after exercise: immediate soreness and delayed localized soreness, which does not appear until 24 to 48 hours after activity. Currently, muscular soreness is explained by at least five possible mechanisms that may work together or independently of one another: the damaged or torn muscle hypothesis, the damaged connective tissue hypothesis, the hypothesis of metabolic accumulation or osmotic pressure and swelling, the lactic acid hypothesis, and the hypothesis of localized spasm of motor units. Regardless of the causes, everything that is known of muscle physiology tends to support the need for warm-up, cool-down, and stretching as prudent preventive measures.

Chapter 10

Special Factors in Flexibility

Besides those already discussed, there are a number of additional factors that can affect one's potential degree of flexibility and suppleness. A few of these factors are age, gender, body build, laterality (handedness), training, and circadian rhythms, all of which are discussed in this chapter.

Children and Flexibility Development

Conflicting data exist concerning the relationship between age and flexibility, especially the increase or decrease of flexibility during the growing years. The complexity is compounded because studies often focus on specific joints or on specific populations involved in various athletic disciplines. In addition, lack of standardized testing procedures makes it difficult to compare the various studies. Consequently, the literature must be read carefully and in total. Generally, the research seems to indicate that small children are quite supple and that during the school years flexibility decreases until about puberty, then increases throughout adolescence. After adolescence, however, flexibility tends to level off and then begins to decrease. Although flexibility decreases with age, the loss appears to be minimized in those individuals who remain active.

Flexibility Changes in Young Children

Gurewitsch and O'Neill (1944) carried out one of the earliest studies and found gradual declines in flexibility from ages 6 to 12 and then increases through age 18. Kendall and Kendall (1948) administered two flexibility tests to some 4,500 children from kindergarten to 12th grade. The tests were toe touching and touching the forehead to the knees in a long-sitting position. They found that at age 5, 98% of the boys and 86% of the girls could perform the toe-touch test. Beginning at age 6, there was a sharp decline in these percentages, so that by age 12 only 30% of both sexes could perform this test. After about age 13, the percentage who were successful gradually increased each year through age 17. At age 5, only 15% of the girls and 5% of the boys could touch their foreheads to their knees. This percentage did not change appreciably in either group through age 17 (see Figure 10.1, a and b).

Hupprich and Sigerseth (1950) investigated a group of girls 9 to 15 years of age and reported no significant differences among them in six different flexibility test items. However, it did appear that there was a trend toward decreasing shoulder, knee, and hip flexion from ages 12 through 15. Leighton (1956) measured the flexibility characteristics of boys 10 to 18 years of age. He reported decreases in flexibility during ado-

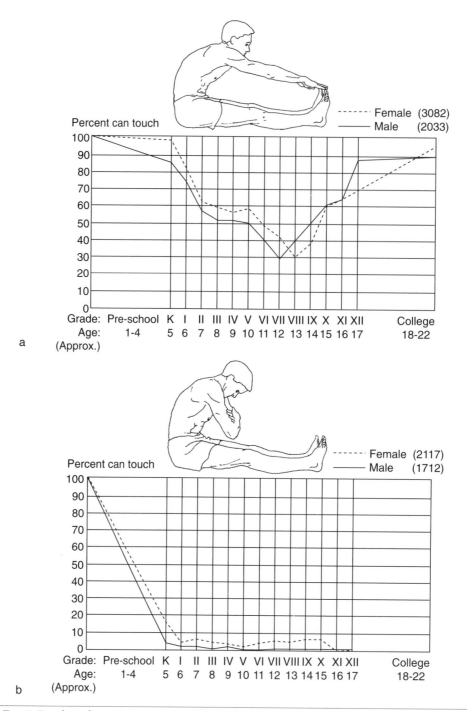

Fig. 10.1. (a) Test 1: Touching fingertips to toes ($N = 5,115$). (b) Test 2: Touching the forehead to the knees in a long-sitting position ($N = 3,829$).
Reprinted from Kendall and Kendall (1948).

lescence. One year later, Buxton (1957) found decreases in both girls and boys from age 6 to 12 and then increases through age 15. Soon afterward, Burley, Dobell, and Farrell (1961) reported that there were no significant age group differences in several flexibility measures among seventh- through ninth-grade girls. Clarke (1975)

reported flexibility decreases beginning at age 10 for males and age 12 for females. Milne, Seefeldt, and Reuschlein (1976) found significant decreases in flexibility between kindergarten and second-grade children. Krahenbuhl and Martin (1977) found a decrease in shoulder, knee, and hip flexibility between the ages of 10 and 14. A study of shoulder flexibility by Germain and Blair (1983) indicated an increase at 5 to 10 years of age and then a steady decrease with age thereafter. An investigation by Docherty and Bell (1985) found a significant decrease in trunk and neck extension, shoulder and wrist elevation, and sit-and-reach flexibility between 6 and 15 years of age. Koslow (1987) undertook an investigation involving 320 males and females ranging in age from 9 to 21 years. Shoulder flexion-extension was greater in the 13-year-olds than in the 9-year-olds of both sexes. Males and females ages 17 and 21 years were significantly more flexible than 9- and 13-year-old males and females using the modified sit-and-reach test to evaluate lower extremity flexibility. A decrease in flexibility was even found between 5- and 6-year-olds (Gabbard and Tandy 1988).

According to Sermeev (1966), flexibility is not developed identically in various age periods and not equally for various movements. Nonetheless, M.L. Harris (1969b) is of the opinion that one age is as good as another to study the structure of flexibility as long as the study is kept within a limited age range. However, Corbin and Noble (1980) suggest that when evaluating the flexibility of children and adolescents, growth (especially individual differences in growth) should be considered. Of significant interest, Pratt (1989) found that maturational age as measured by Tanner staging was better correlated with strength and flexibility for the lower extremity than was chronological age.

One's degree of flexibility clearly depends on a multitude of interacting factors. In the area of athletics and dance, flexibility relates to the level of preparation and training (M.J.L. Alexander 1991; Chatfield et al. 1990; Klemp, Stevens, and Isaacs 1984; Nelson, Johnson, and Smith 1983; Sermeev 1966). As would be expected, the higher the qualification requirements for many sports and events, the greater the mobility of the athlete. For laypeople, the quality and quantity of one's activities, both occupational and avocational, is of chief importance (Salminen et al. 1993). Although flexibility did decrease with age, the loss appeared to be minimized in those individuals who remained active.

Increased Tightness of Children Growing Into Adolescence

Several suggestions have been made to explain the decline in flexibility experienced by children growing into adolescence. One explanation previously mentioned is that during periods of rapid growth bones grow much faster than the muscles stretch. As a result there is an increase in muscle-tendon tightness about a joint (Kendall and Kendall 1948; Leard 1984; Micheli 1983; Sutro 1947). Another hypothesis is that the decrease in flexibility, especially in the hamstrings, is directly related to the prolonged sitting position in school (Milne and Mierau 1979; Milne, Mierau, and Cassidy 1981).

The mechanics of sitting have been investigated by Pheasant (1986, 1991). In brief, most people are comfortable when sitting with a backward rotation of the pelvis so that the superior iliac spine lies well behind the pubis. "If you palpate the hamstring tendon (just behind the knee), you will find that they are slack. Sit up straight and they tighten" (Pheasant 1991, 105). Consequently, over an extended period of time the hamstrings will shorten to take up the slack. An extension of this proposition is that decreases in flexibility and increased tightness could be the result of a less physically active population that is instead watching television, talking on the telephone, playing computer games, and working at desks.

Critical Periods of Flexibility Development

Is there a critical period during which stretching is most effective in developing flexibility? A *critical period* is the period of time following the age when one becomes capable of performing a particular function effectively, when changes are most likely to occur at rapid or optimal rates. Flexibility can be developed at any age given the appropriate training; however, the rate of improvement will not be the same at every age, nor will the potential for improvement.

Sermeev's (1966) research on the mobility of the hip joint of 1,440 athletes, 10 to 30 years old, of both sexes and 3,000 children and adults not participating in sports demonstrated that mobility in the hip joint is not developed identically at various ages and not equally for various movements. Specifically, he observed that the greatest improvement occurs between the ages of 7 and 11. However, by 15 years of age the indices of mobility in the hip joint are maximal; in later years that amount decreases.

This information does not mean that a stretching program has no effect after the critical period has passed or that one critical period determines all potential. The question, then, to be asked is, Can the effects of the lack of stretching and consequent tightness during the critical period (i.e., the growing years) be counteracted by engaging in stretching programs after the critical period has passed? This question is relevant for individuals in late adolescence or adulthood.

There is evidence that even senior adults benefit from exercise programs for developing ROM (Bell and Hoshizaki 1981; Dummer, Vaccaro, and Clarke 1985; Frekany and Leslie 1975; Germain and Blair 1983; Hopkins et al. 1990; Morey et al. 1989; Rikli and Busch 1986; Van Deusen and Harlowe 1987). Common sense and research suggest that it is likely that maintained or increased use of full joint range could help maintain ROM and offset some of its age-related loss (Bassey et al. 1989). In general, it is reasonable to conclude that the longer one waits to start on some type of flexibility program after adolescence, the less likely there will be an absolute improvement.

Gender Differences in Flexibility

Evidence suggests that, as a general rule, females are more flexible than males (Allander et al. 1974; Gabbard and Tandy 1988; Haley, Tada, and Carmichael 1986; M.A. Jones, Buis, and Harris 1986). Although conclusive evidence of this is lacking, several factors, including anatomical and physiological differences, may account for the difference in flexibility between the sexes.

Anatomical Gender Differences

One anatomical factor that allows the female human body a greater range of flexibility is the difference between the pelvic regions of men and women. Men's pelvic bones are generally heavier and rougher; the brim is not as rounded; the cavity is less spacious; the sacrosciatic notch, pubic arch, and sacrum are narrower; and the acetabula are closer together than women's. Generally, because most women have broader and shallower hips than men, they have a greater potential for ROM in the pelvic region (Figure 10.2, a and b). In particular, the shallowness of the female pelvis permits a greater degree of joint play.

However, even among women there are various pelvic types, and each has its own influence

on ROM (Figure 10.3). The most commonly quoted and described pelvic classification system was developed by Caldwell and Moloy (1933). It describes four main groups based on the shape of the pelvic brim.

1. The *gynecoid* pelvis is the most common pelvis type. Occurring in 50% of all women, this pelvic type, which permits the easiest vaginal birth, is characterized by a round or slightly oval pelvic inlet; the subpubic angle, or pubic arch, is almost 90°.

2. The *android* pelvis resembles the male pelvis. This type is found in about 20% of women. It is characterized by a heart-shaped brim, a wedge-shaped pelvic inlet, and a subpubic angle between 60° and 75°. This pelvis shape, also called the "funnel" pelvis, produces difficulty in delivery, because the baby's head frequently becomes arrested transversely in the midpelvis.

3. The *platypelloid* or *flat* pelvis is the least common pelvic structure among men and women. This type of pelvis is found in less than 5% of those examined. It is characterized by a kidney-shaped brim and a narrow anteroposterior diameter. During labor, rotation of the baby's head may be restricted, and deep transverse flattening of the head may occur.

4. The *anthropoid* pelvis is found in about 20% of women. It has an oval brim, a larger anteroposterior diameter, and a smaller transverse diameter compared with the other types of pelvis. Generally, the pelvis is so large that labor is easy.

In addition to pelvic differences, women usually have a greater range of extension in the elbow. This ability is the result of women having a shorter upper curve of the olecranon process of the elbow than men (Gelabert 1966).

Corbin (1980) also suggests that girls have greater potential for flexibility after puberty in such areas as trunk flexion because of their lower center of gravity and shorter leg length compared with boys. Corbin and Noble (1980) suggest that differences in regular activity between the sexes may also account for their flexibility differences.

Hormonal Effects of Pregnancy on Flexibility

Flexibility is also affected by pregnancy (Abramson, Roberts, and Wilson 1934; Bird, Calguneri, and Wright 1981; Brewer and Hinson

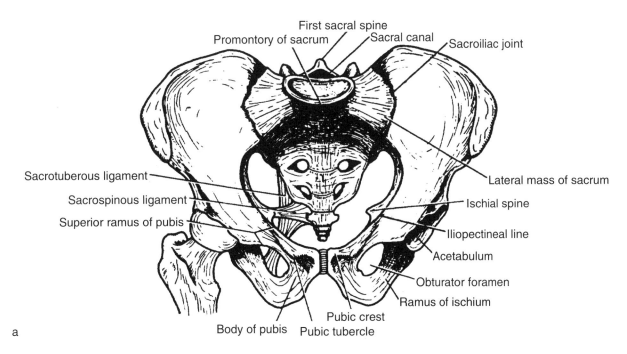

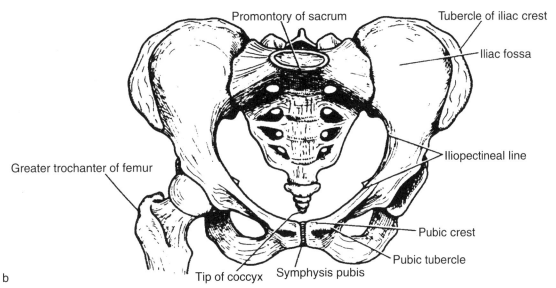

Fig. 10.2. (a) The male pelvis. (b) The female pelvis.
Reprinted from Snell (1992).

1978). As a result of changes during pregnancy, joint laxity and flexibility increase. According to Beighton, Grahame, and Bird (1989) and McNitt-Gray (1991), the changes in the pelvic joint during late pregnancy may arise from both local and systemic causes. Local causes include the weight of the uterus on the pelvic brim and other biomechanical factors, such as modifications in the center of mass and changes on mechanical loading; systemic causes are presumably circulating hormones. The hormone most commonly thought to be responsible for these changes is *re-*

laxin (discussed later). After childbirth, the production of relaxin decreases, and the ligaments tighten up again. However, Beighton, Grahame, and Bird (1989) point out that whether these changes should be attributed to relaxin, progestogens and estrogens, or altered steroid metabolism remains undetermined.

Estrogen

Collagen constitutes approximately one-third of the total mass of the body (Hall 1981). Despite

| Gynecoid | Android | Flat | Anthropoid |

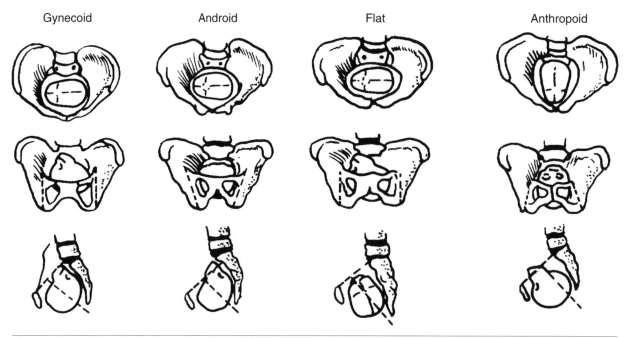

Fig. 10.3. Diagrammatic representation of the four parent pelvic types and the influence of the characteristic pelvic variations upon mechanisms.
Reprinted from Danforth and Ellis (1963).

this fact, little work has been done to establish the relationship between collagen and sex hormones (Brincat et al. 1987). Usually, the research involves mice or rats, and human studies are related to skin and bone loss in females. There is an almost total absence of research correlating the effect of estrogen on human muscular fascia, joint capsules, ligaments, and tendons in nonpregnant women. Research in humans has primarily focused on the postmenopausal decrease of bone density and skin moistness and thickness.

Relaxin

Relaxin is a polypeptide hormone that has to date been shown to have three main biological actions. These actions include inhibition of uterine contraction, elongation of the interpubic ligament, and softening of the cervix. During pregnancy, the cervix undergoes modifications that allow sufficient dilation for the passage of the fetus at birth. The hormonal influences that bring about softening of the cervix are as yet poorly understood. Nonetheless, several schemes have been postulated by Wahl, Blandau, and Page (1977) and Lowther (1981) to account for the changes in the pubic symphysis of pregnant women. A detailed review of relaxin can be found in the work of Bryant-Greenwood and Schwabe (1994).

Hormone Effects on Newborns

The only research in the literature on the relationship between estrogen and joints in newborns deals with congenital dislocation of the hip. Andren and Borglin (1961) suggested that congenital dislocation of the hip could be the consequence of abnormal estrogen metabolism in the fetus during the perinatal period. However, Aarskog, Stoa, and Thorsen (1966) criticized the work of Andren and Borglin (1961) and found no supporting data in their study. Later, Thieme et al. (1968) also determined that this hypothesis was not supported.

Other Effects of Pregnancy on Flexibility

The tremendous biological changes that take place in pregnant women have significance for various specialized health care providers, such as podiatrists, orthodontists, chiropractors, and physical therapists. Recent evidence indicates that peripheral joints, such as the feet, teeth, fingers, and knees experience increases in joint laxity during pregnancy (Alverez et al. 1988; Block et al. 1985; Calguneri, Bird, and Wright 1982; Danforth 1967). Ligament laxity in the lower back and pelvis has been linked with sacroiliac dysfunction (DonTigny 1985) and changes in the pubic symphysis (DonTigny 1985; Mikawa et al. 1988). This laxity has implications not only for patients, but also for health care providers who specialize in back disorders (e.g., chiropractors, physical therapists, osteopaths, and medical doctors specializing in orthopedics). Regarding potential cause and treatment, P.L. Williams and colleagues (1989, 518) write:

> During pregnancy, the pelvic joints and ligaments are relaxed and capable of more extensive movements. This relaxation renders the locking mechanism of the sacro-iliac joint less restrictive and permits greater rotation. This change may allow alterations in the diameter of the pelvis at childbirth. The less the locking mechanism the more the strain of weight bearing falls on the ligaments leading to frequent occurrence of sacro-iliac strain after pregnancy. After childbirth, the ligaments become tightened up but in some cases the locking may occur in the position of rotation of the hip bones adopted during pregnancy. This so-called subluxation of the sacro-iliac joint causes pain by the unusual tension which it imposes on the ligaments and the reduction by forcible manipulation may be attempted.

Body Build and Flexibility

Numerous attempts have been made to relate flexibility to factors such as body proportions, body surface area, skinfold thickness (obesity), and weight. However, the results of such research have been inconsistent. What is almost unanimously agreed upon is that flexibility is specific (Dickenson 1968; M.L. Harris 1969a, 1969b). That is, the amount or degree of ROM is specific to each joint. Therefore, ROM in the shoulder is not correlated with ROM in the hip, and ROM in one hip or shoulder may not be highly related to ROM in the same joint on the opposite side. Furthermore, flexibility is not merely specific to the joints of the body, but is also specific to individual joint movements. This concept of specificity of flexibility is based on the fact that different musculature, bone structure, and connective tissue are involved in different movements of a joint. There is no evidence, therefore, that flexibility exists as a single general characteristic of the human body. Thus, no single composite test or joint action mea-

sure can give a satisfactory index of the flexibility characteristics of an individual (M.L. Harris 1969a, 1969b).

Body Segment Lengths and Flexibility

Following is a brief summary of studies on the relationship between body build and flexibility. Several investigators have found that body build as determined by segmental length is not significantly correlated with toe-touch flexibility (Broer and Gales 1958; Harvey and Scott 1967; Mathews, Shaw, and Bohnen 1957; Mathews, Shaw, and Woods 1959). In direct contrast, Wear (1963) found that for those people with extreme body types, the relationship of trunk-plus-arm length to leg length was a significant factor in the performance of the toe-touch test. Specifically, people with a longer trunk-plus-arm measurement and relatively short legs have an advantage over those with long legs and relatively short trunk-plus-arm measurements (Broer and Gales 1958). It has also been contended that the ability to touch the toes with the fingertips may be considered normal for young children and adults; however, between the ages of 11 and 14, many young adolescents who show no signs of muscle or joint tightness are unable to complete this movement. Thus, as shown in Figure 10.4, apparently limited flexibility occurs gradually over the same period of years during which the legs become proportionally longer in relation to the trunk (Kendall and Kendall 1948; Kendall, Kendall, and Boynton 1970; Kendall, Kendall, and Wadsworth 1971). However, Harvey and Scott (1967) found that no significant difference existed between means of the best bend-and-reach scores and excess upper body length (trunk-plus-arm length minus leg length) or the ratio of the trunk-plus-arm length to leg length. When prone back extension and supine back extension were compared with trunk length, no significant correlation was found (Wear 1963).

However, questions persist regarding bias for individuals with extreme arm-leg length differences and other extreme body dimensions. A.W. Jackson and Baker (1986) investigated the validity of the sit-and-reach test. They found moderate support ($r = .64$) for the test as a measure of hamstring flexibility and less support ($r = .28$) for the test as a measure of low back flexibility. In another study, A.W. Jackson and Langford (1989)

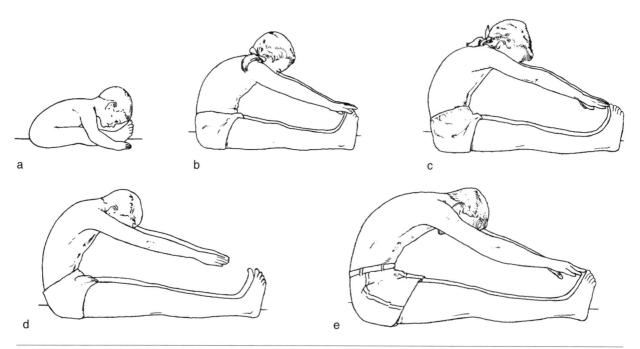

Fig. 10.4. Normal flexibility according to age level: Infant (a), young child (b), child (c), adolescent (d), and adult (e). Reprinted from Kendall, Kendall, and Wadsworth (1971).

also investigated the validity of the sit-and-reach test. They found good support ($r = .89$ for males and $r = .70$ for females) for the test as a measure of hamstring flexibility. In contrast, there was less support ($r = .59$ for males and $r = .12$ for females) for the test as a measure of low back flexibility.

One possible confounding factor is the difference in individual scapular abduction during the sit-and-reach test. It was estimated that scapular abduction may account for 3 to 5 cm of variation in the final sit-and-reach score (Hopkins 1981). Consequently, Hopkins (1981) and Hopkins and Hoeger (1986) have proposed a modified sit-and-reach (MSR) test to administratively negate the effects of shoulder girdle mobility and proportional differences between arms and legs. As can be seen in Figure 10.5, the MSR test establishes a zero point for each individual on the finger-to-box distance (FBD) based on proportional differences in limb lengths. Research studies by Hoeger et al. (1990) and Hoeger and Hopkins (1992) have found that the MSR test does help control for disparities. Normative data and flexibility fitness categories for the MSR test have been reported (Hoeger 1991; Hoeger, Hopkins, and Johnson 1991).

Body Weight and Somatotype Effects on Flexibility

Weight, somatotype, skinfold thickness, and body surface area have all been investigated in terms

of their relationships to flexibility. McCue (1963) found very few significant relationships between overweight and underweight body builds and flexibility. In a similar study, Tyrance (1958) found few significant relationships between flexibility and three extremes in body build: thinnest underweight, fattest overweight, and most muscular. Correlations between flexibility and somatotype were also generally found to be insignificant (Laubach and McConville 1966a, 1966b).

In terms of lean body mass as calculated by skinfold measurements, flexibility differences were again found to be insignificant (Laubach and McConville 1966a). An attempt was made to find a relationship between body surface area and flexibility. The results of the study by Krahenbuhl and Martin (1977) were significantly inversely related or not related at all depending upon the body parts tested. Gabbard and Tandy (1988) examined the relationship of body fatness to the performance of 5- and 6-year-old males and females on the sit-and-reach flexibility test. The data suggested that body fat at four measured sites had little to do with flexibility for either sex.

Racial Differences in Flexibility

The relationship between race and motor performance has been investigated. The term *race* im-

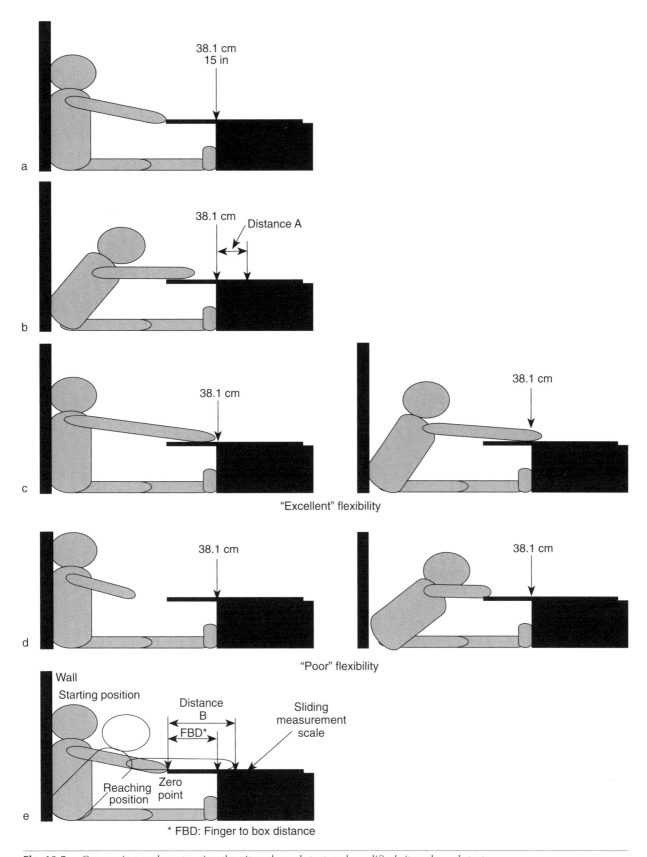

38.1 cm
15 in

a

38.1 cm   Distance A

b

38.1 cm

38.1 cm

c

"Excellent" flexibility

38.1 cm

38.1 cm

d

"Poor" flexibility

Wall
Starting position

Distance
B

FBD*

Sliding
measurement
scale

Reaching
position

Zero
point

e

* FBD: Finger to box distance

Fig. 10.5. Comparing and contrasting the sit-and-reach test and modified sit-and-reach test.
(a) Starting position for the sit-and-reach test. (b) The standard sit-and-reach test. (c) "Excellent" flexibility on the standard sit-and-reach test. (d) "Poor" flexibility on the standard sit-and-reach test. (e) The modified sit-and-reach test.
Reprinted from Hoeger and Hopkins (1992).

plies membership in a group in which there are substantial genetic similarities among individuals (Malina 1988). C. Milne, Seefeldt, and Reuschlein (1976) compared 553 black and white children in kindergarten, first grade, and second grade. The grade-race interaction effect indicated that white children were generally more flexible than black children, but the only significant difference ($p < .01$) was at the second-grade level. In a later study, M.A. Jones, Buis, and Harris (1986) tested 2,546 black and white children in grades 2, 4, and 6. Racial differences in flexibility across sexes and grades were not substantiated.

Dominant Laterality and Flexibility

Human handedness has been a source of curiosity for centuries. One of the earliest recordings is found in the Bible (Judges 20:16), where it is mentioned that the 26,700-man army of Benjamin had 700 left-handed soldiers. Many people tend to favor a dominant side in their chosen sports or activities. As a consequence, they often possess greater strength, coordination, balance, and proprioceptive awareness on one side. Reasons for unilateral development are unknown, although theories exist.

Lateralization Versus Mixed Dominance

Sometimes dominance may be mixed; that is, no clear hand preference exists. For example, a baseball player may bat left-handed and throw right-handed, or a right-handed diver or gymnast may twist to the right side (right-handed people normally twist to the left side because the dominant right arm is used to thrust or wrap across the body). Occasionally, some athletes exhibit bilateral skills despite the unilateral nature of their activities. Some examples are a baseball switch-hitter who can bat from either side of the plate or a boxer who can jab equally well with either right or left hand. In some disciplines, bilateral emphasis is possible—equal execution by opposing limbs can occur (e.g., dribbling a basketball, leg kicks in the martial arts, and dribbling and kicking in soccer). In contrast, a few disciplines and activities, such as swimming and power lifting, require bilateral development.

A variety of studies have provided evidence of the effect of dominant laterality on the normal musculoskeletal system. Hand grips are stronger on the dominant side (Haywood 1980; Lunde, Brewer, and Garcia 1972), and bone density is reportedly greater on the dominant side in the lower radius (Ekman, Ljungquist, and Stein 1970) and in the os calcis (Webber and Garnett 1976). Dobeln (personal communication, cited in Allander et al. 1974) found that the radioulnar width in 434 males aged 16 to 27 (including 307 subjects aged 19 to 21 years) was greater in the right side ($p = .001$). Muscles of the leg and forearm on the dominant side tend to be larger, more dense on computer tomographic scan, and stronger than on the nondominant side of normal people (Merletti et al. 1986; Murray and Sepic 1968). Furthermore, bone density and muscle mass also have been found to be greater in the dominant arm of tennis players (Chinn, Priest, and Kent 1974).

In a related study, Mysorekar and Nandedkar (1986) observed that human beings have a tendency to incline their heads predominantly to one side or the other. They investigated whether dominance in the atlantooccipital articulations would account for this phenomenon. The researchers found that the right side has a tendency to have larger facets or condyles. Since the difference was not statistically significant, it could not be stated that there was a clear right-side dominance.

One area of research that has received attention is the relationship between dominant laterality and ROM. However, only a few studies have involved general populations. Allander et al. (1974) found reduced mobility in the right wrist in comparison with the left in both sexes. The researchers believed that this observation was "in accordance with the higher level of exposure to trauma of the right hand in a predominantly right-handed population." In addition, their study found restriction of movement in the rotation of the left hip joint compared with the right ($p = .001$ for males and $p = .05$ for females). It was suggested that this observation might be relevant to the position of the body at work. Kronberg, Brostrom, and Soderlund (1990) determined that the average angle for humeral head retroversion was 33° on the dominant side and 29° on the nondominant side in 50 healthy subjects, regardless of gender. A larger retroversion angle was consistent with an increased range of shoulder external rotation. Nonetheless, the study found only slight ROM differences between the dominant and nondominant shoulders.

Effect of Lateralized Athletic Skills on Flexibility

Most of the research regarding ROM and laterality pertains to individuals involved in athletics. Chandler and colleagues (1990) found that tennis players' internal shoulder rotation was significantly tighter on the dominant side than on the nondominant side and that their range of external shoulder rotation was significantly greater on the dominant side than on the nondominant side. Research by Chinn, Priest, and Kent (1974) substantiated that both male and female tennis players displayed significant decreases in flexibility in internal shoulder rotation of the playing arm. In addition, they found that both sexes had significant decreases in radioulnar pronation and supination of the playing arm.

A study of baseball players (Gurry et al. 1985) found no significant differences in the flexibility of the right and left sides. In contrast, Tippett (1986) found a significantly greater hip flexion on the kick leg than on the stance leg and a greater internal hip rotation of the stance leg than of the kick leg of baseball pitchers. According to Tippett, "the results appear to be products of the pitching mechanism or the pitcher himself, just as specific upper extremity motion, strength, and anatomical characteristics have been found specific to pitchers" (p. 14).

Koslow (1987) examined 320 male and female students of specific ages (i.e., 9, 13, 17, and 21 years) for bilateral flexibility of shoulder flexion-extension and of the lower extremity (by a modified sit-and-reach test). Little difference was found between the dominant and nondominant shoulders of the 13-, 17-, and 21-year-old females. In contrast, shoulder range measurements for the males significantly decreased for the same age groups. Dominant shoulder joint flexibility measures of the 17- and 21-year-old females were significantly greater than those of the 17- and 21-year-old males. It was suggested that the reason for the males' decrease in dominant shoulder flexibility with age may relate to their activity patterns in such a way as to inhibit increases in flexibility; specifically, males may exhibit a more forceful and mature (effective) throwing pattern as compared with females across all ages. In the same study, it was found that the flexibility measures of the nondominant lower extremity of the 17- and 21-year-old males were significantly greater than the same measures of the dominant lower extremity. For the females, a very small and insignificant increase of flexibility in the nondominant leg was found for all the age groups except the 9-year-olds.

In another study (Bonci, Hensal, and Torg 1986) of static and dynamic range of the glenohumeral joint of male and female athletes, it was found in both sexes that the dominant arm had approximately 5% more motion compared with the nondominant arm. Furthermore, dynamic ROM averaged 25° more than static motion. In addition, an analysis of the effect of a modified Bristow surgical procedure for recurrent dislocation or subluxation of the shoulder demonstrated that static and dynamic ROM were significantly reduced by surgery. Henry (1986, 17), commenting on the paper of Bonci, Hensal, and Torg (1986), stated that the main point to remember is that "postoperative range of motion in the dominant shoulder compared to the range of motion in the nondominant side can be misleading due to the increased range of motion of the dominant shoulder prior to surgery."

Warming Up and Cooling Down

Warm-up may be defined as a group of exercises performed immediately before an activity, which provides the body with a period of adjustment from rest to exercise. Warm-up is designed to improve performance and reduce the chance of injury by mobilizing the individual mentally as well as physically. Analogous to warm-up is cooldown (also called warm-down). *Cool-down* may be defined as a group of exercises performed immediately after an activity that provides the body a period of adjustment from exercise to rest.

Warming Up

Warm-up may be divided into two broad categories: passive and active. *Passive* warm-up incorporates the use of an outside agent or modality (e.g., hot baths, infrared light, ultrasound). In contrast, *active* warm-up is self-initiated. Active warm-up can be further divided into formal and general warm-up. *Formal* warm-up includes movements that either mimic or are employed in the actual performance activity. For example, a baseball player will throw a ball or swing a bat to warm up. In contrast, *general* warm-up consists of movements not directly related to those employed in the activity itself. These movements may include light calisthenics, jogging, or stationary bicycling. The nature of the warm-up depends on the individual's needs but should be intense enough to increase the body core temperature and cause some sweating, but not so intense as to cause fatigue (Karvonen 1992; Kulund and Tottossy 1983; McGeorge 1989; Shellock and Prentice 1985; Taunton 1982). The effects of warm-up will ultimately wear off. How soon will depend on a number of factors such as clothing, exercise intensity, and specificity of the warm-up. Hardy, Lye, and Heathcote (1983) found that passive warm-up was significantly more effective in increasing hip flexion than active warm-up.

An important distinction should be made here between warm-up exercises and flexibility exercises. *Flexibility exercises* are those exercises that are used to increase the ROM of a joint or set of joints progressively and permanently. Flexibility exercises should always be preceded by a set of mild warm-up exercises, because the increase in the tissue temperature produced by the warm-up exercise will make the stretching both safer and more productive (Sapega et al. 1981). However, an increase in temperature also involves a reduction in tensile strength of connective tissue, and thus more ruptures might be expected after warming up. Increased temperature, however, seems to involve an increase in extensibility also, and this greater extensibility is a plausible explanation for the fact that warming up does indeed prevent ruptures (Troels 1973).

Benefits associated with warming up include the following:

- Increased body and tissue temperature
- Increased blood flow through active muscles by reducing vascular bed resistance (The vessel bed is not a fluid and therefore not viscous. Vasodilation is the explanation for the decreased resistance.)
- Increased heart rate, which will prepare the cardiovascular system for work
- Increased metabolic rate
- Increases in the Bohr effect, which facilitates the exchange of oxygen from hemoglobin
- Increased speed at which nerve impulses travel, and thereby facilitation of body movements
- Increased efficiency of reciprocal innervation (thus allowing opposing muscles to contract and relax faster and more efficiently)
- Increased physical working capacity
- Decreased viscosity (or resistance) of connective tissue and muscle

- Decreased muscular tension (improved muscle relaxation)
- Enhanced connective tissue and muscular extensibility
- Enhanced psychological performance

In addition to the above effects, Kopell (1962) is of the opinion that some fatalities associated with exercise may have been avoided if adequate warm-up had occurred. Barnard, Gardner, Diaco, McAlpin, and Kattus (1973) and Barnard, McAlpin, Kattus, and Buckberg (1973) have suggested that warm-up can also prevent ST segment depression (an electrocardiographic abnormality). This abnormality is sometimes seen in healthy people at the beginning of fast running performances.

Viscosity Effects

Viscosity is defined as resistance to flow, or an apparent force that prevents fluids from flowing easily. Connective tissue and muscular viscosity might be partially responsible for restricting movement (Leighton 1960). We know that temperature has an inverse effect on viscosity; that is, as the temperature of the body tissues increases, fluid viscosity decreases, and vice versa. This reduced viscosity includes the viscous relaxation of collagenous tissues (Sapega et al. 1981). The mechanism behind this thermal transition is still unknown. However, it has been suggested that the collagen intermolecular bonding becomes partially destabilized, enhancing the viscous flow properties of collagenous tissue (Mason and Rigby 1963; Rigby et al. 1959). This reduced viscosity in turn decreases resistance to movement and results in increased flexibility.

Probably the most common method of elevating body temperature and reducing tissue viscosity is warm-up exercise. Other methods include heat packs, hot showers, diathermy, ultrasound, and massage. Viscosity has no long-term effect on the improvement of one's flexibility. Rather, its effects relate to various physiological factors that exist at the moment when stretch is being developed (Aten and Knight 1978).

Effect of Warm-Up on Injury Rates

Several studies have raised questions about the ability of warm-up exercise to increase flexibility and reduce the risk of injury. Williford and colleagues (1986) investigated the effects of warming up the joints by jogging and then stretching on increasing joint flexibility. Their results did not support the claim that warming up the muscle by jogging prior to stretching results in significant increases for all of the joint motion angles evaluated. In a study of 1,680 runners, the Ontario cohort study found that runners who say they never warm up have less risk than those who do, and runners who use stretching "sometimes" are at apparently higher risk than those who usually or never use it (Walter et al. 1989). However, in an interview of Grana by Finkelstein and Roos (1990), readers were cautioned that the study's findings probably reflect "the terrible number of variables that you can't control" in such a study. In a more recent study, van Mechelen et al. (1993) randomly studied 316 subjects in a 16-week experiment. Subjects were randomly split into an intervention (159 subjects) and a control group (167 subjects). Injury incidences for control and intervention subjects were 4.9 and 5.5 running injuries, respectively, per 1,000 hours of running exposure. Therefore, warm-up, cool-down, and stretching exercises were found not to reduce the running injury incidence.

Further confounding the controversy regarding the supposed benefits of warm-up was a study by Strickler, Malone, and Garrett (1990). They investigated the effects of passive warming on biomechanical properties of the musculotendinous unit of rabbit hindlimbs heated to different temperatures (35° C and 39° C) and then subjected to controlled strain injury. Their investigation found the force at failure was greater at 35° C than at 39° C, and the difference in energy absorbed by the muscles before rupture at different temperatures was not statistically significant. Obviously, the relationship among warm-up, stretching, flexibility, and injury is extremely complex, and additional research is needed to resolve these uncertainties.

Murphy (1986, 45) points out a dangerous misconception that relates to the order of stretching and warm-up in an exercise program:

> Some health clubs and fitness instructors have encouraged athletes to stretch *before* warming up. Their reasoning: Cold muscles, they claim, are like plastic, and stretching them results in a more permanent stretch, as opposed to stretching the muscles when they are warm and pliable like a rubber band.

This method is *not* supported by any research. In actuality, it is an invitation to probable injury.

Stretching should *always* be preceded by a period of warm-up.

Cooling Down

Cool-down may be defined as a group of exercises performed immediately after an activity, which provides the body a period of adjustment from exercise to rest. Although cool-down may serve as an additional effort to improve flexibility, its main objective is to facilitate muscular relaxation, promote the removal of muscular waste products by the blood, reduce muscular soreness, and allow the cardiovascular system to adjust to lowered demand. It is recommended that stretching be incorporated immediately after the main part of a workout and cool-down period, because tissue temperatures will be highest (Sapega et al. 1981).

Karvonen (1992) has suggested that cool-down is also important in reaching an emotional balance after the possible disappointment of a poor performance. In particular, when the next competition or performance soon follows, it is possible to begin the preparation for it during the cool-down from the initial performance. Furthermore, Karvonen points out that the cool-down period may be the most beneficial time for the coach to give feedback because it is given soon after the performance.

Strength Training and Flexibility

Many misconceptions and stereotypes still exist regarding the relationship between strength training and flexibility. Many coaches and athletes believe that strength gains may limit flexibility or hinder suppleness, or conversely that substantial gains in flexibility may have a deleterious effect on strength (Hebbelinck 1988). But the belief that weight training causes a "muscle-bound" condition is false. A. Jones (1975) points out several possible reasons why such beliefs persist: Certain individuals with large muscles lack a degree of flexibility; large muscles can be developed while doing absolutely nothing to improve one's flexibility; and activities that build large muscles can produce a loss of flexibility. However, the size of a person's muscle has very little or nothing to do with flexibility, and if strength training is properly conducted, it can in fact actually help to increase flexibility. This last point deserves special attention. The research of several investigators (Leighton 1956; Massey and Chaudet 1956; Wickstrom 1963; Wilmore et al. 1978) demonstrates that weight training does not decrease flexibility and in some instances actually improves it. Thus, with proper training, one can improve overall strength and flexibility as long as the training is technically correct.

There are two key principles in developing flexibility with resistance techniques. First, the entire muscle or muscle group must be worked through its full range of motion. Second, there must be a gradual emphasis on the negative phase of work. *Negative work* or *eccentric contraction* takes place when a muscle is stretched (i.e., elongated) while it is contracting. This eccentric contraction is associated with the lowering phase of a resistance exercise.

During negative work, the number of contracting muscle fibers decreases. Since the workload is shared by a smaller number of muscle contractile components, the tension in each one increases. Consequently, the excessive stress and tension produces a greater stretch on the involved fibers, resulting in enhanced flexibility. One should remember, however, that eccentric training is also associated with muscle soreness.

Circadian Variations in Flexibility

The quantitative study of biological phenomena that fluctuate periodically over time is called *chronobiology*. The term *diurnal* is frequently used for a rhythm whose period is one day. Conroy and Mills (1970) prefer the term *circadian* to indicate a period of approximately 24 hours. This term is derived from the Latin (*circa* = about; *dies* = day). Most physiological functions exhibit circadian rhythmicity: maximum and minimum function occur at specific times of day. The influence of circadian rhythms on many physiological and behavioral variables has been well established. In humans, circadian rhythms are expressed by oscillations in various physiological systems, including blood pressure, body temperature, heart rate, hormone levels, and tremors. In addition, alertness and responsiveness to either internal stimuli (e.g., neurotransmitters, electrolytes, or metabolic substrates) or external stimuli (e.g., environmental factors, drugs, or food) oscillate as a function of circadian rhythms (Winget, DeRoshia, and Holley 1985). It is not uncommon for individuals to recall periods of

stiffness related to specific times of the day as well as stiffness following activity or inactivity (Gifford 1987). Our concern in this section is the interrelationship of time of day or night to flexibility.

Research Regarding the Diurnal Rhythm of Flexibility

It is one thing to say that people perceive greater stiffness after sleeping or at different times during the day, but it is another thing to determine if there is a quantifiable decrease in ROM. One of the earliest observations that flexibility varies with the time of day was reported by Osolin (1952, 1971), cited by Dick (1980) and Bompa (1990). The highest amplitude of movement seems to be available between 1000 and 1100 and between 1600 and 1700, while the lowest amplitude likely occurs earlier in the morning. According to Osolin (1971), the reason "seems to lie with the continuous biological changes (CNS and muscle's tonus) which occur during the day." Gifford (1987) citing the work of Stockton and colleagues (1980) found the greatest improvement of suppleness was between 0800 and 1200. However, no details were given.

O'Driscoll and Tomenson (1982) measured cervical movements at 0700 and 1900 hours. They recorded greater ranges in the evening than in the morning. One year later, Baxter and Reilly (1983) reported a "time of day" effect for trunk flexibility in 14 young swimmers, best at 1330 and poorest at 0630. Gifford (1987) investigated the circadian flexibility in five different areas taken every 2 hours over a period of 24 hours using 25 normal subjects between 25 and 32 years of age. The ability to bring the fingertip to the floor while standing on a wooden platform revealed that maximum stiffness occurred in the morning at or prior to rising from bed. Maximum flexibility occurred between midday and midnight. Maximum stiffness for lumbar flexion was recorded during the hours of sleep, with flexibility increasing from 0600 through the day. Lumbar extension displayed a rise from maximum stiffness during the early hours to maximum flexibility around 1400, before gradually stiffening again toward evening. With the passive straight-leg-raising test, minimal scores occurred when the majority of the subjects were either recumbent or relatively inactive (2200–0800). Last, glenohumeral lateral rotation indicated an overall rise in ROM through the day and a decrease during the early hours of the morning. More recently, Russell, Weld, Pearcy, Hogg, and Unsworth (1992) conducted a study of 10 young adults who were tested every 2 hours over a 24 hour period. The results showed a significant decrease in flexion, extension, and lateral bend for the lumbar spine after sleep and a significant increase in the afternoon compared with measurements taken between the hours of 0200 and 0730 (Figure 10.6).

Circadian Variation in Human Stature and Disk Height

For some time it has been recognized that the stature or height of the human body fluctuates throughout the day. However, it was not until the mid-1970s that this fluctuation in stature was investigated in detail. These bodily fluctuations are important because of their potential influence on posture, ROM, mechanical efficiency, risk of injury, perception of stiffness, and low back pain. Among the factors influencing this fluctuation in bodily stature are the effects of posture, occupation, movement, load, age, disease, trauma, and nutritional status of the vertebral disks.

Early Research on Stature Variation

Kazarian (1975), in a perusal of the literature, showed that as early as 1897 Bencke had pointed

out that the vertebral column becomes shorter during the day and regains its normal length throughout the night. Later, De Puky (1935) presented the first detailed paper dealing with the oscillation of body length. He investigated 1,216 subjects from ages 5 to 90 and found that the physiological curves of the vertebral column become more curved over the course of the day. Consequently, there is a decrease in the vertical length of the body. During the night, the vertebral column recovers its original form, lengthening the body again. The average daily fluctuation of the body length is 15.7 mm, and the smallest fluctuations were found in people over 50 years old. De Puky also observed an interesting phenomenon that may have relevance for certain medical practitioners: When patients got up after being confined to bed, they seemed to have grown because of the swelling of the intervertebral fibrocartilage. However, in the surgical ward, this often failed to happen because the pain of the illness or postoperative pain caused defensive rigidity of certain muscles.

Early Research and Theories Concerning the Disk's Fluid Content

Puschel (1930) investigated the water content of two fibrocartilaginous components of the vertebral disk—the annulus fibrosus and the nucleus pulposus—in relation to age. He reported that in a newborn the water content of the nucleus pulposus

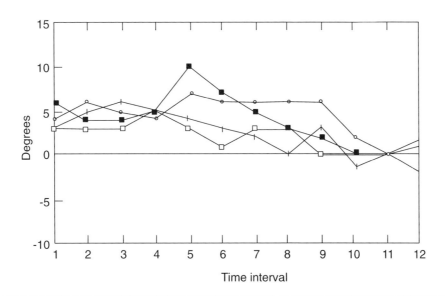

Fig. 10.6. Mean change in movement relative to time of day. Time interval 1 = 0800–0930; 2 = 1000–1130; 3 = 1200–1330; 4 = 1400–1530; 5 = 1600–1730; 6 = 1800–1930; 7 = 2000–2130; 8 = 2200–2330; 9 = 0000–0130; 10 = 0200–0330; 11 = 0400–0530; 12 = 0600–0730. ■ = flexion; + = extension; ○ = lateral bend; □ = axial rotation.
Reprinted from Russell, Weld, Pearcy, Hogg, and Unsworth (1992).

was 88% (by weight) and decreased to 69% by age 77. The annulus fibrosus declined in water content from 78% percent at birth to 70% by age 30.

Based on Puschel's and De Puky's findings, J.R. Armstrong (1958) postulated a theory that could explain their results. First, the intervertebral disks can be considered as an osmotic system in which a free exchange of fluid occurs through the semipermeable cartilaginous end plates of the disks. During the day, when the vertebral column is vertical and the disks are subjected to dynamic muscular forces and the gravitational force of body weight, fluid is squeezed out (disk dehydration). Then, during sleep, the disks are rehydrated, because the osmotic pressure exceeds disk compression when the vertebral column is horizontal. Therefore the disks absorb fluids from the surrounding area.

Circadian Variations in Stature

Stature decreases throughout the day. As previously stated, De Puky (1935) reported an average circadian oscillation of 15.7 mm. Later studies by Reilly, Tyrrell, and Troup (1984) and Tyrrell, Reilly, and Troup (1985) found an overall mean circadian variation of 19.29 mm, or 1.1% of stature. Fifty-four percent of the diurnal loss in stature occurred in the first hour after rising, and approximately 70% was regained during the first half of the night. Similarly, an average decrease of 14.4 mm, or 0.83%, was reported by Leatt, Reilly, and Troup (1986). They also found that 38.4% of the height loss occurred in the first 1.5 hours after rising and 60.8% within 2.5 hours of rising. The height lost during the day was regained completely during sleep, with 68% recovered during the first half of the night's sleep.

However, Foreman and Linge (1989) and van Dieën and Toussaint (1993) point out that spinal length needs to be measured independently from the length of the lower extremities. In particular, Foreman and Linge (1989) confirmed the suspicion that heel pad shrinkage may contribute to the change in total body stature. Their study found that compression of the heel pad soft tissue averaged 4.4 mm and that a period of 2 min is needed for the heel pad to compress sufficiently before measurements are taken.

Another issue that has generally not been appreciated is the effect of diurnal height variations in the measurement of growing children. Strickland and Shearin (1972) analyzed the differences in A.M. and P.M. heights of 100 children. The mean difference was 1.54 cm, with a range of variation from 0.80 to 2.8 cm. According to

Strickland and Shearin, this finding is significant because "if an interval measurement includes an occult error secondary to a diurnal variation, then a projected yearly growth rate can be subjected to a considerable error" (p. 1024).

Factors That Influence Circadian Stature Variation

Gravity, as discussed in the preceding sections, is only one of a variety of factors that can influence circadian stature. Other significant factors are exercise, occupation, age, and disease. These topics will be reviewed in the following sections.

Effects of Exercise on Stature

The vertebral column is subject to loading by gravity, changes in motion, truncal muscle activity, external forces, and external work. One of the earliest observations of the effects of physical activity on stature was by Forssberg (1899; cited by Corlett et al. 1987). He discovered that cavalry recruits lost more body height after riding at a hard gallop than when riding at a more sedate pace. Fitzgerald (1972) found that significantly greater losses of height occurred when healthy young male adults carried shoulder loads of 9 kg with the trunk erect than when unloaded. Leatt, Reilly, and Troup (1986) investigated the effect of a 6K run on nine novice runners and a 25K run by seven trained runners. The mean height loss was 3.25 mm for the novices and 2.35 mm for the trained group over the first 6 km of their run. The mean shrinkage during the 19 km that followed was 7.8 mm. Wilby and colleagues (1987) investigated the effects of two 20-min weight-training circuits on 10 females from 20 to 30 years old. The exercise regimen was conducted twice a day: in the morning immediately upon rising and again after 2200. The mean loss of height from circuit training was 5.4 mm in the morning and 4.3 mm in the evening. The influence of bounding and jumping exercises, commonly referred to as *plyometrics*, was investigated by Boocock and colleagues (1988) in two test sessions at least 5 days apart using eight male subjects ages 20 to 26. The exercise consisted of 50 standing broad jumps performed in sets of five with 15-s recovery between each set. The first day's exercise session was followed by standing for 20 min and the second day's session was followed by involved gravity inversion at an angle of 50° to the vertical. "When the exercise period followed standing, a mean loss in height of 1.69

mm was found compared to 3.49 mm when following by gravity inversion" (p. 1634). The researchers concluded that the benefits gained by unloading the spine are short lived.

Effects of Occupation on Stature

The direct influence of occupation on stature also has been investigated. Foreman and Troup (1987) evaluated eight female and four male nurses throughout two working shifts. The mean total losses in height were 10.2 mm for the early shift and 9.8 mm for the late shift. Furthermore, "there was a significant correlation between loss of stature and both the total duration of lean/stoop postures and the total duration of lifting" (p. 48). Sitting in a chair for just 5 min has also been found to result in shrinkage of the spine (Magnusson et al. 1990). The average mean shrinkage was 4.53 mm for 15 females. This has implications for individuals whose occupation requires extensive sitting, especially with poor posture (e.g., computer operators, secretaries, and assembly line workers). Accordingly, McGill and Brown (1992, 43) advise that it might be prudent for "those who experience prolonged full flexion postures to stand and walk for a few minutes prior to performing demanding manual exertions." This advice is based on research showing that the lumbar spine recovers more rapidly and completely from cyclic loading of short duration, allowing periodic recovery, than from prolonged loading using the same force (Koeller, Funke, and Hartman 1984; Twomey and Taylor 1982).

In another study, Botsford, Esses, and Ogilvie-Harris (1994) designed a test on eight male subjects using two protocols. In one protocol, the volunteers were in the supine position for 6 hours before magnetic resonance imaging (MRI). In the second protocol, the same group was tested one week later, after spending 4 hours standing and 3 hours sitting before MRI. Three-dimensional MRI was then carried out on the L3-4, L4-5, and L5-S1 disks. The results showed that

> volume height and AP (anterior-posterior) diameter of the lumbar intervertebral disks decreased significantly after the protocol of a day's activity. The mean decrease in disk volume at the L3-4 level after standing was 21.1%. At the L4-5 level, it decreased a mean of 18.7%, whereas at the L5-S1 level, there was a 21.6% mean decrease. The mean simulated diurnal volume decrease in the lower three lumbar disks is 16.2%. (p. 935)

Furthermore, their investigation documented that the bulk of the height loss is caused by fluid loss, the contribution from radial bulging being minimal, if any. The implications of these findings will be discussed later.

Effect of Age and Disease on Stature

Age and disease have been found to influence stature. It is well known that there is a decrease in the range of spinal movement with aging. For example, Twomey and Taylor (1982) determined that the amount of flexion creep (see chapter 5) is age dependent. With a standard load, creep was greater in the older vertebral column than in the younger.

In investigations of diseased spines, Hindle and Murray-Leslie (1987) observed that diurnal stature loss was significantly reduced in subjects with ankylosing spondylitis (fusion of the vertebrae). Hence, the absence of stature variation might be a useful indicator of this pathological condition. The relationship between diurnal behavior of the spine and idiopathic scoliosis (spinal lateral curvature of unknown origin) has been investigated by Beauchamp and colleagues (1993). They reported an average diurnal increase of curvature in moderate and severe adolescent idiopathic scoliosis. In the opinion of the investigators, the variation was clinically significant, in that it could serve as an indicator of curve progression in the treatment of this disorder, but not statistically significant.

Recovery of Stature

As was pointed out previously, recovery from spinal shrinkage occurs with bed rest. The question is, Can recovery be facilitated more quickly or effectively? Goode and Theodore (1983) demonstrated that a group of female subjects could adjust their height upward between 7 and 36 mm when standing tall as compared with relaxed standing. Theoretically, applying a tensile force on the spinal column should enhance recovery from spinal shrinkage (Boocock et al. 1990; Boocock et al. 1988; Kane, Karl, and Swain 1985; Nosse 1978). Badtke, Bittmann, and Lazik (1993) recently demonstrated that positioning subjects in a specially developed extension apparatus could produce in 8 min the same gain in spinal column length as 2 hours of rest in bed. In contrast, Pope and Klingenstierna (1986) reported that the increase in height is greater with lying down quietly than with traction. Recovery of height can also be achieved by adopting the Fowler position (i.e., supine with legs on a stool and with hips and knees flexed to achieve minimal spinal loading). In the study by Wilby et al. (1987), 20 min reclining in the Fowler position resulted in a 4.5 mm and 3.4 mm gain in body length in the morning and evening, respectively.

Eklund and Corlett (1984) made the significant finding that if short periods of unloading of the spine are allowed in a heavy job, a substantial recovery can take place during these rest pauses. Consequently, the total shrinkage or disk compression is diminished. Implementing appropriate rest pauses in occupational or athletic situations may potentially serve to reduce the risk of injury. Astronauts' experiences with weightlessness further substantiate that unloading or a reduction of gravity influences body stature. Kazarian (1974) has reported that astronauts measure from 5 to 10 cm taller upon return to earth than when they left.

Influence of Sleep on Flexibility

People often feel stiff after sleeping. In the following sections, we explore possible causes for this phenomenon.

Influence of Sleep on Increased Sensitivity

One possible explanation for waking with stiffness is that during sleep there is a temporary change in the sensitivity of the Pacinian corpuscles, joint mechanoreceptors, muscle spindles, or Golgi tendon organs. Specifically, the respective receptors' sensitivity settings might be tem-

porarily "reset" during the period of inactivity or sleep. Lee and Kleitman (1923) and Tuttle (1924) have demonstrated a reduction of the amplitude of the patellar tendon reflex (knee jerk) in humans during sleep. Hormone effects may also influence spinal processes, as suggested by Tyrer and Bond (1974), who demonstrated diurnal variation in physiological tremor, which they hypothesized to be primarily due to changes in circulating catecholamines among other possible explanations. Research by Wolpaw, Noonan, and O'Keefe (1984) and by Wolpaw and Seegal (1982) has documented that the amplitude of the spinal stretch reflex in monkeys is subject to diurnal rhythm (i.e., altered excitability function by time of day). Winget, DeRoshia, and Holley (1985) cite a dissertation (Freivalds 1979) that found that the minimum Achilles tendon reflex sensitivity (ms) occurred between 2138 and 0845. Additional research is required to determine whether the decreased body temperature during sleep can influence the various proprioceptors' stretch response thresholds.

Influence of Sleep on Vertebral Disks

As previously pointed out, research has demonstrated that during sleep the spine is only lightly loaded and the disks swell by uptaking the body's tissue fluid. Consequently, there is an increase in total body length and the fibers of the disk are under more tension (Botsford, Esses, and Ogilvie-Harris 1994). However, throughout the normal

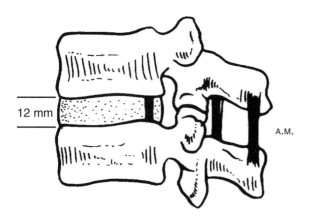 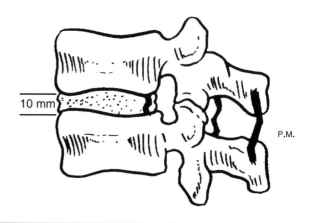

Fig. 10.7. (A.M.) Motion segment with three bands or ties representing the structures that resist forward bending movements; these are (from left to right) the annulus fibrosus, the intervertebral ligaments of the neural arch, and the back muscles and lumbodorsal fascia. (P.M.) Creep loading reduces disk height and gives slack to the three ties. The annulus is affected most because it is the shortest tie; the muscles and fascia are affected least, because they are the longest tie. Thus, creep loading reduces the motion segment's resistance to bending and transfers bending stresses from the disk (especially) and intervertebral ligaments onto the back muscles and fascia.
Reprinted from Adams, Dolan, and Hutton (1987).

activities of the day, the extra fluid is rapidly expelled from the disk. Adams, Dolan, and Hutton (1987) have identified three significant implications of diurnal variations in the stresses on the lumbar spine: (1) this swelling accounts for the increased stiffness in the spine during lumbar flexion upon awakening; (2) lumbar disks and ligaments are at greater risk of injury in the early morning; and (3) ROM increases later in the day.

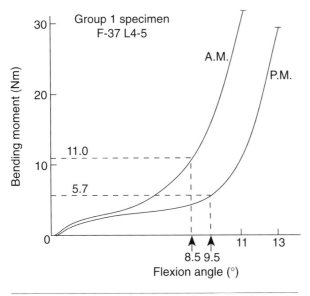

Fig. 10.8. Bending stiffness curves for a typical motion segment before (A.M.) and after (P.M.) creep loading. Reprinted from Adams, Dolan, and Hutton (1987).

As explained in Adams and colleagues' (1987) model, creep loading reduces the disk height and brings the vertebrae closer together throughout the day (Figures 10.7 and 10.8; Tables 10.1 and 10.2). In turn, this disk compression produces slack in the annulus fibrosus, in the intervertebral ligaments of the neural arch, and in the back muscles and lumbar fascia. This slackening explains why there is a small amount of extra flexion (5%) in the afternoon. However, during sleep the disks swell, increasing disk height and spreading the vertebrae. Consequently, this swelling results in increased stiffness in the morning. Furthermore, this change in fluid content of the disks affects the strain on the fibers of the annulus and may affect the likelihood of injury in the postsupine state.

Table 10.1. Comparison of Average Range of Flexion in Cadaver Spines and Living People in Early Morning (A.M.) and Late Afternoon (P.M.)

	Range of flexion of the lumbar spine	
	A.M.	P.M.
Cadaver spines	65°	77.5°
Living people	50°	55°
Margin of safety	15°	22.5°

Table 10.2. How Bending Stresses on Disk and Ligaments Decrease in Live Subjects in Course of a Day

Specimen No.	Bending moment resisted (Nm)					
	A.M.		P.M.		% reduction	
	Disk	Ligaments	Disk	Ligaments	Disk	Ligaments
1	2.8	7.0	0.7	3.4	76	52
2	4.9	11.8	1.6	7.3	67	39
3	3.9	9.7	0.8	6.0	81	37
4	3.2	7.8	0.8	4.9	75	37
5	6.7	16.4	1.6	9.8	76	40
6	4.4	10.9	0.4	2.7	92	75
7	3.9	9.7	1.0	5.5	75	44
8	4.5	11.0	1.2	5.9	73	46
9	2.1	5.0	0.4	3.6	79	29
Averages	4.0	9.9	0.9	5.5	77	44
	(±1.3)	(±3.3)	(±0.4)	(±2.1)	(±7)	(±13)

Arthritis and Morning Stiffness

Morning stiffness is a frequent complaint among patients with rheumatoid arthritis (RA). Several explanations have been put forward to explain this phenomenon. Perhaps the most plausible is an accumulation of fluid in and around joints as a result of fluid retention during sleep (J.T. Scott 1960; Wright and Johns 1960). However, one study employing a diuretic in the treatment of morning stiffness failed to find any difference in either the severity or duration of stiffness (Magder, Baxter, and Kassam 1986). Additional research in this area is needed to identify the actual cause(s) of morning stiffness and effective treatments for the cause and not the symptom.

Summary

There are a number of factors that can affect one's potential degree of flexibility. Among them are age, gender, body proportions, weight, dominant laterality, warm-up, activities, and time of day. Research substantiates that flexibility is specific to each joint. In general, flexibility can be developed at any age given the appropriate training; however, the rate of development and potential for improvement is not the same at every age.

Flexibility is affected by gender: Females are generally more flexible in the pelvic region. ROM is also affected by relaxation of the ligaments during pregnancy. The effects of body segment lengths, body weight, somatotype, race, laterality, warm-up and cool-down, strength training, and circadian variations on flexibility have also been investigated. Through a proper understanding of these relationships, misconceptions and stereotypes can be eliminated along with their potential deleterious consequences.

Chapter 11

Social Facilitation and Psychology in Developing Flexibility

The discipline of *psychology* is associated with attempts to describe, explain, and predict behavior. According to Sage (1971), "social facilitation examines the consequences upon individual behavior of the sheer presence of others" (p. 470). The field of *social psychology* is concerned with how and why the behavior of any person affects the behavior of another (Sage 1971). In this chapter, we will explore four issues related to the influence of psychology on the development or reversal of flexibility and ROM: the influence of an audience, mental concentration, psychosomatic conditions, and compliance with prescribed stretching programs.

Effects of an Audience on Developing Flexibility Through Stretching

No matter how often an athlete says he or she does not pay attention to the audience or to feedback from teammates, there are times when that athlete cannot escape their influence. The same holds true for someone who is working out with a friend or for a patient rehabilitating with a health care practitioner.

Many athletes, such as gymnasts, swimmers, and track and field athletes, perform on their own for all practical purposes. Nevertheless, these sports still involve dynamic social relationships, because they involve interaction with coaches, teammates, opponents, and frequently with fans and spectators. For people involved in activities such as cheerleading, dancing, or team sports, the interactions with one's comrades and the audience are obvious. These social factors may well affect the development of flexibility and ultimately the performance itself.

Because the people who may influence the athlete—friends, parents, peers, strangers, authority figures—have different relationships to the athlete, they also vary in their potential for affecting the athlete's behavior and psychological state. They may be perceived as positive, neutral, or negative influences, depending on the individual's past associations and experiences with them.

Ramifications of Social Facilitation

The audience may be passive and do nothing to encourage or discourage the performer, or it may be active and verbal, giving either encouraging or disparaging remarks. Research on the effects of a passive audience on individual performance has yielded contradictory results. In some studies performance was impaired, while in others it was improved. According to Sage (1971, 471), "The confusion that arises out of these contradictory findings on social facilitation and a passive audience does not seem to lead to any fruitful generalizations." However, Zajonc (1965), after a careful analysis of the research findings, uncovered a rather subtle consistency. In general, Zajonc's research found that performance is facilitated but learning is impaired by the presence of spectators.

The motivational effects induced by spectators may be learned, for they are likely a function of positive or negative experiences associated with being observed or evaluated. The anxiety level of the individual must also be considered in such instances. Research indicates that the level of a person's anxiety parallels the level of perceived stress in a given situation.

How, then, does social facilitation with an audience affect potential development of flexibility? Misconceptions and stereotypes regarding extreme flexibility in men are one example of social facilitation's negative influence. The ability of a man to perform a split, for instance, or some other skill of extreme suppleness may be perceived negatively by an audience. For very young children, such a situation may present a very real conflict and a source of potential anxiety and psychological stress. Boys who wish to participate in activities such as dance may be discouraged from doing so. Toufexis (1974) states that potential boy dancers "must surmount not only physical difficulties but psychological ones." Male dancers often confront stereotypes about their sexuality (Schnitt and Schnitt 1989; Toufexis 1974). However, Schnitt and Schnitt (1989) state that recent changes in the public perception of sex roles may be responsible for males entering the dance field in larger numbers and at an earlier age.

Social facilitation affects people's decisions to continue participating in sports. In a study of attrition in children's sport, R.E. Smith (1986) has proposed a theoretical framework to explain the process of sport withdrawal. In reviewing Smith's framework, Gould (Gould and Weiss 1987) distinguishes between sport burnout and sport dropout: "Burnout-induced withdrawal is defined as the psychological, emotional, and physical withdrawal resulting from chronic stress, whereas dropping out results from a change of interests and/or value reorientation" (p. 71). Based on the works of others, Gould (1987, 72) explains the process of dropping out:

> The decision to participate and persist in sport is a function of costs (e.g., time and effort, anxiety, disapproval of others) and benefits (e.g., trophies, feelings of competence) with the athlete

constantly trying to maximize benefits and minimize costs. Thus, interest and participation is maintained when the benefits outweigh the costs, and withdrawal occurs when costs outweigh benefits. However, behavior is not fully explained by a simple rewards-minus-costs formula. The decision to participate and persist is mediated by the athlete's minimum comparison level (the lowest criteria one uses to judge something as satisfying or unsatisfying) and the comparison level of alternative activities. Consequently, someone may choose to stay involved in sport even if costs are exceeded by rewards because no alternative opportunities are available. Similarly, an athlete who perceives that the rewards outweigh costs in a program may discontinue involvement because a more desirable alternative activity is available.

The key to the question of how an audience affects development of flexibility is the extent to which the individual values peer approval over personal goals. To avoid the potentially negative effects, it may be prudent to conduct practice sessions during the early stages of learning in privacy. In this way, peer pressure from either an active or a passive audience can be eliminated. It may be appropriate for the instructor to explain the factors that determine one's flexibility, thereby mitigating the influence of negative peer perceptions. Last, it may help to instill into students an understanding and appreciation of the rewards in partaking in the chosen discipline.

Effects of Coaction in Developing Flexibility Through Stretching

Coaction with teammates, that is, engaging in the same activity or task while in view of one another (Sage 1971), during the stretching or warm-up period just before a practice session or performance can be a definite aid in the development of flexibility. When teammates (or coactors) stretch and warm up together, they often provide each other with learning cues and thus serve as guides or models for one another. That is, they can reinforce correct responses to achieve optimum flexibility and warm-up.

However, coaction can also elicit the desired response through negative means. Social pressure may be imposed in practice, requiring capitulation or ostracism. Such an example is illustrated by Counsilman's (1968) concept of the *hurt-pain-agony approach* as employed in swimming. It suggests that unless one is willing to pay the price of the highest levels of discomfort, one is not likely to excel in sports. Pride is fostered when swimmers push themselves hard during the agony phase of exertion; furthermore, other team members will develop contempt for a laggard or one who does not "put out" in practice.

If suffering pain or discomfort becomes an everyday experience, shared by all members of the team, the aversion to it tends to subside. Consequently, the more the athletes engage in unemotional talk about their discomfort and pain, the more acceptable their discomfort becomes. Thus, they develop mental as well as physical callousness to pain. In short, athletes come to accept some degree of pain as a natural and necessary part of attaining their goals. Such an approach may be practical for such competitive disciplines as body building, swimming, and running, but it is definitely not ideal or practical for developing flexibility.

Theoretical Aspects of Mental Training

Mental training includes all psychological methods to improve performance. In flexibility training there is a need for the targeted muscles to relax during the stretching phase and for the body segments to move through the desired ROM at the desired velocity with the desired accuracy. Two mental training techniques that may be employed in a flexibility training program include *imagery*, or *visualization*, and *self-hypnosis*. They can be used for both tension management and performance enhancement. Mental training can theoretically facilitate the development of flexibility on two levels: a decreased motoneuron activation, resulting in greater relaxation, and altered programming levels of the motor system. The most illustrative research on the relationship between mental training and stretching is in the area of biofeedback and the use of imagination to enhance strength gains.

Cybernetic Stretch

One psychological approach to the development of flexibility is the *cybernetic stretch*, a technique developed by Bates (1976) as a direct adaptation

from Dr. Maxwell Maltz's highly recommended book *Psycho-Cybernetics* (1970). The basic approach here is "mind over matter." In the preface, Maltz states: "The 'self image' sets the boundaries of individual accomplishment. It defines what you can and cannot do. Expand the self image and you expand the area of the possible" (p. ix).

The psychocybernetic method consists of learning, practicing, and experiencing new habits of thinking, imaging, remembering, and acting in order to bring about success and happiness in achieving particular goals. Psychocybernetics holds that the human brain, nervous system, and muscular system are together a highly complex "servomechanism" used and directed by the mind. If you hold a picture of yourself long enough and steadily enough in your mind, you will be drawn toward it, and you must clearly see a thing in your mind before you can do it.

According to the psychocybernetic philosophy, experiencing success is the key to functioning successfully. Confidence is built upon the experience of success. When we first begin any undertaking, we are likely to have little confidence because we have not yet learned from experience that we can succeed. Fortunately, the nervous system cannot tell the difference between an imagined experience and a real experience. In either case, it reacts automatically to information given to it. Therefore, visualizing successful performance can build confidence and help enhance actual performance.

As described by Bates (1976), cybernetic stretch consists of two steps: the mental practice step and the direct practice step. Following Maltz's guidelines, the first task is to select a specific goal. To facilitate visualizing the goal, the "creative automatic mechanism" must be provided with facts. "Physiologically, a 50 percent increase in muscle length is possible if no inhibitions to stretch are operative; therefore your goal of 'making it flat' in the side split exists" (Bates 1976, 240). Of course, this assumes the absence of any structural limitations. It is essential to know that the goal is attainable and practical.

Next, by the use of imagination, one sets up mental images that one's "servomechanism" will work to fulfill. To do so properly, a mental practice period of 30 min each day for at least 21 days is recommended. The setting should be quiet, comfortable, and relaxing. The key to the mental practice step is making the image as real and as vivid as possible. As Bates (1976, 241) points out,

"It is most important that you see yourself successfully and ideally completing the flexibility action."

The final step is direct practice. Bates (1976, 240–241) writes:

> Skill learning of any kind is accomplished by trial and error, mentally correcting aim after an error, until a successful motion is achieved. Your servo-mechanism achieves its goal in the same manner, it remembers the successful responses and forgets the past errors. Stretch slowly, keeping spindle firing to a minimum, up to the point of pain; ease off slightly, causing spindles to stop firing briefly and allowing the muscle to relax. The servo-mechanism remembers that position and the absence of muscle contraction that opposes holding that relaxed position, if you are supplying it with the "end result" or goal.
>
> Relax while you maintain your held position; you must allow your servo-mechanism to work rather than force it to work. Connections exist on both alpha and gamma motor neurons from higher centers such that sensory information to these motor neurons may be offset by information from the higher brain centers. While relaxing, your servo-mechanism is finding the pathway and the degree of inhibition to maintain in order to achieve your goal.
>
> Proceed further forward when you have learned to reduce the tension at your present level. As increased stretch positions are achieved it is helpful to have a partner maintain your position, after you have eased off slightly. Initially, this aids in allowing the subject to relax, that is, concentrate on one thing at a time. In fact, it is often advisable in the very beginning for the partner to passively assist in increasing the range of motion, allowing for the easing off, and then maintain the subject's position.

Psychosomatic Factors

The idea that certain ailments and diseases may have psychosomatic aspects has been recognized for thousands of years. In the Bible we read: "A soft heart is the life of the flesh: but envy is the rottenness of the bones" (Proverbs 14:30) and "A merry heart doth good like medicine: but a broken spirit drieth the bones" (Proverbs 17:22). In recent times, there has been growing recognition and acceptance of psychosomatic disorders, which are physical disorders of the body that are caused or complicated by psychological factors. Two physical disorders of presumably psychogenic origin that potentially affect range of motion are myofascial trigger points (small nodules of spastic or degenerative muscle tissue that serve as focal points for referred pain and other noxious reflexes) and arthritis (Asterita 1985; McFarlane, Kalucy, and Brooks 1987). The growing recognition of the importance of this area is evident by the number of published articles, books, and journals that deal exclusively with this topic, including the *Journal of Psychosomatic Research*, the *Journal of Psychosomatic Medicine*, and *Psychosomatics*.

Psychology of Compliance in Preventive and Rehabilitative Programs

The history of patient compliance problems dates back at least 2,500 years to Hippocrates, who reported that patients often lied about taking their medicines and that, when treatment then failed, the physician was blamed by patients and their families (Ulmer 1989). With the rise of professional interest in the study of patient compliance, descriptive, anecdotal, and self-report approaches developed to facilitate compliance (Cousins 1979). Eventually, these approaches evolved into quantitative evaluations of carefully planned compliance interventions and outcomes (Ulmer 1989).

In the following sections, attention will be primarily devoted to athletes and nonathletes recovering from injury and in need of rehabilitation. However, it should be noted that compliance for the healthy individual is equally important in the maintenance of good health. Compliance is an economic concern for individuals and for corporations. For the ill and the healthy, it is also a matter of potential longevity and quality of life (Hilyer et al. 1990; Locke 1983).

Definition of Compliance

Webster's Dictionary defines *compliance* as "acquiescence to a wish, request, or demand" or "a disposition or tendency to yield to the will of others." Compliant behavior may be defined as a class behavior resulting from a specific set of cues and consequences (Ice 1985). Researchers who have studied health behavior have employed a number of other words for this concept: adherence, obedience, cooperation, concordance, collaboration, and therapeutic alliance (DiMatteo and DiNicola 1982).

Importance of Compliance

Compliance is important on a variety of levels. At the economic level, client compliance is vital to the financial success and livelihood of the proprietors and employees of health care businesses, including fitness and health clubs, yoga schools, medical and allied health care institutions, and medical care providers. Without client compliance (e.g., registering or signing up for classes, attending appointments, and receiving services), there is no income. Thus, there is an ulterior financial motive when the client is told to adhere to a given practice or recommendation. Perhaps for this reason many clients do not trust the sincerity of the provider and hence fail in compliance.

Patients' noncompliance with prescribed treatment has long been the bane of the clinician and health care professional. Compliance and noncompliance affect patients, the health care provider, and society as a whole. When patients fail to carry out their instructions and programs, the health care provider's experience and expertise are nullified (Fisher, Domm, and Wuest 1988). Noncompliance interferes with the practitioners' therapeutic efforts. Obviously, failure to adhere to directions can exacerbate the condition of the patient. As a consequence, the practitioner may needlessly order a renewed round of diagnostic evaluations or prescribe another second-choice treatment regimen. Most important, it may perhaps take longer for the patient to recover (DiMatteo and DiNicola 1982; Fisher, Domm, and Wuest 1988; Johnson 1991). Conversely, when patients comply, treatment outcomes improve dramatically.

Noncompliance is also important because of its potential concomitant cost to the health care system and the economy. Compliance is very important in preventive measures—those that seek to forestall, reduce the severity of, or prevent the occurrence of undesired consequences. Failure to follow directions adds to society's costs through lost work time, productivity, and income. It also increases expenses to insurance companies, which in turn pass on costs in the form of increased insurance premiums to the public. Patients' failure to keep medical appointments is expensive because clinician and clerical staff time is wasted (Sackett and Snow 1979). If patients drop out of treatment, their histories, physical exams, and tests must be repeated when they seek care in another medical setting (DiMatteo, Prince, and Taranta 1979; Kasteler et al. 1976). Then, if treatment fails or diagnoses are delayed, the question may arise as to who was responsible for the failure. Too often, this confusion results in malpractice issues (Ulmer 1989).

Factors Contributing to Compliance and Noncompliance

A variety of factors influence the compliance or noncompliance of a patient, including such things as age, intelligence, medical knowledge, state of anxiety, mood, social support, self-motivation, economic factors, perceived exertion, discomfort or pain tolerance, and available time (Ice 1985; Ley 1977; Milberg and Clark 1988; G. Miller et al. 1977). Another factor is a patient's ability to remember advice dispensed by health practitioners. Common sense dictates that patients cannot be expected to comply with advice or information that they cannot remember (Ice 1985).

Given that recall is vital for optimal compliance, how can it be facilitated? Research indicates that the way in which medical information is presented to a patient may affect recall (Ice 1985). An experiment by Ley (1977) found that recall after oral, visual, or written presentation was not significantly different. However, the investigation revealed that the information given earliest in the presentation was retained better than that provided later. "In clinical practice, this research suggests placing instructions and advice first and stressing their importance will reduce forgetfulness and increase recall" (Ice 1985, 1833).

Compliance: A Matter of Faith

What does one actually desire when compliance is sought from another? The answer is an act of faith! Belief is commonly defined as a state or habit of mind in which trust or confidence is placed in some person or thing. We may define compliance as an action based upon a belief. All the belief that one holds is useless unless something concrete follows—there must be an action. This is true for almost any situation in which the compliance of another is sought. Doctors, therapists, athletic trainers, teachers, even baby-sitters all want the same thing: action and not just words. But to gain a patient's compliance, a health care provider must gain that patient's trust.

Practical Strategies for Securing Compliance

Over the years, numerous practitioners and researchers have proposed various strategies to improve compliance. Although there are no guaranteed methods, there are several important do's and don'ts for health care providers. Two obvious reminders are that there is no such thing as an average person and that no two people are alike. Table 11.1 presents one example of a summary of suggestions for improving communication with patients.

Summary

The mind sets the boundaries of individual accomplishment and defines what one can and cannot do. Accordingly, if one can expand the self-image and mind, one can expand the "area of the possible." However, being social in nature, we are affected by the presence of people around us. This influence may be perceived as positive, neutral, or negative.

A major determining factor of the success of a flexibility training program or a rehabilitative program is the compliance of the patient or athlete. Compliance is action based upon belief. Numerous theories have been proposed to explain the nature of compliance and potential strategies that facilitate compliance.

Table 11.1. Suggestions for Improving Communication With Patients

Satisfaction	Short waiting time
	Be friendly rather than businesslike
	Some talk about nonmedical topics
	Listen to patient
	Find out what worries are
	Find out what expectations are—if not to be met, say why
Selecting content	What does patient want to know
	What are the patient's health beliefs:
	Vulnerability
	Seriousness
	Effectiveness
	Costs and barriers
	What do you want the patient to know
	What motivating communications help
Understanding and memory	Avoid jargon
	Use short words and short sentences—simplification
	Encourage feedback
	Increase recall
	Primacy
	Stressed importance
	Explicit categorization
	Specific rather than general
	Repetition
	Written back-up
	Readability
	Physical format:
	Letter size
	Color
	Quality of print and paper

Chapter 12

Stretching Concepts

Traditionally, many sports and disciplines have accepted the *hurt-pain-agony* approach to training. This philosophy has been widely adopted and widely proselytized. However, this philosophy is due to a lack of knowledge about normal ROM, the causes of restricted motion, and the most effective and efficient methods of increasing flexibility, among other things.

Why do people find it so difficult to motivate themselves to stretch regularly? Many people lack knowledge about proper stretching and how it should be done. Because many physical educators and coaches teach the philosophy that unless stretching hurts, it is not doing any good, few physical educators present an approach to stretching that could be useful and enjoyable in everyday life. Anderson (1978) addressed this issue with reference to runners. He argues that the painful experience, which many runners believe is the correct approach to stretching, is not the approach that leads to everyday benefits and enjoyment. Another practical explanation is that many people are just too busy with everyday activities such as work and raising a family. This can be a particular problem for health care providers, who may instruct a patient to perform a series of exercises as either a preventive or rehabilitative measure, with which the patient fails to comply.

Consequently, the task that we face is one of *reeducation*. What needs to be taught is that stretching is both beneficial and potentially enjoyable. It must also be stressed that the quality of stretching, not the quantity of stretching, is what ultimately determines the degree of flexibility. If one wishes to obtain optimal development of flexibility, the hurt-pain-agony concept should be discarded.

Homeostasis

Homeostasis may be defined as the maintenance of a steady state. Organisms have means of maintaining steady states in their internal environments, which are, in large measure, a product of the organism and controlled by it, and also in their external environments. Stressful environmental factors (such as overwork) may alter the steady state of an organism. When an organism's ability to maintain homeostatic control is exceeded, injury or death may result.

The concept of homeostasis can be extended to the cellular and even subcellular level. Thus, within certain limits, the cell is capable of adjusting to varying demands. However, like the organism as a whole, its adaptive capability may be exceeded, and cellular injury or death may follow.

One's response to stress depends in part on one's ability to adapt oneself to new conditions. During or following stress, the functioning of the homeostatic mechanism may change, and the individual may enter a new state. This process is called *adaptation*. Research indicates that adaptive responses for increased flexibility involve both functional and structural changes. Consequently, there can be quantitative as well as qualitative improvement in performance. However, for such changes to occur, one's homeostatic state must be overloaded.

The Overstretching Principle

Doherty (1985, 425) suggests that "if we accept the word *overloading* as related to building strength in muscles, then overstretching should be acceptable in building flexibility." This *overstretching principle* is the physiological principle on which flexibility development depends. According to this principle, when the body is regularly stimulated by an increasingly intense stretching program, it will respond with an increased ability to stretch. Therefore, the body adapts to the increasing demands placed on it.

Flexibility is simply a result of stretching. No other factor is more important in the development of flexibility in a healthy person. Stretching may be applied either manually (i.e., by oneself or a partner) or by machine. Increased flexibility is achieved by implementing a movement that exceeds the existing range of possible motion (A. Jones 1975). Consequently, flexibility is best acquired by stretching up to the edge of discomfort. Needless to say, discomfort is a subjective matter and will vary from person to person.

Retention of Flexibility

The question of what happens to the flexibility of joints when a stretching program ceases has not received the attention that other aspects of stretching programs have received (Zebas and Rivera 1985). An investigation by Möller, Ekstrand, Öberg, and Gillquist (1985) compared the retention of flexibility in several treated muscle groups 0, 30, 60, and 90 min after the stretching procedure. The increased flexibility remained for 90 min for most of the muscle groups. In a subsequent study, Möller, Öberg, and Gillquist (1985, 52) found "the effect of stretching done at the start of the session persists over the training session and up to 24 hours." In reviewing the literature, Zebas and Rivera (1985) point out that in a number of studies attention has primarily been focused on the hip joint, and in all cases a significant amount of flexibility was retained in the hip joint. Specifically, their review found that hip flexibility was retained after 3 weeks (Long 1971), 4 weeks (Tweitmeyer 1974), 8 weeks (McCue 1963), and several months (Riddle 1956). Other significant flexibility retention was found in the neck joint (McCue 1963; Turner 1977) and back (McCue 1963). A retention of flexibility 4 weeks after cessation was also found in the study by Zebas and Rivera (1985). However, they point out that "even though flexibility was retained from the pretesting period

through the retention period, there were significant losses of flexibility from the posttesting period to 2 weeks after the cessation of exercise" (pp. 188–189). They also point out one major limitation of such longitudinal measures: The activities outside of the class could not be monitored or controlled.

Requisite Knowledge for Stretching

The methods of stretching employed in the disciplines of athletics, dance, physical therapy, and yoga can vary considerably. However, certain knowledge is required in all of these disciplines. A basic knowledge of the normal neuromuscular mechanism, including motor development, anatomy, neurophysiology, and kinesiology is very helpful, if not essential. Furthermore, whatever the method of stretching used, one should be thoroughly familiar with the structure and function of the joint in question. One should know not only the degree of limitation of motion, but also which tissues are responsible for the limitations.

Joint Flexibility Limitations

Range of motion at a joint, and thus flexibility, is restricted primarily by five factors:

1. Lack of elasticity of connective tissues in muscles or joints
2. Muscle tension
3. Lack of coordination and strength in the case of active movement
4. Bone and joint structure limitations
5. Pain

To increase ROM at a joint, stretching procedures must therefore do at least one of three things: (1) increase the extensibility of connective tissues in muscles or joints, (2) reduce muscular tension and thus produce relaxation, or (3) increase the coordination of the body segments and the strength of the agonistic muscle group (Table 12.1). Generally speaking, loss of motion due to abnormal bone and joint structure is beyond the scope of traditional stretching procedures.

Table 12.1. Theoretical Model of Approaches and Courses of Action to Improve Range of Motion

Approach	Psychological conditions	Courses of action	
		Physical	Psychological
Decrease resistance of target area	Lengthen connective tissue	(a) Prolonged stretch (b) Contract target area while under stretch	
	Relax myotatic reflex	(a) Reciprocal inhibition	(a) Mind-set (gamma bias)
		(b) Accommodation	(b) Biofeedback (monitored inhibition)
		(c) Heat, ice, massage, exercise fatigue, etc.	(c) Relaxation training
		(d) Strength training	
Increase strength of opposing muscles	Muscle loading of opposing muscles	(a) Isometric (b) Concentric (c) Eccentric	(a) Motivation
	Facilitation techniques	(a) Successive induction (proprioceptive neuromuscular facilitation)	(a) Learning: recruitment, coordination, synchronization

Reprinted from Hartley-O'Brien (1980).

Other Principles of Stretching

Following are some principles that should be observed when developing flexibility. These principles are not necessarily the final word but do represent some of the more important points to remember when undertaking a flexibility training program.

Safety

Safety always comes first. Although the coach, instructor, or trainer is ultimately responsible for the safety of the participants, participants should also be involved in the prevention of injury. Safety requires attitudes, skills, and knowledge about the control of potential hazards. The American Alliance for Health, Physical Education, and Recreation (1968) advocates a simple four-step approach to safety issues: (1) know the hazards, (2) remove the hazards when feasible, (3) control the hazards that cannot be removed, and (4) create no additional hazards.

Medical Examination

Ideally, a medical examination should be obtained before undertaking any exercise program. Such an examination may reveal that certain types of stretching exercises are contraindicated (Rusk 1977). An example of contraindications for therapeutic muscle stretching (TMS), "specific muscle stretching performed, instructed, or supervised by a therapist in patients with dysfunctions of the musculoskeletal system," has been developed by Mühlemann and Cimino (1990, 255):

1. Lack of stability. TMS is contraindicated if joint integrity or stability is jeopardized or decreased by any (pathologic) process.

2. Endangered vascular integrity. Pathologic processes or drugs (e.g., anticoagulants) can endanger vascular integrity or facilitate bleeding.

3. Inflammation or infection in and around the involved structures.

4. Acute injury to the soft tissues and muscles. If performed without sufficient time for healing, TMS must be postponed until scar formation is sufficient for moderate tensile loads to be tolerated.

5. Diseases of the soft tissues and muscles. Contraindications can be relative (i.e., TMS can or cannot be administered dependent on the actual condition of the tissue, the operator's skills, the patient's cooperation, and so forth) or absolute (as in conditions such as myositis ossificans).

6. Lack of patient compliance and excessive pain or reaction. Any therapeutic maneuver is contraindicated if the patient cannot or does not want to tolerate its application. If the pain during TMS is not tolerated even though TMS is administered skillfully and as painlessly as possible, then TMS maneuvers should not be used. Patients may be taught self-stretching exercises instead, the performance of which should be supervised, and, later, controlled periodically.

7. When common sense says "NO."

Identifiable Goals

One should define one's goals before beginning a flexibility program and have an idea of the time it will take to reach the desired degree of flexibility. For example, the goal may be the ability to place the palms flat on the floor with legs straight after 6 weeks of stretching. Whatever the goals may be, they should be realistic.

Individualized Program

Ideally, all exercises should be designed to fit an individual's specific needs. However, one is often expected to fit into a group or team in a flexibility program. The question then arises, Should a coach insist that a given stretch be held for a specific time, or rather encourage each athlete to sustain the stretch until his or her individual threshold or objective is fulfilled?

The answer to this question depends on a number of factors. Ideally, one should have already warmed up and stretched out on one's own before participating in the team stretch. However, doing so is not always possible or even desirable if the individual does not have the knowledge to

warm up and stretch safely. In most instances, the team approach is the most appropriate course to follow. At least some stretching is guaranteed if one participates in a group, and a team program also fosters camaraderie and team spirit. At the end of the team workout, each individual can concentrate on those muscles that need additional stretching.

However, if one is stretching in a class at a fitness or health club, one should listen to one's own body and either participate with the class or hold the stretch as individually appropriate. In such a class, there may be a wider range of abilities, and stretching beyond one's safety limit is a real possibility, especially for beginners. Instructors should educate class members about which and to what degree exercises should be attempted. In addition, instructors should tell their students that there is nothing wrong with stopping and resting in the middle of a class session or modifying an exercise. Adaptation is particularly appropriate in the case of fatigue, pain, or excessive difficulty with a given exercise. It is vital that the instructor constantly monitor all members of the class during the workout for potential complications.

Keep Accurate Records

A well-planned program is also a recorded one. Records should include the date and time of exercise; types of exercises performed; exercise intensity, duration, and frequency; and self-evaluation before, during, and after the program. A number of devices can be used for measuring and evaluating ROM, ranging from the sophisticated and expensive to the simple and inexpensive. They include radiography, photography, schematography, outline tracing, goniometers or protractors, electrogoniometers, tape measures, performance charts, and visual observations. The value of record keeping may be purely motivational, or it may reveal positive or negative patterns in the training program (Uram 1980).

Expect Gradual Progress

The development of flexibility takes time; it does not develop overnight. Therefore, be sure to set realistic goals and remember that it is necessary to begin with easy exercises before advancing to more difficult ones. Plateaus, or periods of no apparent progress, are part of the learning process.

Comparing and Competing

Do not attempt to compare yourself to others. Improvement and progress are important, not competition with someone who may be at an entirely different level of ability. No two people are alike: Some may develop flexibility rapidly; others may take a longer period of time to reach the same level (Figure 12.1).

Clothing and Positioning

Wear loose and comfortable clothes when working out. Because a warmed muscle is believed to be more flexible and pliant, people often wear sweat suits and wool socks. Position yourself as comfortably as possible to reduce muscle tension and make the stretching more enjoyable.

Attitude

A positive mental attitude is important. The mental, physical, and spiritual aspects of life are inseparable from one another. Without a positive mind set, the best of all possible results will never be achieved in a flexibility training program.

Relaxation

Relaxation is the opposite of tension. Tension originates in contracted muscles and results in inflexibility, an insufficient oxygen supply, and fatigue. The ability to relax is important because it decreases tension and its negative consequences, thus allowing one to function more effectively and efficiently. If you want to learn to relax, learn to listen to your body. Stretch slowly

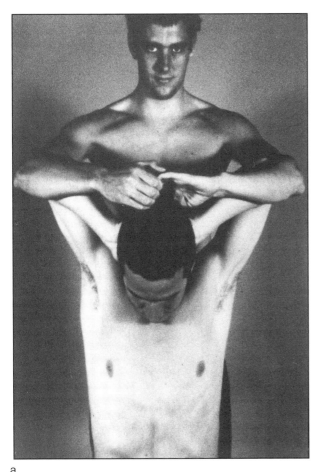

a

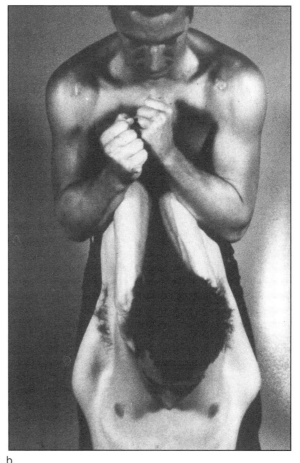

b

Fig. 12.1. Comparing degrees of flexibility in different individuals. Each swimmer was able to perform at peak efficiency. If the individual in (a) tried to equal the limits of flexibility of the individual in (b), he may have overstretched musculotendinous units beyond their effective ranges. (a) An NCAA division II gold-medal winner in the 100-yard freestyle. (b) An NCAA division II gold-medal winner in the 200-yard butterfly.
Photo courtesy of J.V. Ciullo, M.D.

and exhale gently at the moment of maximum stretch. Do not hold your breath. Concentrate on, and be totally aware of, the task at hand to ensure the deepest relaxation.

Warm-Up and Cool-Down

Warm-up and cool-down exercises improve performance and reduce the chances of injury. The most important advantages of both active and passive warm-ups are increased muscle temperature, reduced muscular viscosity, decreased muscular tension, and more extensible tissue. See chapter 10 for more information about warm-up and cool-down.

Isolate the Muscle

For stretching to be most beneficial, the proper muscle group must receive the activity, and compensation by other muscles and structures (e.g., the spine) reduced. For example, the anterior tilt position was determined to be more important than stretching technique (PNF or static stretching) for increasing hamstring muscle length (Sullivan, Dejulia, and Worrell 1992).

Application of the SAID Principle

According to Wallis and Logan (1964), strength, endurance, and flexibility training should be based on the principle of *specific adaptation to imposed demands* (SAID). That is, one should stretch at a velocity not less than 75% of the maximum velocity through the exact plane of motion, through the exact range of motion, and at the precise joint angles used while performing skills in a specific activity. For example, high leg kicks emulate punting a football. For movements performed at rapid velocity, a slow stretch should precede the application of the SAID principle.

Application of the Overstretching Principle: Stretching Duration, Frequency, Timing, and Intensity

The physiological principle on which strength development depends is the *overload principle*. Its analogue for flexibility is the *overstretching prin-*

ciple. The difference between the two is that the latter uses stretch while the former uses resistance—usually weight. Overstretching is a function of the duration, frequency, timing, nature, and intensity of the stretch.

Most programs recommend holding each stretch for 6 to 12 s. However, 10 to 30 s is also commonly recommended. Bandy and Irion (1994) compared the effectiveness of 15, 30, and 60 s of static stretching of the hamstrings. Their study revealed that 30 and 60 s of stretching were more effective at increasing hamstring flexibility than stretching for 15 s or no stretching at all. "In addition, no significant difference existed between stretching 30 seconds and for 1 minute, indicating that 30 seconds of stretching the hamstring muscles was as effective as the longer duration of 1 minute" (p. 845). Madding et al. (1987) compared the effectiveness of a 15-s, 45-s, and 2-min passive stretch to increase hip abduction ROM in 72 male subjects. No significant mean difference between the three groups was demonstrated. Based on this data, the authors concluded that it was "reasonable to stretch 15 seconds in athletic settings where immediate increases in abduction ROM are desired" (p. 416). Research by Borms et al. (1987) suggests that a duration of 10 s for static stretching is sufficient for improving hip joint flexibility. According to Bates (1971), 60 s of maintained stretch is optimal for increasing and retaining flexibility.

There also appears to be a difference of opinion regarding the most effective frequency or number of repetitions (C.A. Smith 1994). Taylor et al. (1990) experimented using rabbit extensor digitorum longus and tibialis anterior muscle and tendon units. They found that the greatest change in muscle and tendon length occurred in the first four stretches. Further stretching did not result in significant increases in length.

As a general rule, you should stretch at least once a day for maintenance of flexibility. Such daily workouts are feasible if interest and motivation can be maintained (Rasch and Burke 1989). However, empirical evidence suggests that stretching at least twice a day is preferable. The best times appear to be in the morning after awakening (to eliminate morning stiffness and energize oneself) and in the afternoon or early evening after the day's work. However, the best time to stretch is when you feel as if you want to.

Several options are possible for the placement of the stretching program within a workout: before or after an exercise program or both. Opinions on the specific placement of stretching exercise are usually based on an intuition. In investigating this question, Cornelius, Hagemann, and Jackson (1988) found that adherence to a static flexibility program will produce gains in joint range of motion regardless of the placement of the flexibility routine. Their findings refute claims that specific placement of stretching exercises within a workout session makes a difference in increasing ROM. They found instead that placement was more relevant for "other objectives such as increasing tissue temperature and reducing tissue discomfort that might be affected by specific placement of stretching" (p. 236).

The intensity of the stretch should also be up to you. Although stretch may produce some discomfort (especially for beginners), it should not be so great a discomfort as to cause pain. As a general rule, if your muscle begins to quiver and vibrate, if pain persists, or if ROM decreases, you have stretched too much, and either the force or the duration of the stretch should be decreased. Discomfort and pain are subjective matters, so there is no absolute answer about where to draw the line. The best advice is to use common sense: Train, don't strain.

Mechanics

The individual must use proper mechanics and techniques when stretching to achieve optimal results. Applying proper mechanics involves identifying and isolating those muscles and tissues to be stretched and using the appropriate exercise to fulfill that goal. Correct technique reduces the risk of injury and the impairment of performance.

Stretch Reflex

Generally speaking, laypeople should use slow or static methods of stretch. Sudden or painful movements may elicit a stretch reflex, causing the muscle to contract (see chapter 6). Therefore, ballistic stretching should be avoided, especially during the early stages of a program. On the other hand, it is recognized that certain sports and disciplines necessitate ballistic stretching. For individuals engaged in those activities, it is strongly recommended that they first thoroughly warm up then progress from passive or static stretching to dynamic sports-related movements.

Anticipation and Communication

During passive stretching, partners should communicate with each other. It is the responsibility of the person being stretched to inform the partner when the stretch becomes unpleasant or painful. It is the responsibility of the person applying the stretch to anticipate how much overstretch should be employed. This activity is a two-way process.

Appropriate Injury Management

If an injury should occur, one should determine to the best of one's knowledge the extent of the damage. As a general rule, rest, apply ice and pressure, and elevate the injured part of the body, then seek appropriate medical care. The sooner an injury is treated, the earlier rehabilitation can begin and the faster the recovery will be. Again, a good rule of thumb is to use common sense.

Enjoyment

Stretching should be enjoyable and satisfying and create a sense of well-being. Enjoyment and pleasure are a matter of satisfying one's motives. However, stretching has the potential to involve varying degrees of pleasantness or unpleasantness. When stretching ceases to be enjoyable, it becomes self-defeating. To paraphrase Iyengar (1979), stretching can be compared to an electric current: Your muscles and connective tissues are the filament of the light bulb that is your body. When the proper flow reaches the bulb, it glows. So, too, can one's body and mind be illuminated.

Summary

Homeostasis is defined as maintenance of a steady state. In order to develop flexibility, one's homeostatic state must be exceeded by added stress to enter a new state, in a process called adaptation. Overstretching is the physiological principle on which flexibility development depends: When one stretches regularly, the body will respond with an increased ability to stretch. For stretching to be successful, a movement must actually exceed the existing range of motion.

Before engaging in a stretching program, one should have some knowledge about anatomy, physiology, and the structure and functions of joints. In addition, there are a number of important principles to observe when developing flexibility: Safety always comes first; expect gradual progress; warm up and cool down; and use appropriate medical treatment in case of injury.

Chapter 13

Types and Varieties of Stretching

Coaches and teachers of sports, dance, yoga, and other highly specialized physical activities have long recognized the need for more than normal flexibility in certain joints or groups of joints. To help the participants under their direction achieve this flexibility, they have developed special stretching exercises and drills, which can be broadly classified into two categories: ballistic and static. In addition, a variety of stretching devices and machines have been developed to facilitate the development or maintenance of flexibility.

Traditional Classifications of Stretching

Ballistic stretching is usually associated with bobbing, bouncing, rebounding, and rhythmic motion. Often the terms *dynamic*, *fast*, *isotonic*, or *kinetic* are used to refer to this kind of stretching. In contrast, *static* stretching involves the use of a position that is held and that may or may not be repeated. Synonyms for static stretching are *isometric*, *controlled*, or *slow* stretching.

Regardless of the method employed, the possibility of stretching beyond one's safety limit depends on a variety of factors, including the intensity of the stretch; the duration of the stretch; the frequency, or number of movements performed in a given period; and the velocity or nature of the stretch.

Ballistic Stretching

One of the most controversial topics in sports science is the relative value of ballistic versus static stretching programs for developing flexibility. The controversy is complicated by the lack of research on ballistic flexibility. Ballistic stretching is difficult to assess because of the need for elaborate equipment and technical expertise in measuring the force that is required to move the joint through its range of motion at both fast and slow speeds (Stamford 1981). There is, however, a considerable amount of research indicating that both ballistic and static methods are effective in developing flexibility (Corbin and Noble 1980; Logan and Egstrom 1961; Sady, Wortman, and Blanke 1982; Stamford 1981; Weber and Kraus 1949).

Arguments Supporting Ballistic Stretching

There are four major arguments supporting ballistic stretching, based on its following advantages: development of dynamic flexibility, effectiveness, team camaraderie, and interest. Most important, ballistic stretching helps to develop dynamic flexibility. Because most activities and movements are dynamic in nature, ballistic stretching permits specificity in training and warm-up. For example, ballistic training has been time-tested in various martial arts.

In terms of effectiveness, a study by Vujnovich and Dawson (1994) demonstrated that ballistic stretch following static stretch appears to be more effective than static stretch alone in reducing alpha motoneuron pool excitability, which correlates with increased flexibility. However, these results should be interpreted with caution considering the size of the static and ballistic stretching groups—14 and 5 people, respectively. A practical advantage of ballistic stretching is its use during team stretching and warm-up, for it can be easily practiced in unison to a beat or cadence, thus promoting team camaraderie. Finally, ballistic stretching can be less boring than static stretching (Dowsing 1978; Olcott 1980).

Arguments Against Ballistic Stretching

There are four major arguments against ballistic stretching. These arguments involve the following disadvantages: inadequate tissue adaptation, soreness resulting from injury, initiation of the stretch reflex, and inadequate neurological adaptation.

When muscle and its supporting connective tissues are rapidly stretched, they are not given adequate time to adapt. All living tissues are characterized by the presence of time-dependent mechanical properties, including *stress-relaxation* and *creep* (see chapter 5). If tissues are stretched too rapidly, lasting flexibility cannot be optimally developed. Research has demonstrated that permanent lengthening is most effectively achieved by lower force, longer duration stretching at elevated temperatures (Laban, 1962; Light et al. 1984; C.G. Warren, Lehmann, and Koblanski 1971, 1976).

Ballistic stretching should be avoided also because it generates rather large and uncontrollable amounts of angular momentum. This can be demonstrated by swinging the arms horizontally in an extended position. Consequently, when the movement reaches its limit and suddenly stops, the angular momentum can often exceed the absorbing capacity of the tissues being stretched. Practical examples are improper or uncontrolled swings in such disciplines as baseball and golf.

A logical extension of the first argument concerning tissue adaptation is the hypothesis that ballistic stretching can result in soreness or injury. Obviously, if a tissue is stretched too fast, it can be strained or ruptured. In either event, the result is pain or impairment of ROM. As an example, imagine a 3-cm rubber band rapidly stretched to a length of 6 to 8 cm. Under those conditions, the rubber band will probably rupture. However, if the rubber band is slowly stretched through the same range, it is less likely to break. The mechanical explanation is that the

rubber band is not required to absorb the same amount of energy per unit of time. However, if progressively stretched, all tissues will ultimately reach a point of rupture, regardless of velocity.

A third argument against ballistic stretching concerns the stretch reflex. If a sudden stretch is applied to a muscle, a reflex action is set into motion that causes the muscle to contract. As a result, muscular tension will increase, making it more difficult to stretch out the connective tissues and defeating the very purpose of the stretching procedure. Generally, for stretching to be safest, the contractile elements of the muscle should be totally relaxed.

Finally, it can be argued that ballistic stretching does not allow adequate time for neurological adaptation to take place. For example, Walker (1961) found that the amount of tension for a given amount of stretch is more than doubled by a quick stretch as compared with a slow stretch. Similarly, Granit (1962) reported that a pull on a muscle with a given force produced an efferent impulse frequency of more than 100 impulses per second within 1 s after the stretch. However, with a slower increase in muscle length until the same force was applied, a peak volley of only 40 impulses per second was produced within 6 s. This reduced motoneuron firing frequency reduces the tension in the muscle.

Implementing a Safe Ballistic Stretching Program

If ballistic movements are to be a part of a stretching program, how should they be implemented? Zachazewski (1990) recommends a *progressive velocity flexibility program* (PVFP). As with all programs, the PVFP is preceded by a warm-up. Then, over a course of time, the individual goes through "a series of stretching exercises in which the velocity and range of lengthening are combined and controlled on a progressive basis" (p. 228). This gradual program permits the muscle and musculotendinous junction to progressively adapt to functional ballistic movements. Hence, this will reduce the risk of injury. Zachazewski (1990, 228) briefly describes the program as follows:

> The athlete progresses from an environment of control to activity simulation, from slow-velocity methodical activity to high-velocity functional activity. After static stretching, slow short end of range (SSER) ballistic stretching is initiated. The athlete then progresses to slow full

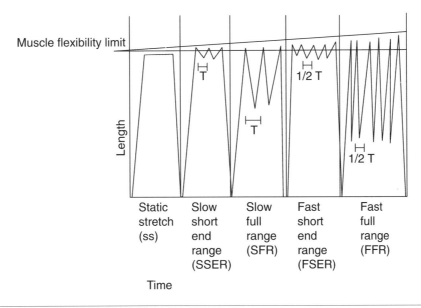

Fig. 13.1 Progressive velocity flexibility program.
Reprinted from Zachazewski (1990).

range stretching (SFR), fast short end range (FSER) and fast full range (FFR) stretching. Control and range are the responsibility of the athlete. NO outside force is exerted by anyone else. [see Figure 13.1 and Table 13.1]

Table 13.1. Progressive Velocity Flexibility Program

Static stretching
↓
SSER—Slow, short end range stretching
↓
SFR—Slow, full range stretching
↓
FSER—Fast, short end range stretching
↓
FFR—Fast, full range stretching

Reprinted from Zachazewski (1990).

Static Stretching

Static stretching involves a position that is held for a period of time and that may or may not be repeated. The key qualities of static stretching are maximum control, little or no movement, and minimal to no velocity of movement. The pros and cons of static stretching are reviewed in the following sections.

Arguments Supporting Static Stretching

Traditionally, there appears to be general agreement that static or slow stretching is preferable to ballistic stretching. Static stretching has been used for centuries by practitioners of hatha-yoga and is time proven. Static stretching is scientifically based and has been proven to be effective in enhancing ROM. Other advantages of static stretching are that it meets the typical restraints of limited funds and time and requires less space. Static stretching can be performed anywhere. Furthermore, some argue that static stretching is required for the optimal development of static flexibility (i.e., specificity of training). Research by Thigpen (1984) demonstrated that short bouts of static stretching reduced electrical activity within the muscle, which theoretically facilitates stretching. According to de Vries (1966, 1986), static stretching is preferable to the ballistic method because it requires less energy expenditure, it will probably result in less muscle soreness, and it can provide more qualitative relief from muscular distress. A number of additional claims are commonly made about static stretching, but they are not supported by research.

Arguments Against Static Stretching

At first glance, the arguments against static stretching may not seem as substantive as those against ballistic stretching. On a superficial level, some claim that static stretching is boring. A more persuasive argument against static stretching is that it may be practiced exclusively, at the expense of ballistic exercise (Schultz 1979). Because the vast majority of activities and movements are ballistic in nature, static stretching is not the optimal technique for specificity of training. An optimal blending of both stretching methods is the solution to this problem (Corbin and Noble 1980; Dick 1980; Schultz 1979; Stamford 1981).

Murphy (1991) carried out a critical and substantive review on the shortcomings of static stretching. His investigation revealed that the supposed usefulness of static stretching usually was attributed to one of five causes: (1) it aids warm-up, (2) it aids cool-down, (3) it helps relieve postexercise delayed-onset muscle soreness, (4) it helps enhance athletic performance, and (5) it helps prevent injury. However, the literature provides very little support for these notions. In fact, clinical research as well as neuromuscular physiological principles indicate that these rationales for static stretching are incorrect.

First, Murphy points out that since the very nature of static stretching is passive, it does nothing to increase core or peripheral temperatures. Hence, it does not aid as a warm-up. Second, again because it is passive, static stretching does not facilitate the redirection of blood flow away from the muscles that have been exercised and therefore cannot aid in cool-down. Third, the original notion that static stretching relieves delayed muscle soreness as originally proposed by de Vries (1961a) has not been reproduced in the studies of McGlynn, Laughlin, and Rowe (1979) and Buroker and Schwane (1989). Furthermore, research by Abraham (1977) found that static stretching only provided relief for 1 to 2 min after active exercise. Fourth, there are no scientific studies to substantiate the claim that static stretching improves athletic performance. In fact, Iashvili (1983) showed that passive flexibility as developed by static stretching has a relatively low correlation to the level of sports achievement, whereas active flexibility has a relatively high correlation. Last, Murphy's careful search of the literature failed to support the notion that static stretching reduces injury. In elaborating on this point, Murphy (1991, 68) writes:

> While it has been shown that the lack of "flexibility" is highly correlated to increased injury rate (Ekstrand and Gillquist 1982, 1983), it has never been shown that SS [static stretching] as a means of establishing flexibility does anything to prevent injury. Rather, as Iashvili (1983), Mora (1990), and Gajda (personal communication) have pointed out, SS can actually increase chances of muscular injuries, even if it is done "properly." (Iashvili 1983)

Furthermore, research by Wolpaw (1983) and Evatt, Wolf, and Segal (1989) has demonstrated that an individual can downtrain, or reduce the amplitude of, the stretch reflex. The stretch reflex is an important protective mechanism for the muscles and the joints that it controls (Radin 1989). With this downtraining, athletes may be prone to stretching beyond their safety limits, causing injury.

In addition to the issues posed by Murphy, one more challenge can be raised. It is often reported that an advantage of static stretching is its facilitation of two physical characteristics of soft tissues: stress-relaxation and creep. The question that needs to be answered is, What is the minimum amount of time necessary for these actions to take place in a living person? Stress-relaxation and creep take place during sustained traction of 10 to 20 minutes. If it requires this amount of time for stress-relaxation and creep to develop, then this argument for static stretching is not valid in a nonclinical setting because "compliance may decrease if durations of stretching are too long, particularly in people with muscle tightness" (Bandy and Irion 1994, 58).

Additional Classifications

In addition to the foregoing traditional categories of stretching, there is another way to classify stretching or exercises for the maintenance of ROM, based on who or what is responsible for the range of motion (Figures 13.2 and 13.3). The movement can be further analyzed as to whether it is free or resistive. In the following sections, several categories of stretch are discussed. Among several of the more well-known types are passive, passive-active, active-assisted, and active.

Passive Stretching

In *passive* stretching, as the name implies, the individual makes no contribution to generating the stretching force, as in the absence of active contraction (i.e., voluntary muscular effort). Rather, the motion is performed by an outside agent (see Figure 13.3a). This agent may be either a partner or special equipment such as traction equipment. Irrgang (1993) divides passive exercise into *physiologic* or *accessory* components. He further divides passive physiologic exercise into ROM and stretching. *Passive physiologic ROM* is motion that occurs within the unrestricted range of motion—

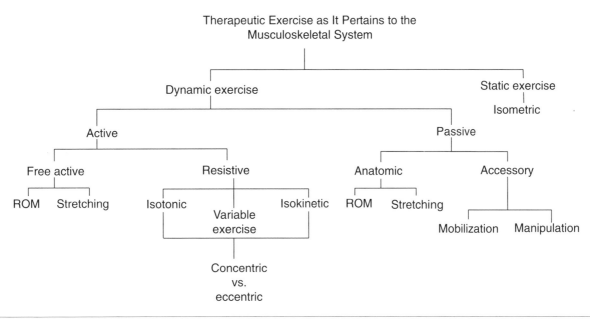

Fig. 13.2. The categorization of therapeutic exercise in the treatment of the musculoskeletal system.
Reprinted from Irrgang (1993).

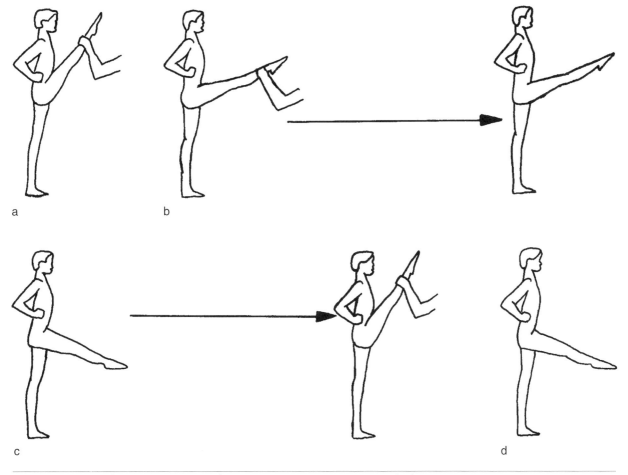

Fig. 13.3. Types of motion. (a) Passive. (b) Passive-active. (c) Active-assisted. (d) Active.
Reprinted from Alter (1988).

the normal ROM for a given joint. In contrast, *passive physiologic stretching* incorporates movements beyond the restricted range—the available ROM at a specific joint with restricted, or limited, motion—which are executed in an attempt to increase motion.

Passive accessory motions are those motions or movements that the individual is not capable of producing by voluntary muscle contraction. They are usually performed by a health care practitioner to increase joint play. Passive accessory movement is traditionally classified as mobilization or manipulation. In chapter 14, these topics will be discussed in detail. For now, these terms will simply be defined. *Mobilization* involves low-velocity, medium- to high-amplitude passive movements of one or more joints, sometimes in graded oscillations. In contrast, *manipulations* use a sudden, high-velocity, low-amplitude thrusting technique at the end of the available range of motion.

With the passive stretching technique, forced motion restores the normal ROM when it is limited by the loss of soft tissue extensibility. Its effect on muscle is to lengthen the elastic portion passively. The greater length will then allow greater ROM in the affected joints. Passive stretching is indicated either because the agonist, or prime mover, is too weak to move the joint, or because attempts to inhibit the antagonistic muscle are unsuccessful.

According to Dowsing (1978) and Olcott (1980), passive stretching with partners provides several additional benefits:

1. Teammates counting for each other ensure that repetitions are completed. Furthermore, the individual tries harder to complete the repetitions because the partner is always watching.
2. The coach is free to walk around to help with corrections. Once a correction is made, that partner can help future partners avoid the same mistakes.
3. A greater feeling of progress exists when partners can recognize improvement in others and let them know it.
4. Exercises performed with partners tend to promote the teammates' concern for one another.
5. Tandem exercises are more enjoyable.

However, when implementing partner flexibility exercises, both partners need to be totally familiar with each exercise. Because each partner is working the other's body, each must listen to the other's signals for stopping and holding the stretch. Just one mistake by a partner can wipe out all the benefits of a flexibility training program.

Passive stretching may not be the optimal technique in treating tightness (Cherry 1980) or in attempting to regain muscular range of motion, especially after injury (Jacobs 1976). According to Jacobs, there appear to be at least four reasons why passive stretching is contraindicated. First, extreme stretch could cause the Golgi tendon organs (GTOs) to fire. Second, passive stretching can be painful. Third, there is no retention of flexibility because the muscular imbalance is not eradicated by the GTO's short-lived inhibitory message. Consequently, there is no motor learning and no improvement in the capacity for active motion of the tight muscle or its antagonist. Fourth, if passive stretching occurs too rapidly, the muscle spindle complex may be activated, and the resultant stretch reflex would initiate contraction of the muscle, thus defeating the very purpose of the procedure.

Passive-Active Stretching

Passive-active stretching is only slightly different from passive stretching. Initially, the stretch is accomplished by some outside force. Then the individual attempts to hold the position by contracting the agonistic muscles isometrically for several seconds (see Figure 13.3b). This approach strengthens the weak agonist opposing the tight muscle.

Active-Assisted Stretching

Active-assisted stretching is accomplished by the initial active contraction of the agonistic group of muscles. When the limit of one's flexibility is reached, the range of motion is then completed by a partner (see Figure 13.3c). The advantage of this method is that it can activate or strengthen the weak agonist opposing the tight muscle and help to establish the pattern for coordinated motion.

Active Stretching

Active stretching is accomplished by the voluntary use of one's muscles without aid (see Figure 13.3d). Irrgang (1993) divides active exercise into two major classes, free active and resistive, each with its own components. *Free active* exercise or stretch "occurs when muscles produce movement without application of additional external resistance" (p. 82). Free active exercise comprises range of motion exercise and stretching. *Active ROM* exercises "include those movements within the unrestricted available range of motion and are produced by voluntary contraction of the individual's muscles" (p. 82). ROM exercises are performed to maintain the current level of motion, whereas *stretching* exercises are designed to enhance or increase motion.

Active exercises to increase flexibility can also use resistive strategies. *Resistive* exercises are defined by Irrgang (1993) as "those exercises in which the individual utilizes voluntary muscle contractions to move against an applied resistance" (p. 82). The resistance may be mechanical, as in the case of isokinetic machines, or manual. Examples of resistive exercise to enhance ROM are PNF and muscle energy techniques (MET). Resistive exercises may include concentric or eccentric contractions.

Research by Iashvili (1983) has verified that active ROM values are lower than passive ones, but active flexibility has a higher correlation to the level of sports achievement (*r* = .81) than does passive mobility (*r* = .69). In addition, Iashvili also found that when using stretching exercises primarily, the coefficient of correlation between active and passive movements varies within the limits of .61 to .73. However, when using strength and combined exercises (active and passive), the coefficient of correlation increases to .91. Therefore, it can be concluded that the relationship between passive and active flexibility is dependent on the training methods (Hardy 1985; Iashvili 1983; Tumanyan and Dzhanyan 1984).

Total range of motion is the combination of active and passive ranges of motion (see Figure 13.3c). If passive stretching exercises are used to develop flexibility, then mainly passive flexibility will be developed. Consequently, there is a reduction in the passive inadequacy zone (Figure 13.4). However, the greater the difference between the ranges of active and passive movement in a joint, the greater is the likelihood of an injury (Iashvili 1983). To avoid such risks, strength exercises in the active inadequacy zone are recommended. They will reduce the passive inadequacy and increase the zone of active mobility.

Tumanyan and Dzhanyan (1984) compared four training methods. The control group in their study showed no changes in active or passive flexibility. The second group, which used stretching exercises alone, increased by approximately

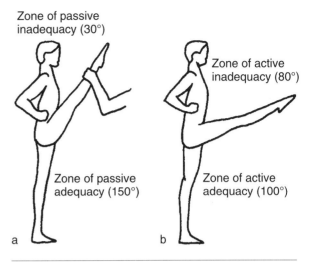

Fig. 13.4. Flexibility zones. (a) Zone of passive inadequacy (30°). Zone of passive adequacy (150°). (b) Zone of active inadequacy (80°). Zone of active adequacy (100°).
Reprinted from Alter (1988).

the same amount in active and passive flexibility. However, the flexibility difference between the active and passive flexibility remained unchanged. The third group, which used strength exercises alone, increased only in active flexibility. The fourth group, which used both strength and stretching exercises, had the greatest gain in active flexibility along with an increase in passive flexibility. Consequently, as active and passive flexibility increased, the difference between them decreased.

If active stretching increases active range of motion, does the duration of isometric contraction also affect flexibility? A study by Hardy (1985) found that it did. Larger gains in active flexibility were associated with longer periods of isometric contraction in the active muscle group.

Active stretching can be either ballistic or static. According to Matveyev (1981), ballistic exercises should be performed in a series, with a gradual increase in the size of the movements. The number of repetitions in a series usually ranges from 8 to 12. Repetitions should cease when the amplitude of the movements decreases due to fatigue. Well-trained athletes may perform as many as 40 or more repetitions with maximum amplitude. Static stretch training is characterized by a gradual increase in holding time from a few to dozens of seconds.

Although both active and passive exercises contribute to the improvement of flexibility, their effects on active and passive flexibility are different. When should one type of exercise be preferred over the other? Passive stretching is preferred when the elasticity of the muscles to be stretched (antagonists) restricts flexibility, but active stretching is preferred when the weakness of those muscles producing the movement (agonists) restricts flexibility. Therefore, one should know the elasticity of the antagonists and the strength of the agonists at the joints in question (Pechtl 1982).

Proprioceptive Neuromuscular Facilitation

Proprioceptive neuromuscular facilitation (PNF) may be defined as a method of "promoting or hastening the neuromuscular mechanism through stimulation of the proprioceptors" (Knott and Voss 1968, 4). PNF is more than a technique, it is a philosophy of treatment whose basis is that all human beings, including those with disabilities, have untapped existing potential (Adler, Beckers, and Buck 1993). PNF was developed in the late 1940s and early 1950s by Herman Kabat. In the development of PNF techniques, maximal resistance throughout the range of motion was emphasized, using many motion combinations related to primitive movement patterns and postural and righting reflexes (Voss, Ionta, and Meyers 1985). These motion combinations include isometric, concentric, and eccentric contractions, along with passive movement. PNF may be applied manually by oneself or an assistant, or non-manually. Today, PNF techniques are commonly used for rehabilitation and in such areas as athletic training.

Basic Neurophysiological Principles of PNF

PNF techniques are based on several important neurophysiological mechanisms, including facilitation and inhibition, resistance, irradiation, and reflexes. *Facilitation*, or *facilitatory techniques*, is designed to increase motoneuron excitability. Examples of facilitatory PNF techniques are any stimuli that increase the depolarization (increase the excitability) of motoneurons or cause the recruitment of additional motoneurons. In contrast, *inhibitory techniques* are designed to decrease excitability. That is, they initiate stimuli that hyper-

polarize (reduce the excitability of) motoneurons or result in a drop in the number of actively discharging motoneurons (F.A. Harris 1978; Knott and Voss 1968; Prentice 1983). Although inhibition is the opposite of facilitation, they are inseparable from one another: A technique that promotes facilitation of the agonist, or prime mover, simultaneously promotes relaxation or inhibition of the antagonist. Thus, there is an overlapping effect on both opposing muscle groups (Knott and Voss 1968). However, inhibitory techniques are of greatest relevance to increasing flexibility. The underlying assumption is that by inhibiting motoneurons to antagonistic muscles these muscles will be more relaxed and therefore will provide less active resistance to the intended agonist movement.

Facilitation and inhibition produce muscular *resistance* (i.e., active contractions). *Maximal resistance* was originally defined as the greatest amount of resistance (opposing force) that can be applied to an isotonic contraction or an active contraction allowing full range of motion to occur (Knott and Voss 1968). Today, many PNF instructors consider the terms *optimal* or *appropriate* more accurate (Adler et al. 1993). Maximal resistance produces overflow, or *irradiation*, from stronger to weaker patterns of movement. Thus, irradiation may be defined as the spread of excitation in the central nervous system that causes contraction of synergistic muscles in a specific pattern (Holt n.d.; Surburg 1981).

The effectiveness of PNF techniques also involves the stretch reflex. As discussed in chapter 6, the stretch reflex involves muscle spindles, which are sensitive to a change in length as well as to the rate of change in length of the muscle fiber. GTOs, which detect changes in tension, may also be activated by extremes of passive stretch. Both receptors help produce changes in the excitability of motoneurons that cause muscles to relax under specific conditions. In addition, efforts to increase range of motion by moving the joint to its physiological extreme will excite not only the muscle spindles and GTOs, but also sensory endings in the joint itself.

Benefits of PNF Techniques

People who endorse PNF techniques claim that PNF offers a wide range of benefits. The particular benefits depend on the technique employed. Regarding ROM, research by numerous investigators (M.A. Moore and Hutton 1980; Prentice

1983; Sady, Wortman, and Blanke 1982; Tanigawa 1972) found that PNF techniques produced the largest gains in flexibility, as compared with other forms of stretching. This effectiveness has also been claimed by other researchers (Beaulieu 1981; Cherry 1980; Cornelius 1983; Cornelius and Hinson 1980; Hartley-O'Brien 1980; Hatfield 1982; Holt n.d.; Holt and Smith 1982; Holt, Travis, and Okita 1970; Perez and Fumasoli 1984; Sullivan, Markos, and Minor 1982; Surburg 1983).

Among other potential benefits of PNF are greater strength, greater balance of strength, and improved stability about a joint (Adler et al. 1993; Cherry 1980; Hatfield 1982; Holt n.d.; Knott and Voss 1968; M.A. Moore 1979; Sullivan, Markos, and Minor 1982; Surburg 1981, 1983). Since flexibility without strength may predispose the individual to joint injury, specific PNF techniques may be useful in preventing athletic injuries by developing both qualities together (M.A. Moore 1979).

PNF techniques also have been claimed to improve endurance and blood circulation (Adler et al. 1993; Cailliet 1988; Knott and Voss 1968; Sullivan, Markos, and Minor 1982; Surburg 1981) and to enhance coordination (Adler et al. 1993; Knott and Voss 1968; Sullivan, Markos, and Minor 1982; Surburg 1981). Proponents further claim that PNF techniques result in superior relaxation of the muscles (Cherry 1980; Holt n.d.; Knott and Voss 1968; Prentice 1983; Sullivan, Markos, and Minor 1982; Tanigawa 1972). However, it should be noted that not all PNF techniques produce the same positive results (Condon 1983; Condon and Hutton 1987; Etnyre and Abraham 1984, 1988; M.A. Moore 1979; M.A. Moore and Hutton 1980).

Controversy About PNF Techniques

Although PNF techniques offer many potential benefits, they also have disadvantages. For instance, most methods require a well-motivated individual (Cornelius 1983; M.A. Moore and Hutton 1980). Another drawback reported by M.A. Moore (1979), M.A. Moore and Hutton (1980), and Condon and Hutton (1987) is that certain PNF stretches are perceived as *more* uncomfortable and painful than static stretch. Of greater significance, it is proposed that various PNF techniques are sometimes more dangerous than static stretching, because PNF stretching actually occurs with more tension in the muscle. In particular, the hold-relax technique, which employs an isometric contraction of the antagonist at its extreme range, applies an additional stretching force to the structures in series with that muscle, such as the tendon and its attachment. PNF procedures therefore need to be more closely monitored if the chance of soft tissue injury is to be minimized. Furthermore, most PNF exercises are designed as partner stretches and if done incorrectly can cause injury (Beaulieu 1981; Cornelius 1983).

Another disadvantage of PNF techniques is the possibility of the *Valsalva phenomenon*, which elevates systolic blood pressure and has obvious implications for hypertensive individuals (Cornelius 1983; Knott and Voss 1968). The Valsalva phenomenon is an expiratory effort against a closed glottis (holding the breath and bearing down), which can occur during the performance of an isometric or heavy resistance exercise. The process begins with a deep inspiration followed by closure of the glottis and contraction of the abdominal muscles. Consequently, there is an increase in intrathoracic and intraabdominal pressures, which leads to decreased venous blood flow to the heart and a decreased cardiac output, followed by a temporary drop in arterial blood pressure and an increase in the heart rate. When expiration finally occurs, an increase in blood pressure follows, which may reach levels of 200 mmHg or higher. Finally, there is a rapid venous blood flow into the heart and a subsequent forceful heart contraction. The higher the maximum voluntary isometric contraction utilized during a PNF procedure, the greater the probability of the Valsalva phenomenon.

Individuals with a history of coronary artery disease or high blood pressure should avoid the possibility of this phenomenon occurring. These people may run an increased risk of heart attack or cerebral vessel rupture (H.H. Jones 1965). Another danger is herniation of abdominal contents if a weakness or defect in a muscular or fascial layer of the abdominal wall is present (H.H. Jones 1965). However, a review of the literature by Fardy (1981) indicated that the risk of the Valsalva phenomenon occurring during isometric exercise is less than has been presumed. Nevertheless, preventive measures should be incorporated into an exercise program to reduce potential risks. These measures include exhaling during heavy resistance exercise and breathing rhythmically during other exercises.

Experiments by Eldred, Hutton, and Smith (1976) and Suzuki and Hutton (1976) challenge some of the ideas supporting the neurophysiological basis of PNF. Specifically, these studies

Table 13.2. Comparison of Stretching Methods

Author (year published)	Equal periods	Measurement device	Joint measured	Terms	Methods (ROM attained)	Control group used (ROM)	Gender of subjects	Greatest ROM	Statistically significant
Cornelius & Hinson (1980)	Yes	Leighton flexometer	Hip	OPI 3 & 6PI 3 & 6PIC	SS (89.3°) CR (100.6°) CRAC (103.4°)[a]	No	M	CRAC	Yes[d]
Etnyre & Abraham (1986)	Yes	Goniometer	Ankle	SS PNF1 PNF2	SS (0.4°) CR (2.6°) CRAC (5.6°)[b]	No	M	CRAC	Yes
Hardy (1985)	Yes	Leighton flexometer	Hip	OPI 3 & 6PI 3 & 6PIC	SS (12.7°) CR (13.0°) CRAC (20.3°)[b]	Yes (-1.0°)	F	CRAC	Not determined
Hartley-O'Brien (1980)	Yes	Leighton flexometer	Hip	Ballistic Relaxation Passive PNF Active PNF	Ballistic (18.1°) SS (21.4°) CR (17.7°) CRAC (16.6°)[b]	Yes (16.9°)	F	SS	No
Holt & Smith (1983)	Yes	Goniometer	Hip	SS ICO 3S	SS (8.4°) CR (11.6°) CRAC (14.8°)[b]	Yes (0.2°)	M	CRAC	Yes
Holt, Travis, & Okita (1970)	Yes	Sit & reach	Hip	Fast Stretch Slow Stretch IA-CA	Ballistic (0.75°) SS (0.75°) CRAC (2.10°)[c] (in.)	No	M	CRAC	Yes
Lucas & Koslow (1984)	No	Sit & reach	Hip	Dynamic Static PNF	Ballistic (2.7°) SS (2.9°) CRAC (3.3°)[b] (in.)	No	F	CRAC	No
Medieros et al. (1977)	Yes	Goniometer	Hip	SS Isometric	SS (5.7°) CR (7.3°)[b]	Yes (0.6°)	M	CR	No
Moore & Hutton (1980)	Yes	Goniometer	Hip	SS CR CRAC	SS (133.7°) CR (132.8°) CRAC (136.8°)[a]	No	F	CRAC	No
Sady, Wortman, & Blanke (1980)	Yes	Leighton flexometer	Hip, trunk, & shoulder	Ballistic SS PNF	Ballistic SS CR (10.6°)[b]	Yes (3.4°)	M	CR	Yes
Tanigawa (1972)	Yes	Tape measure & triangulation	Hip	SS PNF	SS (7.1°) CR (15.9°)[b]	Yes (1.4°)	M	CR	Yes

[a]Total range of motion. [b]Pre-post gain. [c]Reach gain. [d]No difference between CR & CRAC.
OPI = a passive flexibility maneuver of the agonist; PI = passive flexibility maneuver, MVIC (maximum voluntary isometric contraction) of the agonist passive static maneuver; 3 & 6 PI = passive flexibility maneuever with either a three or six second MVIC; PIC = passive flexibility maneuver; MVIC of the agonist concentric contraction of the antagonist-passive static flexibility maneuver; 3 & 6 PIC = same as the above but with either a three or six second MVIC; SS = static flexibility; CR = contract relax; CRAC = contract-relax agonist-contract; ICO = isometric contraction only; 3S = method of increasing flexibility by a series of isometric contractions of the muscles to be stretched (muscles start in a lengthened position), followed by concentric contractions of the opposite muscle group together with light pressure from a partner; IA-CA = isometric contraction of the agonist (IA), followed by a concentric contraction of the antagonist (CA).
Reprinted from Etnyre and Lee (1987).

have found that a static contraction preceding a muscle stretch facilitates contractile activity through a lingering after-discharge of the spindles in the same muscle. Furthermore, contrary to traditional views, it has been demonstrated that a muscle is initially more resistant to change in length after a static contraction (J.L. Smith, Hutton, and Eldred 1974). Supposedly, this is because the GTOs are only momentarily depressed following sustained contractions of muscle on stretch. These issues will be dealt with in greater detail later in this chapter.

Last, Etnyre and Lee (1987) raise questions about the difficulty of interpreting comparative data from the large number of studies utilizing various stretching methodologies. In reviewing the research, Etnyre and Lee state:

> Although it appears PNF methods produce the most favorable results, investigations to determine the efficacy of various flexibility techniques have differed greatly in methodology, experimental design, and procedures, making direct comparison difficult. Contradictions and controversies exist in the comparative literature over the effectiveness of static stretching and PNF methods. Discrepancies have been attributed to varied training programs, measurement instrument differences, and inadequate controls (Hardy 1985; Sady, Wortman, and Blanke 1982). Differences in administration of stretching methods reported in the comparative research include length of time for each session, number of sessions per week, and number of weeks of treatment (Lucas and Koslow 1984). Also, the experimental designs have varied in whether treatments were administered to the same group or separate groups. (pp. 185–186)

This comparison problem is illustrated in Table 13.2. The need for well-designed and carefully implemented studies cannot be overemphasized.

One Plane–Single Muscle PNF Techniques

Prior to the development of PNF techniques, paralyzed patients had been rehabilitated using a method that emphasized one motion, one joint, and one muscle at a time (Voss, Ionta, and Myers 1985). An example of a single-plane-of-motion stretch is manually stretching the patient's triceps brachii muscle. PNF techniques also can employ this same strategy of stretching in a single plane of motion. The advantage of this technique is its ease of mastery as compared with the more com-

plex spiral-diagonal patterns covered in the next section. Single-plane PNF techniques are effective but not optimal. Nonetheless, excellent facilitation can be obtained by using various single-plane PNF strategies without ever using a diagonal mass movement (Kabat, McLeod, and Holt 1959).

Spiral and Diagonal-Plane (Rotary) PNF Techniques

Normal, functional human movement is not performed in one motion, by one joint, or by one muscle at a time. Rather, movement occurs through mass movement patterns or spiral-diagonal patterns. Recognizing this point, Kabat and Knott developed techniques that use natural patterns of movement and thus stimulate the nervous system more effectively in the rehabilitative process (Voss, Ionta, and Myers 1985). *Mass movement patterns* are defined by Voss, Ionta, and Myers (1985, 1) as "various combinations of motion . . . [that] require shortening and lengthening reactions of many muscles in varying degrees." A common example of the spiral-diagonal function in sport is swinging a golf club. The spiral-diagonal character of normal movement patterns arises from the design of the skeletal system and the placement of the muscles on it. The muscles spiral around the bones from origin to insertion, and, therefore, when they contract they tend to create a spiral motion. An example of free movements demonstrating PNF patterns for the lower extremity can be seen in Figures 13.5 and 13.6.

Line of Movement

PNF techniques using a particular movement pattern assume a starting position with the major muscle components in their completely lengthened state, where the fibers of related muscles may be subjected to the maximal stretch for facilitation. This starting position is termed the *lengthened range*, the *range of initiation*, or the *stretch range*. A pattern of motion that is optimal for a specific "chain" of muscles allows these muscles to contract from their completely lengthened state to their completely shortened state when the pattern is performed through the full range of motion.

As previously mentioned, because most muscles lie diagonally between origin and insertion, their optimal function will be obtained by

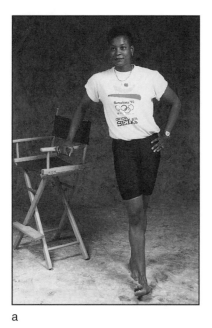
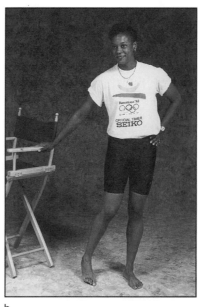
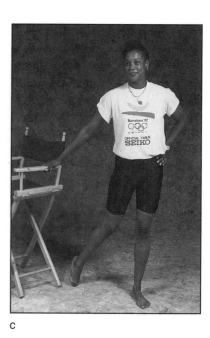

a   b   c

Fig. 13.5. Free movements demonstrating PNF patterns for the lower extremity. D1 extension (toe-off): (a) initiation, (b) midphase, and (c) end position. D1 flexion (soccer kick): (c) initiation, (b) midphase, and (a) end position. Reprinted from McAtee (1993).

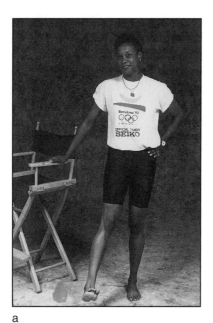
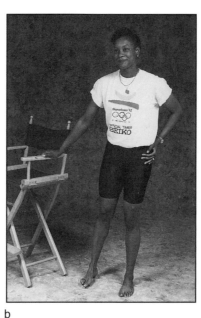
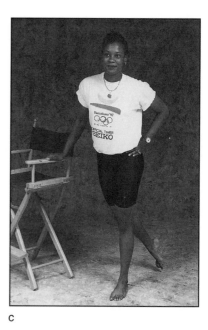

a   b   c

Fig. 13.6. Free movements demonstrating PNF patterns for the lower extremity. D2 extension (turnout): (a) initiation, (b) midphase, and (c) end position. D2 flexion (snow plow): (c) initiation, (b) midphase, and (a) end position. Reprinted from McAtee (1993).

contracting in a diagonal and frequently spiral direction (Kabat, McLeod, and Holt 1959). This diagonal line of movement is referred to as the *groove* of the pattern. It is the optimal line of movement produced by the maximal contraction of the major components in proper sequence from their lengthened state to their shortened state (Voss, Ionta, and Myers 1985).

Motion Components

Each diagonal or spiral pattern is composed of three component motions of the joints or pivots of action that participate in the movement. The three components of the diagonal or spiral pattern are flexion or extension, motion toward and across the midline or across and away from the midline, and rotation. The motion component that places the most stretch on a muscle determines its primary action component. The other components are considered secondary and tertiary action components.

PNF therapy uses two different spiral-diagonal patterns for each extremity (arm or leg). They are named diagonal 1 (D1) and diagonal 2 (D2). Figure 13.7 diagrams the PNF patterns for the lower extremities. The patterns are named according to the proximal pivot at the hip. Table 13.3 describes specific movements in the D1 and D2 patterns for the lower extremities. Figures 13.5 and 13.6 show the starting, midphase, and terminal positions for the D1 and D2 patterns.

Specific PNF Techniques

PNF involves a variety of techniques that promote specific results. They may combine isotonic and isometric (both concentric and eccentric) contractions in different combinations. They may also involve contractions of agonistic and antago-

nistic muscles. The following descriptions of PNF techniques are based on the works of Knott and Voss (1968), Sullivan, Markos, and Minor (1982), and Surburg (1981).

Repeated Contractions

Repeated contractions (RC) involve contracting the agonistic muscle group until fatigue is evident in the performance of a specific motion (Figure 13.8a). In the less advanced form of RC, only isotonic contractions are used. RC may be preceded by an isotonic contraction of the muscles of the stronger antagonistic pattern to facilitate the weakened musculature. After an initial isotonic contraction, the more advanced form of RC is performed against resistance with resultant overflow to a weak pivot action. Then the individual is instructed to hold an isometric contraction until active effort is felt to be lessening in power. Resistance is increased at the weakened pivot, the individual is instructed to pull again, and the isometric contraction becomes an isotonic one. RC helps to develop strength and endurance and promotes ease of impulse transmission through the central nervous pathway.

Rhythmic Initiation

Rhythmic initiation (RI) involves voluntary relaxation, passive movement, and repeated isotonic contractions of the major components of the agonistic pattern (Figure 13.8b). With this tech-

Table 13.3. Lower Extremity Movement Patterns for PNF D2 Pattern

Body part	Moving into flexion		Moving into extension	
	Starting position	Terminal position	Starting position	Terminal position
Hip	Extended Adducted Externally rotated	Flexed Abducted Internally rotated	Flexed Abducted Internally rotated	Extended Adducted Externally rotated
Knee	Extended	Flexed	Flexed	Extended
Position of tibia	Externally rotated	Internally rotated	Internally rotated	Externally rotated
Ankle and foot	Plantar flexed Inverted	Dorsiflexed Everted	Dorsiflexed Everted	Plantar flexed Inverted
Toes	Flexed	Extended	Extended	Flexed
Hand position[a]	Right hand on dorsilateral surface of foot Left hand on anterolateral thigh near patella		Right hand on medioplantar surface of foot Left hand on posteromedial thigh near popliteal crease	
Verbal command	Pull		Push	

[a]For right leg
Reprinted from Prentice (1990).

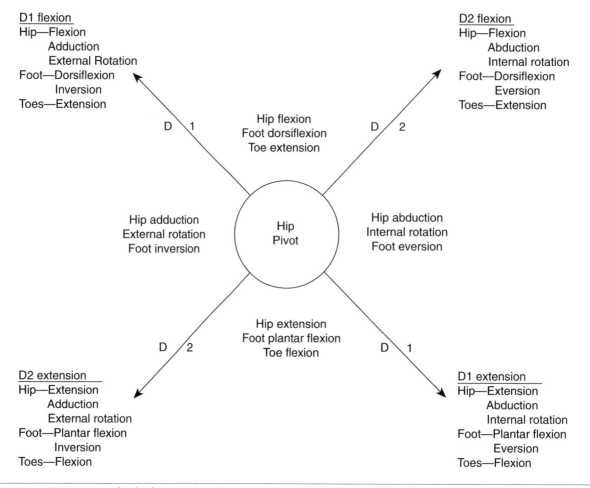

Fig. 13.7. PNF patterns for the lower extremities.
Reprinted from Prentice (1990).

nique, passive, active-assisted, active, and resistive exercises are progressively executed. RI is used to improve the ability to initiate movement.

Slow Reversal

Slow reversal (SR) involves an isotonic contraction of the antagonist, followed by an isotonic contraction of the agonist (Figure 13.8c). This technique may be used to improve action of the agonistic muscles, facilitate normal reversal of antagonistic muscles, and develop strength of antagonistic muscles. Resistance is always graded to allow movement through as much active range as possible.

Slow Reversal–Hold

Slow reversal–hold (SRH) involves an isotonic contraction of the antagonist, followed by an isometric contraction of the antagonist, followed by the same sequence of contractions by the agonist (Figure 13.8d). It may be applied to the stronger pattern, because it may have a facilitatory effect

on the weaker antagonistic musculature. SRH is used to achieve the same beneficial effects as the SR technique.

Rhythmic Stabilization

Rhythmic stabilization (RS) alternates between an isometric contraction of an agonistic pattern and an isometric contraction of the antagonistic pattern (Figure 13.8e). The strength of the contractions is gradually increased as the range of movement is progressively reduced during the entire sequence. RS results in increased holding power, local circulation, and later relaxation.

Contract-Relax

Contract-relax technique (CR) involves a maximal isotonic contraction of the antagonist against a resistance from a point of ROM limitation, followed by a period of relaxation. Next, a partner moves the limb passively through as large a range as possible to the point where limitation of ROM is felt (Figure 13.8f). Then the process is repeated.

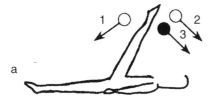

a

1. Isotonic contraction of antagonist.
2. Isotonic contraction of agonist.

3. Isometric contraction of agonist.

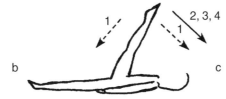

b

1. Passive stretch of agonist.
2. Active-assistive contraction of agonist.
3. Active contraction of agonist.
4. Active-resistive contraction of agonist.

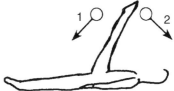

c

1. Isotonic contraction of antagonist.
2. Isotonic contraction of agonist.

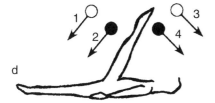

d

1. Isotonic contraction of antagonist.
2. Isometric contraction of antagonist.
3. Isotonic contraction of agonist.
4. Isometric contraction of agonist.

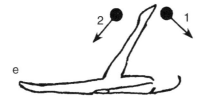

e

1. Isometric contraction of agonist.
2. Isometric contraction of antagonist.

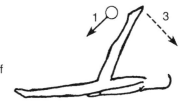

f

1. Isotonic contraction of antagonist.
2. Relaxation.
3. Passive stretch of antagonist.

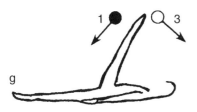

g

1. Isometric contraction of antagonist.
2. Relaxation.
3. Isotonic contraction of agonist against minimal resistance.

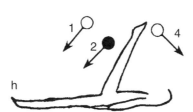

h

1. Isotonic contraction of antagonist.
2. Isometric contraction of antagonist.
3. Relaxation.
4. Isotonic contraction of agonist.
5. Relaxation.

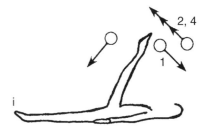

i

1. Isotonic contraction of agonist.
2. Eccentric contraction of agonist.
3. Relaxation.
4. Eccentric contraction of agonist.

Fig. 13.8. PNF procedures. (Isotonic contraction = open circle; isometric contraction = closed circle; passive stretch = dotted line; active stretch or contraction = solid line; eccentric contraction = line with arrows.) (a) Repeated contraction (RC). (b) Rhythmic initiation (RI). (c) Slow reversal (SR). (d) Slow reversal–hold (SRH). (e) Rhythmic stabilization (RS). (f) Contract-relax (CR). (g) Hold-relax (HR). (h) Slow reversal–hold–relax (SRHR). (i) Agonistic reversal (AR). Reprinted from Alter (1988).

A similar technique, contract–relax agonist–contract (CRAC), is identical to CR except that during the final stretching phase the agonist is concentrically contracted. CR is used to improve ROM. According to some, the CR method presents a greater chance of injury compared with static stretching and the hold-relax technique (discussed next) because of the gradual increase of tension within the muscle.

Hold-Relax

Hold-relax (HR) is an isometric technique that is effective when ROM has decreased because of

muscle tightness on one side of a joint. This technique employs an isometric contraction of the antagonist followed by a period of relaxation. Then the limb actively moves against minimal resistance through the newly gained range to the new point of ROM limitation (Figure 13.8g).

Slow Reversal–Hold–Relax

Slow reversal–hold–relax (SRHR) involves an isotonic contraction of the antagonist, followed by an isometric contraction of the antagonist, a brief period of voluntary relaxation, then an isotonic contraction of the agonist (Figure 13.8h). SRHR facilitates normal reversal of the antagonistic muscles and develops strength of the antagonistic muscles.

Agonistic Reversal

Agonistic reversal (AR) employs movement isotonically through a ROM with a resistance. At the end of the concentric range, a slow, controlled, rhythmical sequence of eccentric and concentric contractions of the same muscle is repeated a number of times (Figure 13.8i). AR is used to promote both concentric and eccentric contractions of a movement pattern.

Neurophysiology of PNF Techniques

Having briefly described the major PNF techniques, we will now analyze in detail their neurophysiological basis. It will soon become apparent that, while there are many theories, there is much we still do not know. PNF stretching techniques that employ "active muscle contractions to minimize active resistance and overcome passive resistance to stretch is best assessed through careful consideration of the effects of the components of the stretching procedures on neural activity and passive structures in the limb" (Condon 1983, 13). Because PNF stretching techniques include several components in a variety of possible combinations, these components will be considered independently. The major components are static stretch, relaxation, contraction of the antagonist, and contraction of the agonist.

Static Stretch

A slow static stretch will normally result in low levels of EMG activity during most of the stretch, demonstrating lower motoneuron excitability. At the initial application of stretch, dynamic discharge of the muscle spindles in the antagonistic muscle will facilitate its alpha motoneuron pool. Once the elongation phase ceases and the stretch is maintained, the dynamic portion of the muscle spindle discharge should lessen and subside (Burke, Hagbarth, and Lofstedt 1978; Condon 1983; M.A. Moore and Hutton 1980; Vallbo 1974a). During a very slow stretch, it is possible that high sensitivity of Ia afferents to small increases in muscle length may be maintained through selective activation of the gamma static neurons (Matthews 1981). However, Vallbo's (1974b) studies of spindle afferents in humans have failed to demonstrate significant gamma activity during passive stretch.

Theoretically, during the maintained stretch, autogenic inhibition by the GTO could occur through the Ib pathways. However, slow passive stretch is not an optimal stimulus for GTOs (Burke, Hagbarth, and Lofstedt 1978; Houk, Singer, and Goldman 1971). Another possible source of autogenic inhibition during stretch is small muscle afferents (Rymer, Houk, and Crago 1979). Because the static stretch requires no voluntary effort, supraspinal input would be expected to be minimal (Condon 1983). A subject's ability to voluntarily relax the muscle while it is being stretched could reduce the central drive to the alpha motoneurons and would lower the background motor activity upon which peripheral contributions summate (Moore and Hutton 1980). Phillips is quoted in Condon (1983, 14) as pointing out that "the corticospinal tract has the potential for very potent transmission to alpha motoneurons." But "if a person chose to resist a stretch for any number of reasons, which may include attempts to minimize pain or maintain a posture, he/she is certainly capable of overriding spinal inputs and discharging alpha motoneurons" (Condon 1983, 14).

Relaxation

The relaxation component can follow or precede a static stretch or contraction of an agonist. This component can be completely passive. As in the static stretch component, one can also facilitate or inhibit the process voluntarily (via supraspinal mechanisms), depending on the quality of concentration on the desired end product. Respiratory, imagery, eye movement, and gravity techniques can further assist relaxation (see chapter 8).

Contraction of the Antagonist

Original simple reflex theories suggested that muscle relaxation will follow a prior contraction of the same muscle. It has been hypothesized that contracting a muscle under stretch causes the GTOs to begin to discharge, causing relaxation, or that the Renshaw cell synaptic connections may inhibit muscle contraction (Condon 1983). Another theory is that the isometric contractions somehow alter the manner in which the muscle spindles respond to stretching conditions by decreasing the afferent flow of impulses from these proprioceptors (Holt n.d.). Consequently, this decrease in muscle spindle firing would tend to enhance greater ROM by offering less resistance to stretch.

However, these concepts have been challenged by several investigators (Condon and Hutton 1987; Etnyre and Abraham 1988; M.A. Moore 1979; M.A. Moore and Hutton 1980). Although a contraction of an antagonist should theoretically facilitate relaxation or inhibit subsequent contraction of the antagonist, the opposite results are seen. That is, the contraction may instead leave the muscle in a more excitable state. A hypothesis to explain this phenomenon has been proposed, based on peripheral and central neural factors. The interested reader is encouraged to review the works by Condon (1983), Condon and Hutton (1987), M.A. Moore (1979), and M.A. Moore and Hutton (1980) for a detailed review of this subject.

The lingering discharge (facilitation) of a muscle being stretched resulting from a preceding contraction of the same muscle challenges a basic and fundamental concept of stretching. Spinal segmental neural circuitry and functional interactions are known to be much more complex than commonly depicted. The preceding discussion and the issues addressed in chapter 6 serve to emphasize that simplistic notions concerning reciprocal inhibition during muscle

stretch should be discarded (M.A. Moore and Hutton 1980).

These findings have several implications: Complete muscle relaxation is *not* a requisite for effective stretching; greater muscle relaxation is *not* associated with greater range of motion (Ostering, Robertson, Troxel, and Hansen 1990); and claims that techniques similar to CRAC promote relaxation of the muscle to be stretched should be viewed with some skepticism. If comfort, time, or learning difficulties are important considerations, static stretch may be preferred since it is more comfortable and elicits less resistive activity than the other types of stretching. Further research into the details of how these stretching techniques really work is needed (Condon 1983; Condon and Hutton 1987; Etnyre and Abraham 1988; M.A. Moore 1979; M.A. Moore and Hutton 1980).

Contraction of the Agonist

The effects of reciprocal innervation are used to justify an agonist contraction during stretch. Specifically, contraction of the agonistic muscles (e.g., quadriceps) is thought to induce relaxation of the antagonistic muscles (e.g., hamstrings) through reciprocal inhibition (Figure 13.9). Thus, when

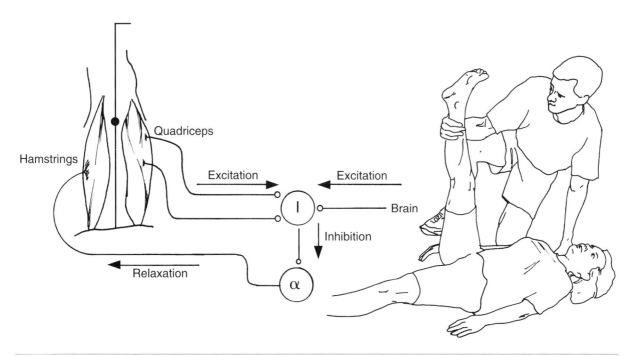

Fig. 13.9. Partner-assisted flexibility training. Using the Hold–Relax–Agonist Contract technique, the partner maximally stretches the hamstrings while the subject (lying down) attempts a submaximal concentric activation of the quadriceps muscle group (I = inhibitory neuron, α = alpha motoneuron).
Reprinted from Enoka (1988).

motoneurons of the agonistic muscle receive excitatory impulses from afferent nerves or from the brain motor centers, the motoneurons that supply the antagonistic muscles are inhibited (e.g., if the quadriceps contract, the hamstrings must relax). So, during an agonist-contract procedure, reciprocal Ia inhibition of the antagonist would be favored by both spinal and supraspinal inputs. Therefore, an agonist contraction theoretically would be expected to produce lower levels of contractile resistance in the antagonist than would occur in a static stretch procedure (Condon 1983).

In contrast, research by Condon and Hutton (1987), M.A. Moore (1979), and M.A. Moore and Hutton (1980) found that an agonist contraction significantly increased EMG activity in the antagonistic muscle. Therefore, the antagonistic muscle was apparently not relaxed after prior contraction of its agonist. However, they suggested that active reciprocal inhibition may still occur in a muscle but not be apparent. The reciprocal inhibition effects may be masked by excitatory input from other pathways, resulting in a net excitatory effect to the antagonist. Later, Etnyre and Abraham (1988) suggested that the appearance of cocontraction between antagonistic muscles was actually a result of intermuscular electrical cross-talk (i.e., cross-talk between the electrodes). Therefore, the apparent electrical activity in the antagonistic muscle may actually be an artifact of the activity in the agonistic muscle (the likelihood of this is greater when the two opposing muscles are small and close together).

Another potential advantage of a voluntary contraction of the agonist is the reduction of discomfort arising from the muscles under stretch. M.A. Moore and Hutton (1980) interviewed subjects after their experiment utilizing the CRAC method. The subjects reported that they tended to associate the discomfort with the preliminary contraction of the antagonist while it was in the stretched position, rather than with the hamstring stretch phase during the agonist contraction. Moore and Hutton have suggested that the voluntary contraction of the agonists tends to mask discomfort arising from the antagonistic muscles under stretch.

Other Stretching Techniques

In addition to PNF, there are several other methods used to facilitate muscle relaxation to enhance and restore movement. Three such methods are muscle energy, strain-counterstrain, and functional techniques. All three methods were developed by osteopaths. To paraphrase Goodridge (1981), these techniques should not be considered a panacea, but an addition to one's store of professional resources.

Muscle Energy Techniques

Muscle energy was a technique developed by Fred L. Mitchell, Sr., between 1945 and 1950. *Muscle energy technique* (MET) is defined as a form of osteopathic manipulative treatment in which the patient actively uses his or her muscles, on request, "from a precisely controlled position in a specific direction, against a distinctly executed counterforce" (Goodridge 1981, 67). MET appears to be similar in many ways to the CR, HR, and AR methods of PNF. In particular, the neurophysiological basis of MET is the same as that of the PNF methods.

However, there are several important differences. One major difference is the degree of force or counterforce. Pounds of force may be utilized in dealing with large muscles (e.g., the hips), but only ounces of force should be used when weaker, shorter, and smaller muscles are being treated (Goodridge 1981). Others state that no more than perhaps 20% or 25% of a patient's strength should be employed (Chaitow 1990; Lewit 1991; Stiles 1984). A second major difference is the localization of the resisting force. This factor is considered to be more important than the intensity of the force. In MET, "localization depends on the operator's palpatory proprioceptive perception of movement (or resistance to movement) at or about a specific articulation" (Goodridge 1981, 71). Last, there is a difference in the terminology used, such as barrier (i.e., resistance) and localization. According to Goodridge (1981, 68), resistance can be visualized as a gate in one of three positions—open, partially closed, or closed:

> The striking bar on a gatepost represents an end point much like that of a bony ridge in the body's skeletal system [Figure 13.10, left]. A wet rope attached to that gate might restrain its range of motion and prevent it from closing; and when the rope has dried and is shortened, it offers further restraint to motion, somewhat resembling that of a muscle that is shortened [Figure 13.10, center]. If the gate has springing type hinges, they will produce greater initial resistance to movement than ordinary hinges, requiring initial force to overcome the spring resistance be-

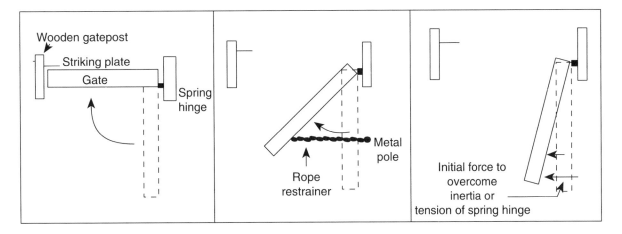

Fig. 13.10. Superior view of swinging gate at three positions: (left) abduction against an end point (striking plate); (center) restraint of abduction by shortened muscles, as by drying of a previously wet rope; (right) initial restraint of abduction by short muscles or ligaments, as by tension of a spring.
Reprinted from Goodridge (1981).

fore the gate is moved [Figure 13.10, right]. A similar proprioceptive sensation may be perceived as one initiates passive abduction of a patient's hip. This restraint may be muscular or ligamentous and voluntary or involuntary.

Strain-Counterstrain

Strain-counterstrain is a technique first introduced and characterized by Lawrence Jones (L.H. Jones 1964, 1981). Two factors commonly associated with a reduction in movement following injury are the presence of spasm and localized areas of tenderness. These tender points are often referred to as *trigger points*. When the position of part of the body is distorted because of muscular spasm, any attempt to stretch or elongate the muscle meets increased pain and spasm. In an attempt to reduce movement, the muscle remains in a guarded state of contraction or spasm. By so doing, the adjacent joint is moved to the position that maximally shortens the muscle containing the tender spot. This position creates a sense of ease or comfort.

Jones found that moving a joint further into the direction of its distortion, actually exaggerating the guarded position, facilitated an immediate release of the muscle in spasm. To do so usually requires moving the opposing muscle to, or close to, a position of strain (Laxton 1990). The joint is held in this position for 90 s. When the muscle relaxes, the joint is very slowly returned to its neutral position. In effect, the malfunctioning agonistic muscle spindles are turned off by applying a mild strain to their antagonists, a "re-

lease by positioning." It is thought that this position may mimic the position in which the original strain was experienced. In addition to this treatment technique, L.H. Jones (1981) also discovered that the tender point also vanished or was markedly reduced if the tender point was pressed lightly while in the position of greatest ease.

Functional Technique

The functional technique was developed by Harold Hoover (1958). Similar to strain-counterstrain, the goal is to reduce the exaggerated muscle spindle discharge from facilitated segmental muscles. The position of spontaneous release is the same as in strain-counterstrain, and so is the direction of movement toward ease and comfort. However, the functional technique differs in that the end position is one in which the tensions of tissues around the joint are equal. This position is termed *dynamic neutral* (Hoover 1958). Contraction or relaxation is indicated by checking the texture of the tissue.

One neurophysiological explanation of the cause and treatment of the movement problem following injury has been postulated by Korr (1975). When the gamma motoneuron discharge to the muscle spindle is excessive, the result is a sustained contraction of the intrafusal fibers (i.e., muscle spindles). In turn, this activity keeps the primary endings firing continuously, which maintains the extrafusal fibers (i.e., muscle) in a state of contraction, leading to high resistance to stretching. Any lengthening of the facilitated muscle causes the muscle spindle to fire and therefore creates more tension. By reducing the hyperactive spindle responses from the facilitated segmental muscles, the muscle can be stretched. This reduction is accomplished by passively positioning the facilitated muscle so that it is shortened, which reduces the afferent discharge from the primary endings of the muscle spindle. Subsequently, the central nervous system decreases the gamma motoneuron discharge.

Traction

The term *traction* is derived from the Latin word *tractio*, the act of drawing or pulling. *Traction* is defined as a technique in which a longitudinal tensile force is applied to a part of the body to stretch soft tissues or separate articular surfaces (Jaskoviak and Schafer 1986). Traction may be regarded as a form of mobilization, since it involves the passive movement of joints by mechanical or manual means (Saunders 1986). Traction is usually administered as an adjunct to other therapies, including heat, massage, various types of manipulation and mobilization, and exercises.

Traction has been used since the beginning of recorded history. Hippocrates, along with other Greek and Roman physicians, recognized the importance of traction for treating patients with spinal disorders (such as scoliosis) and fractures. It is reasonable to presume that any treatment modality that has remained a viable clinical choice for several thousand years must have some successful therapeutic effect (Rath 1984).

Types of Traction

Numerous types of traction are currently available. They are usually categorized as mechanical or manual (in which the therapist utilizes a special belt, harness, or strap). Within these two main categories are additional subclassifications. The selection of the type of traction depends on a number of factors, including therapeutic objectives, patient's condition, ease of use, durability and maintenance, cost, and safety. Seven types of traction will be discussed in the following sections.

Self-Treatment

Self-treatment comprises a series of techniques, proposed by McKenzie (1981, 1983), employing repeated movements and sustained positions to centralize or abolish the patient's symptoms. An example is having the patient lie supine with the head, neck, and upper torso extended over the edge of the treatment table. Then the patient allows the cervical spine to extend and distract in an inverted position. Self-treatment places a major emphasis on educating the patient about proper posture to avoid aggravating and perpetuating the symptoms.

Positional Traction

Positional traction involves a particular body position, combined with rolls, sandbags, pillows, and blocks, to create a tensile force on the desired structure(s). This technique usually incorporates lateral truncal bending. Consequently, only one side of the spinal region is affected or stretched (Jaskoviak and Schafer 1986; Saunders 1986).

Manual Traction

The tensile force created with *manual traction* is directly produced by the therapist. It can be applied by direct contact with the patient or by use of special belts, harnesses, head halters, and straps. Manual traction offers several advantages as well as disadvantages when compared with mechanical traction. One advantage is that the therapist can use manual traction as a means of assessing the patient's potential response prior to the use of mechanical traction (Rath 1984). Another advantage is that the therapist can adjust the amount, duration, and angle of application of tension based on tactile feedback from contact with the patient. For some patients, it may be more difficult to relax with manual than with mechanical traction because the exact amount of manual force to be applied cannot be anticipated (Saunders 1986). For other patients, the "laying of hands" inherent in manual traction may result in greater relaxation. Unlike mechanical traction, manual traction requires the continuous concentration of the therapist when working with the patient. Any sudden twist or turn may exacerbate a previously existing condition. Furthermore, it is more physically demanding for the therapist.

Continuous Mechanical Traction

Continuous mechanical traction, as its name suggests, is traction force applied in a single direction in a continuous manner. The duration may range from a few minutes up to several hours.

With long-duration traction, only small weights are generally used. Experimental findings by Colachis and Strohm (1965) suggest that a constant pull causes no more vertebral separation after 30 or 60 s than it does after only 7 s.

Intermittent Mechanical Traction

Intermittent mechanical traction is another form of traction using a device that alternately applies and releases tension over a period of time. Consequently, during the period that tensile force is not applied, there is time for the muscles to relax and thus reduce their fatigue. This technique is thought to facilitate vascular flow, lymph drainage, and mechanoreceptor stimulation and to reduce edema.

Autotraction

Autotraction is a back traction treatment accomplished on a bench of a special design. The bench consists of two sections that can be individually angled and rotated. The patient applies the traction by pulling with his or her own arms on an upper bar while the pelvis is fixed by a belt and the feet are braced or supported against a lower bar.

Gravity Traction

One of the more popular techniques available to the general public is *gravity traction*. This technique employs special boots or straps that attach to the pelvis or to the ankles. Then the patient hangs from a frame in an inverted position. About 50% of the body weight exerts a tractive force on the spine. Supposedly, this force provides sufficient pull to distract or separate the lumbar vertebrae from one another.

Indications for Traction

Traction has two broad purposes: *mechanical* (e.g., to elongate tissues and separate joint spaces) and *therapeutic* (e.g., to relieve pain and muscle spasm). The specific applications depend on the type of traction applied. The most commonly cited purposes for traction are to stretch the musculature, to stretch fibrotic tissues and break adhesions, to separate or stretch joints, to promote distraction and gliding of joint facets, to lessen or eliminate muscle spasm, to restore blood and lymph circulation, to dissipate edema or congestion in an area, to lessen or eliminate pain, to trig-

ger proprioceptive reflexes, to maintain muscle tone, to reduce and immobilize fracture, to prevent fracture deformity (i.e., to regain normal alignment), to straighten spinal curves, to regain normal body or spine length, and to promote the return of a herniated disk's nucleus.

Contraindications for Traction

As with all forms of mobilization therapy, certain contraindications need to be recognized. Contraindications to traction are in part determined by the type and degree of injury sustained by the patient and the mode of traction being used. Traction has the capacity to aggravate and further complicate existing conditions and symptoms. Several of the main contraindications for traction are acute traumatic syndromes, cancer or malignancy, spinal cord compression, osteoporosis, rheumatoid arthritis, joint instability, acute inflammation, infectious diseases (e.g., tuberculosis), cardiovascular disease, pregnancy, and relative age (Hinterbuchner 1980; Jaskoviak and Schafer 1986; Kisner and Colby 1990).

Actions Prior to Implementing Traction

All forms of mobilization present a degree of risk. In order to reduce or eliminate such risks a number of precautions should be taken. According to Hinterbuchner (1980), as a general rule traction should not be administered until three prerequisites have been implemented: a complete medical work-up of the patient, a definitive diagnosis of the condition, and the establishment of specific indications for traction. Hinterbuchner describes a complete work-up as consisting of "a careful history, physical examination, and diagnostic radiographies." With the spine in particular, the X-ray views must be anteroposterior, lateral, and oblique.

Principles of Traction

The following list of general principles for the application of traction has been culled from Downer (1988), F.A. Harris (1978), Hinterbuchner (1980), Jaskoviak and Schafer (1986), and Saunders (1986).

- Explain to the patient what will be done during the treatment.

- Make sure sanitary factors have been addressed (i.e., the surface should be clean, disinfected, and, if necessary, sterilized).
- Traction force must be great enough to effect a structural change at the targeted area or structure.
- Place the patient in a position that will most optimally affect the final outcome.
- Secure all attachment halters, straps, or other traction connections.
- Make sure there is ample protection for the skin.
- The magnitude of the traction should increase and decrease slowly.
- The duration of the treatment should be tailored to the patient.
- Undertreatment is better than excessive magnitude or duration.
- Monitor the patient continuously.
- Discontinue treatment with the start of dizziness, nausea, undue discomfort, or other adverse sensory changes (e.g., numbness).
- Allow a period of transition after the treatment (i.e., time for the patient to rest).

Parameters of Traction

The application of traction has three significant parameters: magnitude, angle of pull, and duration.

Magnitude of Traction

Magnitude refers to the amount of tractive force that must be applied in order to achieve the optimal results. This force is commonly measured in weight or poundage. In general, the longer the treatment, the smaller the weight, and the shorter the treatment, the heavier the weight. Additional factors that determine magnitude include the medical condition being treated, the region of the body being treated, the physical status of the patient, and patient tolerance. It is always safer to start with a minimal tensile force to prevent the risk of exacerbating an existing condition.

Angle of Pull

A significant factor that can determine the effectiveness treatment is the *angle of pull*, which may vary from horizontal to vertical. The angle of pull is determined by such things as the body region being treated (e.g., cervical versus lumbar spine), the positioning of the other parts of the body, and patient tolerance.

Duration of Traction

The *duration* of the therapy will be determined by several factors, the most important of which are the medical condition being treated, the physical status of the patient (e.g., age, the presence of inflammation, or stage of healing), and patient tolerance. Other factors include the mode of traction being employed and the clinical expertise of the therapist. According to Hinterbuchner (1980, 191), a review of the literature reveals "a great deal of variation in the magnitude and duration of the tractive force required to achieve optimal results with minimum discomfort to the patient."

Nontraditional Stretching Devices

In this section, we will define as *nontraditional* those devices that are primarily targeted toward the nonmedical community. Among the targeted groups are athletes, practitioners of the martial arts and yoga, dancers, laypeople, and members and staff of health and fitness gyms. However, these devices may also be utilized by the medical community in clinical or hospital settings.

Descriptions of various stretching devices are recorded by Hippocrates. The function of these inventions was essentially orthopedic or therapeutic. There is no doubt that stretching devices have also been used as a means of torture, as discussed in chapter 1. The earliest known description of the use of stretching machines in the arts was written by Noverre (1782–1783). His letter dealt with the use of a device called the *tourne-haunch* (i.e., hip, hindquarter) to assist the ballet dancer in improving his or her turnout:

> I avoid mentioning the tourne-haunch, a clumsy and useless invention, which, instead of producing good effect, serves only to lame those who use it, by giving a distortion to the waist, much more disagreeable than what it was intended to remove.
>
> The simplest and most natural means are those which reason and good sense ought to adopt;—and of these, a moderate, but continual exercise is indispensible: the practice of a circular motion or turning of the legs, both inwardly and outwardly, and of boldly *beating* at full extent from the haunch, is the only certain exercise to be preferred. It insensibly gives freedom, spring, and pliancy; while the motions acquired by using the machine, have more an air of constraint,

than of that liberty and ease which should find conspicuous in them. . . .

No more can a dancer hope to attain the perfection of his art, if for one half of his life he is confined in shackles? I repeat it again, sir, that the use of the machine, is hurtful: for natural or innate defects are not to be overcome by violence; it must be the work of time, study and application. (pp. 71–73)

Only 50 years after Noverre's warning, the utilization of the tourne-hanche was cited by Kirstein (1939) as part of Alberic Second's *Les Petits Mystères de l'Opéra* (1844). In this opera, Gavarni, a dancer, complained, "Each morning the Master imprisoned my feet in a grooved box. There, heel to toe, and knees turned outward, my martyred feet became accustomed to remain in a parallel line. It is called 'turning oneself out' (*se tourne*)" (p. 67).

Since the writing of Noverre, the need to improve ROM has become increasingly recognized and appreciated among the general population. In recent years, a number of inventors and entrepreneurs have attempted to meet the demand for an "elixir" to enhance ROM. Consequently, an increasing number of professional instruments and training aids have proliferated in the marketplace. Most have been targeted primarily to athletes and laypeople for training, rehabilitation, and physical fitness management.

Stretching Devices and Machines

Stretching machines range in technical sophistication, from the simplest to the most high-tech. Simple equipment uses balls, ropes, and sticks. Usually, these devices are relatively easy to use and are inexpensive. Machines that are more complex and substantial are often correspondingly more expensive. High-tech machines require a substantial ($500 or more) investment of money. Such machines may have power motors, possess special features (e.g., a modulating stretch), or stretch multiple parts of the body. A unique and effective example of the latter is StretchMate (Figure 13.11).

The Rack System

The need for flexible groin and hamstrings muscles is essential for success in dance, gymnastics, and the martial arts. Various stretching

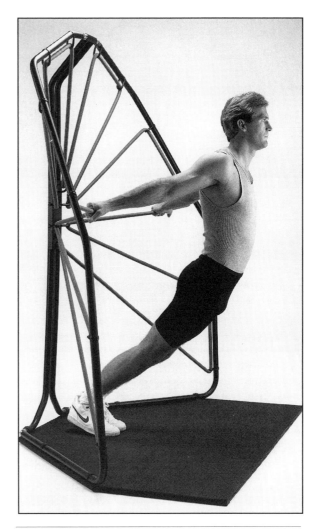

Fig. 13.11. StretchMate.
Photo courtesy of Fred Dolan.

machines have been invented to facilitate the ability to perform splits in all directions and high leg kicks. Many of these devices superficially appear to follow a similar "rack" design. However, there are distinct differences. Because the rack system is probably the most popular and widely promoted device on the market, we will look at this design in more depth.

The first part of the rack that needs to be examined is the frame. It can be constructed of steel, aluminum, or plastic. The quality and gauge of these materials will determine to a major extent the rack's useful life expectancy. Attached to the frame is a pair of leg decks, which are often padded. Some racks have a seated back while others do not. If the rack comes with a seated back, one should determine how many positions are available and whether it can be adjusted while stretching. Similar determinations should be made re-

---

Factors to Consider in Evaluating Stretching Devices

Several factors need to be considered before prudently acquiring any stretching device. The first factor to take into consideration is safety. Can the device be used with a minimal risk of injury? The problem here is that most people do not have the expertise to make such an evaluation. The knowledge of a certified athletic trainer, physical therapist, or physician should be sought. Professional endorsements in advertisements must be read with caution. A famous athlete's or celebrity's endorsement of a product is no guarantee of its effectiveness or safety.

Second, ask if the device does what it claims or provides a free trial with a money-back guarantee. Rarely are any studies published demonstrating the efficacy of such devices. A third factor to consider is the ease of operation or "user friendliness" of design. Does the machine require special training? Is it bulky, heavy, and large (making it difficult to store)? The product's warranty in case of damage should also be considered. How long does the warranty last, what is necessary to get a temporary replacement, and how long does it take to get a replacement? Consider the materials and components that make up the machine. How sturdy is the device, and how will it stand up to wear and tear? The final consideration is commonly the first—the cost.

---

garding the leg supports. Two accessories that come with some racks are the sidebar and the T-bar and handle, which assist the individual during the stretch. One of the most important components is the stretching mechanism, which may utilize a crank mechanism, worm drive, hydraulic system, or electric system. Each of these mechanisms has its own advantages and disadvantages (e.g., simplicity, durability, possibility of leaking, cost). An important safety component is the presence of a release mechanism to provide the user with a means to disengage the applied stretch to prevent possible injury. Last, the measuring device permits the user to quantify in some way the degree of stretch. Other factors to consider before purchasing include the types of stretches permitted, the angle of stretch permitted, its ease of use, safety, weight, and dimensions.

Summary

Special stretching exercises and drills have been developed to achieve flexibility. Regardless of the method employed, overstretching may be produced in several ways, determined by the amount or intensity of stretch, the duration of the stretch, the frequency of movements performed in a given period, and the velocity or nature of the stretch. Stretching techniques to increase ROM include static, ballistic, passive, active, PNF, muscle energy, strain-counterstrain, functional, traction, and nontraditional modalities. Additional research is necessary to identify the optimal method for a given person.

Chapter 14

Mobilization, Joint Play, Manipulation, and Chiropractic Adjustment

*S*tedman's Medical Dictionary defines manipulation as "any manual operation or maneuver." However, as Nyberg (1993, 22) points out, the term "takes on different meanings among health practitioners and lay people." Consequently, the ambiguity and lack of clear definition "results in communication problems which ultimately lead to misconceptions." In this chapter we will explore a wide variety of manipulation procedures, with special attention to nonthrust mobilization and thrust manipulation. In addition, we will examine the difference between a *manipulation* and *chiropractic adjustment*.

Mobilization

Mobilization involves low-velocity, medium- to high-amplitude passive movements of one or more joints. The technique may be applied with an oscillatory motion or a sustained stretch. The technique chosen will depend on the nature of the abnormal movement and the goal of the treatment (to decrease pain or increase mobility). Mobilization maneuvers are commonly passive but are under the patient's control, who may prevent them from taking place (Kranz 1988). Currently, two systems of grading dosages for mobilization are widely recognized. However, Grieve (1991) points out that "like 'grades' of anything and everything, the values overlap to a degree, and in practice minus or plus signs are used to indicate this modification."

Maitland's Grades of Movement

In 1965, Geoffrey D. Maitland, an Australian physical therapist, was preparing a lecture for the Chartered Society of Physiotherapy's 1966 Congress (Maitland 1979). One of the objectives for the paper was to describe the different amplitudes of passive movement that could be used at treatment under specific circumstances, and the positions in a range of available movement in which they could be used. Maitland developed a system based on five grades (Figure 14.1). Grades I–IV refer to *mobilization*, whereas grade V refers to *manipulation*.

Grade I. Small-amplitude rhythmic oscillations are performed at the beginning of the range of motion.

Grade II. Large-amplitude rhythmic oscillations are performed within the range, not reaching the limit.

Grade III. Large-amplitude rhythmic oscillations are performed up to the available motion.

Grade IV. Small-amplitude rhythmic oscillations are performed at the limit of the available motion.

Grade V. A single passive movement beyond the available motion that is not under the control of the patient; it may be regional or localized.

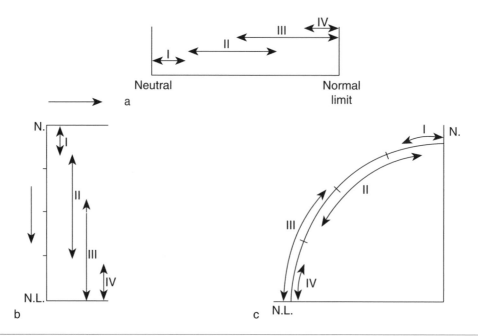

Fig. 14.1. The position and amplitude of grades of mobilization, represented (a) horizontally, (b) vertically, and (c) on the rotation range, of available excursion of the movement in normal joints.
Reprinted from Grieve (1991).

Kaltenborn's Grades of Movement

Freddy M. Kaltenborn has also developed a system of joint-play techniques. Similar to John Mennell, a well-known American physician who advocates manipulative therapy, Kaltenborn believes "the mechanical reason for decreased movement is often because the normal proportion of rolling and gliding is missing in the joint" (Kaltenborn 1989, 3). Hence, he is of the opinion that "it is more rational to first examine for normal gliding and if necessary restore gliding with joint mobilization before continuing with other treatment methods" (p. 3).

His technique utilizes three types of movements. The first is *translatoric gliding*, which is movement performed parallel to the treatment plane. The movement is rectilinear, or in a straight line. The second movement is *traction*, a passive, rectilinear bone movement at a right angle and away from the treatment plane. The third type of movement is *compression*. It is performed by moving a bone perpendicularly and toward the treatment plane.

Based on these movements, Kaltenborn developed three grades in his system of movement. The system describes only joint-play techniques that distract or glide the joint surfaces. Grade I traction involves an extremely small amplitude

of joint movement. The joint is merely *loosened*, and there is no appreciable joint separation. Hence, joint traction does not place stress on the capsule. Instead, it equalizes cohesive forces, muscle tension, and atmospheric pressure acting on the joint. Grade II traction and gliding employ sufficient traction or gliding of the joint surfaces to tighten the tissues around the joint. Kaltenborn calls this "taking up the slack." Grade III traction and gliding utilize an amplitude large enough to place a stretch on tissues crossing the joint. This movement can only occur after the slack has been taken up.

According to Kaltenborn (1989, 46), the following rationale are the appropriate indications for traction and gliding:

Traction

Grade I.   To relieve pain

             Always used while performing gliding mobilizations

Grade II.   To relieve pain (the slack is not completely taken up)

             To test the joint-play movement (traction-test)

Grade III.   To increase mobility (traction-mobilization)

             To test the joint-play movement (traction-test)

Gliding

Grade II.   To test the joint-play movement (glide-test)

Grade III.   To increase mobility (glide-mobilization)

To test the joint-play movement (glide-test)

Joint Play

As has been previously discussed, joint movement may be either active or passive. *Active or functional movement* is carried out by the individual. However, the range of voluntary movement is only part of the range of normal movement at any joint. *Passive* movement, which cannot be carried out by the individual, can involve

- a rolling of one bone surface on another,
- a shifting or sliding movement of one joint surface against the other,
- a rotation,
- a compression or decrease of the joint space between the bone articulations, or
- a distraction (a separation or pulling apart of joint surfaces).

As explained by Mennell (1960, 18), "the range of voluntary movement is entirely dependent on the integrity of a normal range of involuntary movement." Mennell refers to this passive movement as *joint play*. The importance of joint play is of both academic and clinical interest (Lewit 1991). Mennell (1960, 22–23) elaborates:

It is because of the movements of joint play that we rarely suffer from fracture-dislocation around the ankle when we stub our toes or stumble, and rarely sustain fractures about the wrist when we fall on our outstretched hands, and seldom tear our ligaments when we catch onto something moving away from us. Joint play saves us a thousand times a day from bone, joint, and muscle injury; it allows the tissues around the joints to act as shock absorbers before the full brunt of the force of the lifting or other force is transmitted to the ligaments and joint capsule.

According to Mennell, *dysfunction* "is a loss of one or more movements of an involuntary nature which occurs at any synovial joint" (p. 29). The performance of the voluntary movements at that joint depends on the integrity of these involuntary movements. Although "the loss of voluntary movement in a joint at which no joint or muscle disorder is demonstrable by the usual clinicopathological methods" (p. 27) is common, Mennell is of the opinion that this loss of voluntary movement is often a result of the loss of joint play. Hence, "because the lost movements are primarily involuntary, they can only be restored by their being reproduced by a manipulator." In the following section, we will describe various methods and degrees of manipulation.

Manipulation

The definition of manipulative procedures (e.g., "the therapeutic application of the hands in patient care," Greenman 1989, vii) tends to vary among the various disciplines that use manual medicine, such as chiropractic, osteopathy, and physical therapy (Szmelskyj 1990). Methods or techniques of manual manipulation have been periodically categorized and defined by various authors (Figure 14.2), but there are no uniformly agreed upon classifications (Buerger 1984; Grieve 1991; Haldeman 1983; Kimberly 1980; Kranz 1988; Nyberg 1993; Prentice 1990; Stonebrink 1990; Szmelskyj 1990). A simply structured schema of multidisciplinary modes of manual therapy has been offered by Kranz (1988; Figure 14.3).

Why Manipulation Works

Since the development of chiropractic and osteopathy, numerous hypotheses have been developed to explain the proposed mechanism of action of manipulative therapy. Janse (1975) has provided a concise and detailed description of seven hypotheses. Haldeman (1978) developed a broader list of 14 theories of proposed mechanisms of action. The interested reader is encouraged to review these works and the cited references in their entirety.

Contraindications for Manipulation

As mentioned previously, all forms of manual therapy carry certain risks. Disasters can often be prevented through the recognition of contraindications to spinal manipulative therapy (SMT). Many lists of such contraindications are found in the literature (Kleynhans 1980). These contraindications reiterate the importance of knowledge about the mechanisms of action of the

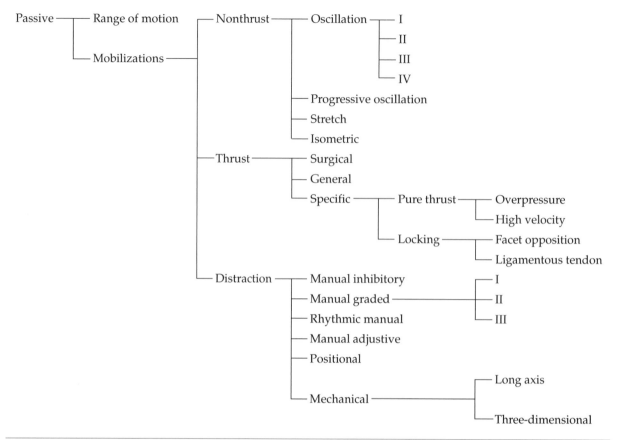

Fig. 14.2. Mobilization: A Classification.
Reprinted from Prentice (1990).

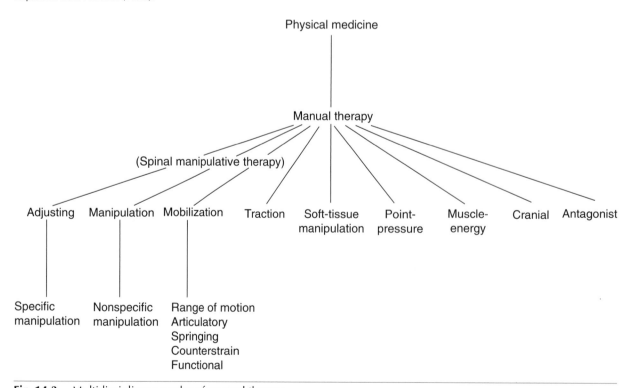

Fig. 14.3. Multidisciplinary modes of manual therapy.
From "Chiropractic Treatment of Low-Back Pain," by K.C. Kranz, 1988, *Topics in Acute Care and Trauma Rehabilitation* **2**(4), p. 47-62.
Copyright © 1988 Aspen Publishers, Inc. Reprinted by permission.

various forms of SMT and of a good understanding of the exact nature of the patient's response to SMT.

Thrust Techniques

In this section, we will adopt the definition given by Sandoz (1976, 91) for a chiropractic adjustment as

> a passive manual manoeuvre during which an articular element is suddenly carried beyond the usual, physiological limit of movement without however exceeding the boundaries of anatomical integrity. This usual but not obligate characteristic of an adjustment is the thrust which is a brief, sudden and carefully dosed impulsion delivered at the end of the normal passive range of movement and which is usually accompanied by a cracking noise.

This description corresponds to *grade V mobilization* in Maitland's system. It is important to recognize that this definition is void of any reference to objective or philosophy and treats chiropractic adjustment as synonymous with thrusting manipulation. In the following section, these issues will be raised to differentiate between the traditional view of a chiropractic adjustment and a thrusting manipulation procedure.

The Difference Between a Chiropractic Adjustment and a Thrusting Manipulation

There is a great deal of ambiguity regarding the definition of a manipulation and of a chiropractic adjustment. The three major chiropractic organizations—the American Chiropractic Association (ACA) [the most "liberal" of the three], the International Chiropractors Association (ICA) [seemingly more moderate, but nonetheless with straight convictions], and the Federation of Straight Chiropractic Organizations (FSCO) [the most "fundamentalist" of the three]—do not agree on a definition of an adjustment. Since the inception of chiropractic, there has existed within the profession two broadly defined philosophies or schools of thought: straights and mixers. The terms *straights* and *mixers* were coined by B.J. Palmer, the son of the founder of chiropractic, and his associates (Dye 1939). The term *straight* was applied to those who adhere strictly to the origi-

nal principles of Palmer chiropractic in locating the cause of disease at the spine and providing relief by adjusting the spinal column only (J.S. Moore 1993). This gave birth to the phrase *specific, pure, and unadulterated chiropractic,* or S.P. & U. chiropractic. The most "straight of straight" chiropractors are commonly referred to within the profession as "super-straight" or as "purpose-straight" by its adherents (Keating 1995). Straights "view chiropractors as primary health care providers, concerned with one kind of condition, subluxation, affecting a limited portion of the anatomy, the spinal area and using one form of corrective care, the adjustment" (Gelardi n.d.). In contrast, Winterstein (1989, 1) points out that

> the chiropractic doctor is a *primary care, first contact physician.* As such, (s)he must recognize the need for other forms of treatment when indicated, always in the best interest of the patient. Consequently, mixers use other conservative means which may include, but are not limited to nutritional counseling, physiological therapeutics, and acupuncture.

Consequently, mixers do not limit themselves to spinal adjustments. Of the three major chiropractic organizations, only the ACA recognizes "physiotherapeutic methods and procedures as adjunctive therapy" (e.g., traction, diathermy, ultrasound, massage; American Chiropractic Association 1991, 3). The practical significance of this statement is that, just as MDs vary in their philosophies and practices (some prefer non-invasive treatments such as medication, others favor invasive treatments like surgery), chiropractors vary also. Therefore, prospective patients should carefully consider the factors mentioned previously before selecting their primary care physician. The key components and distinguishing features of a manipulation in the eyes of the traditional chiropractic profession are that it does not imply precision, specificity, or the correction of vertebral subluxation (World Chiropractic Alliance 1993). Instead, its goal is solely to increase range of motion. For example, Strauss (1993, 72), a straight chiropractor, states:

> Manipulation is putting a bone through a hyper range of motion. Its purpose is to increase mobility. Again, we must return to the intention or the objective which we are trying to accomplish. Manipulation is done to enable a joint to go through a greater range of motion than it presently is able. It may be increasing the range of motion more toward its maximum or it may be increasing the bone's range of motion to a greater degree than it was intended to have.

In the eyes of a traditional chiropractor, an adjustment of the vertebral column consists of the specific application of precise forces in order to facilitate the body's correction of the vertebral subluxation (American Chiropractic Association 1991; Federation of Straight Chiropractic Organizations n.d.; International Chiropractors Association 1993; World Chiropractic Alliance 1993). Stated another way, the purpose of an adjustment is the repositioning of a malpositioned vertebra. In further elaborating on this point, Strauss (1993, 72) writes:

> It is very possible that in the process of manipulation, in increasing the range of mobility of a joint, an adjustment may be given. It is also possible that by giving an adjustment the range of motion of a vertebra will increase, however, the increase in the range of motion of a vertebra is not the objective of the adjustment, it is merely an effect of correcting a vertebral subluxation as any symptomatic or physiological change is the effect of correcting a vertebral subluxation.

The Stages of an Adjustment or Manipulation

According to Sandoz (1976), the phases of a typical adjustment can be illustrated graphically using a central arc (Figure 14.4). The central arc on each side of the neutral position represents the *active range* of movement of a joint in plane. Active spine motions may include flexion-extension, lateral bending, or rotation. When the joint is mobilized passively, the range of movement is slightly increased in both directions. At the end of this *passive range* of movement the slack has been eliminated. Here, a resistance is felt, called the *elastic barrier of resistance*. In ordinary joint play and mobilization, the joint is passively moved back and forth in both directions up to the elastic barriers of resistance. This passive motion coincides with Maitland's grade IV mobilization.

If mobilization is forced beyond the elastic barrier of resistance, a sudden give is felt, a cracking noise is perceived, and the range of movement is slightly increased beyond the usual physiological limit. Sandoz (1969, 1976) cites Terrier (1959, 1963), who calls the added range of movement the *paraphysiological space* or zone. Terrier adopted this term because the range of movement is more than physiological without being pathological, since no capsular damage is present yet. Hence, the paraphysiological space represents the last margin of safety for the joint.

At the end of the paraphysiological space of movement, a second ultimate barrier of resistance is encountered. This limit is formed by the joint's ligaments and capsule. It is called the *limit of anatomical integrity*. Forcing the movement beyond this barrier (into the pathological zone) would damage the ligaments and capsule. This damage could range from a sprain to complete rupture.

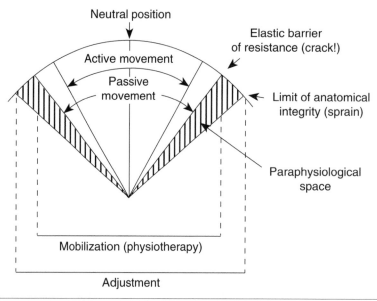

Fig. 14.4. Schematic representation of the range of movement in mobilization and adjustment of a normal diarthrodial joint. In passive mobilization, the range of movement is limited by the elastic barrier of resistance. When the movement is forced beyond the elastic barrier, one enters into the paraphysiological space. At the end of this space, one encounters the barrier of anatomical integrity of the joint.
Reprinted from Sandoz (1976).

In summary, when adjusting or manipulating a joint, it is possible to distinguish three zones of movement:

1. The zone of physiological movement, subdivided into active and passive movement
2. The paraphysiological zone of movement
3. The pathological zone of movement

Separating these three zones of movement are two barriers of resistance: the elastic barrier, an initial resistance that can be overcome without damage, and the limit of anatomical integrity, a second barrier of resistance that cannot be exceeded without soft tissue damage.

The Nature of the Cracking Sound

In many cases an *articular noise* or *crack* is commonly heard during a high-velocity thrust adjustment or manipulation. Almost three decades ago, Sandoz (1969, 47) stated, "we must admit that we know little about the exact nature of the crack." Unfortunately, in the subsequent years, our knowledge about this phenomenon has progressed very little. To date, a systematic investi-

gation of the causes and characteristics of spinal adjustment or manipulative cracks has never been undertaken. Only the finger joint has been investigated, perhaps because the finger's anatomy and physiology are less complex than the spine's.

In 1947, Roston and Haines, two British anatomists, published their research in the metacarpophalangeal joint. Their results revealed three phenomena that occurred simultaneously at the moment the elastic barrier is passed (i.e., movement into the paraphysiological space): (1) a sudden separation of the articular surfaces evidenced by the discontinuity in the tension increase curve, (2) a cracking noise, and (3) the appearance of a radiolucent cavity (interarticular shadow) in the joint space. These phenomena can be explained as follows. In normal joints, there regularly exists a small negative pressure of 40 to 60 mm of water in joints (Lepique and Sell 1962). This suction maintains the cartilage surfaces in apposition and is one of the factors that maintains stability of the joint. When axial traction is applied to a joint, the soft tissues (e.g., synovial folds, meniscoids, and even to a certain extent the articular capsule) tend to invaginate toward the center of the joint because the joint

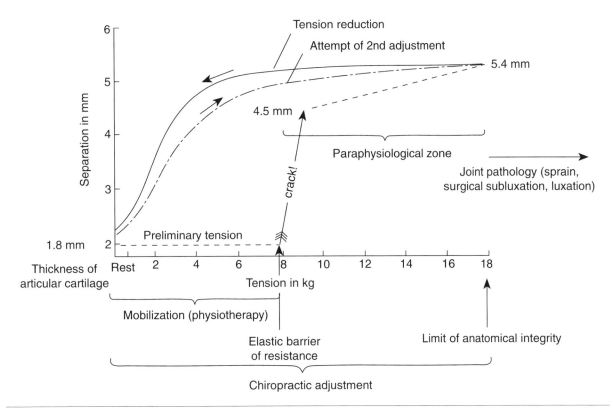

Fig. 14.5. Composite graph of the effect of an adjustment of a carpometacarpal joint under axial stretch. Reprinted from Sandoz (1976).

cavity is airtight. When the limit of possible invagination is reached, an elastic resistance is felt. Research has demonstrated that up to the elastic barrier of resistance, the behavior of the joint is an elastic one. Thus, if the traction is released before the crack occurs, the joint surfaces elastically return to their original position. On the other hand, if the joint surfaces are forced beyond the elastic barrier of resistance (i.e., beyond the limit of possible invagination of the soft tissues), gases are suddenly released from the synovial and tissue fluid to form a radiolucent cavity visible on the radiograph. Unsworth, Dowson, and Wright (1971) analyzed the gas content of synovial fluid and found it to be carbon dioxide (constituting 80% of the gas volume), nitrogen, and oxygen. The extraction of gases from the tissue fluids is a complex phenomenon known to physicists as *cavitation*. "The energy released by this phenomenon is thought to be responsible for the cracking noise" (Sandoz 1976, 99; Figure 14.5).

After cracking, the joint surfaces are maximally separated. If the joint is then left alone, the bubble of gas breaks up and slowly redissolves into the tissue fluids. At the same time the articular capsule slowly returns to its original length. The *refractory period* or *latent period* is the time during which a second crack cannot be elicited. This period lasts approximately 15 to 20 min. Roston and Haines (1947) explain the inability to crack in the refractory period as follows: When the tension is released after cracking, the large space contracts to a small gas nucleus. Upon renewal of the tension it will expand again. This expansion prevents the sudden decrease of pressure in a gas-free joint cavity, which is essential to the production of the cracking sound.

Based upon the research, Sandoz (1976, 99–100) points out a few practical consequences:

1. After an adjustment, the range of active and passive movement of a joint is temporarily increased, the paraphysiological space being added to the range of passive movement.

2. This gain in the range of movement does not only occur in the direction in which the joint was adjusted, but in all other directions as well. This enhanced motion can be explained by the disappearance of the normal coaptative forces of the joint.

3. After an adjustment and during the refractory period, a joint is consequently unstable and particularly susceptible to trauma. The habit of having the patient lay down for twenty minutes after an adjustment is physiologically sound.

4. After an adjustment with cracking, it may seem useless and even dangerous to attempt a second adjustment. One must keep in mind that during the refractory period, the first and sole barrier of resistance encountered is the barrier of anatomical integrity, which obviously, should not be mistaken for the elastic barrier of resistance! However, at times it may seem useful to carefully force the movement well into the barrier of anatomical integrity; this (forcing) is best done when, following an adjustment, the joint is mobilised slowly and repeatedly deep into the barrier of anatomical integrity without using an actual thrust. . . . In many instances, joint cracking is probably a necessary but sufficient condition of a successful adjustment.

Analysis of the Sound

According to Meal and Scott (1986), Wolff (1967) published the first graphic recording of a joint crack. However, no mention is made of the method of recording. His recordings indicated that the duration of the crack was from 0.04 to 0.06 s. In a later investigation, Meal and Scott (1986) found the duration of a crack varied from 0.025 to 0.075 s. Furthermore, their study revealed "that the joint crack is a *double* sound wave and that the separation of the joint surfaces starts between the two sounds." Unfortunately, they were unable to explain the full sequence of events responsible for these sound waves.

Significance of the Sound

For the early chiropractors and osteopaths, the crack was considered to be the tangible acoustic and palpable sign of reduction of a subluxation (Sandoz 1969). Unfortunately, there are many patients and some inexperienced practitioners who think that the crack is the best criterion of a successful maneuver. To quote Mennell (1960), the joint crack is a phenomenon which is "dear to the ear of the bone-setter." Thus, Lewit (1992) quotes Gaymans as saying that there can be a *click addiction* in both the patient and practitioner. In the opinion of Lewit (1992), "this attitude is the real cause of most forceful and harmful manipulations." Yet, is the crack a necessary part of the adjustment or is it incidental to the adjustment? Sandoz (1969), citing Terrier, is of the opinion that the crack is an important indictor for the manipulator. First, the crack indicates that the mobility of the joint is normal and free, at least in the direction of the manipulation. Second, the crack can provide valuable information on the improvement or decline of a case.

An argument against the importance of the click is that there is no relationship between a cracking sound and a successful repositioning of a vertebra. Similarly, in manipulation there is no established relationship between the cracking sound and the breaking of adhesions in the targeted area. The crack is not necessarily a criterion for a successful maneuver. Patients and practitioners must be educated that the presence or absence of a cracking has no relationship with the success or failure of the maneuver.

Effects of Manipulation on Joint Mobility

According to Sandoz (1969), after cracking there was a gain of 5° to 10° in the range of passive movement of the finger metacarpophalangeal (MCP) joint in all directions. The gain in amplitude was pluridirectional. In addition, the active range was also increased, but to a lesser extent. Motion at other joints can be increased by manipulation too. Numerous studies have substantiated an improvement in ROM following either an adjustment (i.e., a specific force applied by a chiropractor) or a manipulation (i.e., a nonspecific force that produces a passive movement of a joint beyond its active limit of motion). Following is a brief review of a variety of these studies.

Several investigators have studied the relationship between spinal manipulation and ROM in the hip and spine. Fisk (1975) demonstrated that spinal manipulation is usually followed by an increase in the angle of straight leg raising. In a 1977 study, Fisk and Rose demonstrated that a significant difference between the right- and left-side hamstring tightness was eliminated by spinal manipulation. One year later Evans et al. (1978) found significant increases in forward flexion during periods in which patients were being treated by spinal manipulation. In another clinical trial, Rasmussen (1979) reported that 12 out of 12 manipulated patients showed increased forward flexion, while only 6 of 12 controls showed any improvement. Using a controlled clinical trial, Fisk (1979) demonstrated that selected patients with unilateral low back pain showed substantial decreases in hamstring tightness as a result of spinal manipulation. Nwuga (1982) reported increased mobility in manipulated patients measured for spine flexion and extension. Nwuga also found a significant increase in lateral flexion and rotation. P.S. Kim et al. (1992) investigated the effect of a single chiropractic manipulation on the sagittal mobility of the lumbar spine in 96 symptomatic patients with low back pain in a double-blind controlled study. The

study demonstrated a mean lumbar range of motion increase of 0.20 cm.

Recently, two studies assessed the effect of manipulation in the cervical spine. Yeomans's (1992) study revealed that post–spinal manipulative therapy (SMT) mobility was significantly ($p < .05$) greater than the pre-SMT data, with exception of the C1 segment of both the male ($n = 22$) and the female ($n = 36$) treatment groups. In another research project, Cassidy et al. (1992) found a post-treatment increase in all planes of ROM utilizing 21 male and 29 female patients.

In contrast to the positive findings of increased mobility via manipulation, several other investigators have been unable to substantiate such gains. Jayson et al. (1981), using a goniometer, and Farrell and Twomey (1982), using a spondylometer, found no effects of manipulation on forward flexion. Using another measure of forward flexion (i.e., distance from the fingers to the floor during maximal forward bending), Doran and Newell (1975) and Hoehler, Tobis, and Buerger (1981) failed to observe any effect of spinal manipulation. Hoehler and Tobis (1982) found that patients with low back pain had diminished anterior flexion and did not appear to be greatly affected by spinal manipulation.

Complications From Spinal Manipulation Therapy

Inherent risks are present in all the healing arts. On a continuum, these risks may range from minor reactions such as a small ache or discomfort up to injury resulting in death. Livingston (1971) has classified complications from spinal manipulative therapy (SMT) as follows:

Accidents—serious impairments, permanent or fatal, resulting from SMT

Incidents—consequences of SMT that are noticeable by their seriousness or their long duration

Reactions—consequences of SMT which are slight and short lived

Indirect complications—consequences of SMT resulting from delayed diagnosis and rational treatment

Several literature reviews have been published dealing with complications resulting from manipulation. These include the studies of Livingston

(1968), Ladermann (1981), Gotlib and Thiel (1985), Terrett (1987, 1988), and Terrett and Kleynhans (1992). Analysis of the data has resulted in the identification of numerous factors contributing to SMT complications, including the following:

- Inadequate diagnostic habits
- Inadequate X-ray evaluation
- Delay in referral and reevaluation
- Lack of interprofessional cooperation
- Ignoring patient intolerances
- Poor technique selection and implementation
- Excessive use of SMT

According to Dvorak et al. (1992), "the most frequent cause of complications is perceived to be the failure or negligence to recognize or respect nonindications." Hence, all things being equal, the greater the number of contributing factors that potentially cause complications from SMT that can be controlled or eliminated, the smaller is the risk of such complications.

Lewit (1992) raises the point that it is unfortunate that the literature does not describe the technique that was responsible for the damage. He states, "this is like describing postoperative complications without giving details of the operation technique used" (p. 196). Another unfortunate fact is that "the literature of medical organizations, medical authors, and respected, peer-reviewed, indexed journals have, on numerous occasions, misrepresented the facts regarding the identity of a practitioner of manual therapy associated with patient injury (i.e., as being a chiropractor)" (Terrett 1995, 208). Thus, to prevent further complications, it is necessary to have all of the facts and information related to the case.

The Post–Spinal Manipulative Therapy Vertebrobasilar Vascular Injury

Critics of SMT emphasize the possibility of serious injury, especially by cervical manipulation (Terrett 1988). As described by Terrett (1990), the usual mechanism of post-SMT vertebrobasilar injury is rotation of the neck, which produces a tear in the intima (lining) of the vertebral artery in the C1-2 or C2-3 region. The tearing produces a thrombus (clot formation) or embolus (traveling clot). The clot occludes either the posterior inferior cerebellar artery (PICA), producing the Wallenberg syndrome, or the basilar artery, resulting in the locked-in syndrome.

Statistical Data on Complications

According to Terrett (1988), vascular accidents following SMT are extremely rare. Cyriax (1978, 110) concluded that the "risk works out to about one in 10 million manipulations, and is no argument against manipulative reduction in suitable cases." Jaskoviak (1980, 213) noted that "over the past 15 years, it is estimated that over five million manipulations have been given in the National College of Chiropractic Clinics without a single reported case of manipulation induced vertebrobasilar artery accident."

There are several difficulties in designing and implementing research on spinal manipulation. Two significant factors are the criteria for internal validity of a treatment study and the criteria for external validity (applicability of the study conclusions to the target population). Deyo (1983) identified seven criteria for internal validity: (1) random allocation of subjects to treatment and comparison groups, (2) minimal patient attrition, (3) blinded assessment of outcome, (4) equivalent cointerventions, (5) patient compliance with treatment regimens, (6) minimal contamination of treatment, and (7) adequate statistical power and appropriate applications of inferential statistics. The criteria for external validity are (1) adequate demographic and clinical descriptions of the patients, (2) adequate description of the treatments, and (3) valid, reliable, and relevant outcome measurements.

Furthermore, Meeker (1991, 19) is of the opinion that SMT is also hampered by "historical and emotional biases blocking the successful execution of even well-designed studies." Chiropractors do not have the financial resources of the traditional medical community, especially the support of the pharmaceutical industry. To make matters more challenging, Meeker points out that randomized, controlled clinical trials can be expensive. For example, one recent SMT proposal to study 300 patients over three years had a "bare-bones" $450,000 budget!

Technical difficulties are also a challenge in assessing the value of an adjustment or manipulation. The thrust to be investigated lasts approximately 0.125 s. To analyze its effect on a living person requires sophisticated technological apparatus, including force detectors that measure the amount of pressure being applied in any direction, high-resolution infrared cameras to track how much a person's body moves when it absorbs a thrust, and a device that measures electrical activity and contractions in a patient's muscles before, during, and after a thrust (Herzog et al. 1993; Weiss 1993). Haas (1990) has developed a chart illustrating seven explicit parameters for calculating the critical force and energy and the factors that determine them, seen in Figure 14.6. In addition to these measurement difficulties, there is no standardization in methodology, experimental design, procedures, and terminology. Consequently, direct comparison of investigations to determine the efficacy of various techniques is difficult.

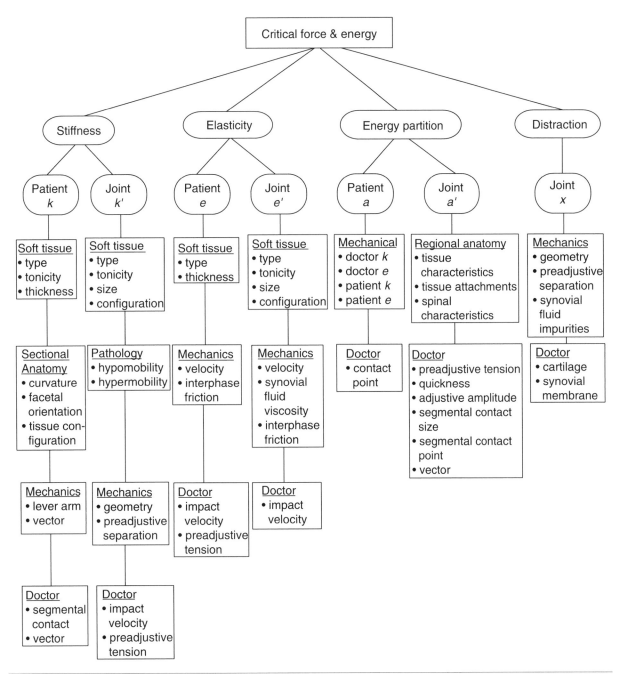

Fig. 14.6. The seven explicit parameters for calculating critical force and energy (k, k′, e, e′, a, a′, x) and their implicit governing factors.
Reprinted from Haas (1990).

The Philosophy of "Straight" Chiropractic

The difficulties in technically assessing the value of an adjustment or manipulation have been discussed in the preceding sections. However, it would be remiss not to briefly discuss the traditional philosophical rationale of a chiropractic adjustment. Straight, or traditional, chiropractors contend that chiropractic cannot be viewed mechanistically (i.e., natural processes such as life cannot be completely explained by the laws of physics and chemistry). Therefore, straights challenge the belief that a spinal adjustment is quantifiable, definable, or open to the critical inquiry of the scientific process (Phillips and Mootz 1992).

Instead, straights believe that chiropractic can only be based on an a priori self-evident truth, namely, that there is a *universal intelligence*, which is manifest in living things as an *innate intelligence*, that provides purpose, balance, and direction to all biological function. This premise requires a "leap of faith" and cannot be tested. Based upon this premise, such chiropractors believe that a subluxation is an interference with the transmission of innate intelligence. The chiropractor through his or her hand and mind introduces into the patient's body a refined and external invasive manifestation of the universal force, directed to the specific area where it is believed the patient's innate intelligence could best use it. The patient's innate intelligence converts the force into an adjustment. Thus, it is the patient who makes the adjustment. This holistic or vitalistic philosophy of chiropractic resists measurement or scientific analysis.

Need for Additional Research

Manipulative therapy is a conservative and alternative method to traditional medical and surgical therapy (Kranz 1988). Research has demonstrated that it is effective in many instances in assisting the patients back to wellness (Inglis, Fraser, and Penfold 1979; Quebec Task Force on Spinal Disorders 1987). Currently, the precise reasons why an adjustment or manipulative therapy provides relief for many conditions have not yet been scientifically explained, although numerous theories exist. The Quebec Task Force on Spinal Disorders (1987) has established four categories of research priorities in the field of spinal disorders: causation (e.g., physical, physiological, and psychological factors), prevention (e.g., designing comprehensive educational and interventional measures), clinical terminology, and clinical management (e.g., identifying the safest and most efficient methods). However, research agendas are only useful if they are put into effect.

Summary

Manipulation can be defined as any manual operation or maneuver. However, because the term takes on different meanings among various groups, this disagreement ultimately leads to misunderstandings. Manipulative therapy is performed among various disciplines, with chiropractic, osteopathy, and physical therapy being the most common ones. According to one classification system, mobilization can be graded on a I to V scale from minimal to maximal. Grade V refers to manipulation. Various benefits are attributed to the use of manipulation by its proponents. Nonetheless, the procedure is not without risks, such as a simple strain, stroke, paralysis, and death. Numerous challenges must be faced in analyzing the complex interactions and results of manipulation and chiropractic adjustment. Last, research is needed to identify its safest and most effective use.

Chapter 15

Controversial Stretches

An aura of controversy surrounds the topic of stretching. Walsh (1985) recalls this statement by Gordon Pirie, British middle distance record holder of the 1950s, "Race horses don't stretch, so why should humans?" In a satirical essay, Frederick (1982) states that the reason behind the increased interest in stretching is a highly skilled platoon of stretchers being trained by the infamous Universal Church of Flexibility. These "stretchees" are charged with infiltrating the running community to spread the gospel of stretching and flexibility. In a more serious vein, orthopedic surgeon Richard H. Dominguez writes that the public has been swept up by a "cult of flexibility" (Shyne 1982). Dominguez believes this trend got started because naturally loose-jointed people would do stretching exercises and say, "Boy, this feels good." Consequently, many others would assume this to be true and follow along. Numerous additional articles have also raised questions about the virtues of stretching and flexibility (Davis 1988; Fixx 1983; Read 1989; Wolf 1983).

The Flexibility Continuum

Although it is commonly assumed that flexibility can reduce the incidence of injury, various authorities and researchers contend that flexibility training might actually increase the risk of injury! In order to understand this point, it is necessary to visualize flexibility on a continuum (Surburg 1983). At one end is no flexibility or movement, as in ankylosis (stiffness or fixation of a joint by disease, injury, or surgery). At the opposite end of the continuum is extreme flex-

ibility or instability, that is, subluxation or dislocation. Between these two extremes lies an optimal level of flexibility that allows efficient execution of movement and diminishes the risk of certain types of injuries.

Potential Disadvantages of Flexibility Training

One concern raised by several authorities (Bird 1979; Lichtor 1972; Nicholas 1970) is that increased joint laxity or looseness increases the likelihood of ligament injury, joint separation, and dislocation. Lichtor (1972) found that individuals with loose joints do not have normal bodily control and coordination. Therefore, such persons are not usually seen in professional sports, having been eliminated early by injury or poor performance. Similarly, another study (Barrack et al. 1983) concluded that joint hypermobility may be a factor in decreased positional sense, which may produce hyperactive protective reflexes and thus increase the risk of acute or chronic injury. Another argument against stretching is that tight-jointed individuals are better protected from severe injury because their characteristically bulky build limits the ROM of their joints. Similarly, some studies have suggested that in looser joints the stabilizing fibrous tissue that resists the impact is so low in quantity and quality that the joints lose their parallelism (i.e., proper alignment) when they are hit, especially when the body or legs are fixed (Nicholas 1970; Sutro 1947).

A vital question that must be addressed is whether joint looseness or flexibility training is potentially detrimental for some individuals. There are numerous authorities who are of the opinion that too much flexibility or ROM can be as dangerous as inadequate flexibility (Barrack et al. 1983; Bird 1979; Corbin and Noble 1980; Nicholas 1970). The literature also contains informal accounts in which it has been reported that international athletes believe that they have become less injury prone once they have stopped or diminished their stretching routines (Read 1989) or that they became more injury prone by participating in a stretching program (Fixx 1983; Walter et al. 1989). This issue will be explored later in greater detail as it pertains to runners.

It is hypothesized that excessive flexibility may destabilize joints (Balaftsalis 1982–1983; Corbin and Noble 1980; Nicholas 1970). For example, Klein (1961) contends that the deep squatting of weight lifters tends to weaken the knee ligaments and hence make the knee more vulnerable to injury. Similarly, Nicholas (1970, 2239) reported that "independent of many other factors responsible for injury in football, an increased likelihood of ligamentous rupture of the knee occurred in loose-jointed football players." However, other researchers (Grana and Moretz 1978; Kalenak and Morehouse 1975; Moretz, Walters, and Smith 1982) found no correlation between ligamentous laxity and the incidence or type of injury. Because so many other factors are involved, a correlation between flexibility and injury is almost impossible to establish.

Another controversial issue is that joint hypermobility may predispose one to premature osteoarthritis. Beighton, Grahame, and Bird (1989, 39) present two possible explanations. First, "the particular collagen structure [that] contributes to hyperlaxity may be identical to that which leads to osteoarthritis." Second, the biomechanical factors associated with hypermobile joints assist in the "pathogenesis of the degenerative change." They believe that the truth may lie in a combination of these two theories because there is evidence to support both hypotheses. However, they point out that "surveys of professional sportsmen show that osteoarthritis tends to develop in those who have had surgery or injuries to a joint, causing incongruity of the articulating surfaces or stretching of the ligaments" (p. 40).

Conversely, some studies have suggested that individuals participating in regular physical exercise may avoid osteoarthritis (Beighton, Grahame, and Bird 1989; Bird 1979; Bird et al. 1980). This view is based on the premise that regular physical exercise may protect lax joints from osteoarthritis by stabilizing joints through increased muscular tone.

Summarizing the research, the following statements can be made:

- Sufficient data are not presently available to conclusively determine whether exercises that stretch ligaments are detrimental to ligaments (Booth and Gould 1975; Corbin and Noble 1980; Craig 1973).
- Restricting athletic participation on the basis of ligamentous laxity testing is not warranted (Grana and Moretz 1978).
- Individuals with loose ligaments need to increase strength through a strength training program. The muscle-tendon unit is the first line of defense in protecting ligaments. Strengthening not only increases muscle but also probably protects the joint ligaments (Javurek 1982; Kalenak and Morehouse 1975; Moretz, Walters, and Smith 1982).
- Individuals with less ROM need to increase their flexibility through a flexibility training program.

Thus, three possible courses of action appear to be prudent based on empirical evidence. First, in joints where excessive flexibility is evident, the ROM should be reduced (Sigerseth 1971). Second, preventive and compensatory exercises should be incorporated into the training program to enhance the strength and stability of the joints (Arnheim 1971; Corbin and Noble 1980; Javurek 1982; Kalenak and Morehouse 1975; Moretz, Walters, and Smith 1982; Sigerseth 1971). Third, a flexibility training program is not indicated when the joint or joints in question are hypermobile (Corbin and Noble 1980; Sigerseth 1971).

Relationship Between Stretching or Warm-Up and Running Injuries

Several attempts have been made to statistically quantify the relationship of stretching or warm-up with the incidence of injury and pain in runners. In one study by Kerner and D'Amico (1983), data were obtained from 540 questionnaires received from an original distribution of 800 surveys. They found that "those runners who warmed up prior to running had a higher frequency of pain (87.7%) than those who did not (66%)" (p. 162). In addition, "the comparison of warm-up time versus frequency of pain revealed that there was a higher frequency of pain as warm-up time increased." In this study stretching exercises were considered inclusively with warming up.

Several years later, Jacobs and Berson (1986) investigated injuries to runners in a 10K race. Of the 2,664 registrants for the National Championships, 550 were asked to complete a questionnaire to which 451 runners responded. They found a positive correlation of injury to stretching. However, Jacobs and Berson caution that "it may be runners who are (already) injured stretch because of their injury" (p. 154). Furthermore, "no time frame was given for the questions on stretching and on other training techniques to assess if or how long runners used these techniques just prior to their injury."

In another study, Walter and colleagues (1988) employed an 80-item questionnaire for 688 adult entrants in a 10-mile road race in southern Ontario. The data revealed that the younger runners in the sample reported stretching more often and for longer periods than older runners. However, the percentage of male runners who experienced an injury during the preceding year was the same for both age groups (56.3%). In contrast, 53.1% of the women less than 30 years of age versus 62.5% of older runners experienced an injury during the preceding year. In evaluating this data, Walter et al. state:

> Because stretching is considered an activity that might prevent running injuries, we might have expected a lower injury rate among the young runners. However, because other factors (e.g., differences in training habits, participation in other physical activities, constitutional factors) may have confounded some of the potential benefits of stretching, it would be presumptuous to question the effectiveness of stretching purely on the basis of our data. (pp. 112–113)

In 1989 Walter et al. monitored 1,680 runners several times over a 12-month period. The data revealed that runners who say they never warm up were found to have less risk for a new injury than those who do. In addition, runners who use stretching "sometimes" were determined to be apparently at a higher risk for new injury than those who usually or never use it. In 1993, van Mechelen et al. initiated a 16-week injury intervention program for 421 male recreational runners. The intervention included warm-up, cooldown, stretching exercises, and health education information. "The intervention did not result in a reduction of running injury incidence expressed per hours of running exposure" (p. 718). As Jacobs and Berson (1986) succinctly point out: "Clearly, further research is needed to determine the risk and benefits of the various factors involved in running."

X-Rated Exercises

Stretching exercises and the development of flexibility should not be considered a panacea to enhanced performance or reduced risk of injury in sport or allied disciplines. Virtually every exercise can present some degree of risk. The possibility of an injury depends on numerous variables, including the individual's state of training, age, previous injuries, structural abnormalities, fatigue, and improper technique.

In the following sections, we will investigate eight controversial exercises that are commonly cited in the literature as being potentially dangerous. Nonetheless, it is recognized that many of these stretches are considered an integral part of dance, gymnastics, martial arts, wrestling, and yoga training. These controversial stretches are (1) the hurdler's stretch, (2) the inverted hurdler's stretch, (3) the deep knee bend (squat or lunge), (4) the standing toe touch, (5) the arch and bridge, (6) the standing torso twist, (7) gravity inversion, and (8) the shoulderstand and the plow.

Hurdler's Stretch

The hurdler's stretch has been traditionally one of the most common exercises to stretch the hamstrings, along with the lower back muscles and related soft tissues (Figure 15.1). It is often cited in texts written by athletic trainers, doctors of exercise physiology, physical therapists, and orthopedic physicians who deal with preventing or rehabilitating injuries (Griffith 1986; Pollock and Wilmore 1990; Roy and Irwin 1983). The name of this stretch derives from its similarity to the position used by a track runner clearing a hurdle. This exercise is performed on the floor with the leg to be stretched straight forward (in hip flexion with the knee extended) and the opposite leg abducted, flexed, and internally rotated at the hip with knee completely flexed so that the heel is next to the buttocks. In yoga, the trianga mukhaikapada pashimottanasana corresponds to the hurdler's stretch.

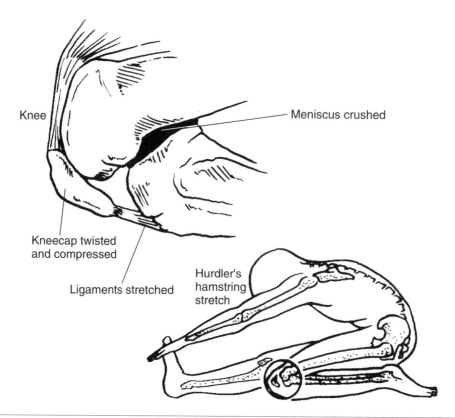

Fig. 15.1. The hurdler's hamstring stretch will stretch the hamstring of the straight leg, but it can damage the bent knee by stretching the front knee ligaments, side-slipping the kneecap, and crushing the rear portion of the meniscus. Reprinted from Cailliet and Gross (1987).

Analysis of Risk Factors

Numerous articles and texts have speculated that the awkward knee position in the bent leg creates a stress point at the medial knee joint (B. Anderson 1980; Beaulieu 1981; Cailliet and Gross 1987; Clippinger-Robertson 1988; Cornelius 1984; Lubell 1989; Peters and Peters 1983; Tucker 1990; Tyne and Mitchell 1983). This problem is further compounded if the knee is externally rotated, allowing the rear foot to flare out to the side, because this position may result in overstretching of the medial collateral ligaments (M. Alter 1990; B. Anderson 1980). Consequently, this exercise is thought to promote medial knee instability. Elaborating upon this point, Cailliet and Gross (1987) cite three major problems associated with this exercise: It stretches the knee ligaments, it can result in twisting and side-slipping of the kneecap, and it can crush the rear portion of the lateral meniscus. Yet another disadvantage is that for most people who have tight hip flexor muscles, the position results in a slight sideways tilting of the pelvis and an improper stretch. When the position is correct, the body's weight is evenly distributed on both tuberosities of the ischium, and both iliac crests are level with the floor (Lasater 1983). Last, the exercise may cause discomfort at the hip joint because "the leg that is tucked behind places the femur in a position of extreme rotation in the joint capsule" (Lubell 1989).

In addition to leg problems, the lower back may also be susceptible to pain or injury when this exercise is incorrectly practiced. According to Lasater (1988a), this asana can cause problems for structural or functional reasons. First, the lumbosacral part of the spine is handicapped because it lacks the same degree of support given by several strong ligaments to other regions of the spinal column. Hence, if the asana is practiced with a rounded spine, the already stressed ligaments can be overstretched, structurally weakening the lumbosacral area. Second, the asana can be complicated by functional factors such as a rounded back caused by the habit of sitting incorrectly in chairs. Therefore, Lasater is of the opinion that practicing the asana incorrectly with excessive rounding of the lumbar spine can further aggravate the problem. However, not a single citation was found in the literature verifying any type of injury caused by performing this exercise.

Risk Reduction

The slight sideways tilting of the pelvis can be easily corrected by placing folded blankets or mats under the lower tuberosity until the pelvis becomes level. However, the problem with the knee remains. Here, the most prudent course is to either change the position of the knee or select an alternative stretch that accomplishes the same goal. The former can be achieved by pointing the foot of the flexed leg along the line of the lower leg. Therefore, the foot is parallel to the thigh of the bent leg (M. Alter 1990; B. Anderson 1980).

Several solutions are available to reduce strain on the lower back. One solution is to perform the stretch from the hip joints with an elongated spine. To assist this process Lasater (1988a) recommends placing the hands on the hip bones to feel the pelvis move forward as the trunk is elongated. If the hip bones do not move and the pelvis is held still, the spine will be overly rounded and the position will be incorrect. A second alternative is to initiate the stretch sitting on a bench or table at approximately crotch-level (Barney, Hirst, and Jensen 1972; Myers 1983). With this technique, the nonstretched rear leg hangs freely over the edge, while the stretched leg is extended on the supporting surface. The trunk is lowered toward the thigh while keeping the upper back extended.

Another effective strategy involves flexing the nonstretched rear leg so that the knee and thigh are brought close to the chest and the foot (rather than the shin) is placed flat on the floor. Then, during the forward stretch, the flexed leg is rotated outward and the thigh is allowed to abduct. Thus, one is free to reach for the toes (Cailliet and Gross 1987). A more popularly cited variation advocated by numerous experts (B. Anderson 1980; Beaulieu 1981; Cailliet 1988; Clippinger-Robertson 1988; Reid 1992; Tyne and Mitchell 1983) is to have the flexed leg fully abducted and rotated so that the outer side of the thigh and calf can rest on the floor, with the heel against the inner side of the opposite thigh. In yoga, the marichyasana and janu sirasana correspond to these two modified hurdler's stretches (Iyengar 1979).

The Single- or Double-Leg Inverted Hurdler's Stretch

The single- or double-leg inverted hurdler's stretch is another exercise commonly cited as potentially dangerous. The exercise is used pri-marily for stretching the quadriceps muscles (Figure 15.2). However, it can also provide a powerful stretch for the anterior structures of the lower leg. In yoga, it is known as the supta virasana, or reclining hero pose (Iyengar 1979; Lasater 1986). There is no doubt that this exercise is quite effective in stretching the hip flexor. Its incorporation in a variety of programs has been recommended by American Academy of Orthopaedic Surgeons (1991), Ehrhart (1976), Griffith (1986), Lasater (1986), O'Donoghue (1984), Reid (1992), Roy and Irwin (1983), Schuster (1988), Sing (1984), C.F. Smith (1977), Weaver (1979), and Wilmore (1982). It has also been suggested that this stretch can drastically decrease the occurrence of debilitating episodes of periostitis (i.e., shin splints; O'Malley and Sprinkle 1986). In addition, it has been suggested that such quadriceps stretching can prevent Osgood-Schlatter disease, an avulsion of the tibial tuberosity in skeletally immature individuals by excessive pull of the patellar tendon (Kulund 1980). However, there is considerable controversy regarding its incorporation in a fitness or training program.

Analysis of Risk Factors

This stretch is thought to place undue stress on the knee by opening the anterior portion of the articulation. Consequently, the exercise is believed to reduce joint stability by overstretching the ligaments, twisting and compressing the kneecap, and crushing the meniscus (M. Alter 1990; B. Anderson 1980; Cailliet and Gross 1987; Cornelius 1984; see Figure 15.2). In addition, Lasater (1986) cautions that pregnant women should avoid prolonged backward bending after the fourth month to prevent a sudden drop in blood pressure due to a compression of the inferior vena cava by the overlying fetus.

Risk Reduction

There are two options for reducing the problems associated with the inverted hurdler's stretches. The first is incorporating alternative exercises that are easier and safer to execute. The second is to learn how to properly perform these stretches with detailed instruction from a competent instructor. The exercises should be mastered in a slow and sequential manner and with correct technique. The most commonly cited warning about technique is to avoid internally rotating the legs and flaring the feet out to the sides (M. Alter 1990; B. Anderson 1980, 1985; Lasater 1986; Luby and St. Onge 1986). Use of blankets, bolsters, mats, or props can fur-

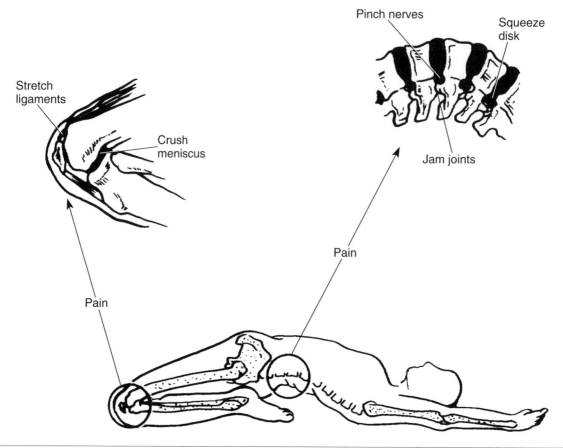

Fig. 15.2. The single- or double-leg inverted hurdler's stretch. This exercise results in overstretching some tissues, crushing others, pinching nerves, and jamming joints.
Reprinted from Cailliet and Gross (1987).

ther facilitate safely mastering this exercise (Lasater 1986; Luby and St. Onge 1986).

The Deep Knee Bend

The deep knee bend (or lunge or squat) is an exercise that can enhance flexibility of the hamstrings, groin, calf, and Achilles tendon. In addition, this exercise can strengthen the muscles of the legs, especially the quadriceps. However, this exercise is potentially dangerous when performed incorrectly. The key factors responsible for initiating an injury are the velocity of the descent, the depth of the descent, and the positioning of the feet. The use of weights can potentially compound the risk of injury (Figure 15.3).

Analysis of Risk Factors

As described by Judy Alter (1983), problems develop when the bend is too deep and goes beyond the place where the muscles hold and control the body's weight. Beyond this point, the ligaments of the knees must bear the sudden and forceful weight. According to J. Alter (1983) and Cailliet and Gross (1987), these exercises can strain the capsule and ligaments, compress the kneecaps, and crush the menisci. Several orthopedic surgeons (Fowler and Messieh 1987; M.D. Miller and Major 1994; Spindler and Benson 1994) point out that hyperflexion with a downward force on the anterior thigh is a common mechanism for posterior cruciate ligament (PCL) tear.

Squatting is a basic component of numerous skills in many disciplines and sports, including baseball, dance, gymnastics, handball, weightlifting, and wrestling. Hence, the avoidance of this exercise is virtually impossible. However, squatting exercises should be avoided by laypeople, especially the middle-aged or elderly. The incorporation of squatting into a fitness or training program must always be evaluated on an individual basis.

Risk Reduction

One option to minimize the degree of risk is to reduce the movement velocity by slowly lower-

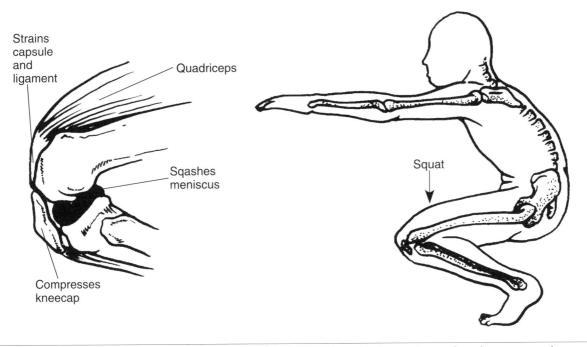

Fig.15.3. Deep knee bends endanger the ligaments of the knee and squash the meniscus. They also compress the kneecap. Partial knee bends, which strengthen the thigh muscles and strengthen the heel cords, are not dangerous. Reprinted from Cailliet and Gross (1987).

ing the body either with the control of the quadriceps, by holding on to something for support, or by squatting with the back against a wall (J. Alter 1983; B. Anderson 1985; Benjamin 1978; Clippinger-Robertson 1988; Fisk and Rose 1977; Luby and St. Onge 1986). The second option is to reduce the depth of the descent. Here, the conservative approach would involve squatting to only a 90° angle at the knee (Clippinger-Robertson 1988). Last, it is recommended that the knees remain over the long axis of the foot (B. Anderson 1985; Benjamin 1978; Clippinger-Robertson 1988).

The Standing Straight-Leg Toe Touch

The standing straight-leg toe touch is perhaps one of the most common stretching exercises. Yet, it is also perhaps one of the most controversial exercises. In yoga, there are three main variations of this exercise: The padahastasana is performed by bending forward and placing one's palms on the floor; the padangusthasana is done by standing and catching the big toe in front of the body; and the uttanasana gives the spine a deliberate and intense stretch by placing the hands on the floor well behind the feet while the upper torso rests on the thighs (Figure 15.4, a–c). The sup-

posed purposes (both correct and incorrect) of these exercises include stretching the hamstrings, stretching the erector spinae (back extensor) muscles, testing flexibility, and exercising the abdominal muscles. The incorrect purpose of these exercises is exercising the abdominal muscles.

Analysis of Risk Factors

It is generally advised that the standing straight-leg toe touch be avoided, especially for people middle-aged or older who have a medical history of back problems (e.g., herniated disk). In addition, it has been suggested that problems are most likely to occur in people with weak abdominal muscles or with tight hamstrings or low back muscles (Falls and Humphrey 1989). Theoretically, the exercise is thought to put stress on the disks and posterior ligaments of the lower back and on the sciatic nerve (J. Alter 1983; M. Alter 1990; B. Anderson 1985; Cailliet and Gross 1987; Coplans 1978; Dominguez, cited in Shyne 1982; Tessman 1980; Zacharkow 1984). The knees may be forced to hyperextend, resulting in permanent deformity, such as loose or "sway back" knees. Also, the exercise is thought to potentially damage the menisci (Cailliet and Gross 1987). For the middle-aged and elderly, there may be an increased risk of loss of balance, resulting in a fall

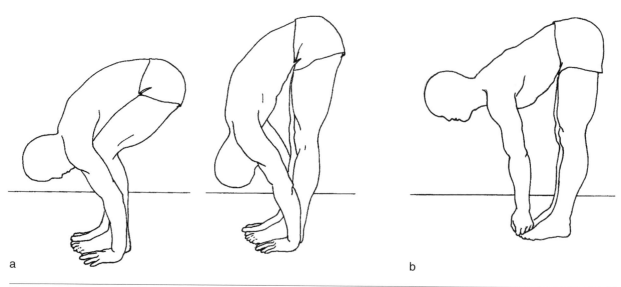

a   b

Fig. 15.4. Variations of the standing straight-leg toe touch.
Reprinted from Alter (1990).

and possible injury (Daleiden 1990; Kauffman 1990). It must be remembered that the higher the center of gravity and the narrower the base of support, the more unstable is the position. This factor can also be compounded, especially in the elderly, by deficient postural control mechanisms (Daleiden 1990; Ochs et al. 1985), diseases (Daleiden 1990; Kauffman 1990), medication (Daleiden 1990; Tideiksaar 1986), and decreased strength (Kauffman 1990; Whipple, Wolfson, and Amerman 1987).

Upon reviewing the literature, one is struck by the question of what and whom to believe. Numerous eminent experts present diametrically opposing views. Some experts contend that the standing straight-leg toe touch is dangerous and should not be practiced at all. In the middle are those experts who provide cautions and warnings about its potential dangers or recommend using safer modifications. At the other extreme are people who either recommend the exercise wholeheartedly or offer no precautions.

Among opponents who contend that the exercise is dangerous and should not be practiced are orthopedic professionals (Berland and Addison 1972; Dominguez and Gajda 1982; Seimon 1983; P.C. Williams 1977); doctors of physical medicine and rehabilitation (Cailliet and Gross 1987; Coplans 1978); a physical therapist (Zacharkow 1984), an athletic trainer (Tyne and Mitchell 1983), a professor of dance (J. Alter 1983), and a professor of physics (Tessman 1980). Equally impressive are the credentials of people who advocate the exercise, including orthopedic surgeons

(Michele 1971; Torg, Vegso, and Torg 1987); medical doctors (Finneson 1980; Friedmann and Galton 1973; Grieve 1988; Kraus 1965, 1970; Shestack and Ditto 1964; Wilkinson 1983), osteopaths (Shuman and Staab 1960; Stoddart 1979); physical therapists (LaFreniere 1979; Shestack and Ditto 1964; Van Wijmen 1986); and chiropractors (Journal of Clinical Chiropractic Editorial Advisory Board 1969). Obviously, there is no consensus regarding the inherent risks and virtues of this exercise.

Risk Reduction

There are several methods that can minimize the degree of risk when using a standing straight-leg toe touch in an exercise program. First, all things being equal, the greater the degree of flexibility and strength, the less is the probability of an injury. Hence, only those individuals with adequate flexibility and strength should incorporate the exercise into their programs. However, in the real world things are seldom equal. Complicating factors to consider include age, condition, injury, and vocation, among others.

One logical strategy to reduce the risk of injury is to slowly and sequentially work up to mastering the exercise. This strategy can include the use of various props or supporting devices. Eventually, by beginning with easier exercises and progressing to more difficult ones, many people should be able to gradually develop the necessary flexibility and strength to successfully and safely master the exercise. Such a sequential program is described by Couch (1979), Carrico (1986), Luby and St. Onge (1986), and Grieve (1988).

Another method of reducing risk requires using correct technique. One school of thought advocates a flat back during the trunk-lowering phase (Couch 1979, Luby and St. Onge 1986). Lasater (1988c) describes the descending position as a gently arching curve and cautions against an overly rounded or overarched spine. Several explanations have been proposed to support keeping a relatively straight back. Bending with a rounded back is thought to put greater stress on the spine, sciatic nerve, and disks, because the back muscles are not supporting the spine. Rather, the back is primarily supported by the ligaments (Luby and St. Onge 1986). Yet another explanation is that "when the back is one unit, 'straight,' no one curve of the back is curving against its natural angle, so the discs and vertebrae are not forced out of alignment" (Couch 1979, 134).

A fourth approach during the descent stage is to slowly and smoothly lower the upper torso, as opposed to rapidly dropping the trunk. The argument against ballistic types of movement involves potentially reducing the risk of injury through two mechanisms. First, by avoiding ballistic movement, the stretch reflex of the erector spinae muscles will not be initiated, thereby reducing the likelihood of back muscle contraction and the risk of opposing muscle tension and strain. Second, ballistic stretching could generate large and uncontrollable amounts of angular momentum. The angular momentum may exceed the absorbing capacity of the soft tissues being stretched and may result in injury. Remember, the greater the amount of energy per unit of time a tissue must absorb, the greater is the stress and likelihood for injury. Hence, ballistic stretching should generally be avoided by nonathletes, especially the middle-aged and elderly.

Another technique to reduce strain during the descent is decreasing any load anterior to the vertebral body. The mechanics of the lumbar spine are such that any increased weight anterior to the vertebral column greatly increases the forces that are exerted on the lumbar spine. Holding the arms outstretched forward and lowering the arms horizontally to the floor increases the anterior load, whereas placing the hands on the hips or thighs during the descent will decrease the anterior load and reduce stress. Strain on the lower back can also be reduced by supporting the hands on the legs or thighs, a chair, a stack of books, or overhead straps or by supporting one-self on a counter with the elbows or outstretched arms (J. Alter 1983, 1986; B. Anderson 1985; Carrico 1986; Couch 1979; Knight and Davis 1984; Lasater 1988c; Luby and St. Onge 1986; White 1983). As one's strength and flexibility increase, one is gradually weaned off the support. Straddling the legs sideways can also reduce the strain. As flexibility and strength increase, the feet can be gradually placed closer together.

A final method that can be used to reduce strain on the hamstrings and lower back is to initiate the stretch from a squatting position. Bend the knees and assume a squatting position. Flex the trunk forward to grasp the toes. Then slowly straighten the legs until a sensation of tightening or stretching is felt. At this point the stretch should be maintained. This technique has been advocated by various authors (J. Alter 1983, 1986; M. Alter 1990; Hossler 1989; International Dance-Exercise Association n.d.; Luby and St. Onge 1986; Tyne and Mitchell 1983; Uram 1980).

Injuries can also develop during the trunk-ascending phase. The most probable cause of injury or pain during this stage is faulty reextension from the flexed position in which lordosis is regained before the pelvis is derotated (Cailliet 1988). Ideally, in reassuming the erect stance, the lumbar spine should act as an inflexible rod, and the back therefore should be straight. With faulty reextension, the upper portion of the body rises too soon so that the lower back arches and the lordosis curve is in front of the center of gravity. This position places excessive stress on the lower back. As further elaborated by Cailliet, the lumbar spine normally is supported by the supraspinous ligaments in full flexion and during reextension until the last 45°. (The reextension to the full upright posture is achieved mostly by pelvic derotation.) During the last 45° of extension, the erector spinae muscles straighten the spine. Hence, the lower back should regain its lordosis last. However, due to the short lever on which the erector spinae muscles act, this phase of reextension is inefficient, requiring a large amount of muscle tension to produce a small amount of movement. Furthermore, when the erector spinae muscles fatigue, the task of maintaining and supporting the excessive load falls on the vertebral ligaments. Once these ligaments give way, the load falls on the joints, and subluxation of the joint results. The International Dance-Exercise Association (n.d.) prefers "rounding the upper torso up" rather than lifting up with a flat back. A similar position is offered by LaFreniere (1979) and J. Alter (1983).

There are two additional variations that can reduce the potential risks associated with the reextension phase. One involves bending the knees after the stretch has been maintained for the desired amount of time. Then, with the knees flexed, one can sit down on the floor. Another variation is to keep the knees flexed while the upper body rises until fully erect. This strategy has been described by several writers (J. Alter 1983; M. Alter 1990; Nieman 1990; Peters and Peters 1983; Tyne and Mitchell 1983).

Biomechanics

The standing straight-leg forward toe touch can be analyzed by two methods. First, it can be evaluated via myoelectric activity of the various muscle groups employed in the exercise. Second, the exercise can be investigated using mathematical models and mechanical analysis.

Myoelectric Activity During Back or Trunk Flexion.
Numerous electromyographic studies have investigated forward flexion and reextension of the trunk. Forward flexion is initiated (during the first few degrees of motion) by contraction of the abdominal muscles (Allen 1948; Floyd and Silver 1950) and then continued passively by gravity. As the upper trunk flexes forward, there is a backward shift of the hips, thus shifting the center of gravity behind the feet. Simultaneously, the pelvic girdle as a unit flexes on the femoral heads while the spinal column bends forward progressively from top to bottom until the L-5 vertebra flexes forward on the sacrum (D. Lee 1989). During the first portion of the flexion, strong myoelectric activity is found in the hip extensor muscles (gluteus maximus, gluteus medius, and hamstring muscles; Okada 1970; Portnoy and Morin 1956). This action stabilizes the pelvis and prevents motion at the hip joints, ensuring that all of the early motion occurs in the spine. As the spine bends forward, there is increased activity of the back muscles proportional to the angle of flexion and to the size of the load carried. The extent and rate at which the flexion proceeds is controlled by the eccentric contraction of the back muscles.

However, as the trunk flexion continues, myoelectric activity of the back muscles markedly decreases. Schultz et al. (1985) determined that EMG activity diminished at 40° flexion of the L-1 vertebra. Eventually, at a certain point during forward flexion called the *critical point*, the myoelectric activity in the back muscles ceases. The critical point does not occur in all individuals or in all muscles.

Schultz et al. (1985) cite Fick (1911) as the first to suggest that the erector spinae muscles need not be active in positions of full flexion. This observation has been confirmed by Allen (1948), Floyd and Silver (1951, 1955), Portnoy and Morin (1956), Pauly (1966), Schultz et al. (1985), and Shirado et al. (1995). Floyd and Silver called this phenomenon *flexion relaxation*. Investigators have reported that some patients with low back pain do not exhibit this phenomenon (Floyd and Silver 1951, 1955; Shirado et al. 1995; Sihvonen et al. 1991).

No research study has determined whether there is a difference in myoelectric activity between the flat-back and the rounded-back techniques. Hence, assuming that with both techniques the same relaxation phenomenon occurs, the argument that the rounded back creates greater stress on the spine may be in question, because the back is supported primarily by the ligaments in either case. This issue needs a detailed investigation to clarify the conflicting claims. A point of particular relevance to weight lifters who perform "morning exercises" (i.e., exercises using weights with the trunk in flexion) is that carrying weights during flexion causes the critical point to occur later in the range of vertebral flexion (Kippers and Parker 1984). It also increases the level of tension in the back muscles, increasing the risk of strain injury. Like the lower back muscles, the gluteus maximus relaxes as full flexion is approached. However, the hamstring muscles are significantly active from the onset and remain active throughout the trunk flexion.

The physiological basis of the critical point is unknown. Floyd and Silver (1951, 134) hypothesized that "stretch receptors in the ligamenta flava and other ligaments are stimulated when these ligaments are stretched, and the afferent impulses from the stretch receptors cause reflex inhibition of the erectores spinae." Kippers and Parker (1984) have also suggested that this muscle relaxation may be due to reflex inhibition initiated by proprioceptors in the lumbar joints and ligaments or in the muscle spindles.

A popular explanation for the flexion-relaxation phenomenon is that in the fully flexed position the trunk flexion moment is resisted by structures other than muscles. That is, the passive resistance to stretching of the ligamentous tissues of the back substitutes for active muscle contractions in the flexed trunk position. Other structures that participate in creating this resistance are the thoracolumbar fascia and skin (Farfan 1973; Gracovetsky, Farfan, and Lamy 1977; Tesh et al. 1985). Since skin is farthest from the bending axis, it can contribute significantly to resisting the bending moment at even moderate stress levels. However, skin resistance is highly dependent on body build. As explained by Tesh et al. (1985, 186), "loose and lax skin of an obese subject would not offer resistance, whereas the tighter skin of a lean subject would contribute considerably more to resisting forward flexion." Furthermore, dermal scar tissue is markedly less extensible than normal skin and can offer a higher resistance to forward bending. Altogether, normal skin can contribute up to 5% of the bending moment developed in full spinal flexion under body weight alone (Tesh et al. 1985).

Myoelectric Activity During Back or Trunk Extension. Extension of the trunk from the flexed to the upright position reverses the sequence of events observed when bending forward (Allen 1948; Donisch and Basmajian 1972; Floyd and Silver 1950, 1955; Morris, Brenner, and Lucas 1962; Okada 1970; Portnoy and Morin 1956). The gluteus maximus comes into action early and probably initiates hip extension together with the hamstrings (Okada 1970). Later, the posterior back muscles become active. It is noteworthy that the extensor muscle activity is greater while the trunk is being raised than while it is being lowered (Okada 1970), because concentric contractions require more muscle active tension than do eccentric contractions. Furthermore, lumbar lordosis increases myoelectric activity of the back muscles (Andersson, Herberts, and Ortengren 1977; Okada 1970).

Mathematical Models and Mechanical Analysis of Trunk Flexion. Estimation of stresses on various parts of the musculoskeletal system during dynamic activities requires a complex model that accounts for such factors as instantaneous positions and accelerations of the extremities, head, and trunk; changes in spinal geometry; and strength variations within different muscle groups and people (Pope et al. 1991). In elaborating on the complexity of spinal modeling, Macintosh, Bogduk, and Pearcy (1993, 889) point out that flexion of the lumbar spine

> causes appreciable elongations of the lumbar back muscles and changes their orientation in relation to the lumbar spine. However, not all changes in orientation are in the same sense; some increase, others decrease. This discrepancy is because of the different orientation of different fascicles of the lumbar back muscles in the upright posture.

Nonetheless, a number of biomechanical models of spinal loading have been developed. These models are based on the notion that the lumbar spine can be thought of as a set of small links with flexible articulations (disks) between them. With proper geometric and physiological data, the forces in each disk during a specific activity can be predicted.

The traditional mathematical model of the spine is one of a simple lever system (i.e., a cantilever model) in which a load carried in front of the body is balanced by the force generated by the spinal muscles. Recently, Aspden (1988) has suggested that the spine should instead be considered as a series of linked rods that function like an arch. This model shows that spinal stresses are not as great as previously calculated.

Regardless of the model, the force, or moment, exerted on the spine when performing a standing straight-leg toe touch is proportional to the weight being moved and its distance from the axis of the body. The moment exerted on any lumbar vertebra is the product of the mass to be lifted and its horizontal distance from the vertebra. Consequently, a proportional increase in the compressive force on the low back is created by increasing the moment (National Institute for Occupational Safety and Health 1981). Moments can be magnified by increasing the weight to be lifted or by increasing the horizontal distance of a constant weight away from the body. This principle is utilized in various exercise regimens, such as body building, power lifting, and weight lifting, in which weights are used to strengthen the back muscles (e.g., dead lifts and the morning exercise). Conversely, moments can be decreased by reducing the mass or by shortening its horizontal distance from the body. Most people should try to decrease the moment of force on the spine when exercising.

Research by Adams, Hutton, and Stott (1980) using 15 cadaveric lumbar spines analyzed the general pattern of ligamentous and disk resistance during flexion. Resistance to the bending moment was calculated as follows:

Structure	Half flexion	Full flexion
Supraspinous ligament	19% on average throughout flexion	
Interspinous ligament	19% on average throughout flexion	
Ligamentum flavum	28%	13%
Capsular ligaments		39%
Intervertebral disk	38%	29%

Adams and Hutton (1986) determined that when people adopt the static, fully flexed posture, the lumbar spine is flexed about 10° short of its elastic limit. They concluded that this restriction in movement is probably due to the protective action of the back muscles and lumbodorsal fascia. However, they emphasized that the margin of safety might be reduced or entirely eliminated during rapid movements. This observation emphasizes the importance of avoiding ballistic stretching for most people performing a straight-leg toe touch.

What posture or technique is optimal in performing a straight-leg toe touch? If we assume that the feet are placed together and parallel and that the knees are straight during trunk reextension, two possible back orientations exist. Some authors recommend what is called a back-bowed-in (BBI; i.e., in normal lordosis), or a flat-back technique. The second technique utilizes the back-bowed-out (BBO; i.e., curved in kyphosis), or a slightly rounded position.

An EMG analysis of lifting from the BBI and BBO positions was performed by Delitto, Rose, and Apts (1987). They found that erector spinae muscle activity during the initial period was greater in the BBI lift than in the BBO lift, and therefore the BBI position may provide optimal protection for the inert structures of the lumbar spine. This observation substantiates the finding of increased myoelectric activity with lordosis during extension (Andersson et al. 1977; Okada 1970).

Most information that may be extrapolated to the standing straight-leg toe touch was obtained from studies of lifting weights. Unfortunately, much of this research is concerned with lifting challenging weights (i.e., heavy to maximum resistance) from the classic squat-lift position with the back nearly vertical. It is difficult to compare the extension phase of the standing toe touch with the squat-lift position, in which the trunk is already in extension and the pelvis in the rotated position. Consequently, the forces acting on the pelvis and spine are not similar.

However, one biomechanical study pertaining to the degree of lordosis during flexion-extension exercises was located. A simple yet intriguing study by Gracovetsky et al. (1989) may provide an interesting solution to the dilemma of how flat the back should be during the exercise. Their investigation indicated that the body naturally assumes the appropriate degree of lordosis or pelvic tilting. Their model hypothesized that for every angle of forward flexion, there is a unique degree of lordosis that will minimize and equal-

ize the compressive stress within the spine. Because the connective tissues cannot contract by themselves, their degree of tension is a result of passive stretching, and is thus controlled mainly by the geometric characteristics of the spine—in particular, the degree of lordosis.

> Thus, when the moment to be balanced is highest (during the first phase of the return to the erect stance), it is advantageous to reduce the lordosis and support the load through ligamentous tension. When closer to the erect stance, the moment is lower, and the lordosis can be allowed to increase. (p. 415) [see Figure 15.5 a–c]

One recognized mechanism that can assist in protecting the lower back during extension involves an isometric contraction of the abdominal muscles throughout the lift. This activity is thought to support the spine both by increasing the intraabdominal pressure and by tensing the thoracolumbar fascia through the attachments of the internal oblique and transverse abdominis muscles (Bartelink 1957; Bogduk 1984).

Rationale for the Standing Toe-Touch Exercise

Based on the previous discussion of risks associated with the standing toe touch, one may ask, What is the practical use of this exercise? How can it be justified? It is not necessary or recommended for the layperson, especially the middle-aged or elderly, because there are safer alternatives that can stretch the same muscle groups. This exercise also is probably not necessary for many sports, but it may be considered essential in several sports and disciplines. In some disciplines, this stretch position actually may be part of a compulsory or optional skill. In 3- and 10-m diving, the deep flexed position is seen in the backward and forward multiple piked somersaults. Divers also use this exercise when pressing to a handstand on the edge of the platform. In gymnastics, this position can be seen in virtually every event.

The Arch and the Bridge

The arch and bridge (Figures 15.6 and 15.7) are two exercises primarily used to enhance the flexibility of the vertebral column and shoulders. They can also facilitate the development of strength in various parts of the body. The result will depend on the variation of the arch or bridge performed and the method of achieving the final

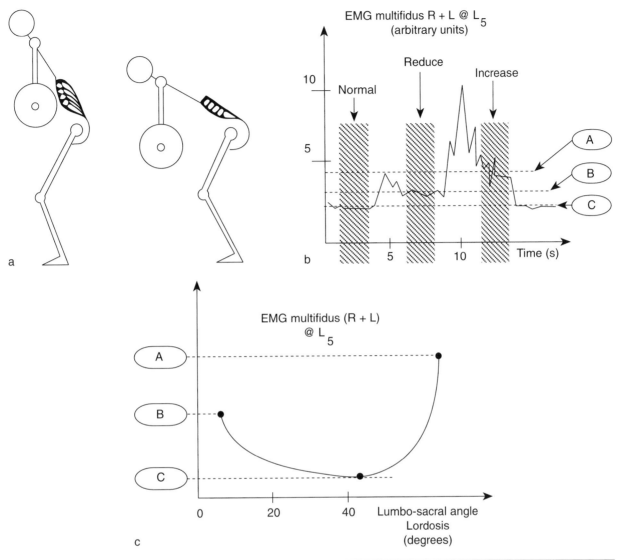

Fig. 15.5. (a) Increased lordosis—ligaments slack. Decreased lordosis—ligaments tighten. (b) The integrated EMG activity is recorded bilaterally and superficial electrodes placed 2 cm to the right and left of the spinous process at L-5. On this graph, the signal from right and left electrodes have been added. The levels corresponding to the most comfortable posture (normal) and reduced and increased lordosis are depicted by arrows. (c) Integrated EMG of multifidus showing relative activity vs. lumbosacral angle (lordosis). A = increased lordosis, B = decreased lordosis, C = normal.
Reprinted from Gracovetsky, Kary, Pitchen, Levy, and Said (1989).

position. Many of these stretches are considered fundamental components of gymnastics, wrestling, and yoga.

Analysis of Risk Factors

Several authorities are of the opinion that various types of arching and bridging exercises can range from potentially dangerous to life threatening. Flint (1964) has criticized the common standing backbend exercise because, if the abdominal muscles are weak and a swayback con-

dition exists, this exercise will exacerbate the condition. Cailliet and Gross (1987) are of the opinion that some arching is acceptable but hyperarching is dangerous. Their argument is that hyperextension of the low back can cause injury by excessively squeezing spinal disks, by jamming together the spinal joints, and by pinching the nerve fibers that emerge from the spinal foramina (openings) to form the sciatic nerve (see Figure 15.6). Similarly, J. Alter (1983) is of the opinion that such exercises will eventually cause pain and result in permanent damage.

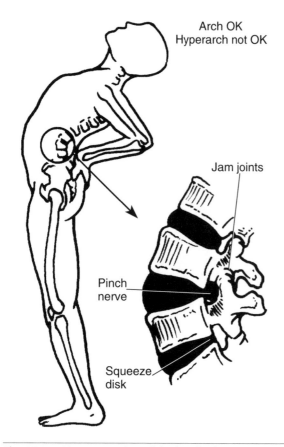

Arch OK
Hyperarch not OK

Jam joints

Pinch
nerve

Squeeze
disk

Fig. 15.6. Hyperextension of the low back can cause injury by excessively squeezing spinal disks (which resemble cartilage), by jamming together the spinal joints, and by pinching the nerve fibers that emerge from the spinal foramina to form the sciatic nerve.
Reprinted from Cailliet and Gross (1987).

The concern of lumbar spine damage to gymnasts as a result of repetitive hyperlordosis and hyperextension (i.e., arching or bridging) has also been addressed by several investigators (Fairbank et al. 1984; Goldstein et al. 1991; D.W. Jackson, Wiltse, and Cirincione 1976; Oseid et al. 1974; Sward, Eriksson, and Peterson 1990). It has been suggested that a result of such continuous insult to the vertebrae is the development of spondylolysis or low back pain. However, Tsai and Wredmark (1993) reported that former female elite gymnasts did not have more back problems than an age-matched control group.

The question that needs to be investigated is whether relatively static skills like the bridge or walkover can cause spondylolysis or whether spondylolysis is the result of chronic overloading during high-impact, weight-bearing activities (such as tumbling passes, vaulting, and dismounts from various apparatus) or of stresses imparted to the body during dynamic skills (such

as giant swings on the horizontal bar, still rings, or uneven parallel bars). A possible solution to this question would be to design a study that compared the vertebrae of three distinct groups that utilize hyperextension: artistic gymnasts, rhythmic gymnasts, and advanced practitioners of yoga.

Perhaps the strongest criticism of this type of exercise was raised by Nagler (1973a, 1973b) and Hanus, Homer, and Harter (1977). It is their medical opinion that the therapeutic value of these exercises for middle-aged people is not sufficient to justify the potential, although rare, risk of vertebral artery occlusion which can be a result of the forceful hyperextension of the cervical spine. The case of a 28-year-old female yoga enthusiast who performed the bridge was described by both Nagler and Hanus et al (1977). During the exercise the woman reported a severe throbbing headache and later was unable to move without assistance. Five days later a craniotomy was performed, and an ischemic infarct (stroke) with secondary hemorrhages was found in the left cerebellar hemisphere of the brain.

Risk Reduction

Before attempting a bridge, one should have the physical requisites of sufficient strength and suppleness. The learner should have the necessary strength to rise up and to support and maintain the position. The student needs adequate suppleness in the hips, lower and upper torso, and shoulders. Proper sequential learning through lead-up drills and exercises, using optimal technique, and the assistance of a knowledgeable spotter can substantially reduce the risk of injury. For the middle-aged and elderly, safer alternatives should be considered.

Rationale for the Arch and Bridge

For some disciplines the bridge is merely a means for conditioning. Yet in other disciplines— including acrobatics, gymnastics, judo, and wrestling— the bridge or a variation thereof may be a required skill. For these disciplines, it is prudent to incorporate an arch or bridge exercise as a part of a regular conditioning program, as long as proper precautions are employed to reduce the risk of injury.

The Standing Torso Twist

The standing torso twist (Figure 15.8) is used in many disciplines, including baseball, discus, golf,

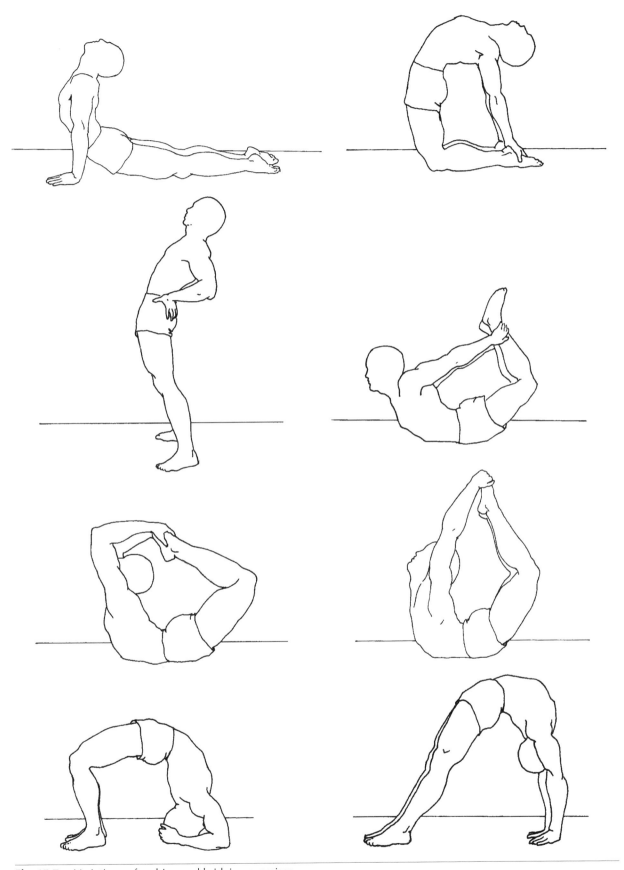

Fig. 15.7. Variations of arching and bridging exercises.
Reprinted from Alter (1990).

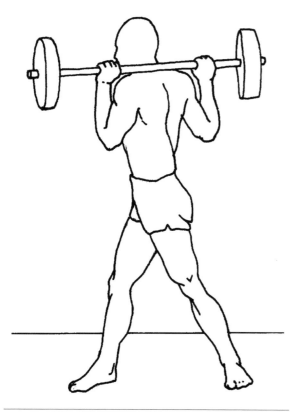

Fig. 15.8. Standing torso twist.
Reprinted from Alter (1990).

and the javelin throw. In the next section, factors related to its risk are discussed.

Analysis of Risk Factors

The potential danger associated with improperly executing the standing torso twist is that its momentum can exceed the absorbing capacity of the tissues being stretched (J. Alter 1983; M. Alter 1990). In particular, it is thought that failure to flex the knees can potentially increase the risk of damage to their ligaments (M. Alter 1990; B. Anderson 1985). Other possible areas susceptible to injury include the muscles, ligaments, and additional soft tissues of the vertebral column.

Risk Reduction

The risk of this exercise can be reduced by performing it with the hands on the hips (Rippe 1990). This position reduces the moment of inertia and consequently requires less muscle activity to rotate the torso and to brake the movement of the trunk. A second alternative is to perform the stretch holding a broomstick across the back of the neck and shoulders while seated in a chair (Yessis 1986). Since the knees are then not bearing weight, momentum and stress on the knees are reduced. Third, if performed standing, the exercise should be executed

with the knees slightly flexed. Last, wearing a lifting belt is recommended for people squatting with weight (M. Alter 1990).

Gravity Inversion

Gravity inversion exercises are traction techniques in which an individual is placed in an inverted position with gravity providing the tractive force (Figure 15.9). A number of gravity inversion products are currently available. Gravity inversion devices can be classified into four major categories: ankle boots that attach to a horizontal bar, oscillating beds that allow moving from a horizontal to a completely inverted position simply by moving one's arms, inversion chairs, and inversion swings. These devices have become increasingly popular in both medical and nonmedical settings.

Analysis of Risk Factors

Ploucher (1982) reported perhaps the first complication observed in two patients who partici-

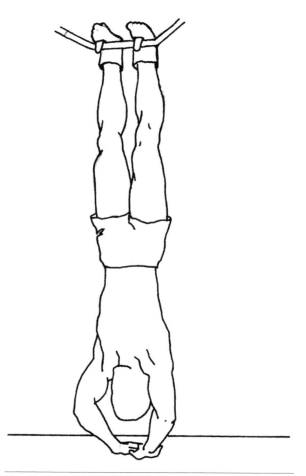

Fig. 15.9. An inversion technique.
Reprinted from Alter (1990).

pated in gravity inversion therapy. A 34-year-old woman and a 44-year-old man suffered periorbital petechiae (i.e., rupture of the blood vessels in the eye). Since Ploucher's observations were reported, several other researchers have expressed concern that inversion exercises may be potentially harmful. Their concern is based on studies that have shown increases in pulse rate and blood pressure in the inverted position (Ballantyne et al. 1986; Heng et al. 1992; Klatz et al. 1983; Leboeuf et al. 1987) and even when moving from a seated to a supine position (Leonard et al. 1983). In addition, increased intraocular pressure has been reported during inversion (Friberg and Weinreb 1985; Klatz et al. 1983; Le Marr, Golding, and Adler 1984; Weinreb, Cook, and Friberg 1984) and during movement from a seated to supine position (Galin, McIvor, and Magruder 1963; Krieglstein and Langham 1975). Another area of concern is the risk of potential retinal tear. Kobet (1985) reported a case of retinal tear without detachment that was presumed to be associated with hanging from gravity boots. There is further speculation that the use of gravity inversion devices could be dangerous for anyone with glaucoma, hypertension, weakness in a blood vessel, or spinal instability or for individuals on anticoagulant drugs or aspirin therapy (Ballantyne et al. 1986; Friberg and Weinreb 1985; Klatz et al. 1983; Leboeuf et al. 1987; Ploucher 1982; Weinreb, Cook, and Friberg 1984).

Despite the preceding findings, proponents of gravity inversion argue that a person's blood pressure rises after any form of exercise. Perhaps of greater significance, de Vries and Cailliet (1985) and Cailliet (1985) are of the opinion that a careful reinvestigation of previous findings have refuted many of the allegations against gravity inversion. Henry (1951), as quoted in de Vries and Cailliet (1985, 127), states:

> Protection against brain hemorrhage is given by the closed box of the skull. This protection is so effective that unprotected animals of human proportions can be exposed to 15 g without rupture of blood vessels, and no case of cerebral hemorrhage has yet been demonstrated following negative acceleration uncomplicated by asphyxia or trauma to the head. It is suggested that the danger of cerebral hemorrhage has been overestimated and that the risks of such accidental exposure of a human to 5 g are vanishingly small.

Consequently, the increases of arterial blood pressure should be of no clinical concern for individuals with a healthy cardiovascular system and without glaucoma.

Risk Reduction

As with all exercise programs, basic good health is a requirement for use of inversion devices. In particular, the medical community, researchers, and some manufacturers recommend that prospective participants should seek medical advice before using these devices (Cailliet 1985; de Vries 1985; Jay and Rappaport 1983; Martin 1982). After medical clearance, the next most important factor is competent supervision (de Vries 1985). Cailliet (1985) points out that those physicians who prescribe the use of gravity inversion need to specify its frequency, duration, indications or contraindications, and whether it is to be used passively or actively with an exercise program. Other factors that could help reduce risk factors include the use of devices that are ergonomically well designed, well constructed, and well balanced (de Vries 1985).

Rationale for Gravity Inversion

It has been hypothesized that gravity inversion may relieve or prevent low back pain via several mechanisms. Among them are stretching of the paravertebral muscles, reduction of muscular spasm, decompression of the spinal segments, relief of nerve entrapment, and relief of neuromuscular tension (Kane, Karl, and Swain 1985; Nosse 1978; Vernon, Meschino, and Naiman 1985). The theoretical basis for gravity inversion's effectiveness relates to the relaxation of peripheral neuromuscular tone. A vagotonic or parasympathetic influence on the cardiovascular system is also considered to cause reflex diminution of peripheral vascular resistance, leading to increased blood flow (Cailliet 1985; de Vries 1985; de Vries and Cailliet 1985). Cailliet (1985) reports that this relaxation is noted by many patients who hang with their head down or who meditate during headstand.

The Shoulderstand and the Plow

Probably the most controversial and potentially dangerous stretches for the cervical region are the shoulderstand and the plow. The former exercise is performed lying supine and raising the legs and torso to a vertical inverted position, with weight borne by the back of the head, neck, and shoulders and the hands placed on the lower back for support (Figure 15.10). In yoga, this asana is called the salamba sarvangasana, which means supporting or propping up the entire body (Iyengar 1979).

The plow is performed very similarly, except that the feet are lowered downward over the head so that the toes rest on the floor. In yoga, this asana is known as halsana, meaning plow position (Iyengar 1979). A variety of plow positions can be performed with various degrees of difficulty and potential risk (Figure 15.10, a–h).

Analysis of Risk Factors

The shoulderstand and the plow are potentially detrimental for several reasons. According to Kisner and Colby (1990), the first problem with these exercises is the forward-head posture. The body's weight creates a strong stretching force involving flexion of the upper thoracic region, a region that frequently tends to be flexed from faulty posture. Hence, the exercise reinforces the faulty posture.

With age comes an almost universal tendency for a forward-head posture to develop (Paris 1990). This forward-head posture is thought to be a consequence of faulty postural habits and awareness, compounded by occupational and recreational activities, and influenced by genetics (Kauffman 1987; Paris 1990). Therefore, Paris (1990) is of the opinion that the forward-head posture should be discouraged, especially in middle-aged and elderly people. This condemnation includes such exercises as the shoulderstand and plow. Instead, exercise and therapeutic programs should emphasize trunk and neck extension.

A second point raised by Kisner and Colby (1990) is that the flexed, inverted position compresses the lungs and heart. This decreases their potential effectiveness by impairing both circulation and respiration. Luby and St. Onge (1986) contend that the plow position also compresses the blood vessels to the brain, upper spinal cord, and chest.

Another interesting argument has been suggested by Judy Alter (1983). It is her hypothesis that these exercises can potentially injure the bones of the cervical region in a gradual way. Her rationale is that when the bones are irritated, in this case by bearing weight in a manner they are not meant to do, the body's response to the irritation is to send calcium to the area. Consequently, the wear-and-tear type of arthritic calcium deposits can and do build up on the neck vertebrae. A search of the literature was unable to substantiate this claim. However, this absence of evidence does not mean that this sequence of events is not plausible. It would make an interesting study to analyze X-rays taken of long-time practitioners of yoga to verify this hypothesis.

The most serious indictments against the shoulderstand and, more so, the plow deal with their potential risk to the vertebral joints. Numerous writers (J. Alter 1983; Beaulieu 1981; Berland and Addison 1972; Luby and St. Onge 1986; Shyne 1982; Tucker 1990; Tyne and Mitchell 1983) suggest that the plow also creates a risk of tearing of the spinal ligaments, injury to the sciatic nerve, and a herniated disk. The more body weight that is supported by the upper vertebral column, the greater the risk. With an additional force from a partner, the results could be disastrous.

Another factor to consider when analyzing the risk factor is age. Children are generally more supple than adolescents, adults, and the aged. However, this fact doesn't mean that the young are not susceptible to injury. The major problem confronting youth during these exercises is a lack of discipline. Horseplay while one is in a compromised position could result in a permanent injury to the vertebral column.

With aging there is an even greater risk of injury, because aging results in a decreased range of motion and a reduced margin of safety due to both quantitative and qualitative changes in the intervertebral disks. Among these changes are a decrease of water content in the nucleus pulposus, from 88% at birth to about 65% to 72% by age 75 (Puschel 1930), an increase in the collagen content of the nucleus pulposus, and a decrease in the concentration of elastic fibers in the annulus, from 13% at the age of 26 to about 8% at the age of 62. Consequently, with aging there is a greater probability of muscular strain, ligamentous sprain, and disk damage. In addition, there is an increased likelihood of osteoporosis in women with aging. The plow could thus be potentially risky because of the compression it places on the bones of affected people. (Clippinger-Robertson, cited in Lubell 1989).

These stretches can be intensified by implementing a number of variations (see Figure 15.10). One method incorporates placing the shins flat on the floor with the knees touching the shoulders. Another technique is to perform this modified position with a twist of the body. However, the greatest degree of potential risk is when the stretch is accentuated by a partner.

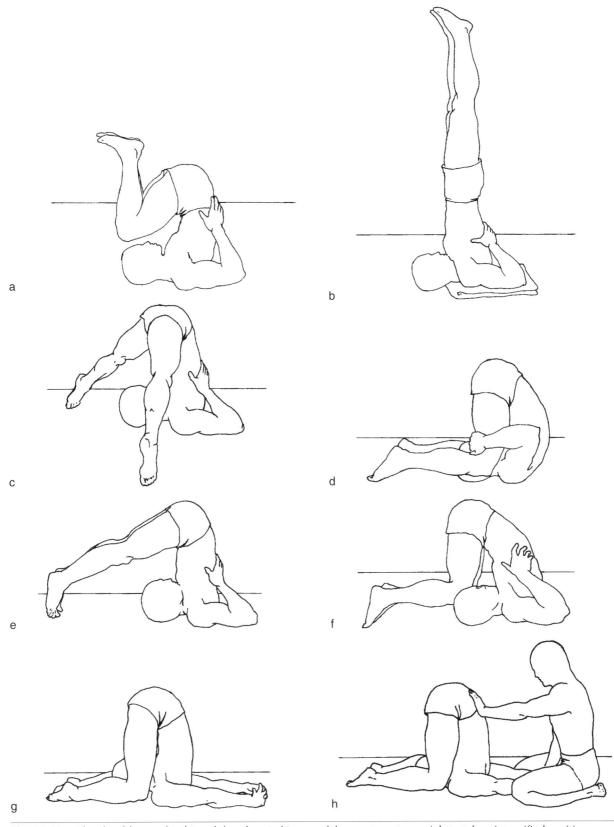

Fig. 15.10. The shoulderstand (a-b) and the plow (c-h), one of the most controversial stretches: intensified positions with a corresponding increased risk of injury.
Reprinted from Alter (1990).

Risk Reduction

The easiest method to reduce the risk of injury is to learn the exercise correctly in sequential stages. The emphasis must be on slowly developing adequate strength to support the body's weight and on increasing suppleness to withstand the tension of the stretch. As the level of fitness improves, the center of gravity can be permitted to move closer to the head, and the feet or shins can be allowed to rest on the floor. Cailliet and Gross (1987, 181) recommend an inverted bicycle modification of this exercise as a part of daily warm-up.

Rationale for the Shoulderstand and the Plow

In certain sports and related disciplines, the plow is considered basic and essential. For example, the skill is considered a requisite in track and field, wrestling, judo, and some martial arts (Alabin and Krivonosov 1987; Krejci and Koch 1979). Being subject to a pinning or submission hold may place one in this position. Consequently, there is no practical way that these exercises can be avoided in some disciplines. However, these exercises should not be practiced in a haphazard manner. Nor should these exercises be part of most conditioning programs. Their practice must be slow, deliberate, and technically precise (B. Anderson 1978; Fitt 1988; Kuprian, Ork, and Meissner 1982; Luby and St. Onge 1986; Peters and Peters 1983; Peterson and Renstrom 1986; Pollock and Wilmore 1990; Ritchen 1975; Roy and Irwin 1983). Two physical therapists conclude, "We like the plow for its benefits, but one must recognize the restrictions of a critical area of the body caused by flexion of the cervical vertebrae. Care must be taken" (Peters and Peters 1983, 33). Luby and St. Onge (1986, 123) concede:

> For the fitness of the average person, this exercise is too complicated. I don't feel one needs to accomplish it. [A well-designed routine can give] you a well-rounded program without the Plow. I recommend this exercise only for the advanced student and only [following specific directions].

No Absolute "No-Nos"

Should one incorporate these controversial stretches into an exercise program or not? There is a tremendous diversity of opinion. This very question was raised in an article by Lubell (1989), who sought the opinion of various experts. Two experts interviewed were Harold B. Falls, PhD, professor of biomedical science at Southwest Missouri State University, and James G. Garrick, MD, orthopedic surgeon and director of the Center for Sports Medicine at St. Francis Memorial Hospital in San Francisco, both editorial board members of *The Physician and Sportsmedicine*. Falls's response was, "There are no absolute no-no's. . . . Everything depends on the individual. There are some exercises that some people can't do, and there are others that some people can do" (p. 191).

In a similar vein, Garrick said:

> Some exercises are discouraged because people look at the movements and say, "Folks shouldn't do that. That looks dangerous." But it's wrong to issue a blanket condemnation of an exercise. There are some people who can and should be doing that exercise. . . . I think it is presumptuous for anyone to say you cannot do this or that. Under those conditions, up to one third of the exercises in the aerobic dance repertoire would be eliminated. (p. 191)

Summary

Flexibility exists on a continuum. At one end is immobility and at the opposite end is joint dislocation. Between these two extremes lies an optimal level of flexibility based on the needs of the individual. The literature is divided as to whether or not joint looseness and flexibility training are potentially detrimental for some individuals. Empirical evidence indicates that stretching should be avoided in hypermobile joints and that instead a strength training program should be initiated. For those people who are physically able, common sense suggests participating in both flexibility and strength training programs.

Stretching exercises are not risk free. However, certain exercises are considered to present a greater degree of risk of injury. They include the hurdler's stretch; the single- or double-leg inverted hurdler's stretch; deep knee bends, lunges, or squats (with or without weights); the standing straight-leg toe touch; the arch or bridge; the standing torso twist (with or without weights); inversion; and the shoulderstand or plow. Authorities disagree over the use of these and other exercises. The major argument in support of their use in athletics and other disciplines rests on the physical demands, technical requisites, and rules of the given discipline. If these exercises are to be incorporated in a training program, appropriate risk reduction strategies should be employed.

Chapter 16

Stretching and Special Populations

From time immemorial, people have searched for the elixir of youth, the magic potion that will restore spent vigor, or at least slow the relentless hands of time (Shephard 1978). The evidence of the effectiveness of wellness and restorative programs for improving strength and endurance is rather extensive, but less abundant in the area of range of motion. In this chapter we investigate numerous topics pertaining to flexibility training programs for geriatric, pregnant, and physically challenged populations.

Flexibility and the Geriatric Population

Aging brings about a loss of flexibility. Stretching exercises can improve flexibility, but the special health concerns of elderly people require precautions to avoid risk of injury. In the following sections, we consider the effects of aging and their consequences for flexibility and stretching programs.

Defining the Elderly

When is a person to be called old? Who are the elderly? Defined in terms of chronological age, the elderly usually include individuals 65 years of age and older. Reviewing the literature, Kramer and Schrier (1990) and May (1990) point out that it has become common to distinguish subgroups of the elderly, such as the *young old* (age 65 to 74),

the *old old*, *frail elderly*, or *aged* (age 75 and older), and the *oldest old* or *extremely old* (85 years of age and older). In contrast, the World Health Organization has adopted the following classification system:

Middle age: 45 to 59

Elderly: 60 to 74

Old: 75 to 90

Very Old: over 90

Whatever classification system is adopted, the elderly constitute a group that is characterized by considerable variation in physiological, mental, and functional capacity. Furthermore, dissimilarities among subgroups are often so pronounced that it can be misleading to consider the elderly as a single group (Hickok 1976; Kramer and Schrier 1990). These dissimilarities include genetic makeup, lifestyle, place of residence, and living arrangement.

Geriatric Demography

The numbers and proportions of older people are increasing in almost every country in the world. Furthermore, there is little doubt that life expectancy will continue to increase. In the United States, people over 65 years of age represent the most rapidly growing group in the population, numbering over 20 million (Table 16.1). Society is being faced with a growing segment of the population who have a greater need for health services and the least capacity to respond to these services. This change places extraordinary

Table 16.1. Selected Statistics on U.S. Population 65 Years of Age and Over, 1985–2080 (middle series projections in thousands)

	1985	2005	2025	2050	2080
Population 65+	28,540	36,275	59,713	68,532	71,630
Percentage of total population	11.9	13.2	20.0	22.8	24.5
Ages (number)					
65-69	9,433	10,106	19,257	17,325	16,951
70-74	7,577	8,304	15,420	14,265	14,977
75-79	5,503	7,246	11,378	12,042	12,820
80-84	3,333	5,287	6,647	9,613	9,917
85-89	1,762	3,141	3,769	7,670	7,681
90-94	720	1,539	2,014	4,775	5,160
95-99	184	520	903	2,066	2,685
100+	28	131	325	775	1,440
Ages (%)	100.0	100.0	100.0	100.0	100.0
65-69	33.0	27.8	32.2	25.3	23.7
70-74	26.5	22.9	25.8	20.8	20.9
75-79	19.3	20.0	19.0	17.6	17.9
80-84	11.7	14.6	11.1	14.0	13.8
85-89	6.2	8.6	6.3	11.2	10.7
90-94	2.5	4.2	3.4	7.0	7.2
95-99	0.6	1.4	1.5	3.0	3.7
100+	0.1	0.4	0.5	1.1	2.0
Sex ratios (male to female)	67.8	69.8	77.1	74.7	76.4
65-69	82.2	87.1	92.0	92.4	93.6
70-74	73.9	80.4	85.7	87.6	89.2
75-79	63.6	70.4	75.7	79.1	81.2
80-84	52.9	59.0	64.2	68.7	71.3
85-89	42.9	47.3	52.3	57.7	61.1
90-94	35.8	35.7	40.7	47.1	51.4
95-99	32.4	26.5	31.2	38.6	45.0
100+	16.7	18.0	20.8	28.8	37.1
Percentage nonwhite of total aged	9.8	12.8	16.2	21.3	26.5

Note. From *Projections of the Population of the United States, by Age, Sex, and Race: 1988 to 2080.* (Current Population Reports, Series P-25, No. 1018) by U.S. Bureau of the Census, 1989, Washington, DC: U.S. Government Printing Office. Reprinted from U.S. Bureau of the Census (1989).

responsibilities on those who are responsible for wellness and restorative programs for the elderly.

Research Dealing With Range of Motion in the Aged

Unfortunately, there has been a limited amount of research on changes in the range of joint motion in the elderly (Munns 1981). Research has shown that ROM decreases with age in the cervical region (Ferlic 1962; Shephard, Berridge, and Montelpare 1990), the shoulder (Allander et al.

1974; Bell and Hoshizaki 1981; Germain and Blair 1983; Shephard, Berridge, and Montelpare 1990), the spine (Einkauf et al. 1986), the spines of women (Battié et al. 1987), the hip (Boone and Azen 1979), the ankle (Shephard, Berridge, and Montelpare 1990; Vandervoort et al. 1992), and the wrist (Allander et al. 1974). In addition, M.L. Harris (1969b) reviewed two doctoral dissertation studies on flexibility in adults. In summary, in 510 men ranging in age from 18 to 71 (Greey 1955) and 407 women ranging in age from 18 to 74 (Jervey 1961), it was found that flexibility decreased with age for most movements.

There also has been a limited amount of research to test the effects of physical activity on the range of joint motion in the elderly. In a study by Frekany and Leslie (1975), 15 female volunteers, ranging from 71 to 90 years old except for one subject who was 55, served as subjects for flexibility measurements. They exercised for one-half hour two times a week for approximately seven months. In addition, the participants were encouraged to exercise on their own as often as possible, preferably daily. A significant improvement in flexibility was found in both the ankles and in the hamstrings and lower back.

Chapman, de Vries, and Swezey (1972) initiated a study to determine the effect of an exercise program on joint resistance (stiffness) of young and old men. The older group consisted of 20 volunteers from 63 to 88 years old. Both groups showed improvement in joint mobility after training. In another study, Gutman, Herbert, and Brown (1977) compared the effects of a Feldenkrais exercise program (i.e., slow therapeutic movement) with a conventional exercise program. Improvements in rotational flexibility were found in both groups. However, there were problems with the test design (Munns 1981).

Munns (1981) employed a 12-week exercise and dance program designed to work on the specific parts of the body to be measured. Twenty subjects over 65 years of age participated in a program that met three times per week for an hour each session. At the end of the program, the range of joint motion of the elderly subjects was significantly improved.

An investigation to determine the effectiveness of PNF flexibility techniques (see chapter 13) for improving hip joint flexibility in older females and to determine if local cold application could enhance the effectiveness of these techniques was carried out by Rosenberg et al. (1985). Thirty-one healthy subjects, ages 55 to 84, participated in the study. It was concluded that PNF flexibility maneuvers enhance hip flexibility in older females to a greater degree than do traditional static stretching techniques and that local cold application had no significant effect on flexibility.

In a more recent study, Raab et al. (1988) investigated the ability of weighted and nonweighted exercises to increase flexibility in 46 women aged 65 to 89 years. The subjects participated in an organized exercise program for one hour, three days per week, for 25 weeks. Similar flexibility increases were found to be achieved through exercise with or without weights for shoulder flexion, ankle plantar flexion, and cervical rotation.

Rationale for Stretching for the Elderly

Properly designed and conducted physical activity programs can increase the range of joint motion of subjects of all ages. Everyday functional pursuits may be limited by a lack of flexibility in major joints. For example, a person may find it difficult to reach something in the cupboard, to comb the back of the head, or even to put on shoes and socks (May 1990). Stiffness in the back or neck could make it difficult or impossible to turn and look backward when backing up a car, increasing the risk of an accident. Programs to increase flexibility can improve everyday functioning.

A second commonly stated rationale for exercising and stretching is to reduce the likelihood of sprains and muscle tears. Of particular importance is the potential for preventing or relieving low back pain by maintaining abdominal strength and low back flexibility through exercise (Pardini 1984). Although numerous testimonials are offered by authorities, no definitive proof has been presented to support this contention. Nonetheless, the Centers for Disease Control and Prevention and the American College of Sports Medicine recommend that people maintain or improve their flexibility to avoid muscle sprains and tears (Pate et al. 1995).

Potential Risks Associated With Stretching in the Elderly

A stretching exercise program can present risks for the geriatric population, in particular, the susceptibility to a fall. Virtually all forms of exercise present the possibility of injury, especially if inappropriate techniques are employed. Numerous factors influence the degree of risk exposure to the elderly. In the following sections, we analyze these risk variables, with special attention to the risk of falling.

Reduced Soft Tissue Elasticity

The application of inappropriate stretching techniques can be potentially hazardous. Three conditions prevalent in the geriatric population require special consideration. First, ligaments, tendons, and muscles in the elderly are less elastic and pliable. Generally, this change is due to decreased water content (i.e., dehydration), increased crystalline orientation, calcification, and the replacement of elastic fibers with collagenous fibers (see chapters 4 and 5). Consequently, these less elastic tissues are potentially subject to an injury such as a sprain or strain.

Osteoporosis and Arthritis

If an elderly person has been bedridden or immobilized or is in an advanced state of deconditioning, osteoporosis may be present. *Osteoporosis* is a bone condition associated with the loss of bone density or mass. Hence, it is sometimes called the bone-robbing disease. This disease is eight times more common in women than in men. Furthermore, it affects primarily small-boned white and Asian women. Because they tend to have greater bone mass than white or Asian women, black women are less likely to suffer from the disorder. Special care must be employed to prevent overzealous stretching that may induce a fracture in people affected with osteoporosis (Hickok 1976; Kisner and Colby 1990).

Another condition that requires special precaution is arthritis, which may occur in two different forms. *Osteoarthritis* is a chronic degenerative disorder that primarily affects the articular cartilage of weight-bearing joints. Treatment for patients with this condition depends on the joints afflicted and the degree of impairment. General treatment goals include decreasing pain, reducing stiffness, and preventing deformities (Kisner and Colby 1990). A program of passive, nonstressful ROM exercises is helpful. However, too much exercise or inappropriate, stressful exercise may aggravate symptoms (Wigley 1984).

Rheumatoid arthritis (RA) is another chronic joint (and systemic) disease, characterized by inflammation of the synovial membrane. The nature of stretching that is prescribed or allowed depends on the degree of inflammation and pain. The rule of thumb is that no strengthening or stretching exercise should cause severe pain at the time the exercise is performed, later pain lasting more than two hours, or increased joint inflammation or excessive pain on the day following the exercise regimen (Swezey 1978).

Reduced Strength

The decline in muscle strength that accompanies aging has long been recognized. Often, this loss of strength is a result of reducing activity, rendering the individual progressively weaker. However, precise strength values reported vary because they depend on many factors. This decrease is known to be due in part to a reduction in the number of muscle fibers and nerve cells (Herbison and Graziani 1995). More important

is the loss of contractile proteins within the muscle cell. Together these factors result in *atrophy*, or loss of muscle mass.

Muscular strength is needed for activities of daily living, as well as for coping with emergencies. Muscular strength must be an important consideration in designing a stretching program for the elderly. Many elderly people may lack sufficient muscular strength to support themselves in an erect stance for a prolonged period of time, resulting in fatigue and a potential fall. Therefore, these seniors have a reduced margin of safety. A logical adaptation is to do mobility exercises on the floor, because there is less chance of a fall. However, many programs for seniors rely on chairs for safe positioning, because many elderly people may lack sufficient strength to rise up from the floor (Rikkers 1986).

Balance and Proprioception Changes

Balance is an important component in some stretching exercises, most notably those that are performed standing. Sensory impairments involving visual, auditory, vestibular, and proprioceptive modalities may affect balance. With progressive degeneration of the proprioceptors due to aging, knowledge of one's position in space can be severely impaired. This ability is further compromised by a reduction in peripheral vestibular excitability. Eventually, these changes in postural stability are manifested as an increase in body sway. With increasing age, the visual contribution to equilibrium becomes the predominant method for assessing body position. Eventually, it too can become compromised. Consequently, the risk of falling increases as the loss of balance becomes increasingly severe.

Medication

Prescribed medications are ubiquitous among the elderly (Ray and Griffin 1990), and numerous sources have associated them with an increased risk of falls (Chapron and Besdine 1987; MacDonald 1985; Stewart 1987). The National Center for Health Statistics, cited by Ray and Griffin (1990), reported in June 1987 that in the United States more than 80% of women and 70% of men 65 years of age and older who live outside nursing homes receive one or more prescription medications at any given time. In nursing homes the prevalence of drug use is even higher. A consistent finding in the studies cited by MacDonald and MacDonald (1977) and by MacDonald (1985) was an increase in fall frequency among people taking more than one drug.

Drugs that are especially apt to predispose a person to falls include ones that induce somnolence (hypnotics), postural hypotension (diuretics, nitrates, antihypertensive agents, and tricyclic antidepressants), and confusion (cimetidine and digitalis; Wieman and Calkins 1986). Stewart (1987) points out that, to further compound matters, very few drugs have precise and narrow ranges of pharmacological effects; rather, many drugs have multiple pharmacological actions. For example, Thorazine, a drug commonly used by nursing home patients, is associated with sedation, decreased blood pressure, decreased motor activity, lowered convulsive threshold, changed EEG patterns, adrenergic blockade, cholinergic blockade, and altered endocrine function. Many drugs can alter functions that may impact the elderly patient's ability to perform stretching exercises and may increase the risk of such exercise programs.

Noncompliance

Another potential risk factor for the elderly is noncompliance. Noncompliance may be due to a variety of factors (e.g., loss of intelligence, decreased ability to remember, lack of a sense of time). The end result of noncompliance with an exercise program could endanger the well-being of an elderly person.

Reduction Risk Strategies for Stretching Exercise Programs for the Elderly

Safety always comes first. A variety of strategies can be implemented to reduce the risk of injury when stretching during an exercise class. In the following sections, several of these strategies will be discussed.

Medical Prescreening

Ideally, the instructor should know of any exercise contraindications for the participants taking the class. In addition, the instructor should know whether any of the participants have any special needs (e.g., auditory or visual impairments). By being aware of participants' physical limitations, the instructor can plan accordingly.

Environment and Facilities

The environment in which the activities are to be performed should be inspected for safety. The area should be large enough to accommodate all participants. There should be no obstructions or obstacles that the participants could kick, hit, or trip over. If the exercises are to be performed in a chair, it should be sturdy yet comfortable. If the exercises are to be practiced on the floor, a non-slip surface should be used. In addition, the carpeting or mat should be well padded to reduce potential discomfort and to cushion landings. Last, there should be adequate lighting and ventilation.

Communication and Instruction

Communication is a major component in instruction. Several factors need to be considered when instructing the elderly. Many elderly people have impaired auditory or visual capabilities. Therefore, the following basic guidelines should be implemented when instructing the older client:

- Eliminate all distracting background noise.
- Face the person to whom you are speaking.
- Talk slowly and clearly.
- Provide concise and simple directions.
- Demonstrate the desired exercise or position. (Remember, if the participants are to mimic your movements while facing you, they will use the opposite arm or leg.)
- Use effective kinesthetic cues.
- Provide time for the elderly to process and internalize the instructions.
- Continually monitor the participants' feedback.

Use a Low Center of Gravity

Another strategy that can be employed in some class settings is lowering the center of gravity of the elderly participants in order to maximize their stability. This modification can be achieved by performing exercises sitting on a chair or resting on the floor (Figure 16.1). However, many senior programs do not include floor exercise for the following reasons: Many older people have real fears about lowering themselves to the floor and getting stuck there; they may not know how to get up safely; and the kneeling position may be uncomfortable for people with arthritis or prior injuries (Rikkers 1986).

Exercise Protocol

Prior to exercising, the participants should be adequately warmed up. The routine should be paced to the ability of the participants. As a general rule, ballistic movements should be avoided since they are potentially more injurious than other types of stretches. Participants should be

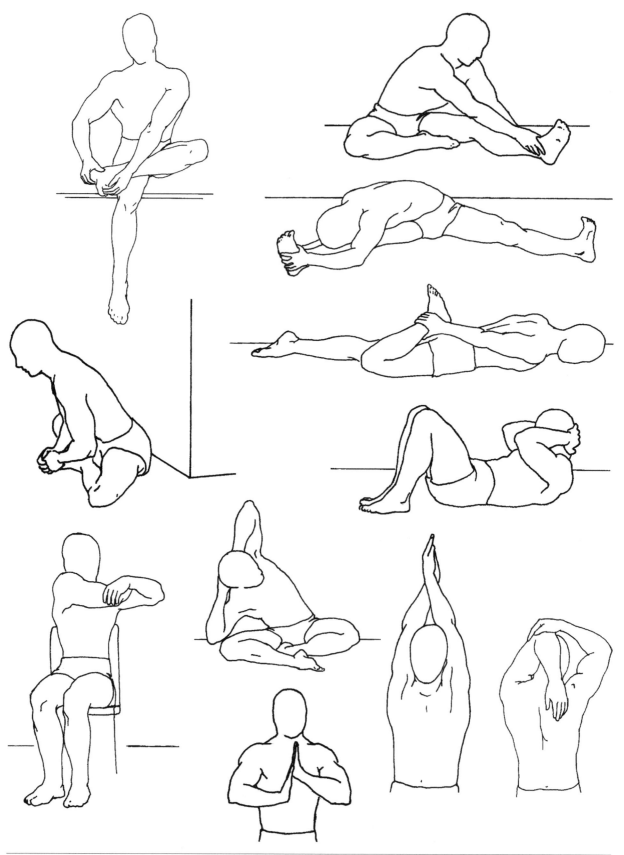

Fig. 16.1. Beneficial stretches for the older athlete. To reduce risk of injury, perform all stretches from a sitting or lying position for maximum balance and support.
Reprinted from Alter (1990).

instructed to breathe naturally during the session and not to hold their breath. Remember, the best form of exercise involves the entire body and is, above all, fun.

Flexibility and Pregnancy

What guidelines for exercise and stretching should women follow during pregnancy and the postpartum period? The American College of Obstetricians and Gynecologists (ACOG) has addressed this question (American College of Obstetricians and Gynecologists 1985, 1994). At the opening of their guidelines, ACOG (1985, 1) cautions women to use common sense and discretion before adopting any exercise program:

> The number and type of exercise programs available now to pregnant and postpartum women have increased dramatically. Some of these programs were designed by nonprofessionals who lack the scientific background to appreciate potential problems and to take steps to minimize their occurrence. A recent review of several exercise programs being marketed to pregnant and postpartum patients revealed medical content that was often inappropriate, inaccurate, or incomplete.
>
> Exercise standards for pregnant women, one of the major subgroups in the general population, have not been set. At present, recommendations for pregnant and postpartum patients are based largely on intuition and "common sense." Little research has been done on the effects of exercise during pregnancy and the postpartum period, and ethical considerations make it almost impossible to define limits of safety.

Risk Reduction During Pregnancy

Perhaps the most prudent and important way to reduce risk during pregnancy is for "all pregnant women [to] obtain an obstetrical and medical examination early in gestation and before engaging in exercise programs" (Mittelmark et al. 1991). Concurrent with the examination the physician should provide specific advice to the patient regarding guidelines for exercise. Mittelmark et al. (1991) state that patients should be educated to recognize and be alert to various symptoms that should signal the patient to stop exercise and contact her physician:

(a) pain of any kind; (b) uterine contractions (at 15-min intervals or more frequent); (c) vaginal bleeding, leaking amniotic fluid; (d) dizziness, faintness; (e) shortness of breath; (f) palpitations, tachycardia; (g) persistent nausea and vomiting; (h) back pain; (i) pubic or hip pain; (j) difficulty in walking; (k) generalized edema; (l) numbness in any part of the body; (m) visual disturbances; and (n) decreased fetal activity. (p. 301)

Factors That Increase the Risk of Injury During Pregnancy

The factors that increase the risk of injury during stretching for pregnant women can be classified as biomechanical or hormonal. The biomechanical factors deal with forces and torques specific to the pregnant body. The influence of hormones renders parts of the body more susceptible to injury.

Biomechanical Factors

Numerous biomechanical factors influence women during pregnancy. One important factor for women contemplating exercise is that total body mass increases throughout pregnancy. This increase in weight is a product of the growing fetus and the mother's retention of fluids, development of fatty tissues, and enlarging breasts. The mother's center of gravity is altered during the later stages of pregnancy because of the increased weight anterior to the body. A change in the center of gravity alters a women's stability and influences the mechanical loading on the body. In particular, greater effort is required of the lower back muscles to prevent the body from falling forward and downward. Therefore, pregnant women should avoid stretching exercises that exacerbate overloading of the back and increase the chance of falls. To improve stability, stretching exercises can be performed while sitting on the ground or on a chair.

Hormonal Factors

As discussed in chapter 10, pregnant women are also influenced by hormonal changes. The loosening of the connective tissues as a result of the hormones estrogen, progesterone, and relaxin may compromise joint stability. This change, in combination with the changes in mechanical loading, may produce serious consequences for the pregnant woman, including increased strain on the sacroiliac and hip joints and, more rarely, separation of the symphysis pubis (ACOG 1985;

McNitt-Gray 1991). Therefore, it is recommended that ballistic movements and deep flexion or extension of joints be avoided and that stretches not be taken to the point of maximum resistance (ACOG 1985). ACOG (1994) points out that, theoretically, hormonal influences may result in generalized increases in joint laxity, thus predisposing the pregnant woman to mechanical trauma or sprains. This hypothesis has been substantiated by objective data only in the metacarpophalangeal joints in a study by Calguneri, Bird, and Wright (1982).

Developing an Exercise Program During Pregnancy

According to ACOG (1985, 1), "The safety of the mother and infant is the primary concern in any exercise program prescribed in conjunction with pregnancy." Therefore, ACOG (1985, 1) is of the opinion that "the goal of exercise during pregnancy and the postpartum period should be to maintain the highest level of fitness consistent with the maximum safety." What must be recognized is that no two women are alike. Some women may be able to tolerate more strenuous exercise than others. Obviously, the guidelines for laywomen will differ from those for highly trained or professional athletes (Mittelmark et al. 1991). For either group, exercise programs should be tailored to meet the individual needs of the patient.

Stretching and Yoga for Pregnant Women

Stretching and yoga exercises are often recommended during and after pregnancy in books and magazines targeted at the general public. One rationale offered by their proponents is to facilitate relaxation. A second justification is to maintain muscle tone and flexibility (Baddeley and Green 1992). A third reason is the popular belief that various stretching and yoga exercises will improve the quality of the labor by loosening the pelvic area and helping prepare the pregnant woman for birth (Tobias and Stewart 1985). Exercise may also help relieve backache and other minor discomforts (Tobias and Stewart 1985). However, ACOG (1994, 4) points out that "no level of exercise during pregnancy has been conclusively demonstrated to be beneficial in improving perinatal outcome."

Flexibility and People With Physical Disabilities

Another population that deserves recognition are people who have impairments and disabilities. An *impairment* refers to any disturbance or interference with normal structure and function of the body. Examples of impairments include loss of an anatomic part, blindness, deafness, cerebral palsy, or spinal cord injury. In contrast, the term *disability* is used to identify the loss or reduction of ability to carry out one's role as dictated by culture or family. Thus, impairments may predispose one to disability.

A variety of pathologies cause disabilities or impairment. Each of these pathological entities may present difficulties in a specific activity or sport. Nonetheless, virtually any individual can participate in some type of stretching program. However, the exercises will need to conform to the limitations and needs of the individual. For many people with disabilities, stretching aids such as balls, ropes, sticks, and wands may be of assistance. Besides being effective in enhancing ROM, such aids can also add creativity, enjoyment, and play to stretching.

Summary

Research has shown that flexibility generally decreases with age. But flexibility can be maintained and improved among most elderly people. However, exercising, and stretching in particular, can present a degree of risk to the geriatric population. Preventive strategies should be employed in exercise programs to reduce the risk of injury to elderly people. Pregnant women are also cautioned to employ common sense and discretion before adopting any exercise program. The most important way to reduce risk is to obtain an obstetrical and medical examination throughout and after the pregnancy. To date, there is no scientific evidence that exercise results in shorter labors, easier labors, fewer complications, or benefit to the baby. People with physical disabilities can also benefit from a stretching program. However, the exercises will need to conform to the limitations and needs of the individual.

— Chapter 17 —

Anatomy and Flexibility of the Lower Extremity and Pelvic Girdle

For our purposes, the lower extremity and pelvic girdle shall be considered to consist of the foot, ankle, leg, knee joint, thigh, gluteal region, iliac region, and hip joint. This chapter contains a description of this anatomical area's structure, function, limits on range of motion, potential for injury, and preferred method of stretching. This chapter describes the flexibility of each region of the lower extremity, beginning with the toes and progressing toward the trunk. (Stretching exercises following chapter 20 are referred to where appropriate.)

The Foot and Toes

The foot is a very complicated structure. It has three major anatomical parts: the hindfoot, consisting of the calcaneus and talus; the midfoot, comprising the navicular, cuboid, and three cuneiform bones; and the forefoot, formed by the metatarsals and phalanges (Figure 17.1). It contains 26 bones (7 tarsals, 5 metatarsals, and 14 phalanges) and four layers of interwoven and overlapping fascia, muscles, tendons, and liga-

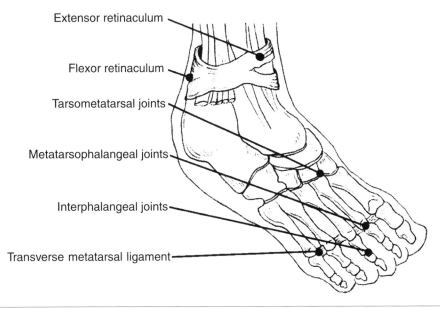

Extensor retinaculum

Flexor retinaculum

Tarsometatarsal joints

Metatarsophalangeal joints

Interphalangeal joints

Transverse metatarsal ligament

Fig. 17.1. The bones and joints of the foot.
Reprinted from Donnelly (1982).

ments. The structure of the foot is similar to the hand, but with differences that adapt it to the functions of weight bearing, shock absorption, and propulsion.

The foot is an elastic, arched structure. The *plantar vault* is an architectural feature that unites all the elements of the foot—joints, ligaments, and muscles—into a single system. It acts as the shock-absorber essential for the flexibility of the foot. However, the curvature and orientation of the vault depend on a delicate balance of muscles (Kapandji 1987). For example, with *pes cavus* (claw feet), there is an unusually high arch, which can result from contractures of the plantar aponeurosis or from the use of shoes with soles that are too rigid (Cailliet 1977; Kapandji 1987). Cailliet recommends exercises for this condition designed to stretch the toe extensors and distal toe flexors. Another problem of the plantar vault is the absence of the longitudinal arch, referred to as *pes planus* (flat feet). Pes planus is usually congenital but may be due to muscle paralysis.

Significance of a Flexible Foot and Ankle

A rigid system absorbs less energy than a flexible one. Such a system is less efficient and more prone to breakdown. On the other hand, a supple foot and ankle absorb energy efficiently, resulting in less chance for injury. For individuals involved in ballet, flexibility in this region is a must, as explained by Hamilton (1978d, 85):

> Flexibility is needed in the instep or midfoot so that the foot in the pointe position becomes the projection of the axis of the tibia (shinbone). This position requires a total of ninety degrees of plantar flexion (combining motion at the ankle and instep), and actually, a few degrees more if the downward movement is going to compensate for the recurvatum most dancers have at the knee [see Figure 17.2]. If this motion is not present, the dancer will not be "all the way up" on pointe or demi-pointe. There is a tremendous difference between being all the way up and almost all the way up in terms of the extra energy required to maintain the pointe position. The result is chronic overstrain of the Achilles and other tendons.

Limits on Foot Range of Motion

The ranges of motion in the foot depend on a variety of things: bony structure, joint articula-

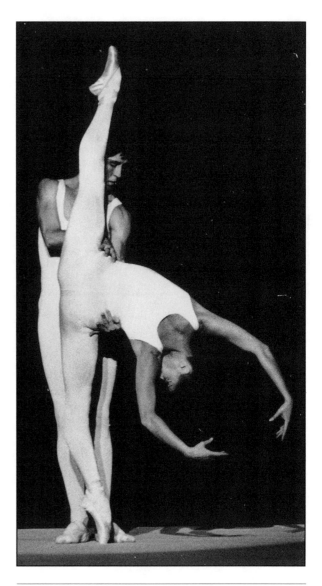

Fig. 17.2. In a pas de deux, Soviet ballerina Galina Shlyapina demonstrates her perfect natural facility for pointe work and turnout.
Reprinted from Warren (1989).

tions, fascia, ligaments, musculature, and tendon support. Like other parts of the body, the foot can become more flexible if its tissues are stretched. But often this part of the body is neglected, for working on flexibility in the foot requires diligence and hard practice.

Interphalangeal and Metatarsophalangeal Joints of the Toes

The interphalangeal (IP) joints are located between the segments of each toe. Each toe has two

IP joints, except for the big toe, which has only one IP joint. The metatarsophalangeal (MTP) joints are located where each toe is attached to the foot; each toe has one MTP joint. Flexion of the IP and MTP joints involves bending the toes toward the sole of the foot. Flexion at these joints has been reported to range from 0° to 90° at the IP joints and from 0° to 35° at the MTP joints (Kapandji 1987). Flexion is produced by both the intrinsic (i.e., muscles that have both origin and insertion within the foot) and extrinsic (i.e., muscles that have their origin outside of the foot) phalangeal flexors. Factors than limit range of motion in the toes are flexor muscle contractile insufficiency, passive tension of the extensor muscle tendons of the toes, and contact of the soft parts of the phalanges.

Extension of the IP and MTP joints involves drawing the phalanges away from the sole of the foot. Extension of the phalanges ranges approximately from 0° to 80°. This movement is produced primarily by the extrinsic extensors of the foot. Factors limiting range of motion are contractile insufficiency and tension of the plantar and collateral ligaments of the toe joints. Extension may also be limited by tight plantar fascia or plantar fascitis (i.e., inflammation of the plantar fascia). Planter fascitis may cause severe pain when running on the balls of the feet.

The plantar metatarsal arch and plantar fascia can be stretched by using either one's own weight or hand. However, the literature is divided over the application of such stretching. J. Alter (1989–1990) is of the opinion that stretching the metatarsal arch and plantar fascia is detrimental or contraindicated. In contrast, a number of sources contend that stretching is recommended (American Academy of Orthopaedic Surgeons 1991; Andrews 1983; Baxter and Davis 1995; Brody 1995; Cantu 1982; Cramer and McQueen 1990; DiRaimondo 1991; Graham 1987; Kraeger 1993; Krissoff and Ferris 1979; Kulund 1980; Lutter 1983; McPoil and McGarvey 1995; Peterson and Renstrom 1986; Subotnick 1979). Additional research is necessary to validate either of these claims. It is agreed that a strength training program must be a part of the management plan.

The Talocrural Joint

The *talocrural*, or ankle, joint is an example of a hinge joint. It is formed by the tibia and fibula (bones of the lower leg) and talus (bone of the

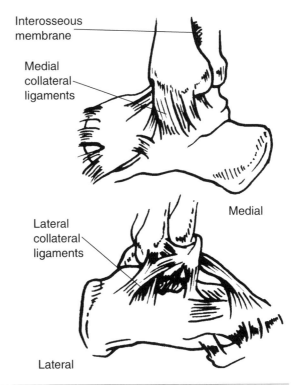

Fig. 17.3. Medial and lateral views of the ligaments of the ankle.
Reprinted from Donnelly (1982).

foot; Figure 17.3). The relationship of these three bones is maintained by a fibrous capsule, ligaments, and musculotendinous structures. The medial collateral ligament, or *deltoid ligament*, of the ankle has four components: the posterior tibiotalar, the tibiocalcaneal, the tibionavicular, and the anterior tibiotalar. The *lateral collateral ligament* comprises three bands: the anterior talofibular, the posterior talofibular, and the calcaneofibular. Because the bony stability is greater laterally than medially (due to the difference in length of the fibula and tibia) and because the deltoid ligament is stronger than the lateral collateral ligament, the joint is predisposed toward inversion (turning in). This fact is of particular importance because the vast majority of all ankle ligament injuries are common inversion sprains, involving tearing structures on the lateral side.

Effects of Excessive Talocrural Stress

The bone structure of an ankle and foot can be modified by excessive stress. For instance, it has been reported that dancers who begin training before age 12 will exhibit architectural changes in the tarsal bones that will allow for increased mobility and plantar flexion of the forefoot (Ende and Wickstrom 1982; Nikolic and Zimmermann 1968). However, excessive stress can also result in decreased range of motion. The formation of spurs on the anterior and posterior lips of the talus limit the range of dorsiflexion and plantar flexion, respectively (Brodelius 1961; Ende and Wickstrom 1982; Hamilton 1978c, 1978d; Howse 1972), which can result in asymmetrical pliés for dancers (Ende and Wickstrom 1982; Schneider et al. 1974). Another problem with excessive stress is osteophytes (small bone spurs) on the tibia impinging on the superior dorsal neck (in front of the ankle), limiting dorsiflexion of the talus. Ankle motion can also be limited by the presence of an extra bone behind the ankle, called an *os trigonum* (Brodelius 1961; Ende and Wickstrom 1982; Hamilton 1978b; Howse 1972).

Limits on Talocrural Range of Motion

The ranges of motion of the ankle depend on its bony structure, joint articulation, fascia, ligaments, musculature, and tendon support. The tissues of the joint are capable of being stretched and its flexibility enhanced, as seen particularly in ballet dancers.

Eversion or Pronation

Eversion, or pronation of the ankle, is turning the sole of the foot so that it tends to move outward and face laterally. This movement is produced primarily by two muscles: the peroneus longus and peroneus brevis. Eversion ranges approximately from 0° to 20°. The factors limiting this motion are evertor contractile insufficiency, passive tension of the deltoid ligaments, passive tension of the tibialis anterior and tibialis posterior muscles, tightness of the medial aspect of the joint capsule, and contact of the tarsal bones with the fibula laterally.

Inversion or Supination

Inversion, or supination of the ankle, is turning the sole of the foot so that it tends to move or face medially. The movement is produced by invertor muscles, primarily the tibialis anterior and tibialis posterior, and is assisted by the flexor digitorum longus, flexor hallucis longus, and medial head of the gastrocnemius. Inversion of the ankle ranges approximately from 0° to 45°. The factors limiting the range of motion are invertor contractile insufficiency, passive tension of ligaments (including the interosseous talocalcaneal ligament, the other tarsal interosseous ligaments, and the calcaneofibular ligament), passive tension of the evertor muscles (peroneus longus and peroneus brevis), tightness of the lateral aspect of the joint capsule, and contact of the tarsal bones with the tibia medially.

Plantar Flexion

Plantar flexion of the ankle is moving the top of the foot away from the front of the shin (i.e., physiological extension of the foot). This movement is produced by plantar flexor muscles, primarily the gastrocnemius and soleus, and is assisted by the tibialis posterior, peroneus longus, peroneus brevis, flexor hallucis longus, flexor digitorum longus, and plantaris. Ankle plantar flexion ranges approximately from 0° to 50°. Factors limiting range of motion are plantar flexor contractile insufficiency, passive tension of the anterior talofibular and the anterior tibiotalar ligaments, passive tension of the dorsiflexor muscles, tightness of the dorsal aspect of the joint capsule, and bone contact of the posterior portion of the talus with the tibia.

Dorsiflexion

Dorsiflexion of the ankle is moving the top of the foot upward and toward the front of the shin (i.e., physiological flexion of the foot). Ankle dorsiflexion is produced primarily by the tibialis anterior and is assisted by the extensor digitorum longus, extensor hallucis longus, and peroneus tertius. Dorsiflexion ranges approximately from 0° to 20°. Factors limiting range of motion are dorsiflexor contractile insufficiency, passive tension of the plantar flexors (especially the gastrocnemius and soleus, but also the tibialis posterior, flexor hallucis longus, flexor digitorum longus, peroneus longus, and peroneus brevis muscles), passive tension of the Achilles tendon, tension of the deltoid and calcaneofibular ligaments, tightness of the posterior aspect of the joint capsule, and bone contact of the talus with the anterior margin of the tibial surface.

It should be noted that dorsiflexion range is greater with the knee flexed than with it extended, due to the influence of a two-joint muscle, the gastrocnemius, which crosses both the ankle and knee joints. When the knee is flexed, this muscle is slack at the knee, allowing it to stretch more at the ankle. However, when the knee is extended, the gastrocnemius is stretched there, allowing it to stretch less at the ankle (passive insufficiency).

Talocrural Injury Prevention

The ankle and foot are susceptible to many injuries, including fascial and ligamentous sprains, muscle strains, tendinitis (inflammation of a tendon or its connective tissue sheath), and stress (incomplete or partial) fractures. Preventive actions include proper conditioning, adequate warm-up and stretching, utilization of proper technique, wearing appropriate shoes, avoiding hard surfaces, resting when fatigued, and avoiding overuse.

The Lower Leg

The *crus*, or lower leg, is the segment of the lower limb between the knee and ankle. It is analogous to the smaller forearm segment of the upper limb. The lower leg is made up of two bones: the tibia, or shinbone, and its smaller companion, the fibula. The two bones are connected together by the interosseous membrane. Surrounding the tibia and fibula are a number of muscles that are susceptible to injury if not adequately stretched before activation. These muscles are all enclosed by a tough connective tissue sheath, the crural fascia.

The Posterior Calf Muscles

The *calf* comprises the muscles in the posterior portion of the lower leg. The calf has three superficial muscles, the gastrocnemius, soleus, and plantaris, plus four deep muscles, the popliteus, flexor hallucis longus, flexor digitorum longus, and tibialis posterior. The gastrocnemius muscle can flex the knee (Figure 17.4). However, the primary function of the superficial muscles is plantar flexion of the ankle; the primary function of the deep muscles is flexion of the toes and inversion of the foot.

The gastrocnemius, the most superficial calf muscle, comprises two portions, or heads, and forms the greater bulk of the calf. The soleus is a broad, flat muscle situated immediately deep, or anteriorly, to the gastrocnemius. Together, they form a muscular mass called the *triceps surae*. The triceps surae contributes 90% of the total plantar

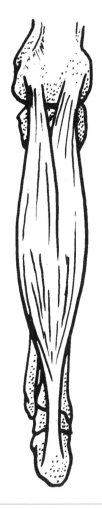

Fig. 17.4. The gastrocnemius muscle. Reprinted from Donnelly (1982).

flexion force of the posterior muscles. The tendons of the gastrocnemius and soleus form the tendo calcaneus, or Achilles tendon.

The tendo calcaneus is the largest and strongest tendon in the body. Its distal end is attached to the posterior surface of the calcaneus. The strength of the tendon approximates 1.24×10^8 N/m² (18,000 psi). Despite the tendon's tremendous strength, it is not invulnerable to injury. The vulnerability of the Achilles tendon will be discussed in the next section.

Injuries to the Posterior Calf Muscles and Achilles Tendon

Pulls or strains of the calf are not uncommon. They can be caused by cold muscles, inadequate warm-up, overuse, fatigue, improper technique, working on a hard surface, or stepping unexpectedly in a hole. A pull of the calf has been dubiously named *tennis leg*, somewhat a misnomer because it often occurs in activities other than tennis. However, it has been demonstrated by surgical exploration that tennis leg is due to a tear of the musculotendinous junction of one of the heads of the gastrocnemius muscle, that is, where the gastrocnemius attaches to the Achilles tendon (Arner and Lindholm 1958; Feit and Berenter 1993; W.A. Miller 1977; Roy and Irwin 1983).

The most common type of injury to the Achilles tendon is tendinitis, most often caused by overuse. Treatment of tendinitis includes rest, ice, mild anti-inflammatory medicines, and appropriate medical assistance. However, the most catastrophic injury to a tendon is rupture. Rupture can be compared to the giving way of an old, frayed rope, because the fibers of a tendon are not straight, but coiled like rope. Treatment consists of either prolonged immobilization in a cast or surgical repair. A preventive approach that includes enhancing both the tendon's flexibility and strength is practical and prudent.

Stretching the Posterior Calf Muscles and Achilles Tendon

The method used to stretch the lower leg's posterior muscles and tendons is virtually identical to the mechanism that often initiates injury. To stretch these muscles, the feet are slowly dorsiflexed from a neutral position with the knee joint in flexion and then in extension. Injury is due to a rapid or ballistic dorsiflexion (Feit and Berenter 1993); prevention of injury is aided by safer slow stretching. Proper stretching of these muscles can be achieved by sitting upright on the floor, kneeling, or standing. In a modified hurdler's stretch position, the stretch is initiated when one pulls up on the toes toward the body. If the toes cannot be reached, a towel may be used (see Exercise #9). Another commonly employed stretch is to stand about 1 m (3 ft) from a wall and lean forward while keeping the heels down (see Exercise #7). One or both legs simultaneously may be stretched in this way.

The Anterior and Lateral Lower Leg Muscles

There are four anterior muscles (on the front of the shin). The tibialis anterior is anterolateral to the tibia and is the major dorsiflexor of the ankle joint and invertor of the foot. The extensor hallucis longus, the extensor digitorum longus, and the peroneus tertius assist in dorsiflexion, and the former two muscles also extend the toes.

There is another set of lower leg muscles, the peroneal group, which are situated on the lateral side of the lower leg. The group consists of the peroneus longus and the peroneus brevis muscles. Both muscles assist in plantar flexion of the feet, but their primary function is to evert the feet.

Injuries to the Anterior and Lateral Lower Leg Muscles

Pretibial periostitis, or shinsplints, is one of the most common injuries to the anterior and lateral regions of the leg. This catch-all syndrome is thought to be most often a microscopic tearing of the attachments of the muscles from the tibia, resulting in tenderness or a dull pain. The etiology of shinsplints has been vaguely attributed to a number of causes, including practicing on hard surfaces, improper warm-up, poor technique, fallen foot arches, improper body balance from low back strain, inherited tendency, lack of flexibility, strength imbalance between the anterior and posterior calf muscles, fatigue, and overuse. Shinsplints can be treated with ice, warm soaks, whirlpool, gentle massage, stretching, taping, reduced activity, or rest, followed later by strengthening. Furthermore, O'Malley and Sprinkle (1986) claim that a deliberate and specialized series of stretching exercises to the anterior aspect of the legs prior to and following physical activity such as running or jogging can drastically reduce (or even eradicate) the occurrence of shinsplints. It has also been suggested that stretching calf muscles will help reduce the possibility of shinsplints (Ellis 1986; Flood and Nauert 1973; Schuster 1978).

Stretching the Anterior and Lateral Lower Leg Muscles

The anterior lower leg muscles can be stretched by slowly plantar flexing. A safe method is to apply a manual stretch by extending the ankle, with one leg crossed over the other while in a sitting position (see Exercise #3). An easily employed method is to stand and lean against a wall with one foot turned under. Then, one's weight is shifted onto the top of the foot to develop the stretch. A method often cited in yoga texts and in numerous sports medicine sources is sitting on the shins with the toes facing back. However, this exercise should be used with caution because of the potential stress placed on the knees by their extreme flexion. Several modifications can reduce the stress, such as sitting on a folded blanket placed on the calves or adjusting the separation between the buttocks and feet. With time, the blanket can be lowered until one is resting on the calves and heels. With increased proficiency, the body weight is gradually shifted backward. Maximum isolation of the tibialis anterior can be achieved from this sitting position by reaching behind, grasping the top portion of your toes (especially the big toe), and pulling them toward your buttocks (see Exercise #4). Once again, go *slowly* and use caution.

The easiest and safest method to stretch the lateral lower leg muscles is to apply a manual stretch by slowly plantar flexing and inverting the ankle, with one leg crossed over the other while in a sitting position (see Exercise #5). A second method is to assume a modified hurdler's stretch position, reach down and grasp the outer portion of your foot (or use a towel if it cannot be reached), and slowly turn the outside of the foot medially. Last, standing on the sole of the feet on an inclined board at a 45° angle is another very simple method to stretch this group.

The Genual Joint

The *genual*, or knee, joint is the largest joint in the body. It is formed by the articulation of three bones: the femur (thigh bone), tibia, and fibula. The knee is an example of a modified hinge joint. The patella (kneecap) glides in front of the femur (see Figure 17.5). Since the bony arrangement of the genual joint is architecturally weak, compensation must be provided by the firm support of muscles and the joint's nine ligaments.

Limits on Genual Range of Motion

The knee moves almost exclusively in flexion and extension. Medial and lateral rotations of the tibia are possible only to a slight degree when the knee is flexed. Consequently, flexion and extension are the motions that will be discussed.

Genual Flexion

Flexion of the knee involves moving the lower leg so as to bring the heel up to the back of the thigh. Flexion can be carried to about 120° with the hip joint extended, to about 135° when the hip joint is flexed, and to about 160° when a passive force, such as sitting on the heels, is introduced. During active movement of the unweighted leg, knee flexion is performed by two sets of biarticular muscles: the hamstrings and the gastrocnemius. Range of motion is limited by

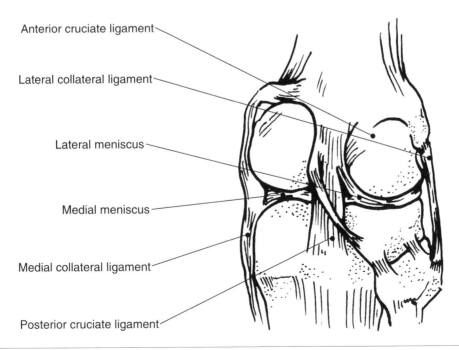

Anterior cruciate ligament

Lateral collateral ligament

Lateral meniscus

Medial meniscus

Medial collateral ligament

Posterior cruciate ligament

Fig. 17.5. The knee.
Reprinted from Donnelly (1982).

flexor muscle contractile insufficiency, passive tension of the quadriceps extensor muscles and their tendon, passive tension in the anterior parts of the capsule, passive tension of the posterior cruciate ligament (with moderate flexion) and both cruciate ligaments (in extreme passive flexion), and contact of the heel and posterior portion of the lower leg with the posterior portion of the thigh and buttocks. Stretches that enhance flexion of the knee will be discussed in the section dealing with the anterior femoral muscles.

Genual Extension

Extension of the knee is the return movement from flexion. Extension beyond 0° has been referred to as *genu recurvatum* or swayback knee. However, the American Academy of Orthopaedic Surgeons (Greene and Heckman 1994) have adopted the term *hyperextension*. Hyperextension is caused by ligamentous and capsular instability or bony deformity. It is one measure for presence of the hypermobility syndrome (Beighton, Solomon, and Soskolne 1973; Carter and Wilkinson 1964; Grahame and Jenkins 1972). Wynne-Davies (1971), in a study of 3,000 Edinburgh children, found that 15% of the three-year-old children could extend their knee beyond 10°. However, this degree of extension was observed in fewer than 1% at six years of age. In two large studies of healthy adult males, the average knee extension was −2° ± 3°. It is normal for adults to have a slight degree of flexion at the knee joint when standing (Greene and Heckman 1994). If hyperextension is present, stretching exercises that further extend the knee should be avoided. Even in nonhypermobile knees, one must be careful not to lock or press back the knee joint when stretching. Instead, bend the knee slightly, and bring it back to a straight, but strong, position. Then raise the kneecaps up toward the thigh (Follan 1981).

Extension of the knee is produced by the powerful quadriceps muscle group, consisting of the rectus femoris, vastus lateralis, vastus medialis, and vastus intermedialis. Factors limiting range of motion are quadriceps contractile insufficiency, passive tension in the hamstring and gastrocnemius muscles, tension of the cruciate ligaments or of the tibial and fibular collateral ligaments, and tightness of the posterior aspect of the capsule. Any abnormal locking of the knee in flexion may also restrict extension and may be due to a mechanical internal derangement, such as a loose body or torn meniscus. The knee is a slid-ing or gliding mechanism. Any foreign object that is interposed between two surfaces will block motion in the same fashion that a wedge beneath a door will hold it fast. Stretches for the knee's extensors will be discussed in the section dealing with the posterior femoral muscles.

The Mechanical and Structural Disadvantages of the Muscles at the Genual Joint

One of the potentially detrimental aspects of the knee joint is that it is partially controlled by two-joint muscles. The hamstrings, which function to flex the knee as well as extend the hip, and the rectus femoris, which extends the knee and flexes the hip, are two examples (Fujiwara and Basmajian 1975; R.E. Jones 1970; Kelley 1971; Markee et al. 1955). Trouble develops when both muscle groups are simultaneously moved to their extremes. The resulting tension on the muscles and tendons may become so great as to cause an injury. Kelley (1971) clearly illustrates how this injury mechanism can happen during the act of sprinting: The passive tension on the rectus femoris must be considerable when the trailing leg is in knee flexion and hip extension. The hamstrings must suffer the same sort of passive stress when a hurdler's leading leg undergoes simultaneous hip flexion and nearly complete knee extension, when a cheerleader or dancer performs high leg kicks, or when a high jumper uses the straddle technique. Stretching exercises for the knee's flexors will be discussed in the section dealing with the posterior femoral muscles.

The Upper Leg

The *thigh* is the segment of the leg between the hip and knee. This limb segment contains a single bone, the femur. The femur is the longest and strongest bone in the body, and is surrounded by a number of muscles called the femoral muscles.

The Posterior Femoral Muscles

The posterior portion of the thigh is made up of three muscles: the biceps femoris, the semitendinosus, and the semimembranosus (Figure 17.6). In lay terminology, these muscles are known as the *hamstrings*. This word evolved from

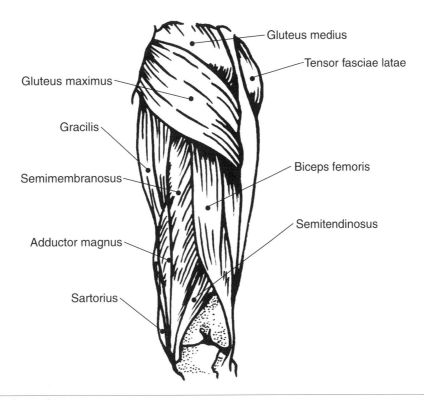

Fig. 17.6. Posterior femoral extensors.
Reprinted from Donnelly (1982).

the Anglo-Saxon *hamm*, meaning "back of the thigh." The biceps femoris is posterior and lateral in the thigh and is so named because it has two heads. The semitendinosus is located posterior and medial in the thigh, and is named for the remarkable length of its tendon: The name literally means that the muscle is half tendon. The semimembranosus lies on the posteromedial aspect of the thigh. It is named for the flattened membranous form of its upper attachment.

The major responsibilities of the hamstrings are to produce both flexion of the knee joint and extension of the hip joint. In flexion at the hip and in leaning forward, they are active in resisting gravity. When the knee is semiflexed, the biceps femoris can act as a lateral rotator and the other hamstrings as medial rotators of the lower leg. When the hip joint is extended, the biceps femoris also laterally rotates the thigh while the other hamstrings act as medial rotators.

The balance of muscle strength between the quadriceps (anterior thigh muscles) and hamstrings is crucial in the prevention of injury. The hamstrings-to-quadriceps torque ratio varies among selected populations. Parker et al. (1983) found that high school football players had a ratio between 47% and 65%. Davies et al. (1981)

reported ratios between 51% and 64.9% for professional football players. Research on healthy soccer players produced an average between 67% and 82%, depending on the speed of the contraction (Stafford and Grana 1984). Gilliam et al. (1979) calculated ratios in the range of 40% to 70% for children between the ages of 7 and 13 years.

Causes and Mechanisms of Injury to the Posterior Femoral Muscles

The hamstring strain, commonly known as a pulled hamstring, is caused by a violent stretch or rapid contraction of the hamstring muscle group, causing rupture within the musculotendinous unit (American Medical Association 1966). The injury is time-consuming to treat, easily aggravated, psychologically devastating, and almost literally a "pain in the butt." A pulled hamstring may occur in the muscle's belly or near the ends of the tendons. Therefore, the pull may occur just below the hip or posteriorly at midthigh level.

For years, numerous people have speculated about predisposing factors that might cause the hamstring muscle group to become strained. Research suggests that a strength imbalance between the hamstrings and quadriceps is such a factor (Burkett 1970; Yamamoto 1993). Currently, researchers are inclined to favor the idea that a decrease from the normal 50% to 70% hamstring-to-quadriceps muscle strength ratio predisposes one to such injuries (Arnheim 1989; Gilliam et al. 1979; Klein and Allman 1969; Liemohn 1978; Parker et al. 1983; Rankin and Thompson 1983; Sutton 1984). However, research by Bozeman, Mackie, and Kaufmann (1986) suggests that a criterion of 75% of the quadriceps strength be adopted. An explanation of the importance of this ratio is based on the fact that during parts of some movements, such as running, both the hamstrings and quadriceps contract at the same time (Burkett 1975). Thus, opposing forces are in action. If one of these forces is greater than the other and resistance is maintained, something must give—usually the hamstring muscles, which are weaker than the quadriceps.

Research by Burkett (1971) has indicated that a strength imbalance between the right and left hamstrings may also initiate an injury. Burkett's study found that a strength difference of 10% or more would likely result in strain to the weaker hamstring. Resistance training could help to maintain these critical strength balances. Clinical studies on the benefits of weight training for hamstring strains have been documented, but no data was presented regarding strength ratios (Gordon and Klein 1987). The problem is that the actual ratios that constitute balance or imbalance have never been accurately defined (Grace 1985). However, theories regarding exact optimal ratios have been presented. In the opinion of Grace (1985, 80), "what constitutes a significant discrepancy depends on the anatomical region, the sport, and the participant's size, age, and sex." Research by Heiser et al. (1984) demonstrated a dramatic reduction in hamstring injuries in collegiate football participants with a specially designed prophylactic rehabilitation program that included correcting the hamstring-quadriceps ratio to 60%. However, Grace (1985, 81–82) points out that "unfortunately the study was retrospective, without concurrent controls with a multifactorial rehabilitation program, therefore the actual relationship between imbalance and injury is unclear."

Another theory that explains the pulled hamstring is based on a neural mechanism. According to Burkett (1975), the cause of the injury could be the asymmetrical stimulation of the two nerves of the biceps femoris (the tibial nerve, which in-

nervates the long head, and the common peroneal nerve, which innervates the short head) by the following mechanisms:

1. The stimulation to the short head is more intense than to the long head, causing an imbalance in the contraction phase.
2. The intensity of the stimulation doesn't change, but the timing of the stimulation to the two different heads is asynchronous.
3. Both 1 and 2.
4. The change from prime mover to stabilizer causes a lag in stimulation.

However, one of the most frequently cited causes of hamstring strain is lack of flexibility. All things being equal, the more flexible a person is, the less the chance of stretch (passive tension) injury. Conversely, the more inflexible a person is, the greater the likelihood of a pull. Klein and Roberts (1976) explain that when the hip flexor muscles are tight and the pelvis tipped forward chronically in an altered posture, the hamstrings are in a state of overstretch because the origin of the attachment on the pelvis is lifted upward and the distance between the origin and insertion of the muscle is lengthened. Consequently, this posture may account for early hamstring fatigue, one of the fundamental causes of hamstring injury.

A more complicated explanation for hamstring tightening that could potentially lead to a pulled hamstring is proposed by Beekman and Block (1975). They point out that during gait, many determinants operate to smooth out the movement of the center of gravity. They are the foot mechanism (eversion), the ankle mechanism (plantar flexion), and the knee mechanism (flexion). These systems are intimately related, so that if one parameter is decreased, the others are increased. If there is the presence of a calcaneal varus (inversion) the foot mechanism is inhibited. The knee is the only determinant that can effectively compensate for the effect of calcaneal varus at heel contact. Consequently, the knee mechanism must be more flexed when the foot contacts the ground. But by so doing the hamstrings do not get properly stretched on each step. As a result, an acquired shortening takes place. Later, this tightness could predispose one to a pulled hamstring. Another explanation is that during exercise muscles swell and shorten. If the muscles are not flexible, they will be more susceptible to strain during the next exercise period. Consequently, there is increased risk of injury.

Among other possible causes of pulled hamstrings are overuse, poor training methods and techniques, lack of endurance, fatigue, structural abnormalities (e.g., lumbar lordosis, leg length discrepancy, or flat feet), poor posture, dehydration, mineral deficiency (e.g., magnesium deficiency), and prior trauma (Corbin and Noble 1980; Hennessy and Watson 1993; Muckle 1982; O'Neil 1976; Taunton 1982).

A review of the literature by Sutton (1984) clearly substantiates that there is probably no single factor that predisposes one to hamstring strain. Furthermore, due to the number of confounding variables, an accurate prediction of which individuals will suffer from hamstring strain is not yet possible with tests currently used. Therefore, more research is still needed. Nonetheless, common sense suggests that one should incorporate lengthening and strengthening programs, as well as control the variables that are thought to predispose one to hamstring strains. An ounce of prevention is worth a pound of cure.

Stretching the Posterior Femoral Muscles

Stretching the hamstrings occurs with flexion of the hip and extension of the knee. This is usually accomplished by lowering the upper torso toward the thighs while sitting or standing with one or both legs extended. Because there is a significant interrelationship among the hamstrings, pelvis, and lower back, the lower back muscles can also be stretched in this manner. A point emphasized by many experts is maintaining an anterior pelvic tilt and an extended upper torso when lowering toward the thighs. The ideal position should form a straight line running from the sacrum to the back of the head (Figure 17.7). However, many untrained people round or slump the upper torso and tilt the pelvis backward rather than forward during the lowering phase. This position raises two significant questions. First, why is it natural to round the upper torso and tilt the pelvis posteriorly during the lowering and stretch phase? Second, is the posture recommended by experts more effective than this more instinctive posture for increasing the stretch and facilitating an improvement in ROM?

Only one study (Sullivan, Dejulia, and Worrell 1992) is known to have partially investigated these questions. The head-to-knee position is commonly performed by flexing the cervical, thoracic, and lumbar spine in an attempt to bring the chin to the knee of the stretched leg or legs. This action could be natural or deliberate. Sullivan, Dejulia, and Worrell (1992, 1387) pos-

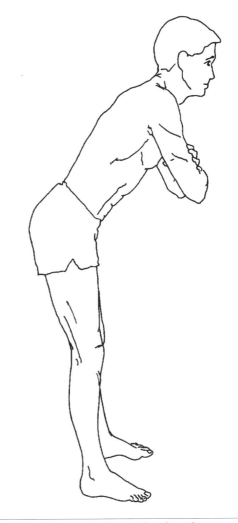

Fig. 17.7. The anterior (forward) pelvis tilt. Reprinted from Donnelly (1982).

tulate that in an anterior pelvic tilt position "the ischial tuberosity (hamstring origin) is placed superiorly and posteriorly, to a position farther from the proximal tibial and fibular hamstring insertions. Thus, greater tension would occur within the hamstring musculotendinous structure." Clinically, the investigators observed that patients immediately felt greater tension (and possibly pain) in the hamstring muscle group when stretching with the back in an extended position. Thus, it may be natural for the body to attempt to compensate for the increased hamstring tension by assuming a back position that results in less musculotendinous tension. In addition, it was suggested that such pelvic compensatory motion may occur due to the combined flexion patterns of the cervical, thoracic, and lumbar spine. This idea is based on Cailliet's (1988) concept of "lumbar pelvic rhythm." As the pelvis rotates posteriorly, the ischial tuberosity becomes displaced anteriorly and inferiorly and positions the hamstring's origin closer to its insertion.

The rounded-back position may be deliberately utilized in an overt attempt to "cheat" in getting the head to the knees. By using this slumping strategy, the spine will not have to go through as much angular or linear displacement when placing the chin on the knees. That is, less range of motion is needed. Hence, the cumulative flexions that occur throughout all the vertebrae can, in effect, create an illusion of a greater degree of hamstring flexibility.

The question remains as to which technique is more efficient in increasing muscle length. In the study by Sullivan, Dejulia, and Worrell (1992), static stretching was compared with the contract-relax-contract PNF technique. The results suggested that "the anterior pelvic tilt position was more important than the stretching method for increasing hamstring muscle flexibility." This conclusion was based on the hypothesis that "this position allows for greater (passive) force within the musculotendinous unit that will increase hamstring muscle length more efficiently" (p. 1388).

The Medial Femoral Muscles: Adductors

The medial portion of the thigh consists of five muscles: the adductor brevis, adductor longus, adductor magnus, gracilis, and pectineus. These are commonly known as the groin muscles, although the word *groin* is applied to the region that includes the upper part of the front of the thigh and the lower part of the abdomen. In medical terminology, the muscles of the medial femoral group are called the *adductor* muscles. The primary functions of these muscles are to adduct, flex, and rotate the thigh. Furthermore, they serve to restrict abduction along with the ligaments of the hips (Figure 17.8).

Causes and Mechanisms of Adductor Injury

Like the hamstrings, the adductors are prone to strain. However, unlike the hamstrings, these injuries are more difficult to manage because they are located in an area that is awkward both to treat and support (due to the proximity of the genitalia). The causes of groin strain are virtually the same as those of the pulled hamstring.

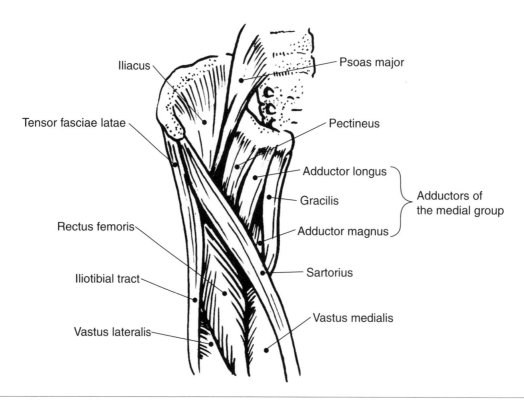

Fig. 17.8. Adductors and flexors of the hip.
Reprinted from Donnelly (1982).

With diligent and disciplined conditioning, the risk of groin strain can be reduced. Here, too, lengthening and strengthening programs and control of the variables that are thought to predispose one to groin strains are prudent.

Stretching the Adductors

Stretching the adductors is possible by abducting the hip, that is, straddling the legs. This position can be performed while standing, sitting, kneeling, or lying, and the knees may be extended or flexed during the stretch (see Exercises #13–16). A method that deserves special attention is the straddle split in a standing position, in which one flexes at the hips and slowly straddles the legs as widely as possible. Biesterfeldt (1974) points out that this technique presents potential risks. Straddle splits apply direct sideways force on the knees. For people who are not fully mature, such forces can, if continued over some time, result in permanent deformity, such as loose and knocked knees. The use of a partner applying pressure on the outside of the knees while standing from behind must be totally avoided.

The Anterior Femoral Muscles: Quadriceps

The anterior portion of the thigh is made up of four quadriceps muscles, the sartorius muscle, the tensor fasciae latae, the gluteal aponeurosis, and the iliotibial band. The quadriceps are commonly known as the *quads*. Each of the quadriceps is named for its respective position. Thus, the rectus femoris is found in front of the femur; the vastus lateralis is located on the lateral side of the femur; the vastus medialis is positioned on the medial side of the thigh; and the vastus intermedialis is situated between the femur and the rectus femoris. The name *sartorius* is derived from the Latin word for *tailor*, after the custom of tailors to sit cross-legged. All the quadriceps function to extend the knee, while the rectus femoris

also produces flexion of the hip. In contrast, the sartorius flexes both the hip and the knee and it rotates the hip laterally and the lower leg medially when the foot is off the ground. The tensor fasciae latae assist in flexion, abduction, and inward rotation of the hip.

Causes and Mechanisms of Quadriceps Injury

Injuries to the anterior thigh are common. Stiffness, soreness, and tenderness are associated with a number of possible causes. One of the most common injuries to the quadriceps is direct trauma. The muscle may also spontaneously cramp, popularly known as a charlie horse. Other potential factors include insufficient warm-up and stretching, overtraining, and fatigue. Here, too, a preventive approach is both practical and prudent.

Stretching the Quadriceps

There are three principal kinds of stretching exercises for the quadriceps: (a) bringing the heel(s) to the buttocks without hip extension; (b) bringing the heel(s) to the buttocks with hip extension; and (c) hip extension with the legs relatively straight (see Exercises #17 and #18). Exercise (a) stretches predominantly the three vasti muscles. Exercise (b) stretches these muscles plus the rectus femoris (a maximal stretch of the rectus femoris can be achieved by a combination of hip extension and knee flexion). Exercise (c) stretches primarily the hip flexor muscles and the anterior hip joint capsule and ligaments, but also the rectus femoris to some extent. For individuals with a medical history of knee problems, only the third method should be used.

Front Split

To perform a technically correct front split, both legs must be straight, the hips squared (facing directly forward, rather than twisted), and the buttocks flat on the floor (Figure 17.9). For aes-

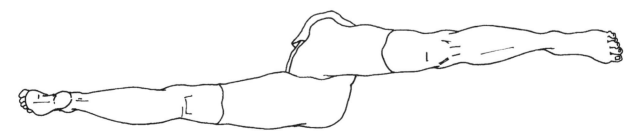

Fig. 17.9. A front split as visualized from below. Notice that the hips are squared.

thetic reasons, some people advocate a slight turnout of the rear hip. However, this rotation usually is carried to an extreme, primarily due to tight hip flexors or improper training. Often, improper training prevents the development of an ideal split. To successfully master a front split, it is necessary to commence from a squared position and slowly lower into the split while maintaining the correct alignment. This movement can be practiced from a modified kneeling position with both hands on the iliac crest. If balance is a difficulty, the split can be practiced between two chairs for support.

The Pelvic Region

The pelvic region can be divided into the iliac (anterior) and gluteal (posterior) regions. These are each discussed in the following sections.

The Iliac Region

The iliac region is so named because of its proximity to the ilium (anterior bone of the pelvis). This region contains three muscles: the psoas major, psoas minor, and iliacus, sometimes collectively referred to as the iliopsoas (see Figure 17.8). The psoas major originates from the anterior surface and lower borders of the transverse processes of all the lumbar vertebrae and is attached to the lesser trochanter of the femur. It serves as the most important flexor of the hip. In front of the psoas major, within the abdomen, is the psoas minor, which is a weak flexor of the hip. The iliacus originates at the iliac fossa (inside the pelvis) and inserts into the lateral side of the tendon of the psoas major. This muscle assists in forward tilt of the pelvis, flexion of the hip joint, and outward rotation of the thigh.

Causes and Mechanisms of Iliac Region Injury

The muscles of the iliac region are susceptible to strain. This injury can significantly impair movement. Without the full use of the iliopsoas, one is unable to maintain an upright posture easily or to move the thigh effectively. Potential factors for strain include insufficient warm-up and stretching, faulty technique, poor conditioning, overtraining, and fatigue.

Stretching the Iliac Region

In order to stretch the iliopsoas, the distance between their origin and insertion must be lengthened (Wirhed 1984). This can be achieved by assuming a kneeling position as shown in Exercise #21. Then, bend the forward leg and lean forward further to pull the trunk and pelvis forward toward the floor. An additional force can be applied by pushing on the buttocks or hip. Another exercise, which should be used only by people who have received instructions from a qualified trainer, can be seen in Exercise #22. However, this must be used with extreme caution.

The Gluteal Region

The gluteal region is often referred to as the buttocks. This region contains nine muscles: three glutei and six smaller, more deeply situated muscles. The gluteus maximus is the largest and most superficial muscle in the region. It is responsible for extension of the hip and assists in outward rotation at the hip. The gluteus minimus is the smallest and deepest of the three gluteal muscles. The gluteus medius is the intermediate muscle, in both size and location. Both of these muscles abduct the hip joint and assist with inward and outward rotation of the thigh. The six remaining muscles—the piriformis, obturator externus, obturator internus, quadratus femoris, gemellus inferior, and gemellus superior—function to produce outward rotation at the hip.

Causes and Mechanisms of Gluteal Injury

Injuries to the gluteal region are common. Like other muscle groups, soreness and strains can occur in this region for a number of reasons, the most common of which are overtraining and the use of poor technique. In addition, the gluteal region is often a target of trauma, especially during falls. As with injuries to the adductor muscles, this area is awkward both to treat and to support.

Stretching the Gluteals

Stretching the gluteus maximus is usually accomplished by applying tension to the hip rotators. The hip is flexed, adducted, and medially rotated. This stretch can be accomplished standing, sitting, or lying (see Exercises #24–31).

The Coxal Joint

The coxal, or hip, joint is perhaps the most striking example in the body of a ball-and-socket joint. It consists of the rounded femoral head, which articulates with the deep, cup-shaped fossa of the acetabulum (socket in pelvis). It is because of the ball-and-socket arrangement that the hip is able to move through a wide range of motions.

Factors Affecting Coxal Stability and Ranges of Motion

Although the coxal joint possesses considerable mobility, its chief function is to provide stability. There are many factors that contribute to the stability of the hip joint and determine its ultimate ranges of motion. These factors are discussed in the following sections.

The Acetabulum

The acetabulum is a somewhat hemispherical cavity that articulates with the femoral head. It is formed from the union of the three pelvic bones: the ilium, ischium, and pubis. When viewed anteriorly, it faces forward, downward, and laterally, a position that enhances stability for weight bearing.

Another factor that assists in creating stability is the acetabular labrum, which is a fibrocartilaginous rim attached to the margin of the acetabulum that increases the depth of the joint and acts like a collar for the femoral head. It improves the fit between the two joining surfaces of the joint and tends to keep the femoral head firmly in place.

Shape of the Pelvis

The shape of the acetabulum is in part determined by the shape of the pelvis. The shape of the pelvis is to a major extent determined by one's gender. The female pelvis differs from that of the male in ways that render it better adapted to pregnancy and childbearing. A woman's pelvis is shallower and shorter, the bones lighter and smoother, the coccyx more movable, and the subpubic arch angle more obtuse. It is also wider and almost cylindrical. As a result, the heads of the femur bones are more widely separated in women. Because the thighs curve toward the center line of the body as they approach the knees, this outward flare at the hips has a tendency to bring the knees of a woman somewhat closer together than a man's. Their broader hips give women a much greater potential for range of motion, such as the ability to do splits and high leg extensions more easily (Hamilton 1978b).

Angle of Femoral Inclination and Declination

The head and neck of the femur form an angle with the shaft of the femur in two directions: the angle of inclination and the angle of declination. The *angle of inclination* is the neck-shaft angle in the frontal plane. At birth, newborns have angles of inclination of almost 150°. However, this angle decreases with age. By adulthood, the average angle is about 135° (Figure 17.10).

When the angle of inclination is larger than 135° in an adult, the resulting deformity is known as *coxa valga* (see Figure 17.10). When the angle is greater than 135°, the range of abduction is increased. In extreme cases, it may reach a straight angle of 180°. With extreme coxa valga, there are no skeletal checks to restrict ranges of motion, thus promoting dislocation (Kapandji 1987; Steindler 1977).

If the angle of inclination is less than 135°, the deformity is termed *coxa vara* (see Figure 17.10). This more acute angulation results in a flaring or widening of the hips. With coxa vara, there is a restriction of the ability to abduct due to impingement of the greater trochanter against the ilium. Furthermore, inward rotation of the femur becomes limited (Steindler 1977).

The *angle of declination* is the measure of the degree of forward angulation of the femur's head in relation to its shaft (see Figure 17.10). In other words, it is the angle between the axis of the femoral neck and the frontal plane. This angle is normally rather high at birth (40°). However, with age, it decreases to about 12° to 15°. The angle of declination is also known as the *angle of anteversion*. A decrease of this angle is called *retroversion* (see Figure 17.10).

An increased angle of anteversion produces an increased internal torsion or medial rotation of the femur and leg, resulting in an in-toeing or a pigeon-toed gait. In contrast, retroversion produces an external torsion or lateral rotation of the femur and leg, resulting in an outward-toeing or duck-toed gait. In ballet, this rotation is referred

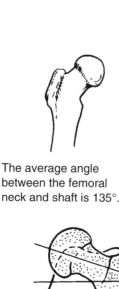

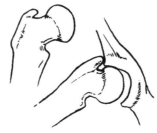

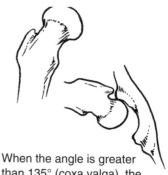

The average angle between the femoral neck and shaft is 135°.

In some individuals this angle is smaller, a condition called coxa vara in which the range of abduction is reduced.

When the angle is greater than 135° (coxa valga), the range of abduction is increased.

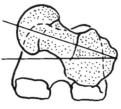

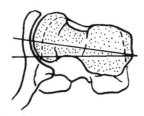

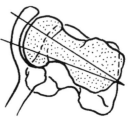

Seen from above, the neck is oriented anteriorly at an angle of 10 to 30°.

When this "anteversion" angle is small, the head fits into the socket well in anatomical position,

and maintains good articular contact even in lateral rotation.

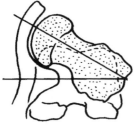

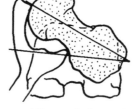

When the anteversion angle is large, the anterior part of the head is more exposed in anatomical position,

and the posterior part loses contact with the socket in lateral rotation.

Lateral rotation is more restricted in these individuals by contact between the neck and the lateral edge of the acetabulum. Curvature and length of the femoral neck also affect mobility at the hip joint.

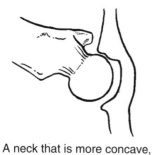

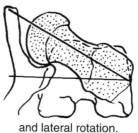

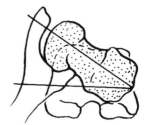

A neck that is more concave, and longer, will facilitate abduction . . .

and lateral rotation.

With a shorter, less concave neck, both these motions are restricted by contact with the edge of the acetabulum.

Fig. 17.10.   Variations of the hip.
Reprinted from Calais-Germain (1993).

to as *turnout*. Turnout is important because it allows one to increase hip abduction range of motion. This technique will be explained in greater detail later. Briefly, the skeletal conditions ideal for ballet (and for certain sports) are a long femoral neck with a small neck-shaft angle of inclination for maximum range of motion, and retroversion for good, natural turnout. Unfortunately, this combination is extremely rare (Hamilton 1978a).

Articular Capsule and Ligaments

Although the bony structure primarily determines the degree of motion of the hip, other factors also play a role. Of these other factors, the most important are the articular capsule and the powerful ligamentous support apparatus. The heavy, fibrous articular capsule, like a sleeve, encloses the hip joint and the greater part of the femoral neck. Integrated into the capsule are the ligaments. At the hip, the principal ligaments are the iliofemoral, ischiofemoral, pubofemoral, and ligamentum teres (Figure 17.11). Their mechanism of checking joint motion will be discussed later.

Muscular Reinforcement and Coordination

The stability of the coxal joint is further enhanced by the muscles that run roughly parallel to the femoral neck. They help keep the femoral head in contact with the acetabulum. These muscles are the piriformis, obturator externus, gluteus medius, and gluteus minimus.

An important factor in range of motion is the role that the muscles play during active stretching, as opposed to the role of their tightness in passive stretch. For example, in active abduction of the legs, the limiting factor may be the lack of strength or coordination of the agonists (i.e., the abductor muscles) to create the movement.

Finally, it must be remembered that resistance of the antagonistic or opposing muscle group and its respective connective tissue sheaths are also a major factor in one's range of motion. Thus, during abduction, the major limitation is tightness of the adductor muscles and their tissue sheaths.

Limits on Coxal Range of Motion

Altogether, there are six major movements of the hip (excluding circumduction): flexion, extension, abduction, adduction, internal rotation, and external rotation. Following is a description of these movements.

Flexion

Hip flexion is defined as a decrease in the angle between the thigh and abdomen. Flexion of the hip with the knee flexed ranges approximately

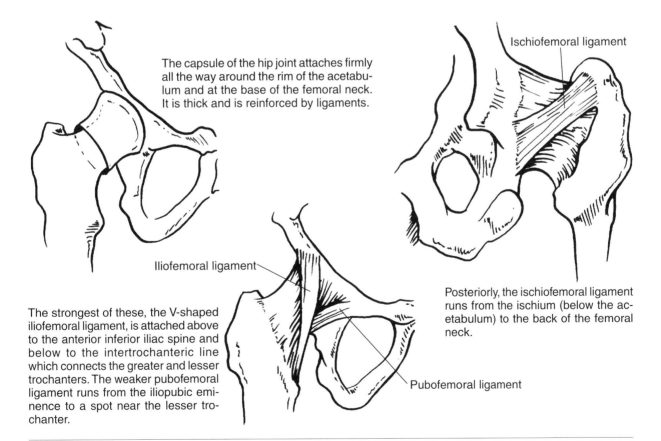

The capsule of the hip joint attaches firmly all the way around the rim of the acetabulum and at the base of the femoral neck. It is thick and is reinforced by ligaments.

Ischiofemoral ligament

Iliofemoral ligament

Posteriorly, the ischiofemoral ligament runs from the ischium (below the acetabulum) to the back of the femoral neck.

The strongest of these, the V-shaped iliofemoral ligament, is attached above to the anterior inferior iliac spine and below to the intertrochanteric line which connects the greater and lesser trochanters. The weaker pubofemoral ligament runs from the iliopubic eminence to a spot near the lesser trochanter.

Pubofemoral ligament

Fig. 17.11. Articular capsule and ligaments.
Reprinted from Calais-Germain (1993).

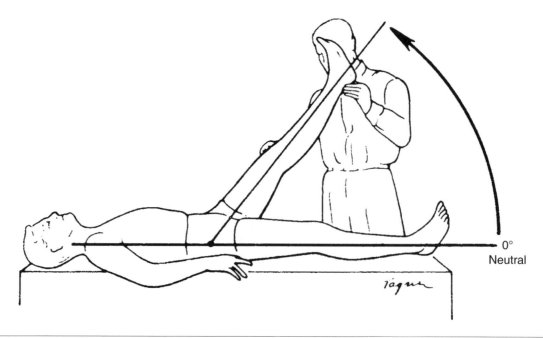

Fig. 17.12. The straight-leg-raising test.
Reprinted from American Academy of Orthopaedic Surgeons (1965).

from 0° to 120°, but with the knee extended, range is usually limited to about 90°. Tests for measuring hamstring muscle tightness include the passive toe-touch test, the passive unilateral straight-leg-raising (SLR) test (Figure 17.12), and the active unilateral SLR test. The SLR test is important because it can also be used as a neurological test to assess lumbar nerve root compression, sciatic nerve normality, and intervertebral disk protrusion (Bohannon, Gajdosik, and LeVeau 1985; Gajdosik and Lusin 1983; Urban 1981).

There are a number of instruments that can be used to assess the SLR test (Hsieh, Walker, and Gillis 1983). However, other studies have found that various factors may influence the results of the test. For example, Bohannon, Gajdosik, and LeVeau (1985) found that posterior pelvic rotation began within 9° from the beginning of leg raising in the passive SLR test and that the angle of pelvic rotation increased in conjunction with the angle of leg raising. Further, in a study of the active SLR test (Mayhew, Norton, and Sahrmann 1983), the findings indicated that the degree of participation of the contralateral hamstrings and abdominal muscles may also contribute to potential variations. In addition to these findings, the pull of the gastrocnemius may influence the degree of movement (Figure 17.13). Hence, to minimize its pull, the ankle should be allowed to plantar flex slightly.

Active flexion of the hip is produced primarily by the psoas major and iliacus and is assisted by the rectus femoris, sartorius, tensor fasciae latae, pectineus, adductor brevis, adductor longus, and adductor magnus. Range of motion is checked by hip flexor contractile insufficiency, contact of the thigh with the abdomen, and passive tension of the hamstring muscles. During flexion, all ligaments are relaxed and slack (Figure 17.14). Thus, they provide no resistance.

Extension

Hip extension is the movement of returning from flexion to the anatomical, or neutral, position. Hyperextension begins when this movement continues beyond the neutral position. Active range of motion is 10° of hip hyperextension with the knee flexed and 20° with the knee extended. Passive hyperextension attains 20° when one lunges forward and reaches 30° when the lower limb is forcibly pulled back (Kapandji 1987). To achieve a true test for the hip flexor muscles (which limit extension), it is necessary to lie with the back flat on a table with one leg flexed at the hip and knee and pulled to the chest, while the other leg (to be tested) is hanging over the table edge from the knee. If the thigh of the tested leg fails to touch the table while the back is held flat, then tightness of the hip flexors is indicated (Kendall, Kendall, and Wadsworth 1971).

Active extension of the hip is produced primarily by the gluteus maximus, semitendinosus, semimembranosus, and biceps femoris muscles.

The straight-leg-raising test for hamstring length is actually a combination of hip flexion and flexion of the lumbar spine. Having the low back flat on the table is a prerequisite to accurate testing.

Normal length of right hamstring, low back, and left hip flexor muscles.

With the low back flat on the table, and the left leg held down to stabilize the pelvis and prevent excessive flexion of the lumbar spine, the right leg with the knee straight can be raised passively to an angle of 80° to 85° hip flexion. This range of motion indicates normal hamstring length.

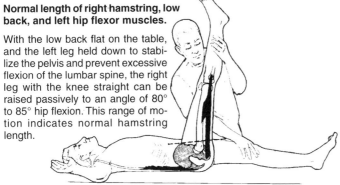

Normal length of right hamstring muscles, short low back and left hip flexor muscles.

Although the right hamstring muscles are normal in length, straight leg raising is restricted because the shortness of the left hip flexor and low back muscles hold the lumbar spine in hyperextension, maintaining the pelvis in anterior tilt when the left leg is held down on the table. To avoid the misdiagnosis of short hamstrings in this case, the left thigh should be allowed to flex sufficiently to flatten the low back, and be stabilized in that position while raising the right leg. Restriction of, or excessive lumbar spine flexion affects the test for hamstring length.

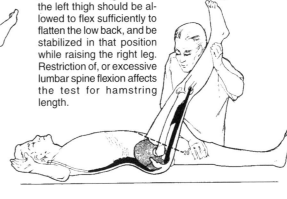

Overstretched right hamstring muscles, normal length of low back and left hip flexor muscles.

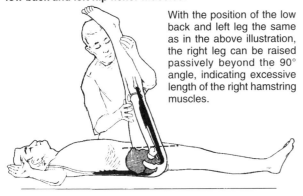

With the position of the low back and left leg the same as in the above illustration, the right leg can be raised passively beyond the 90° angle, indicating excessive length of the right hamstring muscles.

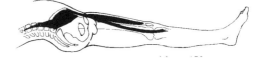

Short right hamstring muscles, normal length of low back and left hip flexor muscles.

With the position of the low back and left leg the same as in the above illustrations, the right leg can be raised passively only to an angle of approximately 50°, indicating a marked shortness of the hamstring muscles.

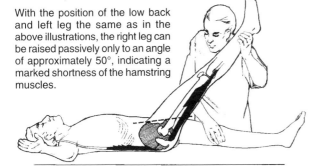

Overstretched right hamstring muscles, short left hip flexor and low back muscles.

The excessive length of the hamstring muscles is obscured because the hyperextended lumbar spine maintains the pelvis in anterior tilt. (See explanation above.)

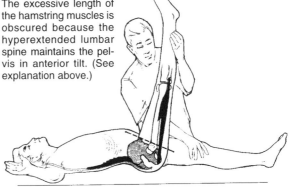

Short right hamstring muscles, overstretched left hip flexor and low back muscles.

The degree of hamstring shortness in this figure is identical with that shown in the left figure directly above. The leg is raised slightly higher than in the other figure due to increased flexion of the lumbar spine.

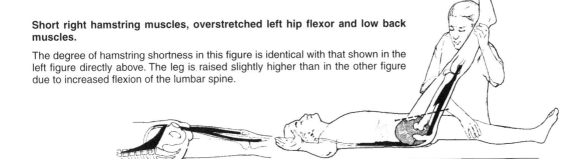

Fig. 17.13. Tests for length of hamstring muscles.
Reprinted from Kendall, Kendall, and Wadsworth (1971).

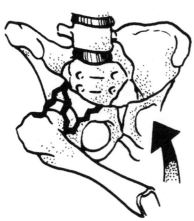

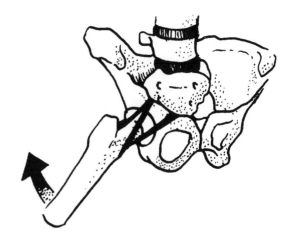

The iliofemoral (both branches) and pubofemoral ligaments become slack in flexion . . .

and taut in extension.

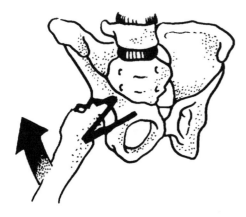

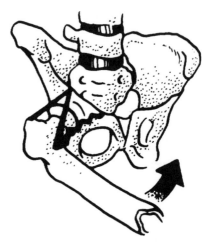

In abduction, the upper iliofemoral is slack while the pubofemoral is taut;

in adduction, the opposite occurs.

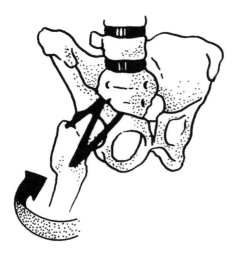

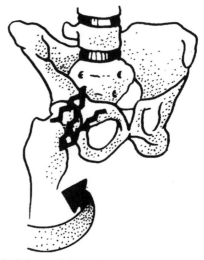

The ligaments all become taut in lateral rotation . . .

and slack in medial rotation.

Fig. 17.14. The iliofemoral and pubofemoral ligaments during various types of movement.
Reprinted from Calais-Germain (1993).

Range of motion is limited by hip extensor contractile insufficiency, passive tension of the hip flexor muscles, locking of the spine that prevents anterior tilting of the pelvis, and tension in all the ligaments (see Figure 17.14). These factors make it difficult, for instance, to execute the rear leg portion of a front split with the hips squared.

Abduction

Abduction of the hip is the movement of the lower limb laterally away from the midline of the body. It is produced primarily by the gluteus medius and gluteus minimus and is assisted by the tensor fasciae latae and the sartorius muscles. In one hip, abduction ranges from 0° to 45°. However, in practice, abduction at one hip is often automatically followed by a similar degree of abduction at the other hip. This opposite hip motion becomes obvious after 30° of abduction in a standing position, when a lateral tilting of the pelvis away from the moving leg can be clearly seen.

To produce 30° of apparent abduction in the moving leg, the pelvis tilts 15° and the hip of the stationary leg abducts 15°. Thus, to produce 30° of apparent abduction, only 15° of hip abduction is required at each hip. Kapandji (1987) points out that as abduction continues, the vertebral column as a whole compensates for pelvic tilt by bending laterally toward the supporting side. Thus, the vertebral column is also involved in movements of the hip.

Abduction of the hip is limited by several elements: hip abductor contractile insufficiency, passive tension of the hip adductor muscles, passive tension of the pubofemoral and iliofemoral ligaments (see Figure 17.14), and bone impact of the femoral neck on the acetabular rim (Figure 17.15). The vertebral column and pelvis can also serve as restraining factors, because the vertebral column is involved in movements of the hip, and any restrictions on the column could in turn restrict compensatory actions required for pelvic tilting.

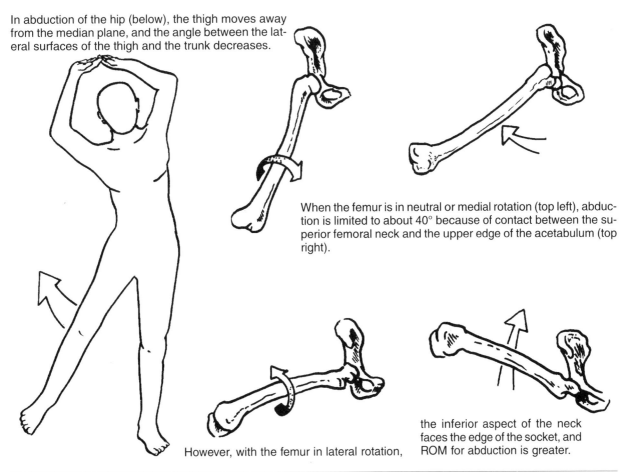

In abduction of the hip (below), the thigh moves away from the median plane, and the angle between the lateral surfaces of the thigh and the trunk decreases.

When the femur is in neutral or medial rotation (top left), abduction is limited to about 40° because of contact between the superior femoral neck and the upper edge of the acetabulum (top right).

However, with the femur in lateral rotation, the inferior aspect of the neck faces the edge of the socket, and ROM for abduction is greater.

Fig. 17.15. The effect of femoral rotation on abduction.
Reprinted from Calais-Germain (1993).

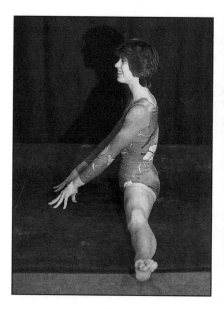 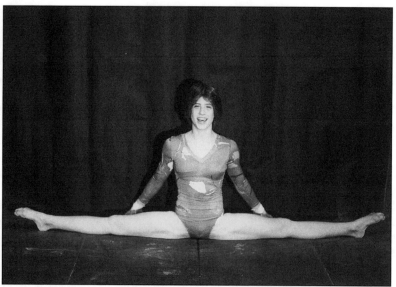

Fig. 17.16. The straddle split. (a) Side view. (b) Front view. Reprinted from Sands (1984).

Can one maximize one's range of abduction? The answer is yes! For example, let's examine the straddle split, as shown in Figure 17.16. This skill can be performed in a static manner on the floor or actively in the air. In either case, when executed to 180°, pure abduction does not take place. After a certain point, hip movement is transferred to the pelvis and thereafter through the spine. The pelvis is tilted anteriorly while the vertebral column is hyperextended. Thus, the hip is put into a position of both abduction and flexion. This serves to reduce and minimize the restraining action of the iliofemoral ligament because during hip flexion this ligament is relaxed (see Figure 17.14).

Another technique used to enhance one's range of abduction is the use of turnout. The rationale for turnout is twofold. First, turnout incorporates a lateral rotation of the hip joint, which results in a relaxing of the ischiofemoral ligament. (However, all the anterior ligaments of the hip become taut, especially those bands running horizontally, that is, the iliotrochanter band and pubofemoral ligament.) The second rationale for the turnout is more significant. Following is a concise explanation by Chujoy and Manchester (1967, 923):

The principle of the turn-out is based on the anatomical structure of the hip joints. In normal positions the movements of the legs are limited by the structure of the joint between the pelvis and the hips. As the leg is drawn to the side, the hip (femoral)-neck meets the brim of the acetabulum and further movement is impossible. But, if the leg is turned out, the big (greater) trochanter recedes (moves posteriorly) and the brim of the acetabulum meets the flat side surface of the hip (femoral)-neck [Kushner et al. 1990; Watkins et al. 1989]. This turn-out allows the dancer to abduct the leg so that it forms an angle of ninety degrees or more with the other leg. The turn-out is not an aesthetic conception but an anatomical and technical necessity for the ballet dancer. It is the turn-out that makes the difference between a limited number of steps on one plane and the possibility of control of all dance movements in space. [see Figure 17.15]

Adduction

Adduction of the hip is the movement of the lower limb toward the midline of the body. This movement is produced primarily by the adductor longus, adductor brevis, and adductor magnus and is assisted by the pectineus and gracilis muscles. Range of motion is limited by adductor contractile insufficiency, passive tension of the abductors, tension of the iliotibial band, and contact with the opposite leg. When the thigh is flexed, the range increases from 0° to 60°. Here, motion is further restricted by tension of the abductor and hip lateral rotator muscles, tension of the iliofemoral ligament, and tension of the ligament of the femur's head.

Internal Rotation

Internal, or medial, rotation of the hip is defined as inward rotation of the femur in the acetabulum toward the midline. This movement is produced by the tensor fasciae latae, gluteus minimus, and gluteus medius. With the knee joint flexed, it ranges approximately from 0° to 45°, and somewhat less with the leg extended. Internal rotation is limited by contractile insufficiency, tension of the hip lateral rotators, and tension of the ischiofemoral ligament with the hip flexed and of the iliofemoral ligament when extended.

Mann, Baxter, and Lutter (1981) contend that stretching the hip by internal rotation is important because it can often eliminate knee pain associated with running. For instance, limited rotation of the hip, pelvis, or back can place more torque on the knee, leg, and ankle during running, especially during the foot-plant phase. Furthermore, if there is an external rotational deformity of the hip, more torque is placed on the knee as the speed is increased and the lower extremity attempts to rotate internally. Hence the importance of stretching the external rotators. The external rotators can be stretched while lying face

down with the body extended and one knee flexed. Then a partner pulls the flexed leg away from the midline.

External Rotation

External, or lateral, rotation of the hip is defined as outward rotation of the femur. This movement is produced by the obturator muscles, gemelli, and quadratus femoris and is assisted by the piriformis, gluteus maximus, sartorius, and adductors. Range of motion is approximately from 0° to 45° with the knee joint flexed. The movement is limited by contractile insufficiency, passive tension of the hip medial rotators, and tension of the iliofemoral ligament. External rotation is seen in many yoga postures, such as the easy posture, perfect posture, and lotus posture, and in ballet when executing a turnout. When the hip is flexed, ROM for external rotation is greater because the iliofemoral ligament is slack (Calais-Germain 1993). Bauman, Singson, and Hamilton (1994) have suggested that loss of external rotation in the hip of ballet dancers may

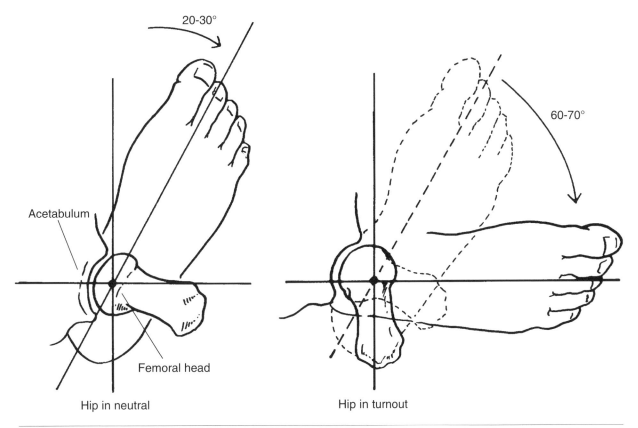

Fig. 17.17.   The dancer's hip turnout. In ideal circumstances, the 90° of desired turnout is achieved by a combination of external rotation at the hip, knee, and ankle joints. Theoretically, the majority of external rotation (60° to 70°) occurs at the hip with the remaining 20° to 30° occurring from the combined outward inclination of the foot, ankle, and knee joints.
Reprinted from Hardaker, Erickson, and Myers (1984).

result from tight, highly developed external rotators, such as the glutei.

The ideal 180° (90° per leg) external rotation demanded of professional ballet dancers is usually achieved with 60° to 70° of external rotation from above the knee and 20° to 30° from below (Hardaker, Erickson, and Myers 1984; Figure 17.17). Regrettably, turnout is often forced at the knees and feet by those who cannot perform sufficient hip lateral rotation. This attempted compensation places increased external torsional stress on the knees and can produce medial knee strain and patellar subluxation. The most common method of forcing the turnout in ballet is called *screwing the knee*. This movement is accomplished by performing a demi-plié (half knee bend), allowing a 180° position of the feet, then straightening the knees without moving the feet (Ende and Wickstrom 1982; Ryan 1976; Teitz 1982). The effect is similar when a football player firmly plants a cleated shoe in the ground and then rotates the leg (E.H. Miller et al. 1975). In addition, forcing the feet into 180° of turnout places stress on the medial aspect of the ankles and feet, potentially leading to pronated feet and flattening of the plantar arches.

Because the turnout at the hip is determined mostly by the bony structure and by the surrounding hip joint capsule and connective tissue, one may wonder to what extent this structure and flexibility can be affected by training. According to Hamilton (1978a), the consensus of medical literature indicates that spontaneous changes in anteversion occur most rapidly from birth to age 8, and that the process is close to completion by age 10. However, it is not completely finished until about age 16. Later attempts to correct anteversion seem to have little effect. Rather, compensatory external rotation deformity is created in the tibia below the knee. Recently, Bauman, Singson, and Hamilton (1994) found that dancers who had excellent turnout also had lower than average femoral neck angles. Consequently, "it appears that the soft tissues, rather than the skeleton, must allow for increased external rotation and turnout at the hip" (p. 61). G.W. Warren (1989, 11), further addressing this issue, succinctly states:

> Very few human bodies possess the capacity for perfect turn out. Students should remember that they are trying to achieve more than the ability simply to turn their legs outward. Their goal must be to develop the muscular strength to *control* and *maintain* their own maximum degree of turn-out *at all times* while they are dancing.

Summary

The lower extremity and pelvic girdle is a complex masterpiece of design. It is capable of numerous types of movement and through various ranges of motion. A host of factors can impede its optimal functioning. Through an understanding of the various structures and functions, optimal performance can be achieved most effectively and efficiently.

Chapter 18

Anatomy and Flexibility of the Vertebral Column

The vertebral column is a truly unique and amazing structure. In lay terms, it is called the backbone, which describes its position in the body but offers little description of its structure and capabilities for movement. In fact, the vertebral column is not a single bone. Rather, it is a stack of 33 bones that are flexibly connected, one above the other (Kelley 1971).

Gross Anatomy of the Vertebral Column

The vertebral column is made up of a series of separate bones, the vertebrae, linked together by cartilage, disks, and ligaments. Altogether, the column consists of 33 vertebrae, which are generally grouped into five divisions:

- 7 cervical vertebrae (neck)
- 12 thoracic vertebrae (rib cage area)
- 5 lumbar vertebrae (lower back)
- 5 sacral vertebrae (base of the spine)
- 4 coccygeal vertebrae (tailbone)

In the adult, the sacrum is a single bone that results from the fusion of the five sacral vertebrae. Similarly, the coccyx is a single bone that results from the fusion of the four coccygeal vertebrae. Therefore, there is a substantial amount of stability and virtually no mobility between the last nine vertebrae.

The structure of the spine can be better appreciated by analogy. The vertebral column can be thought of as a massive transmitting and receiving tower supported by guy wires. The tower is made up of the bony vertebral column, the disks, and the ligaments. The guy wires are the muscles that support the system and hold it erect. The base of the tower is the sacrum and pelvis, and the head is both receiver and transmitter. Another way to visualize the vertebral column is to imagine it as a flexible boom, like the mast of a sailboat.

An important feature of the vertebral column is the presence of four distinct curves when viewed from the side. At birth, an infant's spine has only one long curve. This curve extends over its entire length and is convex posteriorly (C-shaped). However, once the infant starts to raise its head, the cervical curve begins to develop. This anteriorly convex curve is referred to as the cervical lordosis. Later, when the child begins to stand and walk, the lumbar curve develops in the lower back. This curve is also convex anteriorly and is known as the lumbar lordosis. In the adult, the thorax and sacrum retain their original posterior convexity.

Abnormal vertebral curves may be present in some people. Deformities of flexion are called *kyphoses* (see Figure 18.1a). Kyphosis is usually the result of an exaggerated forward bend in the thoracic region. Another deformity is *lordosis*, which is the result of an excessive spinal hyperextension, most commonly seen only in the lumbar area. It is accompanied by a forward protrusion of the abdomen and a backward protrusion of the buttocks (see Figure 18.1b). An abnormal lateral deviation of the spine, seen from the front or back view, is called *scoliosis* (see Figure 18.1c). Scoliosis is almost always primarily in the thoracic region.

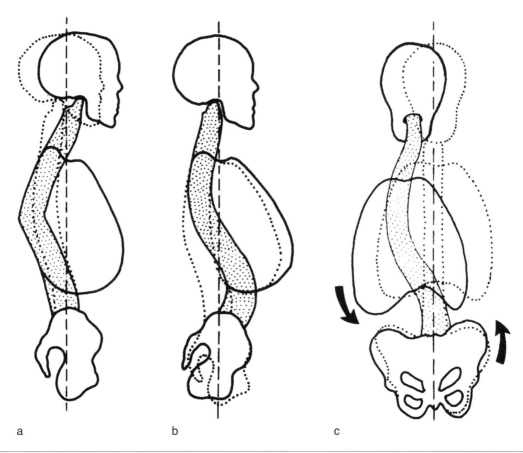

Fig. 18.1. Abnormal curvature of the vertebral column. (a) Kyphosis. (b) Lordosis. (c) Scoliosis.

Function of the Vertebral Column

The vertebral column has a number of different functions. Probably the most important function that it serves is to protect the spinal cord. It also provides a firm support for the trunk and appendages. Thus, it serves as a supporting rod for maintaining the upright position of the body. The vertebral column also provides muscular attachments, serves as an anchor for the rib cage, acts as a shock absorber, and provides a combination of strength and flexibility that affords maximal protection and stability with minimal restriction of mobility.

The Vertebrae

A typical vertebra is made up of two major parts: the vertebral body (found anteriorly) and the vertebral arch (located posteriorly). However, if a

vertebra is dismantled, it is found actually to consist of several fused parts that resemble a house (Figure 18.2). The basic foundation of the house is the vertebral body, the largest part of the vertebra. It is located anteriorly, is cylindrical in shape, and is wider than it is tall. It is the weight-bearing part of the vertebra. The vertebral arch is composed of four smaller structures. Two are the pedicles, which form the supporting sides or walls. They too are built to withstand great forces placed on them. The other two parts are the laminae, which form the roof of the house. Extending from the vertebral arch are three bony processes. Protruding laterally from each pedicle-lamina junction are the right and left transverse processes. They may be thought of as the eaves or wings of the house. Last, there is the midline spinous process protruding posteriorly like a chimney on the roof. The spinous process is the most posterior part of the vertebra. Therefore, its tip is seen when one bends forward.

The direction and degree of vertebral movement is determined by the orientation of the articular processes. In the thoracic region the ar-

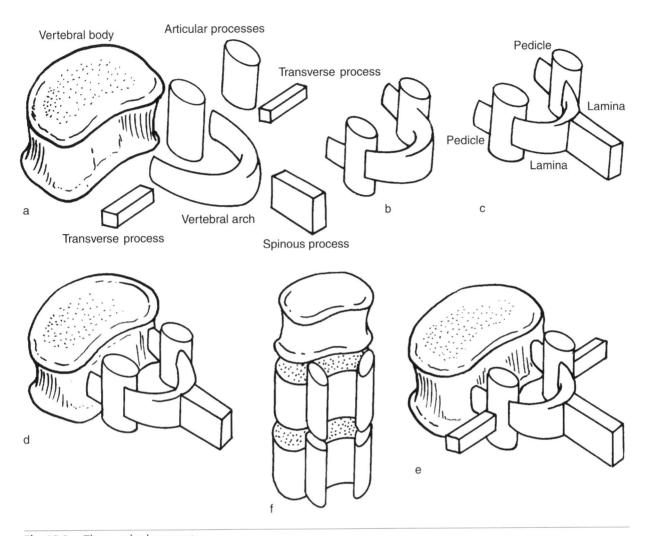

Fig. 18.2. The vertebral segments.
Reprinted from Kapandji (1978).

ticular facets are nearly frontally oriented with the superior and inferior facets facing posteriorly and anteriorly, respectively. This permits rotation and lateral flexion. In the lumbar area the articular facets' orientation is in the sagittal plane and superior facets face medially while the inferior facets face laterally. This orientation allows flexion, extension, and lateral flexion.

The Intervertebral Disks

Between the vertebral bodies and uniting them are 23 intervertebral disks. Altogether, the disks make up approximately one-quarter of the total length of the vertebral column. They function chiefly as hydraulic shock absorbers that permit compression and distortion. Therefore, they allow motion between the vertebrae.

The thickness of the disk is extremely important. The amount of movement that can occur in any region of the vertebral column depends in large part on the ratio between the height of the intervertebral disks and the height of the bony part of the column. Kapandji (1974) concisely describes the significance of the disks. Disk thickness varies with the region of the spine. The regions from thickest to thinnest are the lumbar (9 mm), thoracic (5 mm), and cervical (3 mm). However, more important than the absolute thickness is the ratio of the disk thickness to the height of the vertebral body. In fact, Kapandji states that this ratio accounts for the mobility of the particular segment of the vertebral column because the greater the ratio, the greater the mobility. Thus,

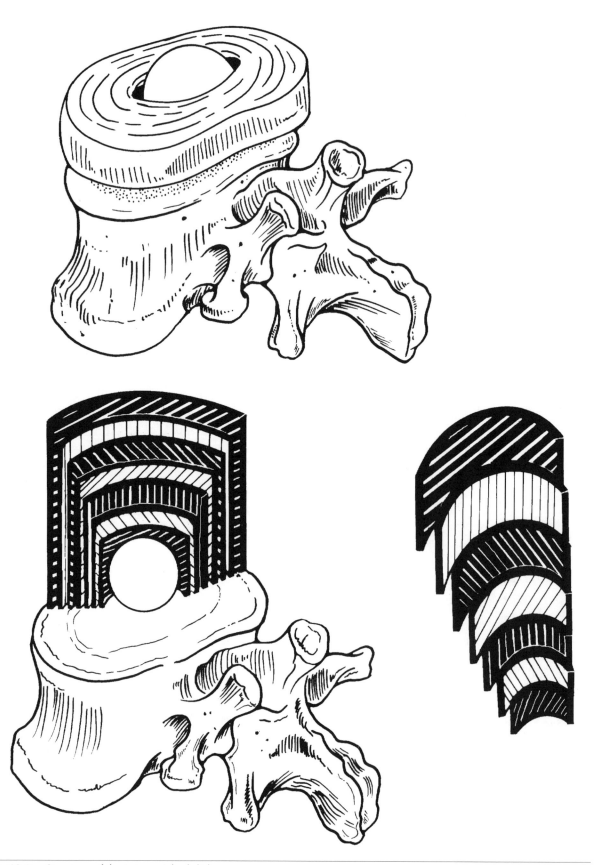

Fig. 18.3. Structure of the intervertebral disk.
Reprinted from Kapandji (1978).

the cervical region is most mobile since its disk to body ratio is 2:5, or 40%. In contrast, the lumbar region is slightly less mobile with a ratio of 1:3, or 33%. The thoracic region is the least mobile with a ratio of 1:5, or 20%. Hence, the disks play a major role in determining the potential range of movement in the back.

The disk consists of two parts: the nucleus pulposus and the annulus fibrosus. The liquid and elastic properties of the nucleus pulposus and annulus fibrosus, acting in combination, enable the disk to withstand great loads (Figure 18.3).

The Nucleus Pulposus

The nucleus pulposus is composed of an incompressible gel-like material that is encased in an elastic container. A protein polysaccharide makes up its chemical composition. The nucleus is strongly hydrophilic; that is, it has a strong affinity to or attraction for water. In fact, it can bind nine times its volume of water (the imbibing pressure of the nucleus has been found to reach 250 mmHg).

According to Puschel (1930), at birth, the water content of the nucleus is 88%. Like all fluids, it cannot be compressed in volume. Furthermore, since it exists for all practical purposes as a closed container, it must conform to Pascal's law: "Any external force exerted on a unit of a confined liquid is transmitted undiminished to every unit of the interior of the containing vessel" (Cailliet 1981, 3). The container can deform in response to the pressure. Thus, the nucleus acts as a hydraulic shock absorber.

When the spine is flexed, the disk becomes wedge-shaped, becoming thinner anteriorly and thicker posteriorly. This deformation allows the vertebrae to come closer together anteriorly and to separate posteriorly, thereby increasing the flexion curve of the spine. Conversely, during spinal hyperextension, the nucleus becomes thinner posteriorly and thicker anteriorly. This deformation allows the vertebrae to come closer together posteriorly and to separate anteriorly, thereby increasing the extension curve of the spine. Thus, deformation of the disks enhances spinal mobility.

Unfortunately, as the nucleus ages, it loses its water-binding capacity. By the age of 70, the water content diminishes to just 66%. The causes and implications of this dehydration are extremely significant. The dehydration appears to be a natural process of aging. It appears to be a by-product of attrition due to continual stress and wear and tear. This water loss can be explained by a decrease in the content of the protein polysaccharide, as well as by the gradual replacement of the gelatinous material of the nucleus with fibrocartilage. Research by Adams and Muir (1976) has demonstrated that with advancing age there is even a change in the molecular size of the proteoglycans in the nucleus pulposus and annulus fibrosus and their specific content, which would be expected to affect the mechanical properties of the disk. Hence, there is a decrease in the fluid content. Last, after the second decade, the disk's vascular supply disappears. By the third decade, the disk, now avascular, receives its nutrition only by diffusion of lymph through the vertebral end plates. This fluid loss can explain the loss of both spinal flexibility and height in the aged, as well as the impaired ability of the aged to regain elasticity in an injured disk (Cailliet 1988).

The chief function of the nucleus pulposus is as a hydraulic shock absorber. Specifically, it serves to receive primarily vertical forces from vertebral bodies, and to redistribute them radially in a horizontal plane. The surrounding annulus fibrosus then resists the created tension. To better understand this action, imagine the nucleus as a movable swivel (Figure 18.4). A summary of these actions is presented in Table 18.1.

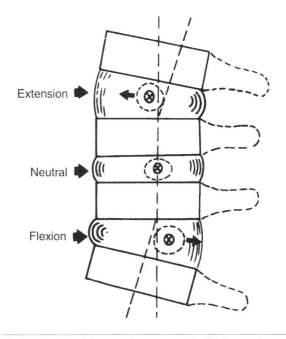

Fig. 18.4. The fulcrum of movement in flexion and extension of the lumbar spine.
Reprinted from Fisk and Rose (1977).

Table 18.1. Functions of the Nucleus Pulposus

Action	Flexion	Extension	Lateral flexion
The upper vertebrae will tilt:	Anteriorly	Posteriorly	Toward the side of flexion
Therefore, the disk will flatten:	Anteriorly	Posteriorly	Toward the side of flexion
Therefore, the disk will enlarge:	Posteriorly	Anteriorly	Toward the side opposite flexion
Therefore, the nucleus will be driven:	Posteriorly	Anteriorly	Toward the side opposite flexion

Note. From: Alter, M.J. (1988). *Science of Stretching* (p. 130). Champaign, IL: Human Kinetics. Copyright 1988 by M.J. Alter. Reprinted by permission.
Reprinted from Alter (1988).

The Annulus Fibrosus

The annulus fibrosus consists of approximately 20 concentric layers of fibers (see Figure 18.3). These elastic fibers are woven so that one layer runs at an angle to the preceding layer so that they seem to cross each other obliquely. This special pattern allows a controlled motion to take place. For example, when a shearing force is applied (i.e., a force that tends to cause one layer of an object to slide over another layer), the oblique fibers in one direction will tighten, while the opposing fibers relax (Figure 18.5).

As stated earlier, the annulus fibrosis receives the ultimate effects of most force transmitted from one vertebral body to another. This function may seem strange because the major loading of the disk is in the form of vertical compression (weight bearing) and the annulus fibrosus is best constructed to resist shear. However, the nucleus pulposus transforms the vertical thrust into a ra-

dial or bulging force. This force is restricted by the elastic and tensile strength of the fibers.

The annulus fibrosus also loses a great deal of its elasticity and resilience with age. In young and undamaged disks, the fibroelastic tissue of the annulus is predominantly elastic. However, with aging or as a result of injury, there is a relative increase in the percentage of fibrous elements. As this change occurs, the disk loses its elasticity, and its hydraulic recoil mechanism decreases. In the older annulus fibrosus, the highly elastic collagen fibrils are replaced by large fibrotic bands of collagen tissue devoid of mucoid material. The disk is therefore less elastic, that is, less able to return to its original shape after being compressed (Cailliet 1988; Panagiotacopulos, Knauss, and Bloch 1979; Walker 1981).

As the disk becomes more inelastic, it becomes more susceptible to injury and trauma. Each episode of trauma sets the stage for extrusion of the nucleus pulposus into the tears of the annulus

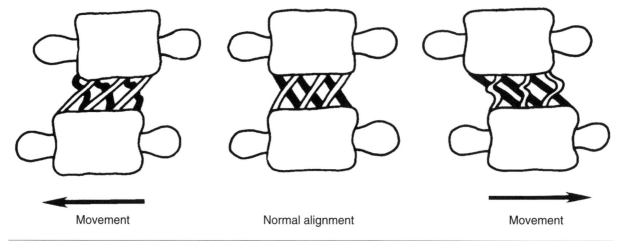

Movement   Normal alignment   Movement

Fig. 18.5.   The elastic fibers of the annulus fibrosus are in part responsible for the controlled motion of the vertebral column. When a horizontal force is applied to the vertebrae, the oblique fibers in one direction will tighten, while those in the other relax.
Reprinted from Alter (1988).

fibrosus. Thus, even a minor stress might tip the scales and result in major injury (Cailliet 1988). Furthermore, due to the reduced vascular supply to the disk with aging, the ability of an injured disk to regain its elasticity is reduced in the elderly. No wonder that herniation, rupture, and bulging of the disk are found more often in the aged than in the young (Cailliet 1988; Panagiotacopulos, Knauss, and Bloch 1979).

The Vertebral Ligaments

Ligamentous structures and other connective tissues also contribute to the stability of the spine (Figure 18.6). Their function is to limit or modify movement occurring at a joint. For maximal stability, ligaments must be short, thick, and strong. However, for maximal range of motion, ligaments need to be long. Ideally, the structures should allow an optimal degree of mobility as well as optimal stability. Hence long, thick, and strong ligaments would be preferred but occur rarely.

How effectively a ligament checks excessive movement depends not only on its length and size, but also on its location and distance from the axis of motion. That is, the greatest strain will fall on those ligaments and structures farthest away from the axis or fulcrum of movement. Conversely, those structures closest to the center of rotation will produce the smallest contribution to checking excessive movement.

Spinal Flexion and Extension

Because the greatest load falls on those ligaments farthest from the fulcrum of movement, the structures limiting flexion (working from the nucleus pulposus outwards in order of increasing contribution) are the posterior annulus fibrosus, the posterior longitudinal ligament, the ligamentum flavum, the facet joint posterior capsule, the intertransverse ligaments, the interspinous ligaments, and the supraspinous ligament. The greatest stress falls on this last ligament. Other structures that may assist in restricting flexion are the

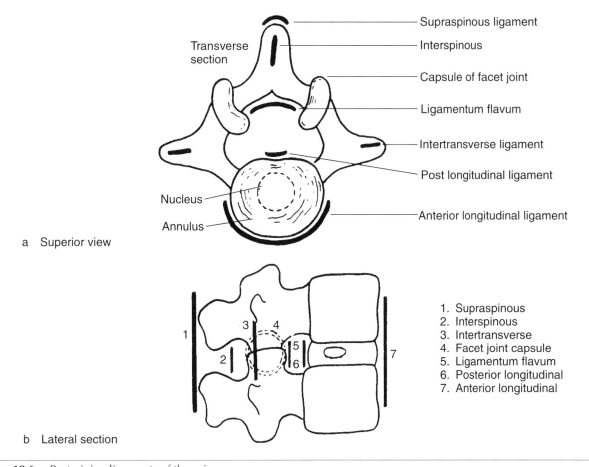

a   Superior view

b   Lateral section

1. Supraspinous
2. Interspinous
3. Intertransverse
4. Facet joint capsule
5. Ligamentum flavum
6. Posterior longitudinal
7. Anterior longitudinal

Fig. 18.6. Restraining ligaments of the spine.
Reprinted from Fisk and Rose (1977).

erector spinae muscles of the lower back and the lower lumbodorsal fascia. The latter is a dense, fascial sheath of connective tissue that encompasses the erector spinae muscles (Farfan 1973; Fisk and Rose 1977). Conversely, spinal hyperextension is limited by the anterior portion of the annulus fibrosus and the anterior longitudinal ligament, supplemented by the abdominal muscles and the fascia (the rectus sheaths).

Lateral Spinal Flexion

Lateral flexion is limited by all ligamentous structures lateral to the midline. Again, the greatest load falls on those structures farthest from the fulcrum of movement. Accordingly, the quadratus lumborum muscle (connecting the upper edge of the pelvis to the lower ribs), erector spinae muscles, abdominal oblique muscles, three layers of lumbodorsal fascia, and the facet capsular ligaments are of major importance, while the intertransverse ligaments are of less importance.

Limits on Range of Motion of the Thoracic-Lumbar Region

The range of movement between any two successive vertebrae is slight. However, the sum total of these movements is of considerable magnitude when the vertebral column is considered as a whole. The ranges of motion of the various regions of the vertebral column depend on numerous factors. Following is a description of the thoracic and lumbar regions of the trunk and their ranges of motion in flexion, extension, and lateral flexion.

Trunk Flexion

Flexion of the trunk is defined as bending or moving the chest towards the thighs. This movement is produced primarily by the rectus abdominis and is assisted by the external and internal abdominal oblique muscles. When trunk flexion is performed from a standing position, it is produced primarily by gravity and controlled by eccentric contraction of the spinal extensor muscles. The rectus abdominis is needed only to perform trunk flexion against gravity, as in the

supine position. Range of motion is limited by trunk flexor contractile insufficiency, tension of the spinal extensor muscles, passive tension of spinal posterior structures (the posterior annulus fibrosus, posterior longitudinal ligament, ligamenta flava, facet joint capsules, intertransverse ligaments, interspinous ligaments, and supraspinous ligaments), bony apposition of the lips of the vertebral bodies anteriorly with surfaces of adjacent vertebrae, compression of the ventral parts of the intervertebral fibrocartilaginous disk, and contact of the ribs with the abdomen. Flexion of the trunk takes place almost exclusively in the lumbar region, due to the unfavorable orientation of the articular facets in the thoracic region.

According to Greene and Heckman (1994) standard methods of measuring joint motion are difficult to apply in the thoracic and lumbar spine. Alternative methods of measurement have been devised and advocated, but without agreement about which method is best. Trunk flexion can be measured using a variety of techniques. Methods of assessing thoracic and lumbar spine motion include visual estimation, skin distraction, goniometric measurements, and inclinometer techniques.

Trunk Extension

Extension of the trunk is returning from flexion to neutral, or anatomical, erect posture. Hyperextension of the trunk is defined as bending dorsally. This movement is associated with an accentuation of the lumbar curvature and is produced by the erector spinae muscles of the lower back. Range of motion is restricted by extensor contractile insufficiency, tension of the anterior abdominal muscles, tension of the anterior spinal structures (annulus fibrosus and anterior longitudinal ligament), and bony contact of adjacent spinous processes and of the caudal articular margins with the laminae.

Trunk Lateral Flexion

Lateral flexion of the trunk is defined as a sideward inclination of the torso. This movement is produced by the external and internal abdominal oblique muscles and is assisted by the erector spinae muscles contracting unilaterally. Range of motion is limited by contractile insufficiency of these muscles, tension of the oblique abdominal muscles on the side opposite flexion, tension

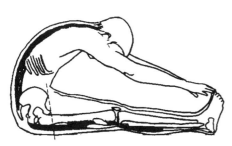

Normal length of back, hamstring, and gastroc-soleus muscles.

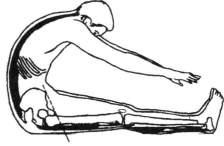

Normal length of back and hamstring muscles, short gastroc-soleus muscles.

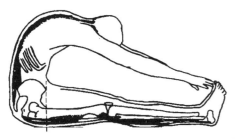

Stretched upper back and hamstring muscles, slightly short low back muscles, and normal length of gastroc-soleus muscles.

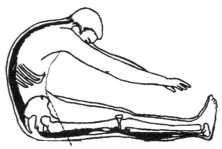

Stretched upper back muscles, slightly short low back and short hamstring muscles, and normal length of gastroc-soleus muscles.

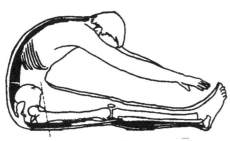

Normal length of back and hamstring muscles, short gastroc-soleus muscles.

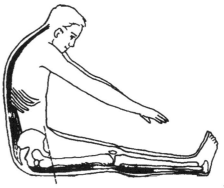

Normal length of upper back, hamstring, and gastroc-soleus muscles, short low back muscles.

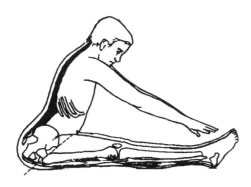

Normal length of upper back muscles, contracture of low back muscles with paralysis of extremity muscles.

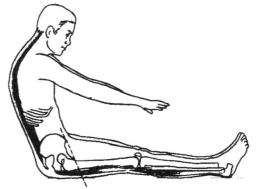

Normal length of upper back muscles, short low back, hamstring, and gastroc-soleus muscles.

Fig. 18.7. Foward-bending test for length of posterior muscles.
Reprinted from Kendall, Kendall, and Wadsworth (1971).

of spinal structures (the annulus fibrosus between the vertebrae, contralateral ligamenta flava, and intertransverse ligaments), interlocking of the articular facets on the side of the movement, and apposition of adjacent ribs.

The Interrelationship of Stretching the Lower Back, Pelvis, and Hamstrings

One of the most commonly performed, least understood, and potentially dangerous flexibility exercises or tests for flexibility of the hamstring muscles and lower back is hip flexion with the knees extended. Although numerous variations exist, this exercise is often performed as a toe touch in one of four positions: from a standing position, from a sitting position, from a hurdler's stretch position, or from a supine position (i.e., a straight leg raise).

When stretching or testing for flexibility, one must be careful to distinguish between tight, nor-

mal, and stretched muscles. Equally important, one must also make sure that only the desired muscle groups are stretched. Often, as will be seen, the true results of flexibility testing are masked or obscured (Kendall, Kendall, and Wadsworth 1971; Figure 18.7). Therefore, some additional knowledge of the structures that are involved is necessary.

Most, if not all, of the forward flexion occurs in the lumbar spine. More specifically, 5% to 10% of flexion is found to occur between L-1 and L-4, 20% to 25% between L-4 and L-5, and 60% to 75% between L-5 and S-1 (Figure 18.8). Furthermore, most of the spinal flexion occurs by the time the trunk is inclined 45° forward. In actuality, total lumbar flexion is limited to the extent of reversing of the lordosis curve (Cailliet 1988). As a matter of fact, Cailliet points out that if a person were to bend forward to touch his or her fingers to the floor without bending at the knees or at the hips, more flexion would be required than is attributed to the lumbar spine. Hence, were this lumbar curve reversal the only flexion possible, one could not bend even half the distance to the floor. Additional flexion must be possible, but how? The answer is that flexion also occurs at the hip joints.

The flexion possible at the hips is attributed to the mobility of the pelvic girdle. If you recall from chapter 17, the hip is a ball and socket formed by the rounded heads of the femurs fitted into the cuplike acetabular sockets. Consequently, the pelvis is capable of rotation around the fulcrum of the two lateral hip joints. This motion can be likened to the action of a seesaw or teeterboard (Cailliet 1988; Kapandji 1974). Therefore, during hip flexion, the anterior portion of the pelvis descends and the posterior aspect ascends. With reextension, the pelvis rotates back to its erect position (Figure 18.9).

Optimal and safe performance when stretching requires a blend of adequate flexibility, strength, and mechanics. For example, when performing hip flexion with the knees extended, several factors may potentially restrict range of motion. The most common causes are tight low back muscles and tight hamstring muscles. Obviously, with tight low back muscles, lumbar flexion is restricted. However, when the hamstrings are tight, the pelvis is restricted from rotating because the hamstrings are attached to the posterior portion of the knee and to the pelvis at the tuberosity of the ischium (Cailliet 1988). Other potentially limiting factors include defects in the disks, ligaments, or bony structure; irregular curvature of the spine; impingement of the intervertebral

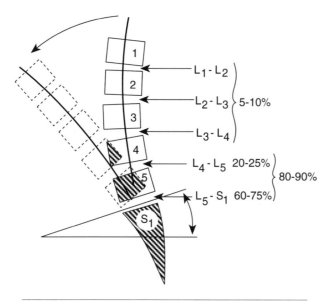

Fig. 18.8. Segmental site and degree of lumbar flexion. The degree of flexion noted in the lumbar spine is indicated as a percentage of total spinal flexion. The major portion of flexion (75%) occurs at the lumbosacral joint; 15% to 20% of flexion occurs between L-4 and L-5; and the remaining 5% to 10% is distributed between L-1 and L-4. The diagram indicates the mere reversal past lordosis of total flexion of the lumbar curve.
Reprinted from Cailliet (1981).

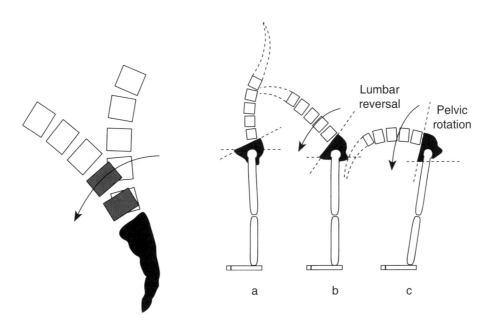

Fig. 18.9. Lumbar pelvic rhythm. With pelvis fixed, flexion-extension of the lumbar spine occurs mostly between the lower segments L-5 and S-1.
Reprinted from Cailliet (1981).

joints (Figure 18.10); sciatic nerve irritation (Figure 18.11); and any muscle imbalance (Cailliet 1988; Walther 1981).

When developing flexibility, safety must always come first. For example, when performing a standing straight-leg toe touch, the body is susceptible to injury and pain. This problem often occurs when tight muscles in the lower back or hamstrings are overstretched (Figure 18.12) and is especially true with ballistic stretching. Faulty mechanics can also initiate injury. The mechanics of the lumbar spine are such that any increased weight anterior to the vertebral column greatly increases the forces that are exerted on the lum-

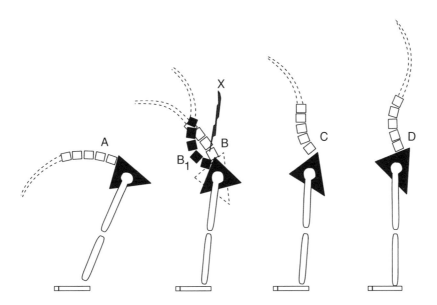

Fig. 18.10. Mechanism of acute facet impingement. (A-D) The proper physiological resumption of the erect position from total flexion with reverse lumbar-pelvic rhythm. (B$_1$) Improper premature lordotic curve that cantilevers the lumbar spine anterior to the center of gravity. This position approximates the facets at X and, coupled with the eccentric leading of the spine, requires greater muscular contraction of the erector spinae group. Facet impingement can occur.
Reprinted from Cailliet (1981).

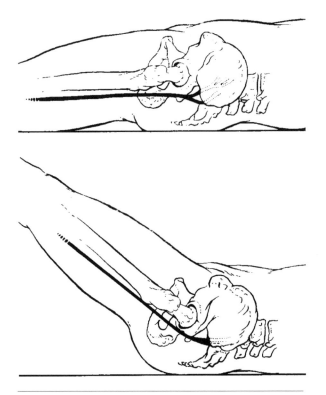

Fig. 18.11. Sciatic nerve irritation. The passive straight-leg-raising test stretches the sciatic nerve as it passes behind the hip joint. If one or several of the nerve roots of the sciatic nerve have been stretched or irritated, the result will be a marked increase in pain.
Reprinted from American Academy of Orthopaedic Surgeons (1985).

bar spine. Consequently, during trunk flexion the resultant forces at the fulcrum, which is the lower lumbar segment, are very high. These forces are increased when one performs the movement with the arms horizontal to the floor. To reduce the strain on the back, place the hands on the hips, as shown in Figure 18.13 (Segal 1983; White and Panjabi 1978).

Research by Schultz et al. (1982) found that twisting and bending the trunk laterally did not load the spine more than positions of forward bending. Lateral bending movements can load the spine moderately, but not nearly as much as the forward flexion movement, for two reasons: The trunk cannot be laterally offset very much, so that the moment imposed cannot become very large, and the lateral abdominal wall muscles act on the spine through a relatively large moment arm, so they need not contract strongly to counterbalance the offset weight moment (Schultz et al. 1982). Nonetheless, the possibility of injury still exists. Segal (1983) points out that in side-bending, when one puts the opposite arm overhead, additional and unnecessary stretch is placed on the lower back muscles on the same side as the extended arm. The risk of injury can be further compounded if the lateral rotation is combined with excessive rotation and flexion or excessive rotation and extension (Garu 1986). When this

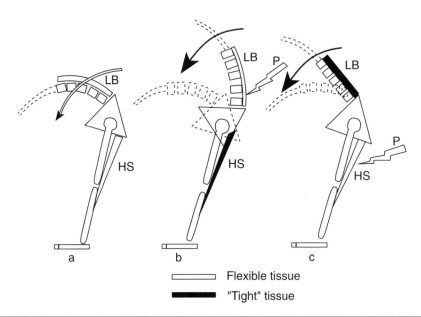

Fig. 18.12. Mechanism of stretch pain in the tight hamstring and the tight low back syndromes. (a) Normal flexibility with unrestricted lumbar-pelvic rhythm. (b) Tight hamstrings (HS) restricting pelvic rotation and thereby causing excessive stretch of low back (LB) resulting in pain (P). (c) Tight low back (LB) performing an incomplete lumbar reversal and thus, by placing excessive stretch on the hamstrings (HS), causing pain (P) in both the hamstrings and the low back as well as a disrupted lumbar-pelvic rhythm.
Reprinted from Cailliet (1981).

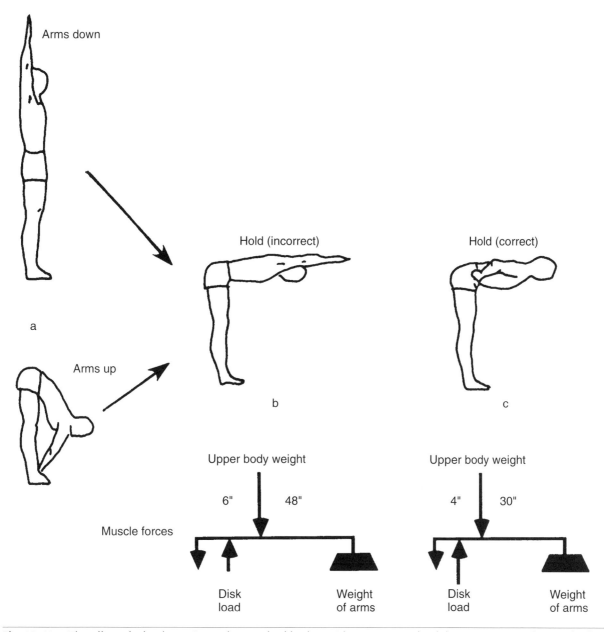

Fig. 18.13. The effect of a load anterior to the vertebral body. (a) The greater any load that is anterior to the vertebral body, the greater the forces exerted on the lumbar spine. (b) Extending or lowering the arms horizontally increases stress on the lumbar spine. (c) Placing the hands on the hips (fulcrum) decreases the load anterior to the vertebral body, reducing stress.

exercise is performed in a ballistic manner, the potential for injury is even greater.

Another potential cause of low back injury or pain is faulty reextension from the flexed position, in which the lumbar lordosis is regained before the pelvis is derotated (Cailliet 1988). Cailliet (1988) recommends that, in reassuming the erect stance, the lumbar spine should act as an inflexible rod, kept straight and fully extended. With faulty reextension, the upper portion of the body rises early, so that the lower back arches and the lordosis curve is in front of the center of gravity (Figure 18.14). Consequently, this position places an excessive stress on the lower back. Remember, pelvic derotation should occur before lordosis is regained when reextending; the erector spinae muscles should straighten the spine and the lower back regain its lordosis during the last 45° of extension. However, due to the short lever arm to which the erector spinae muscles are

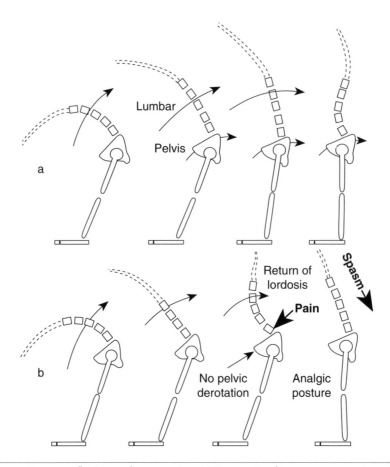

Fig. 18.14.   Proper versus improper flexion and reextension. (a) Proper simultaneous resumption of the lumbar lordosis with pelvic rotation. (b) Regaining of pelvic lordosis with no pelvic derotation, causing painful lordotic posture with the upper part of the body held ahead of the center of gravity.
Reprinted from Cailliet (1981).

attached, this portion of reextension is inefficient and can potentially strain these muscles. When the erector spinae muscles fatigue, the task of maintaining and supporting the excessive load falls on the vertebral ligaments. As further elaborated by Cailliet, the lumbar spine is normally supported by the supraspinous ligament when in full flexion until the last 45° of extension (Figure 18.15).

In contrast, the erector spinae are not active during full trunk flexion. Thus, there is a significant load on the ligaments during trunk flexion, creating the possibility of a sprain or tear of the ligaments. Once the ligaments give way, the load falls on the joints, and subluxation of the joints may result.

A toe touch from a sitting position or modified hurdler's stretch also requires caution, especially when stretching with a partner. Too often, injury occurs when a partner unknowingly imparts a little extra stretch. To prevent such accidents, anticipation and communication must be employed.

The Cervical Vertebrae

The neck's skeletal framework is made up of seven cervical vertebrae. The most well known are the first and second vertebrae below the head, the atlas and axis, respectively. These vertebrae are unique in structure. The atlas directly supports the head and forms a bony ring. The axis features a small upward bony projection that forms a peglike pivot. The atlas rotates around this peglike pivot when the head is turned from side to side. Thus, this structure determines much of the direction and extent of motion of the head.

Movements of the Cervical Region

The cervical region is capable of flexion, extension, lateral flexion, and rotation. This region is

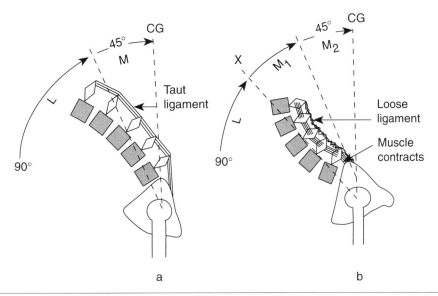

Fig. 18.15. Faulty reextension of the lumbar spine. (a) Correct reextension. Until the last 45°, the lumbar spine (L) is supported by supraspinous ligaments requiring no muscular effort. Muscles normally become active in the last 45° (M) when the carrying angle is close to the center of gravity (CG). (b) Premature lumbar lordosis with pelvis not adequately derotated causes the erector muscles (M_1) to contract before having reached the last 45°. The ligaments loosen, and the muscles take the brunt and contract inefficiently and forcefully, resulting in pain.
Reprinted from Cailliet (1981).

most mobile and shows the freest range of motion of all the vertebrae because the disks are thickest in relation to the height of the vertebral body. The ratio of disk to body is 2:5, or 40% (Kapandji 1974). Furthermore, since the width of the vertebral body is greater than its height or depth, there is a greater capacity for flexion and extension than for lateral bending.

The major determinants of the direction and extent of motion reside in the shape of the vertebral bodies and in the contours and orientations of the intervertebral articulations. The ligaments, fascia, and capsules also provide constraints to motion. When their elastic limits are reached, the tension created causes motion to halt. Following is a brief description of the limiting factors associated with range of motion in the cervical region.

Cervical Flexion

Cervical flexion is defined as moving the head forward to the chest. Typically, when the body is vertical, neck flexion is produced by gravity acting on the head. However, when the body is supine, the head must be lifted against gravity. The primary muscle involved in flexion is the sternocleidomastoid (SCM), assisted by the scalenes, rectus capitis anterior, longus capitis, and cervicis. Flexion of the neck is limited by SCM contractile insufficiency, tension of posterior spinal structures (the posterior longitudinal liga-

ment, ligamenta flava, interspinal ligaments, and supraspinal ligament), tension of the posterior muscles and fascia of the neck, the apposition of the anterior lips of the vertebral bodies with the surfaces of the adjacent vertebrae, compression of the anterior portion of the intervertebral fibrocartilage, and the chin coming to rest on the chest.

Probably the most controversial and potentially dangerous stretch for the cervical region is the plow (see Figure 15.10). In chapter 15, the pros and cons of this exercise were discussed. In brief, the authorities and experts are divided on the issue. For individuals involved in gymnastics, judo, wrestling, and yoga, this stretch may be essential in their discipline. However, for most laypeople and athletes, there are safer alternatives.

Effective stretching of the extensors of the cervical region to increase flexion requires anchoring and stabilization of the scapula and shoulder girdle. This position can be easily achieved lying flat on the floor (see Exercise #42). The key to the stretch is to pull the head off the floor and draw the chin to the chest while keeping the shoulder blades flat on the ground. Once the shoulder blades lift off the floor, most of the stretch is lost. Another effective way to demonstrate the importance of stabilizing the scapula and shoulder girdle is to stand upright while holding a pair of dumbbells or a barbell. With the shoulders de-

Table 18.2. Factors Limiting Lumbar, Thoracic, and Cervical Movement

Factor	Lumbar region	Thoracic region	Cervical region
	Flexion		
Articular facet joint orientation	Sagittal plane (*no* contact/ jamming occurs with flexion)	Frontal plane (contact/ jamming *does* occur with flexion)	45° between frontal and horizontal planes (some sliding occurs with flexion)
Ratio of disk thickness to vertebral body thickness	Thick disks (allow considerable disk wedging prior to vertebral body contact anteriorly)	Thin disks (allow minimal disk wedging prior to vertebral body contact anteriorly)	Moderate ratio (allows moderate disk wedging prior to vertebral body contact anteriorly)
Rib cage	None	Contact of 12th rib with abdomen and incompressible sternum	None
Connective tissue tension	All posterior ligaments, facet joint posterior capsules	All posterior ligaments, facet joint posterior capsules	All posterior ligaments, facet joint posterior capsules
Muscle tension	Spinal extensor muscles (erector spinae and transversospinalis groups)	Spinal extensor muscles (erector spinae and transversospinalis groups)	Neck extensor muscles (erector spinae, transversospinalis, and suboccipital groups)
	Extension		
Articular facet joint orientation	Sagittal plane (*no* contact/ jamming occurs with hyperextension)	Frontal plane (contact/ jamming *does* occur with hyperextension)	45° between frontal and horizontal planes (some sliding occurs with hyperextension)
Vertebral spinous process length	Short process, projects posteriorly (allows much hyperextension prior to impingement)	Long process, projects inferiorly, overlapping like roof shingles (no hyperextension is allowed)	Moderate length, projects nearly posteriorly (allowing moderate hyperextension prior to impingement)
Ratio of disk thickness to vertebral body thickness	Thick disks (allow considerable wedging prior to vertebral body contact posteriorly)	Thin disks (allow minimal wedging prior to vertebral body contact posteriorly)	Moderate ratio (allows moderate wedging prior to vertebral body contact posteriorly)
Rib cage	None	Attachment of ribs to inextensible sternum	None
Connective tissue tension	Anterior longitudinal ligament, facet joint anterior capsules	Anterior longitudinal ligament, facet joint anterior capsules	Anterior longitudinal ligament, facet joint anterior capsules
Muscle tension	Trunk flexor muscles (rectus abdominus)	Trunk flexor muscles (rectus abdominus)	Neck flexor muscles (many)

(continued)

pressed by the weight, look down and slowly bend the head toward the chest as if nodding. The stretch should be felt in the upper back and cervical region.

Cervical Extension

Cervical extension is the returning of the head from the flexed position (the head forward on the chest)

Table 18.2. Continued

Factor	Lumbar region	Thoracic region	Cervical region
	Lateral flexion (side-bending)		
Articular facet joint orientation	Sagittal plane (contact/ jamming *does* occur with lateral flexion)	Frontal plane (*no* contact/ jamming occurs with lateral flexion)	45° between frontal and horizontal planes (some sliding occurs with lateral flexion)
Ratio of disk thickness to vertebral body thickness	Thick disks (allow considerable wedging prior to vertebral body contact laterally)	Thin disks (allow minimal wedging prior to vertebral body contact laterally)	Moderate ratio (allows moderate wedging prior to vertebral body contact laterally)
Rib cage	None	Contact between adjacent ribs on shortened side of trunk	None
Connective tissue tension	Intertransverse ligaments, facet joint lateral capsules	Intertransverse ligaments, facet joint lateral capsules, and costovertebral ligaments	Intertransverse ligaments, facet joint lateral capsules
Muscle tension	Intertransversarii spinal extensor muscles, quadratus lumborum, abdominal obliques on lengthened side	Spinal extensor muscles, intercostal muscles on lengthened side	Neck lateral muscles (many) on lengthened side
	Rotation		
Articular facet joint orientation	Sagittal plane (contact/ jamming *does* occur with rotation)	Frontal plane (contact/ jamming *does* occur with rotation)	45° between frontal and horizontal plane (*no* contact/jamming occurs with rotation)
Rib cage	None	Rib attachments to spine and sternum limit relative motion between adjacent ribs	None
Connective tissue tension	All spinal ligaments somewhat and facet joint capsules	All spinal ligaments somewhat and facet joint capsules	All spinal ligaments somewhat and facet joint capsules
Muscle tension	Back extensor oblique group/transversospinalis group (multifidi, semispinalis, rotatores)	Back extensor oblique group/transversospinalis group (multifidi, semispinalis, rotatores)	Neck rotator muscles (anteriorly: sternocleidomastoideus; posteriorly: splenius, obliquus capitis superior and inferior)

to an upright position. Drawing the head backward beyond the upright position is called *cervical hyperextension*. This movement is produced by several posterior neck muscles (upper trapezius, semispinalis cervicis and capitis, splenius cervicis and capitis, rectus capitis posterior major and minor, obliquus capitis superior and inferior, and interspinales). Range of motion is limited by extensor contractile insufficiency, passive tension of the anterior longitudinal ligament, tension of the anterior neck muscles and fascia, bony approximation of the spinous processes, the locking of the posterior edges of the articular facet, and contact of the head on the muscle mass of the upper trunk. (An effective self-stretch using positioning and gravity can be seen in Exercise #45).

Cervical Lateral Flexion

Cervical lateral flexion may be described as tilting the head so that the left ear moves nearer the left shoulder or the right ear draws closer to the right shoulder. Lateral flexion of the neck is produced by many muscles (the SCM, scalenes, splenius cervicis and capitis, semispinalis cervicis and capitis, rectus capitis lateralis, rectus capitis posterior major and minor, obliquus capitis superior and inferior, intertransversarii, and longus cervicis and capitis) acting unilaterally. Range of motion is restricted by the contractile insufficiency of these muscles, passive tension of the intertransverse ligaments, tension of the neck muscles and fascia on the side opposing flexion, and impingement of the articular processes. Table 18.2 summarizes factors limiting lumbar, thoracic, and cervical movements.

Effective stretching of the lateral portion of the cervical area also necessitates anchoring the shoulder girdle. This stabilization can be accomplished by sitting in a chair grasping its leg or seat base or by holding onto weights. Then the stretch can be applied by pulling on the head with the hand opposite the side of the stretch or by self-positioning and the use of gravity. Once again, if the chair or weights are released, the shoulder on the stretched side will rise and the stretch is dissipated.

Cervical Rotation

Cervical rotation may be described as turning the head and neck so that the face looks over one shoulder. Most rotation occurs at the atlantoaxial joint, that is, between vertebrae C-1 and C-2. Rotation of the head and neck is produced by many muscles (on the opposite side by the SCM, semispinalis capitis and cervicis, and obliquus capitis superior; on the same side by the splenius capitis and cervicis, obliquus capitis inferior, rectus capitis posterior major, and rectus capitis lateralis). Range of motion is restricted by the contractile insufficiency of these muscles, passive tension of ligaments (particularly the atlas ligaments between C-2 and the skull), tension of the opposing neck muscles, and impingement of the articular processes. Table 18.2 summarizes these factors.

Summary

The vertebral column is made up of a series of separate bones, the vertebrae, linked together by cartilaginous disks and ligaments. Together, these components form a structural and functional unit capable of performing its many functions. Among several factors that can determine ROM are the intervertebral disks, the height of the vertebrae, the orientation of the facets, the intervertebral ligaments, and the passive tension of various connective tissues. The optimal efficiency of the vertebral column may be impaired due to aging, attrition, disease, and trauma. ROM of the vertebral column can be maintained or enhanced through purposeful stretching exercises.

Chapter 19

Anatomy and Flexibility of the Upper Extremity

The upper extremity shall be considered here as consisting of the shoulder girdle, shoulder joint, arm, elbow joint, forearm, wrist joint, and hand. It will be described in terms of structure, function, limitation to range of motion, and methodology of stretching.

The Shoulder Girdle and Arm

Each shoulder girdle and shoulder-arm complex is made up of a clavicle, humerus, and scapula bone, plus an attachment to the single midline sternum. In combination, these bony segments articulate at three major joints: the glenohumeral, sternoclavicular, and acromioclavicular joints. According to Kapandji (1982), there are five joints with the addition of the subdeltoid and the scapulothoracic, although neither of these junctions are anatomical joints (Figure 19.1). Although many movements appear to take place in the glenohumeral joint, they often involve simultaneous movement at other adjacent joints. Without the assistance of these joints, movements of the upper limb would be seriously restricted.

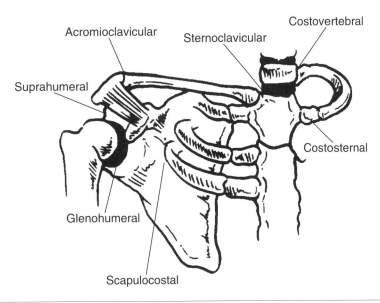

Fig. 19.1. Composite drawing of the joints of the shoulder girdle: glenohumeral; suprahumeral; acromioclavicular; scapulocostal; sternoclavicular; costosternal; costovertebral.
Reprinted from Cailliet (1966).

Gross Anatomy of the Shoulder Girdle

The three major joints that provide motion in the shoulder girdle are the glenohumeral joint, the sternoclavicular joint, and the acromioclavicular joint. Each of these is discussed in the following sections. The scapulothoracic joint, although not a true joint, is very important in shoulder movement and is also described.

Glenohumeral Joint

The glenohumeral, or scapulohumeral, joint is a modified ball-and-socket joint consisting of the humeral head and the shallow glenoid fossa (i.e., cavity) of the scapula. This structure creates one of the most mobile and unstable joints in the human body. The lack of stability is due primarily to its weak bony architecture. The major stability of the joint is provided by the large, enveloping musculature. Its secondary line of support comes from the capsular-ligamentous complexes. These include the glenoid labrum, the fibrous capsule, and the glenohumeral, coracohumeral, and transverse humeral ligaments.

Sternoclavicular Joint

The sternoclavicular (SC) joint is a synovial joint formed by the articulation of the medial end of the clavicle with the first rib and manubrium of the sternum. This joint is the only bony attachment of the entire upper limb to the axial skeleton. The joint is afforded little stability by bony arrangement but is strong because of its ligaments and intervening disk.

Acromioclavicular Joint

The acromioclavicular (AC) articulation is between the acromial end of the clavicle and the medial margin of the acromion of the scapula. The joint obtains its primary stability from the ligamentous binding rather than from its bony architecture. Despite the ligamentous binding, the joint is generally weak and is therefore easily dislocated (Kelley 1971). In addition, the acromioclavicular joint is prone to degenerative changes that can lead to functional impairment.

Scapulothoracic Joint

The scapulothoracic (ST) joint is not a true joint but instead rides on the scapula on the posterior surface of the thoracic cage—there is no articulation of bones. The scapulothoracic joint is considered the most important joint of the shoulder-arm complex, although it cannot function without the scapulohumeral and subdeltoid joints, which are mechanically linked to it (Kapandji 1982).

Description of Shoulder Motion

The clavicular movements that occur at the sternoclavicular and acromioclavicular joints are always associated with movements of the scapula, and movements of the scapula are usually accompanied by movement of the humerus and clavicle. The six scapular movements are elevation, depression, protraction, retraction, and upward and downward rotation. Similarly, movements of the upper arm at the glenohumeral joint are always associated with movements of the scapula and the previously cited shoulder joints. The movements of the glenohumeral joint are best described in relation to the humeral segment moving on the trunk. These arm movements include abduction, adduction, flexion, extension, internal rotation, external rotation, horizontal (transverse) abduction, and horizontal (transverse) adduction.

Arm Abduction

Abduction at the glenohumeral joint is defined as the upward movement of the arm in the coronal (or frontal) plane from anatomical position, that is, raising the arm to the side (Greene and Heckman 1994). The range of abduction at the glenohumeral joint depends on the type of movement and rotation of the humerus. *Active* abduction is limited to about 90°. This limitation is because the greater tuberosity of the humerus will impinge on the acromial process and the coracoacromial ligament. Another reason is a lack of mechanical advantage of the deltoid muscle.

In contrast, *passive* abduction is limited to 120° (Figure 19.2). In order for the greater tuberosity to pass under the coracoacromial hood during arm abduction, there must be simultaneous depression and external rotation of the humerus (Figures 19.3 and 19.4). Thus, when the arm is raised overhead (180° abduction), only two-thirds (120°) of that movement is actually occurring at the glenohumeral joint. However, if the humerus is maintained in internal rotation, it will not abduct beyond 60°, due to earlier impingement. This portion is the *true glenohumeral motion*, as opposed to the scapulothoracic motion (Ameri-

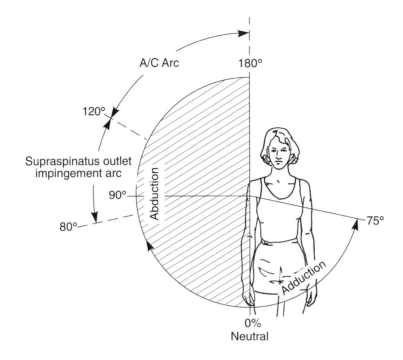

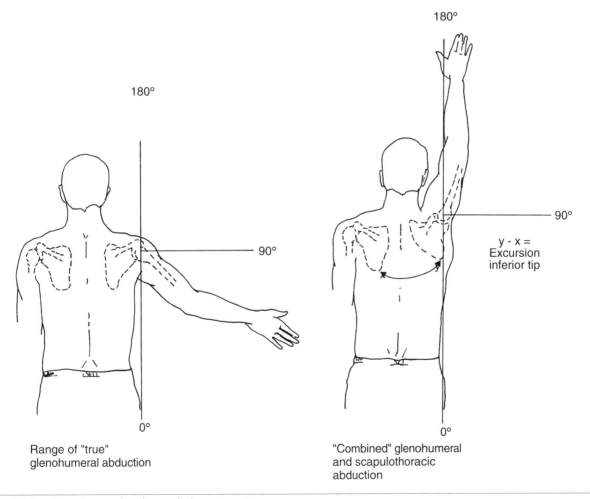

Fig. 19.2.   Glenohumeral and scapulothoracic motion.
Reprinted from American Orthopaedic Association (1972).

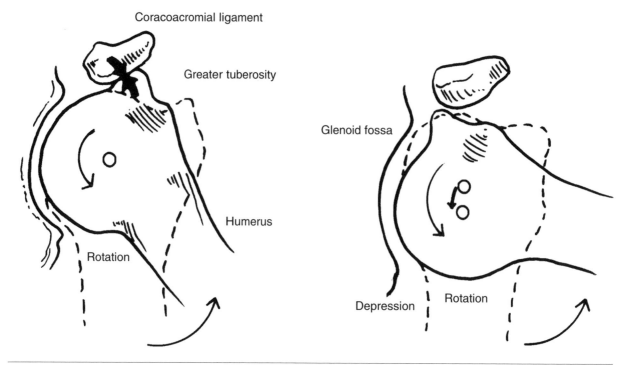

Fig. 19.3. Glenohumeral movement of arm abduction. The incongruity of the articular surface of the head of the humerus and the surface of the glenoid fossa is shown. (left) The greater tuberosity of the humerus impinges on the coracoacromial ligament if rotation is not accompanied by depression of the humerus. (right) Simultaneous depression and rotation in a gliding motion permits the greater tuberosity to pass under the coracoacromial hood during arm abduction.
Reprinted from Cailliet (1981).

can Orthopaedic Association 1985). The remaining 60° of arm motion is achieved by upward rotation at the scapulothoracic joint.

The smooth, integrated movement of the humerus, the scapula, and the clavicle has been termed the *scapulohumeral rhythm*. The intricate interplay of all the articulations of these bones results in coordinated shoulder motion. During the initial *setting phase* (i.e., 30°) of abduction, the motion is mainly glenohumeral with the scapula making very little contribution. The scapula may either remain fixed, move laterally or medially, or oscillate as it seeks stabilization. As abduction continues, the ratio of scapular to humeral motion remains a constant 1° of scapular motion for every 2° of humeral motion (Figure 19.5). Thus, for every 15° of abduction of the humerus, 10° occurs at the glenohumeral joint, and 5° from rotation of the scapula at the scapulothoracic joint. Consequently, if either of these articulations is fixed by injury or disease, the loss of motion is proportionate, with glenohumeral fixation causing twice as much restriction as scapulothoracic fixation (Turek 1984). The muscles primarily responsible for the first phase of action are the deltoid and supraspinatus. Range of motion at the

glenohumeral joint is limited by abductor contractile insufficiency, impingement of the shoulder as a result of the greater tuberosity hitting the superior margin of the glenoid or the acromion, passive tension of the shoulder adductor and internal rotator muscles, passive tension of the inferior portion of the shoulder joint capsule, and tension of the shoulder ligaments.

Another integral component of the abduction of the humerus is the claviculohumeral mechanism. During the first 90° of humerus abduction, the clavicle moves at the sternoclavicular joint with the distal end elevating 4° for every 10° of abduction of the arm. Thus, at 90° of arm motion, the clavicle has elevated approximately 36° at the sternoclavicular joint. In contrast, the motion at the acromioclavicular joint occurs both early (30°) and late (135°–180°) in arm elevation. This motion consists of an upward swing of the scapula on the distal end of the clavicle. Without the cranklike action caused by the clavicle, full 180° abduction of the arm would be impossible (Figures 19.6 and 19.7).

During the second phase of arm motion, abduction ranges from 90° to 150°. This phase can proceed only with contribution of the shoulder

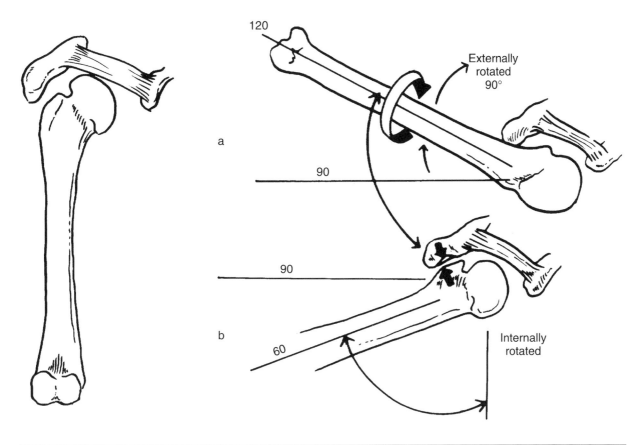

Fig. 19.4. Influence of humeral rotation on abduction range of the glenohumeral joint. (a) Active abduction is possible to 90°, and an additional 30° can be gained passively if the humerus rotates externally approximately through a 90° arc. This abduction range of 120° is possible because the rotation allows the greater tuberosity to pass behind the acromion. (b) With the arm internally rotated, the greater tuberosity impinges against the coracoacromial arch and blocks abduction at 60°.
Reprinted from Cailliet (1981).

girdle. The muscles responsible for this movement are the trapezius and serratus anterior. Range of motion is restricted by contractile insufficiency of the shoulder abductor, scapular upward rotator, and scapular elevating muscles; tension of the shoulder adductor, scapular depressor, and scapular downward rotator muscles (i.e., the latissimus dorsi and pectoralis major); and passive tension of the middle and inferior bands of the glenohumeral ligament. The third phase of arm abduction is from 150° to 180°. To attain a vertical position of the arm, movement of the vertebral column may be required by the exaggeration of the lumbar lordosis (Kapandji 1982). At the end of abduction, all the abductor muscles are in contraction. Limiting factors are the same as in the second phase.

Arm Adduction

Adduction of the glenohumeral joint is defined as returning the humerus from the abducted posi-

tion to its naturally hanging position (i.e., the motion of the arm toward the midline of the body) or beyond. Adduction is produced primarily by the pectoralis major and latissimus dorsi muscles. Movement is restricted when the humerus makes contact with the trunk.

Arm Flexion

Flexion of the arm, sometimes called *elevation* or *forward elevation*, is the upward motion of the arm toward the front of the body. Pure flexion at the glenohumeral joint ranges from 0° to 90°, and if modified, up to 180°. For purposes of analysis, the movement is divided into three phases. The first phase has been called the *setting phase* (Inman, Saunders, and Abbott 1944) and ranges from 0° to 60°. The muscles primarily responsible for this phase are the anterior fibers of the deltoid, the coracobrachialis, and the clavicular fibers of the pectoralis major. Range of motion is limited by their contractile insufficiency, tension

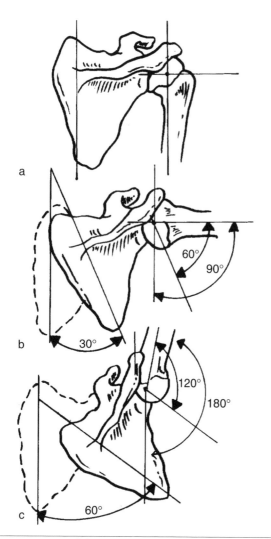

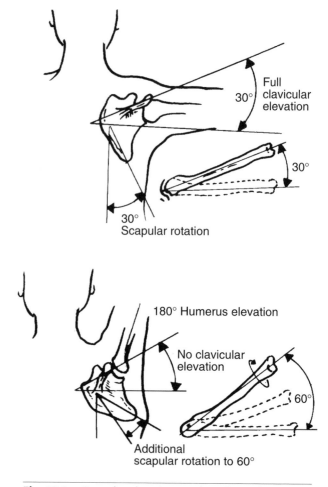

Fig. 19.5. Scapulohumeral rhythm. (a) The scapula and the humerus at rest with the scapula relaxed and the arm dependent, both at 0°. Abduction of the arm is accomplished in a smooth, coordinated movement during which, for each 15° of the arm abduction, 10° of motion occurs at the glenohumeral joint and 5° occurs due to scapular rotation on the thorax. (b) The humerus (H) has abducted 90° in relationship to the erect body, but this movement has been accomplished by 30° rotation of the scapula and 60° abduction of the humerus at the glenohumeral joint, a ratio of 2:1. (c) Full elevation of the arm: 60° at the scapula and 120° at the glenohumeral joint.
Reprinted from Cailliet (1966).

of the coracohumeral ligament and inferior joint capsule, and tension of the teres minor, teres major, and infraspinatus muscles.

The second phase of arm flexion is from 60° to 120°. At this point, as during arm abduction, the scapulohumeral rhythm of the humerus and scapula comes into play. The ratio of motion in the scapulothoracic and glenohumeral joints is a

Fig. 19.6. Scapular elevation resulting from clavicular rotation. The upper drawing shows the elevation of the clavicle without rotation to 30°. The remaining 30° of scapular rotation, which is imperative in full scapulohumeral range, occurs by rotation of the crank-shaped clavicle about its long axis.
Reprinted from Cailliet (1981).

constant 1° of scapular motion for each 2° of humeral motion. So for every 15° of motion of the humerus, the scapulothoracic movement is 5° and the glenohumeral movement is 10°. Again, as in abduction, when either of these articulations is fixed by injury or disease, the loss of motion is proportional, with glenohumeral fixation causing twice as much restriction as scapulothoracic fixation (Turek 1984). The muscles assisting during this phase are the trapezius and infraspinatus. Movement is restricted by contractile insufficiency, tension of the latissimus dorsi and serratus anterior, as well as anything that impedes the scapulohumeral rhythm.

During the final phase, the humerus moves from 120° to 180° of flexion. When flexion is restricted at the glenohumeral and scapulothoracic

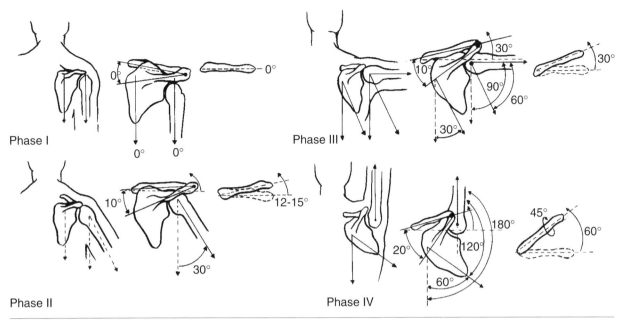

Fig. 19.7. Accessory movement of the scapulohumeral (SH) rhythm other than the glenohumeral movement. Phase I, the resting arm: 0° scapular rotation (S), 0° spinoclavicular angle (angle formed by the clavicle and the scapular spine, SCA), 0° movement at the sternoclavicular joint (SC), no elevation of the outer end of the clavicle (C), no abduction of the humerus (H). Phase II, humerus abducted 30°: outer end of the clavicle elevated 12° to 15° with no rotation of the clavicle; elevation occurs at the sternoclavicular joint; some movement occurs at the acromioclavicular joint as seen by increase of 10° of the spinoclavicular angle. Phase III, humerus (H) abducted to 90° (60° glenohumeral, 30° scapular): clavicle elevated to its final position, no rotation of clavicle as yet, all movement at the sternoclavicular joint, no change in the SCA. Phase IV, full overhead elevation (SH 180°, H 120°, S 60°): outer end of clavicle has not elevated further (at the sternoclavicular joint), but the SCA has increased 20°. Because of the clavicle's rotation and its cranklike form, the clavicle elevates an additional 30°. The humerus through this phase has rotated, but this has not influenced the above degrees of movement.
Reprinted from Cailliet (1966).

joints, movement of the spinal column becomes necessary, which is accomplished by exaggeration of the lumbar lordosis (Kapandji 1982). The muscles responsible for movement and the factors limiting range of motion are the same as in the previous two phases. For a complete 180° movement, the humerus moves 120° at the glenohumeral joint, and the scapula moves upward and forward 60° at the scapulothoracic joint. The 60° of scapular motion would be impossible without the 40° and 20° elevation of the clavicle at the sternoclavicular and acromioclavicular joints, respectively.

Arm Extension

Extension of the glenohumeral joint is the return of the arm from the flexed or elevated position back to anatomical position (arm at the side). *Hyperextension* of the glenohumeral joint is the posterior motion of the humerus in the sagittal plane of the body (i.e., lifting the arm backward and behind the hip). (Greene and Heckman [1994,

6 and 18] of the American Academy of Orthopaedic Surgeons have not adopted this terminology, contending that hyperextension refers only to atypical or asymmetrical motion, such as at the elbow or knee. They point out that extension of the shoulder is sometimes called posterior elevation.) Internal rotation is required for maximum posterior elevation, which ranges up to 60° (Browne et al. 1990). Posterior elevation is displayed in the backswing during bowling. This movement is produced by the deltoid, latissimus dorsi, and teres major and is assisted by the teres minor and long head of the triceps. Range of motion is limited by contractile insufficiency, tension of the shoulder flexor muscles, tension of the coracohumeral ligament, and contact of the greater tubercle of the humerus with the acromion posteriorly.

Arm Internal or Medial Rotation

Internal or *medial* (inward) *rotation* of the glenohumeral joint may be measured by three different methods: rotation with the arm at the side, rotation with the arm in 90° of abduction, and rotation with the arm extended posteriorly. The latter is exemplified by tying apron strings behind one's back. Greene and Heckman (1994) are of the opinion that the abdomen prevents accurate measurement of internal rotation with the arm at the side position. Internal rotation is produced by the scapularis, pectoralis major, latissimus dorsi, and teres major muscles and is assisted by the deltoid muscle. Range of motion is restricted by contractile insufficiency, tension of the superior portion of the capsular ligament, and tension of the external rotator muscles (i.e., infraspinatus and teres minor).

Arm External or Lateral Rotation

External or *lateral* (outward) *rotation* of the glenohumeral joint is also measured by two methods. The first is with the arms at the sides (neutral position), the elbow flexed at 90°, and the forearm parallel to the sagittal plane of the body. The second is from a zero starting position with the arm abducted 90° while aligned with the plane of the scapula and the elbow flexed 90° with the forearm parallel to the floor. Kronberg, Brostrom, and Soderlund (1990) found that a larger angle of humeral head retroversion was consistent with an increased range of external rotation. They also determined the average angle of retroversion was 33° on the dominant side and 29° on the nondominant side. Hence, the dominant side was associated with an increased range of external rotation. Of practical significance, an exaggerated torsion of the humerus might make the glenohumeral joint more vulnerable to instability or dislocation (Brewer, Wubben, and Carrera 1986; Debevoise, Hyatt, and Townsend 1971). External rotation of the humerus is produced by the teres minor, supraspinatus, and infraspinatus. This movement is limited by contractile insufficiency, tension of the superior portion of the capsular and coracohumeral ligaments, and tension of the internal rotator muscles (i.e., subscapularis, pectoralis major, latissimus dorsi, and teres major).

Arm Horizontal Abduction

Horizontal abduction may be defined as moving the humerus laterally and backward with the humerus elevated to a horizontal position. Horizontal abduction ranges approximately from 0° to 30°. This motion is displayed during the cocking or setting phase of a forward stroke with a tennis racquet. Horizontal abduction is produced by the posterior fibers of the deltoid, the infraspinatus, and the teres minor. Range of motion is limited by contractile insufficiency, passive tension of the anterior fibers of the capsule of the glenohumeral joint, and tension of the pectoralis major and anterior fibers of the deltoid muscles.

Arm Horizontal Adduction

Horizontal adduction may be defined as moving the humerus medially and forward with the humerus elevated to a horizontal position. Horizontal adduction ranges from approximately 0° to 130°. This movement is produced primarily by the pectoralis major and anterior fibers of the deltoid. This movement is seen in the follow-through motion executed during a swing of a baseball bat or forward stroke in various racquet sports (e.g., racquetball, table tennis, tennis). Range of motion is limited by contractile insufficiency; tension of the glenohumeral's extensor muscles (i.e., latissimus dorsi, teres major, posterior fibers of the deltoid, and teres minor); and contact of the humerus with the trunk.

Descriptions of Movements at the Scapulothoracic Joint

The scapulothoracic (ST) joint is capable of several types of motion: scapular elevation, scapular depression, abduction of the scapula, adduction of the scapula, and backward extension of the scapula. These movements are discussed in the following sections.

Scapular Elevation

Elevation of the scapula causes the scapula to move upward. This movement is brought about by the upper trapezius, levator scapulae, and serratus anterior muscles. The movement is restricted by contractile insufficiency, tension of the antagonistic muscles, tension of the costoclavicular ligament, and tension of the lower part of the capsule.

Scapular Depression

Depression of the scapula causes the scapula to move downward. Passive depression is brought about by gravity and the weight of the limb. Depression can be active by pressing downward (or resting on the parallel bars). Simple depression, against no resistance, is produced by the pectoralis minor, subclavius, pectoralis major, and latissimus dorsi. Range of motion is limited by contractile insufficiency, tension of the antagonistic muscles, tension of the interclavicular and sternoclavicular ligaments, and the articular disks.

Scapular Abduction (Protraction)

Scapular abduction or *protraction* is defined as the forward movement of the scapula, which is seen in all forward-pushing or thrusting movements. Protraction is produced by the serratus anterior, pectoralis minor, and levator spinae. Range of motion is restricted by contractile insufficiency, tension of the antagonistic muscles, tension of the anterior sternoclavicular ligament, and tension of the posterior lamina of the costoclavicular ligament.

Stretches to facilitate protraction are often frustrating. Usually, motion is directed at the rhomboids. However, shrugging the anterior portion of the shoulders is not very effective. Neither is swinging both arms through horizontal adduction. The most effective stretch for this muscle group requires a partner (see Exercise #41).

Scapular Adduction (Retraction)

Scapular adduction or *retraction* is defined as the backward movement of the scapula and is exemplified by pulling. Retraction of the scapula is produced by the trapezius and rhomboids and is assisted by the latissimus dorsi. Range of motion is limited by contractile insufficiency, tension of the antagonist muscles, tension of the posterior sternoclavicular ligament, and tension of the anterior lamina of the costoclavicular ligament.

Shoulder Complex Injuries, Stretching, and Testing

Injuries to the shoulder girdle and shoulder-arm complex are common. Preventive actions, as for other parts of the body, include proper warm-up, proper exercise technique, and building endurance, strength, and flexibility.

Flexibility should be developed in all directions and through the full range of movement. However, when stretching or testing this region, one must carefully separate shoulder girdle motion from motion in the vertebral column. For example, to achieve a true stretch or to test glenohumeral flexion, one must position the body in hip flexion and lumbar spine flexion. To accomplish this, lie with the lower back on the floor, both legs flexed, and the heels near the buttocks.

Then slowly raise the humerus. Once the lower back begins to arch, the maximum range of flexion has been determined. To facilitate additional stretching, a partner may push down on the ribs to keep the back flat on the floor as glenohumeral flexion continues.

The Elbow Joint and Forearm Region

The elbow is the middle joint of the upper extremity between the shoulder and wrist. The anatomy of the elbow and a description of its movements are discussed in the following sections.

Gross Anatomy of the Elbow

Three bones form the basic skeletal structure of the elbow: the humerus, radius, and ulna. The elbow is classified as a hinge joint. There are actually three articulations at the elbow joint. However, only two of these will be mentioned here. They are the humeroulnar-radial joint, involved solely in flexion and extension in a sliding fashion, and the radioulnar joint, involved solely in pronation and supination (Figure 19.8).

Description of Elbow Movements

There are four major movements that can take place at the elbow joint. These are flexion, extension, pronation, and supination. Following is an analysis of these movements.

Elbow Flexion

Flexion of the elbow is defined as decreasing the angle between the humerus and forearm. The primary flexors of the elbow are the biceps brachii, brachialis, and brachioradialis. The following muscles are considered accessory flexors: the pronator teres, wrist and finger flexors, and radial wrist extensors (Turek 1984). In addition to being a flexor, the short head of the biceps brachii is a major supinator of the forearm. Flexion of the elbow ranges approximately from 0° to 150° when the flexors are hardened by contraction and up to 160° when the muscles are relaxed (Kapandji 1982). Range of motion is limited by contractile insufficiency, contact of the muscles of the upper arm on the forearm, impact

Medial

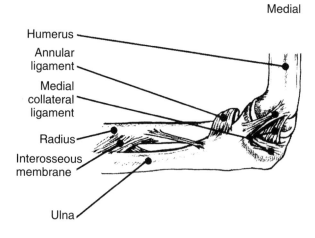

Humerus

Annular
ligament

Medial
collateral
ligament

Radius

Interosseous
membrane

Ulna

Lateral

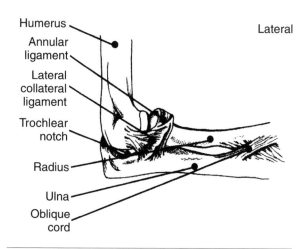

Humerus

Annular
ligament

Lateral
collateral
ligament

Trochlear
notch

Radius

Ulna

Oblique
cord

Fig. 19.8.   Medial and lateral views of the major
ligaments of the elbow.
Reprinted from Donnelly (1982).

of the head of the radius against the radial fossa
and the coronoid process against the coronoid
fossa, tension of the posterior capsular ligaments,
and passive tension in the triceps.

Stretching of the elbow extensors facilitates
motion in the flexion pattern. This can be easily
accomplished by leaning forward with the forearms resting on a table (see Exercise #55). In addition, light dumbbells can be used to increase
both strength and stretch through a slow eccentric contraction. Most often, stretches of the
elbow's extensors concentrate on the short head
of the triceps and ignore the long head. Stretching the long head of the triceps requires flexing
the elbow joint with the humerus in full flexion.
This can be accomplished by placing your elbow
raised about head height against a wall and pulling down on the wrist, using a towel (see Exercise #57), or having a partner apply the stretch.

Elbow Extension

Extension of the elbow is defined as returning
from the flexed position or beyond the zero starting position (the elbow extremely straight). The
primary extensors of the elbow are the triceps
brachii and anconeus. Range of motion from the
zero starting position varies from 0° to 10°. Extension beyond 10° is termed *hyperextension*
(Greene and Heckman 1994). Hyperextension is
one of the measures to determine the presence of
the hypermobility syndrome (Carter and
Wilkinson 1964). Hyperextension is usually more
common in women than in men. This is a result
of a shortened upper curve of the olecranon process in women's arms rather than of loose ligaments in the joint (Gelabert 1966). When this condition is present, stretching should not go beyond
elbow extension. Research by Cummings (1984,
170) investigated whether extension of the elbow
in normal female adults is limited primarily by
muscle or by the ligaments and capsule. It was
concluded that "elbow extension in the normal
adult woman is limited primarily by muscle."
Range of motion is limited by contractile insufficiency; impact of the olecranon process on the
olecranon fossa; tension of the anterior, radial,
and ulnar ligaments at the elbow; and tension of
the flexor muscles (e.g., biceps brachii).

Stretching the flexors of the forearm facilitates
extension of the elbow joint. The dilemma is
how to stretch the biceps when the elbow joint is
extended to 180°. One method is eccentrically
contracting the flexors. However, the most
effective technique is to stretch using either
a doorframe or pole (see Exercise #54). This
stretch is essential for all athletes, especially those
who use a throwing motion, because the throwing motion (especially of a curve ball) causes insult to the biceps tendon. During the throw of a
curve ball, the elbow joint passes from flexion to
extension while supinating the forearm. The biceps is the most important supinator of the forearm. Over the course of a season, the biceps receives thousands of insults. The importance of
stretching the biceps cannot be overemphasized.

Description of Forearm
Movements

There are two main movements of the forearm:
pronation and supination. Each of these is discussed in the following sections.

Forearm Pronation

Pronation may be defined as turning the hand and forearm from the neutral, or thumb-up, position to the palm-down position. Pronation ranges approximately from 0° to 80°. The movement is seen when top spin is applied in racquet sports such as racquetball, table tennis, and tennis. Pronation is produced by the pronator teres and the pronator quadratus. Range of motion is restricted by contractile insufficiency; tension of the dorsal radioulnar, ulnar collateral, and dorsal radiocarpal ligaments; tension of the lowest fibers of the interosseous membrane; and the radius crossing and impacting against the ulna.

Forearm Supination

Supination is defined as the outward rotation of the forearm from the neutral palm down to the palm-up position. Supination ranges approximately from 0° to 90°. The primary supinators of the forearm are the biceps brachii, supinator, and brachioradialis. Range of motion is limited by contractile insufficiency, tension of the volar radioulnar ligament and ulnar collateral ligament of the wrist, tension of the oblique cord and lowest fibers of the interosseous membrane, and tension of the pronator muscles.

Injuries of the Elbow and Forearm

Injuries to the musculotendinous and ligament complex of the elbow have many causes. Strains in particular are commonly associated with activities that demand forceful and repetitive contractions of the forearm muscles. Such injuries are often experienced by tennis, racquetball, and baseball players. Inflammation of the lateral or medial epicondyle is called *epicondylitis*, or *tennis elbow*. The most effective stretching exercise to prevent lateral epicondylitis is to stretch the supinators of the elbow and forearm by grasping a broomstick, golf club, or tennis racquet in a dorsal grip (the back of the hand faces down and the thumb grasps under the handle; see Exercise #59). This stretch can be intensified by hanging from a chin-up bar in a dorsal grip.

Common sense indicates that a preventive approach is the most practical and prudent way to deal with elbow and forearm injuries. This includes proper warm-up, avoidance of sudden, excessive overloading or overuse, optimal technique, and exercises to develop flexibility, strength, and endurance.

The Radiocarpal Joint

The *radiocarpal joint*, or wrist, is commonly classified as an ellipsoid joint. It is formed by the articulation of the distal end of the radius and three of eight carpal bones in the hand. Ligaments bind the carpals closely and firmly together in two rows of four each. The first or proximal row comprises the scaphoid, lunate, triquetrum, and pisiform bones. Only the last carpal does not participate in the formation of the radiocarpal joint. The

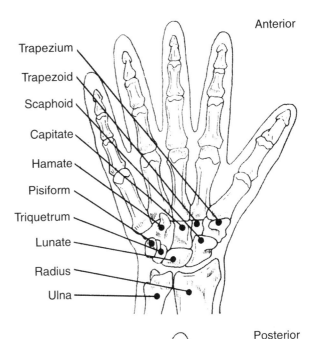

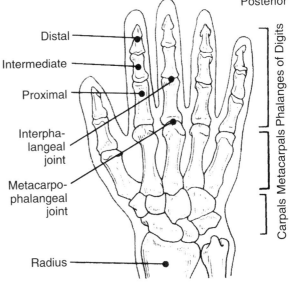

Fig. 19.9.   Bones of the wrist and hand. Anterior and posterior views of the right hand.
Reprinted from Donnelly (1982).

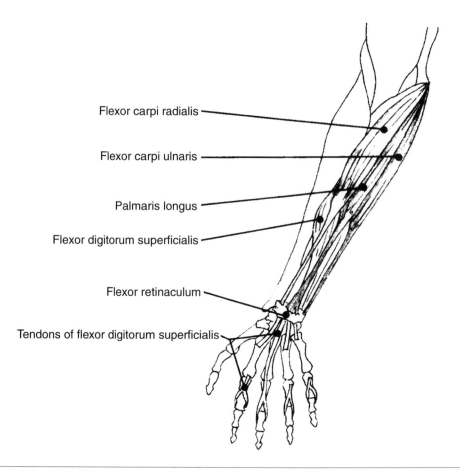

Flexor carpi radialis

Flexor carpi ulnaris

Palmaris longus

Flexor digitorum superficialis

Flexor retinaculum

Tendons of flexor digitorum superficialis

Fig. 19.10.　An anterior view of the flexors of the wrist.
Reprinted from Donnelly (1982).

second, or distal, row is made up of the trapezium, trapezoid, capitate, and hamate bones (Figure 19.9).

Stability of the Radiocarpal Joint

The wrist is a very stable joint. It's stabilized predominantly by the ligaments of the joint and the numerous muscle tendons that pass over it (see Figures 19.10 and 19.11). However, a portion of this stability is also the result of the bony arrangement. The major ligaments of the wrist are the palmar radiocarpal, palmar ulnocarpal, dorsal radiocarpal, radial collateral, and ulnar collateral.

Description of Radiocarpal Movements

The wrist joint allows several active movements. These include flexion, extension, abduction, adduction, and circumduction. All but the latter will be examined in the following sections.

Radiocarpal Flexion

Flexion of the wrist involves drawing the palm toward the forearm and ranges approximately from 0° to 90°. Flexion is greatest when the hand is in the neutral position, neither abducted nor adducted. The chief flexors of the wrist are the flexor carpi radialis, flexor carpi ulnaris, and palmaris longus.

Flexion is limited by contractile insufficiency, tension of the wrist extensor muscles (i.e., extensor carpi radialis longus, extensor carpi radialis brevis, and extensor carpi ulnaris), and tension of the dorsal radiocarpal ligament. Flexion is minimal when the wrist is in pronation (Kapandji 1982). Movement is also diminished when the fingers are flexed, owing to the increased tension of the extensor muscles. Flexion can be facilitated by stretching the wrist extensors (see Exercise #58).

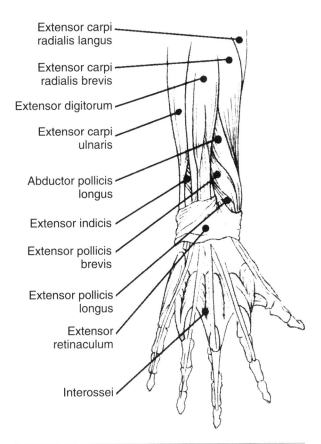

Extensor carpi radialis langus

Extensor carpi radialis brevis

Extensor digitorum

Extensor carpi ulnaris

Abductor pollicis longus

Extensor indicis

Extensor pollicis brevis

Extensor pollicis longus

Extensor retinaculum

Interossei

Fig. 19.11. A posterior view of the extensors of the wrist.
Reprinted from Donnelly (1982).

Radiocarpal Extension

Extension of the wrist occurs when the palm is moved away from the forearm. This ranges from approximately 0° to 85°. Extension is greatest when the hand is in the neutral position. The main extensors of the wrist are the extensor carpi radialis longus, extensor carpi radialis brevis, and extensor carpi ulnaris. Range of motion is restricted by contractile insufficiency, tension of the wrist flexor muscles (i.e., flexor carpi radialis, flexor carpi ulnaris, and palmaris longus), and tension of the palmar radiocarpal ligament. Extension is minimal during pronation (Kapandji 1982). Wrist extension is enhanced by stretching the wrist flexors. This can be achieved by a number of stretches (see Exercise #60).

Wrist Abduction or Radial Deviation

Radial deviation of the wrist is defined as flexion of the hand toward the side of the forearm where the radius bone resides (the side of the thumb). In radial deviation, most movement occurs at the midcarpal joint. It ranges from approximately 0° to 20°. Radial deviation is less than ulnar deviation because of the buttressing effect of the radial styloid process as the carpus becomes mechanically blocked (Greene and Heckman 1994; Volz, Lieb, and Benjamin 1980). In general, the range of radial deviation is minimal when the wrist is fully flexed or extended because of the tension developed in the carpal ligaments (Kapandji 1982). Radial deviation is produced by the flexor carpi radialis, in conjunction with the extensor carpi radialis longus, extensor carpi radialis brevis, abductor carpi radialis longus, and extensor pollicis brevis. Range of motion is limited by contractile insufficiency, tension of the antagonistic muscles, and, when at extreme limits, the radial and ulnar collateral radiocarpal ligaments.

Wrist Adduction or Ulnar Deviation

Ulnar deviation of the wrist is defined as flexion of the hand toward the side of the forearm where the ulna bone resides (the side of the little finger). Ulnar deviation has a range two to three times larger than that of radial deviation. It ranges from approximately 0° to 30°. The greater range of ulnar deviation may be associated with the shortness of the styloid process of the ulna (P.L. Williams et al. 1989). Ulnar deviation is produced by the flexor carpi ulnaris in conjunction with the extensor carpi ulnaris. Range of motion is restricted by contractile insufficiency, tension of the antagonistic muscles, and impingement of the wrist.

Summary

The upper extremity consists of the shoulder girdle, shoulder joint, arm, elbow joint, forearm, wrist joint, and hand. Many types of movements take place in the upper extremity and through various ranges of motion. Often these movements involve simultaneous actions at other adjacent joints. Without the assistance of the appropriate joints and muscles, efficient movement would be seriously restricted. Causes of reduced efficiency of the upper extremity, like those of other parts of the body, include aging, lack of use, disease, and trauma. However, optimal upper extremity efficiency can be maintained or enhanced through purposeful warm-up, stretching, strengthening, and endurance exercises.

Chapter 20

Functional Aspects of Stretching and Flexibility

Numerous factors go into creating optimal performance. Some of these factors are coordination, endurance, power, strength, and mental toughness. In addition to these attributes, flexibility is generally recognized as a crucial factor in skilled movement (Garhammer 1989a). Consequently, flexibility can also play a significant role in determining the final outcome of various performances or competitive situations. Practical, everyday experience substantiates that flexibility enhances and optimizes the learning, practice, and performance of skilled movement. Therefore, some skills may be enhanced more effectively by purposefully increasing or decreasing the range of motion around certain joints until what appears to be optimal flexibility is reached (Hebbelinck 1988; Sigerseth 1971).

Aesthetic Aspect of Skills

From an aesthetic point of view, flexibility is definitely a requirement for skilled movement. But the effects of increased flexibility on sports performance may range from obvious to subtle. For instance, there is an obvious need for excellent flexibility in diving, figure skating, and gymnastics, to mention only a few sports. These disciplines have an aesthetic component, and optimal flexibility obviously enhances performance since it is part of the scoring system (Stone and Kroll 1986). It is flexibility that allows the individual to create an appearance of ease, smoothness of movement, graceful coordination, self-control, and total freedom. Flexibility also helps the individual to perform more skillfully and with greater self-assurance, elegance, and amplitude. This concept of amplitude is further elaborated by George (1980, 7–9):

> Essentially, amplitude refers to the "range" through which a body moves and can be subdivided into two basic types. The first type, "external amplitude," is used to describe the range through which the *total* body unit moves relative to the ground and/or apparatus. . . . However, the "hidden component" that allows the gymnast to take full advantage of technique is her own internal power. . . .
>
> The second type of amplitude, "internal amplitude," focuses upon range of motion *within* the joints of the body. More specifically, it refers to the range through which one or more of the individual body segments move relative to each other. . . . Just as power is the hidden component underlying external amplitude, joint range of motion or *flexibility* is the key factor for obtaining maximum internal amplitude.

Thus, without a supple body, highly skilled performance would certainly be impossible in many disciplines. The difference between good skill and excellent skill is simply a matter of degree. Flexibility can provide the critical difference between average and outstanding performance.

Biomechanical Aspect of Skills

Another factor in skilled movement is the importance of flexibility as a biomechanical parameter.

Biomechanics is the study of the application of mechanical laws to living structures. It examines the forces that act on a body and the effects of these forces. For example, in tennis an increased range of motion allows one to apply forces over greater distances and longer periods of time. Similarly, in gymnastics an increase in distance through which force can be applied improves the potential for a more vigorous and effective kipping action in a forward headkip (George 1980). This greater range can increase velocities, energies, and momenta involved in physical performance (Ciullo and Zarins 1983). There are many skills that depend on a close interaction between internal and external amplitude (George 1980).

Furthermore, flexibility may be needed in lengthening contractions that immediately precede active muscle contraction. An increased range of motion can permit a greater stretch on the involved muscles. As a result, those muscles can produce even greater forces, because a prestretched muscle can exert more force than a nonstretched muscle. Prestretched muscles function with greater efficiency because elastic energy is stored in the muscle tissue during stretching and is recovered during the subsequent shortening (Asmussen and Bonde-Petersen 1974; Boscoe, Tarkka, and Komi 1982; Cavagna, Dusman, and Margaria 1968; Cavagna, Saibene, and Margaria 1965; Ciullo and Zarins 1983; Grieve 1970; Komi and Boscoe 1978). Ciullo and Zarins compare this phenomenon to cocking an air rifle. They point out, however, that A.V. Hill (1961) found that when relaxation of the muscle is allowed to take place between the stretching and shortening phases, the preloaded condition is not taken advantage of and the stored elastic energy is dissipated as heat. Thus, timing is an all-important component of this use of flexibility.

Conversely, just as it might be important in some sports to have a specific degree of flexibility, it might also be equally important in other sports to have a certain degree of stiffness in order to produce maximal performance. To illustrate this point, Öberg (1993) cites an example in which a group of handball players were tested for strength in the thigh muscles, jump performance, and flexibility before and after a set of stretching exercises. The results showed decreased torque in eccentric contractions and in jump performance. Hence, there are activities that can be negatively influenced by stretching. The significant point here is that stretching (if needed)

must be tailored to the needs of the performance and performer. Next, the role of flexibility and stretching in several sports and specific activities will be analyzed.

Jogging, Running, and Sprinting

The general objective in competitive and recreational jogging, running, or sprinting is simply to cover a given distance in the least possible time. This speed is a product of two interdependent factors: *length* and *frequency* of stride. If a runner is to improve his or her speed, he or she must bring about an increase in one or both of these variables without causing the other to be reduced by a comparable (or, worse yet, a more than comparable) amount (Hay 1985). Maximum running efficiency exists only when length and frequency of stride are in optimal proportions. In turn, these factors depend on the weight, build, strength, coordination, and flexibility of the runner (Dyson 1977). Our concern is how optimal flexibility can enhance running times.

Increasing the Length of Stride

One explanation of how flexibility reduces running times is based on the notion that an increase in the body's mobility and joint range will result in a greater length of stride, leading to better performance (Burke and Humphreys 1982). The length of stride is most conveniently measured from the front of the toe print to the front of the succeeding toe print (Slocum and James 1968). One manufacturer of a stretching machine has referred to this greater length of stride as the "geometry of winning." Following is an example from their brochure analyzing a 100-yard dash (TRECO n.d.):

> If a runner has a 96 inch stride it would mean 37.5 strides would be required to run the dash (discounting the shorter starting strides). If this were done in 10 seconds then each stride would have averaged .266 seconds. With no more than a 2 inch increase the 96 inch stride becomes 98 inches. This means that 36.74 strides are now needed to run the 100 yards. If each stride still takes .266 seconds then the 10 second 100 yard dash time will drop to 9.8 seconds. A person running a 9.8 second 100 yard dash will finish nearly 6 feet in front of a 10.0 second runner.

Therefore, on a purely biomechanical level, an increased flexibility in the lower limbs should result in an increased stride length. With all other factors remaining constant, running time should be lowered.

However, stride length is thought to depend on the speed, angle, and height of projection of a runner's center of gravity (Steban and Bell 1978); acceleration of the thigh angle, that is, the angle between the thighs at the moment of first surface contact (Kunz and Kaufmann 1980); hip joint mobility and lower extremity flexibility (Bush 1978); and the power of the runner's legs (Bush 1978; Dyson 1977; Ecker 1971; Robison et al. 1974). The more powerful the leg drive, the greater the thrust against the ground with each step and the longer the stride. In turn, the increase in stride length that results from this forward projection of the body is believed to be the best method for achieving an increase in stride length, since it does not interfere with the mechanical efficiency of the runner's motion. This means that at each

footstrike, the support leg is underneath the runner's center of gravity (Steban and Bell 1978). Attempting to increase stride length by "stretching out" results in overstriding (the support leg being forward of the center of gravity at footstrike). This causes braking on each step, a decrease in stride frequency, and a slower time (Ecker 1971; Robison et al. 1974).

Because the beneficial increase in stride length just described is a result of foot-ground interaction, the importance of stride frequency becomes apparent: Too slow a cadence causes a loss in efficiency of movement, while too great a stride length will decrease the number of strides possible in a given distance, thus reducing momentum.

Another factor that can influence the stride length is the degree of *crossover*, which in turn may be related to flexibility. Crossover is a measure of how far a runner's legs cross over the midline of the body while running (Figure 20.1). This phenomenon is also referred to as *asymmetri-*

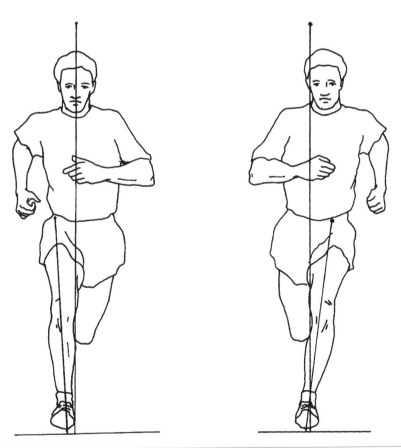

Fig. 20.1.   Excessive upper body torque, which pulls the legs across the midline of the body, is a frequent cause of running injury.
Reprinted from Prichard (1984).

cal leg action. It has been postulated by Prichard (cited by Cailliet 1991; Neff 1987) that these crossover inches can add a substantial extra distance to be run in long-distance races. For example, a typical marathoner takes about 1,000 strides per mile (620 strides/km) or 26,000 strides per race. If the degree of crossover is reduced by 2 inches (5 cm) per stride, the savings are an incredible 4,333 feet (1,320 m)!

What is responsible for runner crossover? One possibility could just be poor technique. However, Prichard (cited by Brant 1987) is of the opinion that crossover can result from any one or combination of three factors: leg length differences, inflexibility of the adductor muscles on the insides of the legs, and *upper body torque* (i.e., tightness in the upper torso). In the opinion of Prichard, upper body torque is most often the result of inflexibility of the shoulders, which in turn results from tightness in the chest muscles. For example, as a runner's right arm goes back, it pulls the left arm across the body. Consequently, the right leg must cross over to the left in a compensating movement (see Figure 20.1). This crossover is referred to as *asymmetrical arm action* (Hinrichs 1990, 1992). Prichard contends that enhancing the flexibility and reducing the stiffness of the upper torso will decrease upper body torque

and increase performance. Furthermore, it is also suggested that another potential detriment of excessive arm movement across the trunk is potential injury to the knees and lower limbs (Brant 1987; Cailliet 1991; Prichard 1984; Volkov and Milner 1990). Further research is needed before any conclusions can be drawn about the actual causes of the asymmetries and whether the runner's performance is helped or hurt by them (Hinrichs 1990, 1992).

Increasing the Range of Force Application

A second means by which flexibility can reduce running times is by increasing the runner's velocity. This is accomplished by increasing the distance or range over which a muscle force is applied. Tolsma (1985) has identified four muscle groups whose enhanced flexibility will increase the range over which a force can be applied. These are the posterior and anterior muscles of the lower leg (ankle plantar flexors and dorsiflexors, respectively), the anterior thigh muscles (quadriceps), and the posterior buttock muscles (gluteals). Following is an analysis based on the work of McFarlane (1987), Slocum and James (1968), and Tolsma (1985).

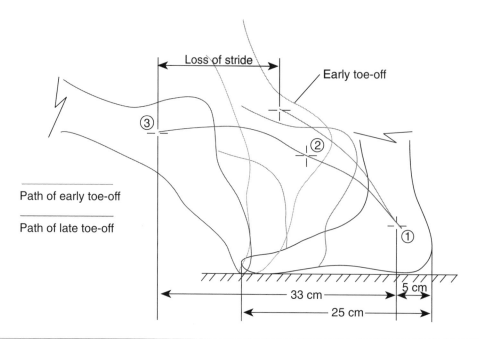

Fig. 20.2. Effect of early and late takeoff on stride length. Early takeoff caused by decreased ankle flexibility results in a shorter stride and more vertical displacement of the center of mass, creating a less efficient running style than later takeoff, which enhances stride length and lessens vertical displacement.
Reprinted from Martin and Coe (1991).

The Ankle Plantar Flexors

The support phase of running is divided into three distinct periods. The *footstrike* period begins when the foot first contacts the ground and continues through the brief moment during which the foot becomes firmly planted. The *midsupport* period starts once the foot is fixed and continues until the heel starts to rise from the ground. Finally, the *takeoff* period commences when the heel starts to rise and continues until the toes leave the running surface. During the midsupport phase, the knee is flexed 30° to 40° as the heel remains on the ground. This position places the posterior muscles of the lower leg in an elongated position. However, if the runner has very short calf muscles, the heel will lift off the ground prematurely. Consequently, the force applied to the ground by contraction of the calf muscles will be through a shorter range of motion (Figure 20.2). Thus, the result is a decrease of force. Accordingly, it is recommended in a warm-up stretching program that the calf be stretched with the knee somewhat bent to simulate the leg position in running during which these muscles are stretched.

The Ankle Dorsiflexors

During the later stages of the takeoff period, the propulsive action of the calf is very important, and the farther the foot can be plantar flexed, the longer this driving force can be sustained. Hence the importance of stretching the anterior portions of the lower leg, ankle, and foot. The difference between the ranges of force application of a flexible and inflexible ankle is shown in Figure 20.2.

The Quadriceps

Flexibility in the quadriceps can also significantly affect running efficiency. During the takeoff period, the hip joint goes through extension. Consequently, the hip flexors (e.g., rectus femoris, iliacus, and psoas muscles) are put on stretch. With enhanced flexibility, the hip flexors can allow a longer application of force to the ground. Once again, the result is the facilitation of force.

The Gluteals

The gluteal muscles of the buttocks can also potentially maximize running efficiency. Their function is extension of the hip joint. During the *forward swing* period of running, the thigh begins to move forward and stops when the hip reaches maximum flexion. It is at this point (i.e., when the knee is brought toward the chest) that these muscles are put on stretch. Theoretically, the higher the knees can be efficiently raised, the greater the range through which a runner can subsequently apply the forces of hip extension. (It should be noted that raising the knee too high will result in reduced efficiency and slower running time.)

Reduced Muscular Resistance

Another advantage of stretching and developing flexibility is reduction of muscular and passive forces that resist motion (de Vries 1963; Tolsma 1985). Hubley-Kozey and Stanish (1990) describe this phenomenon as running without excessive soft tissue resistance, whereas McFarlane (1987) refers to this as running with lower internal muscle resistance. It is known that when a muscle is stretched passively, it opposes stretch by a force that increases slowly at first and more rapidly with increased elongation. The longer or more flexible the muscle, the later in the movement this resistance will be encountered (Tolsma 1985). As a consequence, the resultant force in the muscle being opposed (agonist) will be higher without any additional expenditure of energy and will promote greater local endurance (Kulakov 1989; Tolsma 1985). Research has proven that passive tension can be decreased in subjects irrespective of their flexibility through stretching (Toft et al. 1989).

How Much Flexibility Is Necessary for Running?

Since some degree of flexibility is necessary for optimal running efficiency, we must ask two basic questions. First, how much flexibility is actually required for optimal running? Second, is there any benefit in stretching soft tissues to an extreme range of motion? Specifically, do runners need enough flexibility to perform splits? It is common to witness numerous runners attempting almost contortionistic stretches before a big race. This behavior has been criticized by several leading experts (Dominguez, cited by Shyne 1982; Fixx 1983; Frederick 1982; M.D. Wolf 1983).

Unfortunately, there is little information available for assessing the average ranges of motion required in different athletic activities (Hubley-Kozey and Stanish 1990). Nonetheless, a careful biomechanical analysis of various angles that the legs pass through while running may help to establish a minimal requirement for certain joints. It is generally recognized that distance runners require a much smaller range of motion than do dancers or gymnasts. In a normal running stride, when the hip is flexed, the knee is also flexed. Hence, a long hamstring position is never reached. Consequently, a runner does not need extreme flexibility in the hamstrings (Tolsma 1985). What a runner needs is a range of motion that will permit running without excessive soft tissue resistance (de Vries 1963; Hubley-Kozey and Stanish 1990). Once again, the question of the specific amount flexibility necessary is raised. Research by Prichard (cited by Brant 1987) suggests that recreational runners should have a stride angle of at least 90° and competitive runners at least 100°. The *stride angle* is the composite of two angles: the angle of flexion of the front leg and the angle of extension of the back leg. Additional research is still needed in this area to substantiate the foregoing estimates (Figure 20.3).

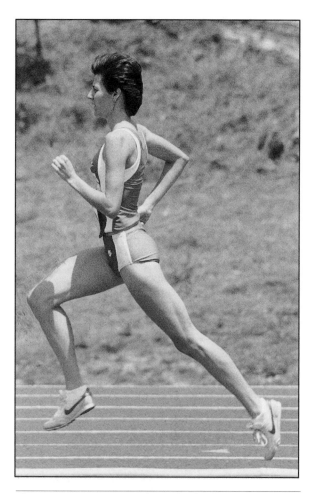

Fig. 20.3. A runner's stride angle should equal 90°—100° would be even better.
Reprinted from Martin and Coe (1991).

Swimming

As with running, the general objective in competitive and recreational swimming is to cover a given distance in the least possible time. Average swimming speed is a product of two factors: the average stroke length and the average stroke frequency (Hay 1985). In turn, stroke length is governed by two forces exerted on the swimmer. The first is the *propulsive force*, which drives the swimmer through the water and is produced by the movements he or she makes. The second is the *resistive force*, which the water exerts on the swimmer in opposition to that motion (Hay 1985). In the sections that follow, we will analyze how flexibility in five specific areas of the body influences swimming.

Increasing the Range of Force Application

As in running, one method by which flexibility can reduce swimming times is by increasing the swimmer's velocity. This improvement is accomplished by increasing the distance or range through which the force is applied. Lewin (1979) has identified five major parts of the body that deserve special attention in developing flexibility to enhance swimming. These areas are the ankles, hips, spinal column, shoulders, and knees. Following is an analysis of these regions of the body.

The Ankles

When swimming the front crawl, back crawl, and butterfly, it is vital to have good plantar flexion of the ankles. The best swimmers use an action in which the legs alternate in an up-and-down (flexion and extension) motion known as the flutter kick (Hay 1985). In the downbeat of the flutter kick, propulsion is produced by the top of the extended foot as hip flexion moves the leg downward. During the upbeat, the sole of the foot applies thrust force as the leg moves from a flexed to an extended position. Cureton (1930), in one of the earliest and most comprehensive studies of the flutter kick, concluded that the up-kick was more effective than the down-kick for propulsion.

Since the application of backward force depends on foot position, flexible ankles are necessary for success in the flutter kick (Broer 1966; Bunn 1972; Counsilman 1968, 1977; Hull 1990–1991; Lewin 1979). In this regard, Robertson

(1960) found significant relationships between ankle flexibility and propulsive force. Thus, in order to improve this type of flexibility, the anterior muscles of the lower leg (i.e., dorsiflexors of the ankles and toes) must be stretched. Research has substantiated the hypothesis that swimmers have more flexibility than nonswimmers in the ankle (Bloomfield and Blanksby 1971; Oppliger et al. 1986).

The importance of dorsiflexing the feet toward the shins is also significant in swimming. This movement is particularly relevant in the breaststroke (Bunn 1972; Counsilman 1968; Hay 1985; Lewin 1979; Rodeo 1984). The most efficient leg action in the breaststroke is called the *whip kick* (Hay 1985). Two explanations have been proposed as to why dorsiflexion enhances the breaststroke. First, during the catch phase the knees are flexed more than 90° with the feet above the buttocks, close to each other, and the ankles everted. At this point the soles of the feet face backward and upward, and the feet are turned so that the toes point laterally (Rodeo 1984). It is when the feet start to spread that ankle dorsiflexion begins. This position presents a large surface to "catch" and push the water backward through the downsweep of the kick (Counsilman 1968; Gaughran 1972; Rodeo 1984). Thus, to the extent that the swimmer cannot do this and the feet remain pointed backward during the power phase, the kick will be correspondingly less effective (Gaughran 1972). A second potential advantage of dorsiflexion has been described by Lewin (1979). He contends that the greater the amplitude of flexion of the foot, the faster the athlete can get a grip on the water in the transition phase between the recovery phase (pulling up the legs) and the power phase (extending the legs). However, the results of an investigation by Nimz et al. (1988) indicate that no outstanding flexibility is necessary for swimming the whip kick.

The Hip Joint

The four Olympic competitive strokes utilize some degree of hip flexion and extension, with the breaststroke incorporating the most motion. Abduction and adduction are another pair of hip movements associated with the breaststroke. In the opinion of Lewin (1979), despite the fact that the full movement amplitude is not used once the swimmer develops an optimal swimming technique, high movement amplitudes in executing straddle movements (abduction) are important for the breaststroker.

The Spinal Column

Often, the literature that discusses the subject of flexibility as related to swimming concentrates exclusively on the ankle and shoulder joints. Flexibility in the vertebral column is also essential for optimal performance. One example is the importance of a flexible back for optimal performance of the breaststroke. As explained by Engesvik (1993), swimmers with very flexible backs look rather like ducks because their shoulders are high above the surface and their hands may recover over the surface, appearing to "hump" over the water. This technique causes less resistance than underwater recovery and improves speed. Lewin (1979, 121) also addresses the importance of spinal flexibility:

> The significance of flexibility of the spinal column is often underestimated in developing an optimum swimming technique. And yet it is an important factor, for it is a necessary condition for adapting the trunk to the changing conditions during a movement cycle in such a manner as to minimize the body's drag in the water and thereby raising the efficiency of the swimming movements. The flexibility (suppleness) of the spinal column in all planes should be developed and improved; flexibility of the spinal column in the sagittal plane is particularly important for the breast and dolphin swimmer, while for the crawl swimmer and backstroker flexibility in the frontal plane is important. It is also essential for being able to twist the body (turning the shoulder line and the hip line in opposite directions around the central body axis). Special attention should be paid to improving the flexibility of the cervical section of the spinal column, because the greater the flexibility of this part of the spinal column, the less detrimental the influences of the movement of the head during breathing on the posture and movement of the trunk and the extremities.

The Shoulder Joint

Another area in which good flexibility is critical for all swimming strokes is the shoulder joint (Counsilman 1968). In the front crawl, limited shoulder flexibility will result in the swimmer recovering the arm with a low elbow. This technique is both incorrect and inefficient (Bloomfield et al. 1985; Counsilman 1968; Hay 1985; Lewin 1979). Furthermore, swimmers with a higher arm recovery seem to have fewer shoulder problems (Greipp 1986). As described by Counsilman (1968), in order to recover the arms and clear them over the water rather than dragging them in the water, the inflexible swimmer must roll the body and make a flatter and wider sweep of the arms during the recovery than a more flexible swimmer. In turn, this poor technique results in a greater reaction or lateral thrust of the legs and initiates an unwanted rotation about the anteroposterior axis that tends to move the body out of alignment in a lateral direction (Hay 1985). Consequently, swimmers with tight shoulders must frequently adopt a two-beat crossover kick to keep the legs in alignment (Counsilman 1968).

The butterfly is another stroke that requires flexibility in the shoulders (Counsilman 1968; Johnson, Sim, and Scott 1987; Rodeo 1985a, 1985b). As the arms leave the water, the palms of the hands face almost directly upward (Counsilman 1968). During this phase the arms are backward in extension and internal rotation. This position decreases the mobility of the upper arms in the shoulder joint (Counsilman 1968). Hence, as soon as the hands leave the water, the swimmer must rotate the arms outward and swing them forward and around. The hands then should enter the water at a point only slightly outside the shoulder line. If, however, the swimmer lacks adequate shoulder flexibility, the shoulder rotation and hand placement in the water will be inefficient. According to Souza (1994, 114), "it is essential that at hand entry the hand enter the water slightly outside of shoulder width to maintain neutral shoulder position allowing movement in mainly the coronal plane."

Shoulder flexibility is also vital in performance of the backstroke crawl. In this stroke, it is most efficient for the swimmer's arm, with the elbow straight, to enter the water in line with and directly over the shoulder (Counsilman 1968) or above and slightly to the side of the shoulder at almost full reach (Hay 1985). Thus, the recovery arm should move in an essentially straight line in the vertical plane (Counsilman 1968, 1977). However, the tighter the shoulder, the farther out of line the arm will enter the water and the less efficient will be the stroke. Deviation sideward from this plane due to limited shoulder flexibility will result in a sideward displacement of the hips and legs. Consequently, the resistance or drag that the swimmer creates will increase (Counsilman 1977).

The Knees

The significance of flexibility of the knees is probably the most underestimated in developing swimming technique. However, the flexibility of the knee joints in connection with the flexibility of the hip joints is particularly significant in the breaststroke. According to Lewin (1979, 120), "the ability to move one's lower legs as far out sideways as possible (abduction) is essential, because this determines the arc of the thrust planes during the power phase of the leg movement."

Reduced Muscular Resistance

As in running, stretching and developing flexibility are thought to reduce the muscular and passive forces that resist motion in swimming. The reader is referred back to the earlier section pertaining to reduced muscular resistance.

How Much Flexibility Is Needed for Swimming?

It should be pointed out that more often than not, swimmers are too flexible rather than insufficiently flexible (Falkel 1988). Marino (1984) cites Douglas (1980), who states that swimming coaches and swimmers appear to be obsessed with the destruction of the anterior capsule of the shoulder joint by often performing damaging passive shoulder stretching exercises. Hence, Marino (1984) addresses the need for coaches and swimmers to realize the distinction between *muscle flexibility* and *capsular laxity*. "Perverse stretching maneuvers such as horizontal abduction of the humerus to the point where the elbows cross behind the back do not promote muscular flexibility, and they do not maintain adequate range of motion" (p. 223). Furthermore, this may actually lead to an increased likelihood of anterior dislocation (Dominguez 1980). Hence, it is not only vital to know how much flexibility is needed for the swimmer, but also which stretches are good or bad.

How much flexibility does a swimmer need? A conservative response is that a swimmer needs range of motion that will permit swimming without excessive soft tissue resistance and that will facilitate optimal technique. Once again, to cite Hubley-Kozey and Stanish (1990, 22), it must be recognized that "there is little information available for assessing the average ranges of motion required by different athletic activities." Therefore, "physicians and therapists (and coaches) must rely on their experience and knowledge of a particular sport and the available literature when suggesting how much an athlete should stretch."

Throwing

One skill that derives its beginning in early childhood is throwing (Corbin 1980). According to Bunn (1972), the skill of throwing is second only to running as the most common element in sport. Lindner (1971) has suggested that throwing motions in various disciplines share a common trait of lateral deviation of the upper part of the body of the throwing arm, which must be considered a natural movement. Several years later, a study by Atwater (1979) corroborated the hypothesis that the throwing angle between the arm and the trunk in projecting a football, javelin, tennis racquet, or baseball are essentially the same. Furthermore, she reported similarity in the nearly completed extension of the forearm at the elbow joint at release or impact as evidence of a commonality of joint and segment actions in sport skills employing the overarm pattern (Figure 20.4). However, M.B. Anderson (1979) has pointed out that slight to moderate spatial-temporal differences between various sport skills require adjustments within the general overarm pattern.

Flexibility is a vital factor in throwing performance. An increase in range of motion permits one to exert muscle forces over greater distances and longer periods of time. Consequently, this ability can increase velocities, energies, and momenta associated with physical performance (Ciullo and Zarins 1983; Northrip, Logan, and McKinney 1983). In short, an increased range of motion can permit a greater prestretch on the involved muscles and thus allow them to produce even greater forces.

Upper Extremity Flexibility Needs

Analysis of athletes who use repetitive throwing movement patterns shows that they are potentially subject to changes in shoulder strength, range of motion, and physical deformation, depending on the quantity and quality of overload. Cook et al. (1987) evaluated dominant and nondominant shoulder ranges of motion in 15 college baseball pitchers. Their research found that the throwing shoulder possessed increased range of external rotation with concomitantly decreased ranges of internal motion. Sandstead (1968) found that throwing velocity was significantly related ($r = .77$) to the range of external shoulder rotation in college varsity baseball players. Similarly, Cohen et al. (1994) demonstrated that numerous flexibility measures—including dominant wrist flexion, dominant shoulder forward flexion, and dominant shoulder internal rotation at $0°$ of abduction—are related to tennis serve velocity. Increased range of shoulder rotation has been shown to be produced merely by warm-up activities that involve the actions of external rotation, as demonstrated by a young athlete photographed by Tullos and King (1973).

Surveying the research, Atwater (1979, 73) insightfully points out:

> Since several anterior shoulder injuries seem to be associated with the position of *maximum* shoulder lateral rotation and since there is a strong positive relationship between throwing velocity and range of shoulder lateral rotation, those pitchers who rely on the delivery of fastballs or those youngsters who practice for hours to increase the speed or distance of their throw, may be most susceptible to anterior shoulder injuries.

An increase in shoulder external rotation and a decrease in shoulder internal rotation, particularly on the dominant side, has also been reported in tennis players (Chandler et al. 1990; Chinn, Priest, and Kent 1974). This adaptation has been explained as a lengthening of the posterior shoulder musculature and capsular structures by the tennis serve or overhead smash (Zarins, Andrews, and Carson 1985). This adaptation occurs because the shoulder is stretched to the extremes of external rotation and abduction during the backswing phase of a serve (Chinn, Priest, and Kent 1974; Nirschl 1973). This critical part of the serve is termed the back-scratch position (Nirschl 1973) in reference to its appearance. It is theorized that the increased range of external glenohumeral rotation allows the muscles producing the arm acceleration to internally rotate the humerus through a wider range for a longer period of time, thereby allowing these muscles to impart added momentum to the ball (Michaud 1990).

Over years of extensive training and competition, repeated insults and microtrauma may produce fibrotic changes in the capsule and ligaments of the posterior shoulder, where the traction stresses of the follow-through are concen-

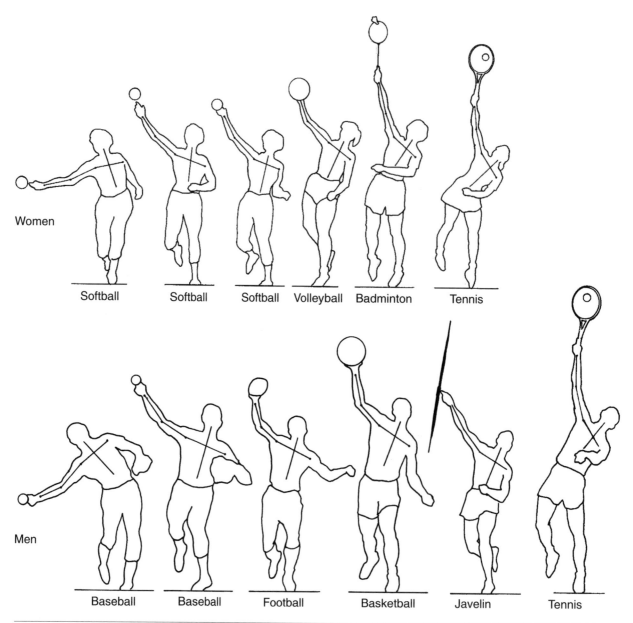

Fig. 20.4. Commonality of overhand throwing patterns. Release position in a variety of unilateral throwing and striking skills is shown for women (top row) and for men (bottom row) with the most extreme overarm skills at the right and the side- or underarm skills at the left. Notice that the spatial orientation of the arm at release in all skills (whether near vertical or horizontal) is determined primarily by lateral trunk flexion toward or away from the throwing arm rather than by shoulder joint action.
Reprinted from Atwater (1967).

trated. Consequently, these fibrotic changes may serve to maintain the overall stability of the joint structure by decreasing capsular distensibility in the posterior portions. Concomitantly, this fibrosis reduces full range of internal rotation reported in a survey of tennis players (Chandler et al. 1990; Chinn, Priest, and Kent 1974).

However, it should be noted that research by Aberdeem and Joensen (1986) discovered a significant difference in range of rotation values at the shoulder joint when comparisons between right and left sides were made of 73 normal right-handed subjects, and this difference was related to handedness. Their findings were that in right-handed people the range of right external rotation will normally be greater than the range of left external rotation and the range of left internal rotation will normally be greater than right internal rotation.

Adaptation as a result of prolonged unilateral training can cause permanent asymmetrical physiological changes in the upper extremity

(Magnusson, Gleim, and Nicholas 1994; Renstrom and Roux 1988). The most common changes in the shoulder are *hypertrophy* (increased muscle mass and humeral bone) and *depression* (low carrying angle of the scapula). Because this physical phenomenon of scapular depression is common among tennis players, it has been dubbed *tennis shoulder*. According to Priest (1989), two possible mechanisms are thought to cause tennis shoulder. First, the muscles that elevate the shoulder, the joint capsule, ligaments, and tendons are recurrently stretched during the serve and overhand smash. When these structures are repeatedly elongated beyond their usual lengths, increased laxity develops in the overloaded shoulder, eventually causing the shoulder to droop (Priest 1989; Priest and Nagel 1976). Second, the greater weight of the playing extremity that has hypertrophied draws the shoulder downward simply through gravitational pull (Priest 1989). Numerous photographs in the literature clearly illustrate this point (King, Brelsford, and Tullos 1969; Priest et al. 1977; Priest and Nagel 1976). In extreme cases scoliosis (lateral curvature of the spine) can develop (Priest 1989; Renstrom and Roux 1988).

Lower Extremity Flexibility Needs

If shoulder range of motion is vital to throwing performance, what about the need for range of motion in the lower extremity? Tippett (1986) investigated lower extremity range of motion between the stance leg and kick leg in 16 college baseball pitchers. His study found ROM of ankle plantar flexion, hip internal rotation, and hip extension to be greater in the stance leg than in the kick leg. Conversely, the kick leg demonstrated greater active hip flexion than the stance leg did. The biomechanical explanation of the interrelationship of the lower extremity's ROM and stage of pitching follows.

1. Internal rotation of the stance leg is facilitated during the *gathering stage*. This rotation allows the trunk to coil on the fixed stanced leg in order to "load" for an efficient transfer of momentum from the leg to the hip, the hip rotators, the torso, and subsequently the arm.

2. The hip flexion of the kick leg corresponds to the flexion of the knee forward and across the body. This movement provides significant momentum to produce significant rotational force on the fixed stance.

3. Finally, during the *drive stage* proper alignment of the kicking leg originates with knee extension, hip abduction, and external rotation. As the pitcher begins striding toward the plate the stance leg provides power via hip extension. It is during this stage that the stance leg displays an increase in hip extension and ankle plantar flexion. "Theoretically, the greater motion can allow for a greater ability for corresponding muscles to generate force" (Tippett 1986, 13).

What flexibility regimen should be followed by athletes who use throwing motion patterns? First, tennis players obviously would benefit from an adequate level of shoulder joint mobility in order to achieve the desired racquet movement during a tennis serve (Bloomfield et al. 1985). Second, prudent athletes who use high velocity throws in their disciplines (e.g., pitchers) must exercise their shoulders for flexibility to allow the range of motion needed in cocking, without producing excessive joint laxity or instability (Boscardin, Johnson, and Schneider 1989). Third, a purposeful exercise program for the nonthrowing extremity should be employed to help prevent asymmetrical development of the shoulders and arms (Priest 1989). Theoretically, failure to develop either sufficient flexibility or strength will result in decreased performance and an increased likelihood of injury.

Wrestling

The importance of flexibility in wrestling performance is mainly theoretical. One argument is that flexibility in the hips and legs permits a wrestler to lower the center of gravity in the defensive position (Sharratt 1984). Consequently, the greater range of motion of the hip will allow for more technique from a defensive position (Song and Garvie 1976). "This can be a chain in thought, that is, this increase in confidence while in the defensive position will allow the wrestler to attack freely and not become pre-occupied by fear of making a mistake and ending up on the bottom only to be pinned" (Song and Garvie 1976, 15). A second factor is that "flexibility enables the wrestler to 'deform' enough to avoid tissue tearing as well as to slip out of positions that would otherwise be disabling" (Kreighbaum and Barthels 1985, 297). For example, the shoulder girdle is often used as a point of attack, particularly when both wrestlers are on the ground. Hence, wrestlers who are tight in the shoulders must go with the move put on them or suffer injury (Sharratt 1984; Figure 20.5). A final factor is that the greater the active flexibility, the better a wrestler is able to wrap the body, arms, and legs around the opponent (Kreighbaum and Barthels 1985). A study by Song and Garvie (1980) of 44 wrestlers training at the Canadian Olympic Training Center reported that there is no significant relationship between flexibility and the different weight classes.

It is interesting that the need for flexibility is also recognized in sumo wrestling. Because sumo wrestling requires considerable speed and agility, stretching encompasses a major component of their training regimen. Even sumo wrestlers weighing 200 kg can master a complete straddle split (matawari), eliminating any doubt that size is necessarily a limiting factor in flexibility.

Weight Lifting, Power Lifting, and Body Building

Three disciplines known for their incorporation of weight training are Olympic-style weight lifting, power lifting, and body building. Olympic weight lifting has two compulsory lifts: the overhead snatch and the clean-and-jerk. Power lifting is competitive lifting of maximal weights with the goal of one repetition maximum (1RM). These lifts include the bench press, the squat, and the dead lift. In contrast, body building is concerned with the development of muscular hypertrophy and definition, body symmetry, and the reduction of body fat (Garhammer 1989b).

Resistance or weight training is also often utilized to strengthen the areas of the body directly involved in performing the skills required in another sport or activity. Such training is valuable for the enhancement of recreational and competitive sport performance.

There is a paucity of evidence concerning the effect of weight training on flexibility, and that which is available is decidedly inconclusive (Wickstrom 1963). Unfortunately, there is still much to be researched on the interrelationship of flexibility and weight training. Theoretically, however, along with reducing the risk of injury, stretching and the development of flexibility are thought to improve the performance of the weight lifter by facilitating the use of optimal technique and enhancing muscular hypertrophy and strength.

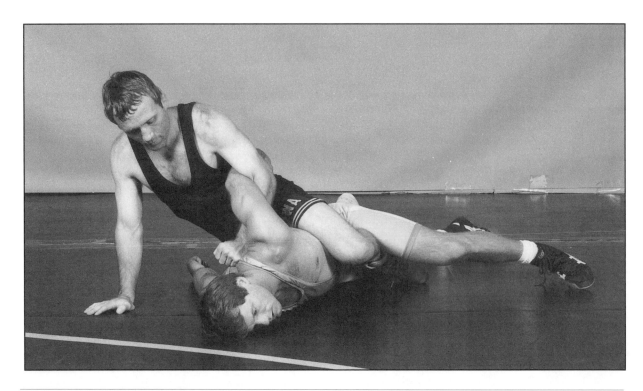

Fig. 20.5. The importance of shoulder flexibility in wrestling. Notice the extreme shoulder hyperextension being forced on the man on the bottom by the man above him.

Facilitating the Use of Optimal Technique

Flexibility or mobility in the joints is an important component of physical preparation in weight training. In lifting the barbell, good flexibility helps in executing the technical elements necessary to establish stable and steady technique of the classic exercises (Dvorkin 1986). For instance, without the requisite flexibility, a lifter will not be able to successfully execute the catch and receiving positions during the snatch lift. It has been suggested that female lifters are more flexible than male lifters and thus learn the technique of weight lifting more readily than men (Giel 1988).

Of greater significance is the consensus of experts that without adequate flexibility the snatch lift cannot be safely performed. This skill requires full shoulder flexibility for external rotation so that a lifter can bail out by "rotating out" if the weight gets behind him or her. This term means that a lifter completely rotates the shoulders from behind the back, getting the weight away from the body where it could cause injury if it were dropped (Burgener 1991; Dvorkin 1986; Kulund et al. 1978). To achieve this specific flexibility, shoulder dislocation exercises with a broomstick are commonly recommended (Kulund et al. 1978; Vorobiev 1987; see Exercise #52).

In addition to shoulder flexibility, lifters need flexibility in the spinal column and elbow joints. Although no substantiating data was presented, Vorobiev (1987) states that high indices of flexibility in the spinal column correlate with high achievement in the snatch lift. According to Vorobiev (1987) a significant (extreme) decrease in mobility in the spinal column can make getting under the barbell (literally) and fixation of the barbell (catching the barbell in a controlled position with the back fairly upright and the bar overhead) in the snatch lift more difficult. It is contended that insufficient flexibility in the elbow joint will result in poor "locking" (elbow extension).

Other areas of the body that require flexibility are the quadriceps, adductors, and the Achilles tendon, which are all stretched during the squat position of the snatch and clean-and-jerk lifts. In the opinion of Webster (1986, 91):

> The need for flexibility in the Achilles and ankles is not well-known and needs greater attention. Tight Achilles and ankles result in the heel raising from the floor, reducing the size of the base and making the lift less stable. Furthermore, the

ability to steeply incline the shins forward, well in advance of the toes, gives a much better position by reducing the tilt of the pelvis, which in turn reduces the lumbar curve.

Hence, it is readily apparent that a certain degree of flexibility is required for optimal performance (Figure 20.6).

Enhancing Muscular Hypertrophy, Strength, and Body Building Performance

Another contention that has appeared in the literature is that stretching a muscle, and specifically its fascia, facilitates muscular hypertrophy (Zulak 1991). The hypothesized mechanism is the reduction of an inhibiting factor that somehow slows muscle growth (i.e., tight fascia does not provide room in which muscle can grow). John Parrillo, a nutritionist and body building expert, is of the opinion that stretching a muscle is not only important, but absolutely essential for body builders to develop "maximum muscle size, shape and separation" (Zulak 1991, 108). Parrillo contends that stretching the fascia is the key to success. His rationale is that "thickened, toughened fascia limits muscle growth and gives a bodybuilder's development a flat appearance" (Zulak 1991, 107). With additional stretching, the muscle underneath the fascia is given greater room in which to grow. According to Parrillo, the best time to stretch the fascia is when the muscles are fully pumped up (full of blood) and after every set.

In addition to the preceding rationale, Parrillo has proposed several other reasons why stretching is advantageous for body builders. First, he is of the opinion that stretching can increase one's strength on a neurological level by as much as 15% to 20%. This improvement is theoretically made possible by raising the GTOs' threshold (see chapter 6). Consequently, one is capable of handling heavier weights and more repetitions. Second, he believes stretching helps to "recharge" the muscles by enhancing the removal of lactic acid that hinders muscular contraction. Third, the loosening effect of stretching is thought to help the body builder breathe better during the workout, increasing the oxygen utilization for improved energy levels. Fourth, stretching may cause muscle fibers to split and increase in numbers (i.e., hyperplasia). Fifth, stretching gives the body a more graceful appearance—essential when posing in a routine. Clearly, clinical testing

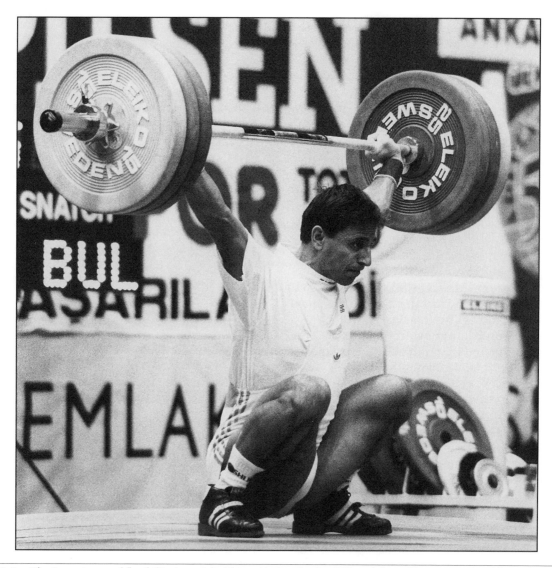

Fig. 20.6. The importance of flexibility in weight lifting. Notice the flexibility of the ankles, groin, shoulders, elbows, and wrists. Yoto Yotev of Bulgaria (155 kg) performs the snatch at the 1994 World Championships in Istanbul. Photo by Bruce Klemens.

under controlled conditions will be necessary to substantiate these various claims.

The Relationship Between Tension and Muscular Hypertrophy

Tension is one of the many important factors involved in the regulation of skeletal muscle size and hypertrophy (Vandenburgh 1987). Studies on developing embryos show that passive stretch plays an important role in muscular development. Stretch has been implicated in such processes as early muscle growth and development (Ashmore 1982; Barnett, Holly, and Ashmore 1980; Holly et al. 1980), denervation hypertrophy (Goldspink et al. 1974), dystrophic muscle (Ashmore 1982; Day, Ashmore, and Lee 1984; Frankeny, Holly, and Ashmore 1983), neurogenic atrophy (Pachter and Eberstein 1985), and compensatory hypertrophy (E. Gutman, Schiaffino, and Hanzliková 1971; Schiaffino 1974; Schiaffino and Hanzliková 1970; Thompsen and Luco 1944). Although it has been known for more than 80 years that mechanical stretching of skeletal muscle increases its metabolic rate, the mechanism involved is still unknown (Vandenburgh and Kaufman 1979). Furthermore, in recent years research has found passive stretching increases DNA and RNA concentrations (Ashmore 1982;

Barnett, Holly, and Ashmore 1980), oxidative enzyme activity in chicken muscle (Frankeny, Holly, and Ashmore 1983; Holly et al. 1980), and proteolytic enzyme activities in chicken muscles (Day, Ashmore, and Lee 1984). Although these findings are interesting, it must be noted that these studies dealt with animals and fowl and not finely conditioned athletes. The applicability of the foregoing research to humans is only speculative. Additional research at the clinical level is needed to substantiate the practical implications of these findings.

Rib Cage Flexibility, Performance, and Respiration

The tissues of the *thoracic cage* have elastic recoil or its reciprocal, *compliance*. The elements responsible for elastic recoil and compliance include the diameter and shape of the chest; the height of the individual; the mass of the musculature; the amount of body fat; the amount of abdominal fluid; and the integrity of the skeletal and muscular systems, the lung tissue, and connective tissue. In individuals with large, heavy, bony frames and heavy musculature, the increased mass of the upper torso muscles will lead to increased stiffness of the relaxed chest wall. Consequently, a greater muscle force may be needed to expand the chest. Similarly, a woman with large breasts or an obese person must exert additional force to lift the added weight with each respiration. Posture can also influence compliance of the chest cage. In individuals with hunched and rounded shoulders or in a head-down posture, the weight of the shoulder girdle pulls down on the chest girdle. Thus, tight and inflexible intercostal or pectoral muscles can decrease chest compliance and may add to the burden of respiration.

Can modifying the chest compliance enhance athletic performance? For some time it has been recognized that a flexible and mobile chest enhances athletic, exercise, and vocational performance. As described by Bowen (1934, 249), "With a mobile chest the muscles can more easily move the amount of air needed in quiet breathing and the subject does not so soon reach his limit in exercise that demands great increase of respiration."

An early study of the relationship between chest girth and vital capacity was undertaken by Louttit and Halford (1930). The test data from 100 boys with an average age of 15.7 years showed little or no relation between chest girth or expansion and vital chest capacity in normal boys. Almost half a century later, Barry et al. (1987) investigated the relationship between lung function and thoracic mobility in 51 normal subjects with ages ranging from 17 to 27 years of age. Statistically significant relationships ($r = .27–.42$: $_p$O .05) existed between the lung function and chest expansion variables. However, this result was in conflict with the findings of Louttit and Halford (1930). Neither lateral flexion of the trunk nor thoracic rotation were significantly related to lung function.

In another investigation, Grassino et al. (1978) demonstrated that restriction of the chest wall compartments is associated with a compensatory increase in the displacement of the abdomen in order to maintain a given tidal volume. Later, Hussain et al. (1985) expanded this study and investigated whether or not the compensatory mechanisms influenced high-intensity cycling performance. Their study found that restricted movements of the rib cage decreased tidal volume, decreased inspiratory and expiratory time, decreased diaphragmatic contractility, increased abdominal muscle recruitment in expiration, and altered the pattern of breathing in normal subjects. Perhaps of greater significance was a reduced exercise time (decreased endurance) in high-intensity exercise.

It is interesting that compliance of the chest wall has rarely been modified as a controlled variable when investigating such problems as asthma, emphysema, adult respiratory distress syndrome (ARDS), and general aging. Instead, there is often a general mention about the use of stretching and mobilization for treating these conditions (Cassidy and Schwiep 1989; Neu and Dinnel 1957; Warren 1968; Watts 1968). A review of the literature was able to locate just one study dealing with stretch gymnastics training in asthmatic children (Kanamaru et al. 1990). This study found that some patients were able to relieve their dyspneic sensation (i.e., difficult or labored respiration) solely by increasing chest flexibility.

This research is potentially significant for three populations: people who have a deformity of the rib cage or respiratory illness, healthy people, and athletes. The question of whether exercises that increase chest expansion and upper torso flexibility improve function for these three categories of people needs to be examined in a clinical setting. To establish the existence of a causal link between chest expansion and lung function, experimental research is required in which chest expansion is deliberately manipulated as an independent variable (Barry et al. 1987).

Summary

Numerous factors go into creating optimal performance, and flexibility is generally recognized as one of these crucial factors. Practical, everyday experience substantiates that flexibility enhances and optimizes the learning, practice, and performance of skilled movement. Since ROM is specific to many disciplines, some skills may be enhanced more effectively by purposefully increasing or decreasing the range of motion around certain joints through a flexibility training program until what appears to be optimal flexibility is reached. It is also claimed that stretching may enhance muscular hypertrophy and improve respiratory function for people with respiratory disorders. These and other claims need to be investigated in order to substantiate any practical implications.

Stretching Exercises

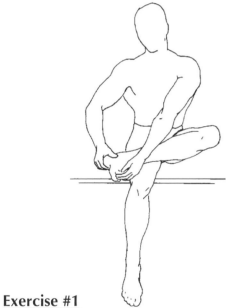

Exercise #1

(Plantar Arch)

1. Sit upright in a chair or on the floor with one leg crossed over the opposite knee.
2. Grasp your ankle with one hand.
3. Grasp the underside of your toes and ball of the foot with your other hand.
4. Exhale, and pull your toes toward your shin (extension of the toes).
5. Hold the stretch and relax.
6. You should feel the stretch in the sole of the raised foot.

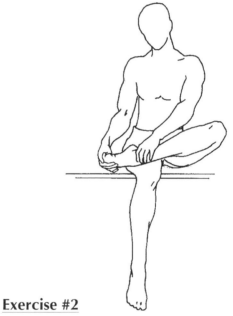

Exercise #2

(Anterior Aspect of the Toes)

1. Sit upright in a chair or on the floor with one leg crossed over the opposite knee.
2. Grasp your ankle and heel with one hand.
3. Grasp the top portion of your foot and toes with your other hand.
4. Exhale, and slowly pull the bottom of your toes toward the ball of your foot (flexion).
5. Hold the stretch and relax.
6. You should feel the stretch on the top of the foot and toes.

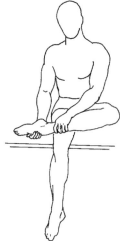

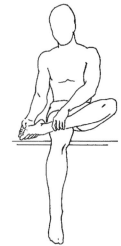

Exercise #3

(Anterior Portion of the Ankle and Lower Leg)

1. Sit upright in a chair or on the floor with one leg crossed over the opposite knee.
2. Grasp your leg above your ankle with one hand.
3. Grasp the top portion of your foot with your other hand.
4. Exhale, and slowly pull the sole of your foot toward your body (plantar flexion).
5. Hold the stretch and relax.
6. You should feel the stretch in the instep and top of the ankle.

Exercise #5

(Anterior and Lateral Aspect of the Ankle and Lower Leg)

1. Sit upright in a chair or on the floor with one leg crossed over the opposite knee.
2. Grasp your ankle and heel with one hand.
3. Grasp the top outside portion of your foot with the other hand.
4. Exhale, and slowly invert your ankle (turn it upward).
5. Hold the stretch and relax.
6. You should feel the stretch in the anterior and lateral aspect of the ankle and lower leg.

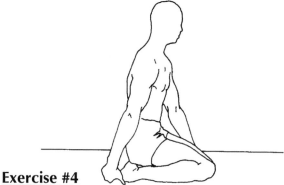

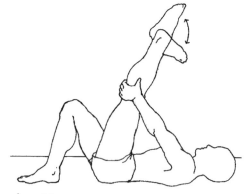

Exercise #4

(Anterior Portion of the Ankle and Lower Leg)

1. Kneel with your toes pointing backward. If this position is uncomfortable, place a blanket under your shins.
2. Exhale, and slowly sit on the top of your heels (if you can).
3. Reach around, grasp the top portion of your toes, and pull them toward your head.
4. Hold the stretch and relax.
5. You should feel the stretch along the shin. The muscle primarily targeted is the tibialis anterior. *Note.* This stretch is used to prevent shinsplints. However, make sure your hips sit on top of the heels and *not* between the feet (The latter position is called W sitting and is bad for the knees). This stretch should be avoided by people with a history of knee problems.

Exercise #6

(Achilles Tendon and Posterior Lower Leg)

1. Lie on your back with the legs extended.
2. Flex one leg and slide the foot toward the buttocks.
3. Raise the opposite leg toward your face and grasp behind the knee.
4. Exhale, and slowly dorsiflex the foot toward your face.
5. Hold the stretch and relax.
6. You should feel the stretch in the Achilles tendon. *Note.* If you have back problems, after the stretch you should flex the extended leg and slowly lower it to the floor.

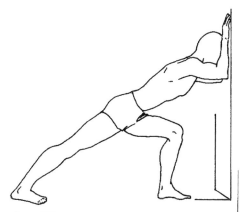

Exercise #7

(The Gastrocnemius and Achilles Tendon)

1. Stand upright slightly more than arm's length from a wall.
2. Bend one leg forward and keep the opposite leg straight.
3. Lean against the wall without losing the straight line of your head, neck, spine, pelvis, rear leg, and ankle.
4. Keep the heel of your rear foot down, sole flat on the floor, and foot pointing straight forward.
5. Exhale, bend your arms, lean toward the wall, and shift your weight forward.
6. Exhale, and flex your forward knee toward the wall.
7. Hold the stretch and relax.
8. You should feel the stretch in the calf and Achilles tendon. *Note.* To stretch the soleus, flex the rear leg at the knee.

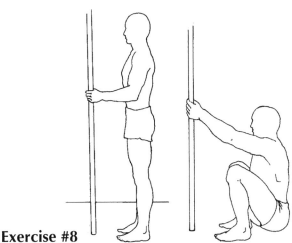

Exercise #8

(Quadriceps)

1. Stand upright, with your feet parallel and about 30 cm (1 ft) apart, holding a pole.
2. Exhale, lean backward slightly, keeping your heels flat on the floor and knees behind your toes, and squat as low as you can.
3. Hold the stretch and relax.
4. You should feel the stretch in the quadriceps.
5. Inhale and return to the starting position. *Note.* This stretch may also be felt in the adductors (i.e., groin) and Achilles tendon of those who are tight in these areas.

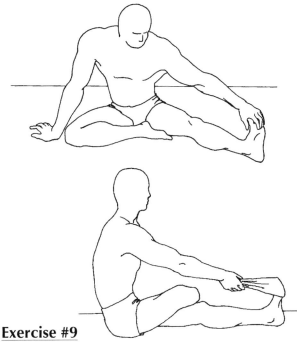

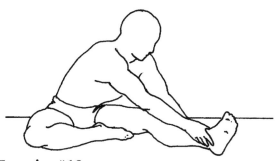

Exercise #9

(Back of the Knee)

1. Sit upright on the floor with the legs straight.
2. Keep one leg straight and bend the opposite leg in until its heel touches the groin of the extended leg.
3. Exhale, lean forward, and grasp your foot.
4. Exhale, keep your leg straight, and pull your foot back toward your trunk.
5. Hold the stretch and relax. *Note.* If you cannot reach your foot, use a folded towel. To intensify the stretch, cross the bent leg and rest the heel on the opposite knee, and then apply the stretch.

Exercise #10

(Hamstrings)

1. Sit upright on the floor with both legs straight and about 90° apart.
2. Flex one knee and slide the heel until it touches the inner side of the opposite thigh.
3. Lower the outer side of the thigh and calf of the bent leg onto the floor.
4. Exhale, and while keeping the extended leg straight, bend at the hip and lower your extended upper torso from the hips onto the extended thigh.
5. Hold the stretch and relax.
6. You should feel the stretch in the hamstrings.

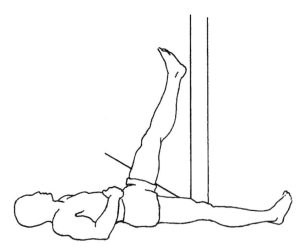

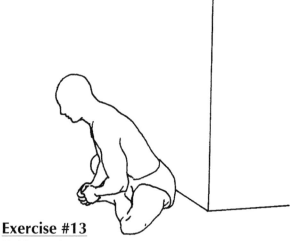

Exercise #11

(Hamstrings)

1. Lie flat on your back in a doorway.
2. Position your hips slightly in front of the doorframe.
3. Raise one leg and rest it against the doorframe, while keeping this knee extended and your bottom leg flat on the floor. To increase the stretch, slide the buttocks closer to the doorframe or lift the leg away from the doorframe.
4. Hold the stretch and relax.
5. You should feel the stretch in the hamstrings. *Note.* To intensify the stretch, use a folded towel wrapped around the foot of the raised leg. By pulling on the towel, the leg can be pulled away from the doorframe and closer to your chest.

Exercise #13

(Adductors)

1. Sit upright on the floor with your buttocks against a wall, your legs flexed and straddled, and heels touching each other.
2. Grasp your feet or ankles and pull them as close to your groin as possible.
3. Exhale, lean forward from the hips without bending your back, and attempt to lower your chest to the floor.
4. Hold the stretch and relax.
5. You should feel the stretch in the groin (adductors). *Note.* A common error is rounding the back.

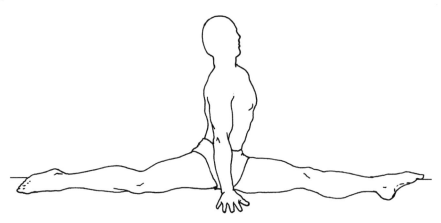

Exercise #12

(Hamstrings)

1. Kneel on the floor with both legs together and your hands at your sides.
2. Lift up one knee and place your foot slightly in front for support.
3. Exhale, bend at the waist, lower your upper torso down onto the front thigh, and place your hands slightly in front of the front foot for support.
4. Exhale, slowly slide your front foot forward, straighten both legs and straighten back into upright position as you extend into the split position.
5. Hold the stretch and relax.
6. You should feel the stretch in the hamstrings. *Note.* A split is one of the more advanced stretches for the hamstrings. To perform a technically correct split, both legs must be straight, the hips squared (facing front, not twisted sideways), and the buttocks flat on the floor. For aesthetic reasons, some people advocate a slight turnout of the rear hip. However, due to tight hip flexors or improper training, this turnout can be too extreme. To increase the stretch one can extend the upper torso and lower the chest onto the forward thigh, or perform the split with the forward leg placed on top of a folded blanket. This latter method should be avoided by the vast majority of even advanced athletes since it can possibly strain the posterior knee.

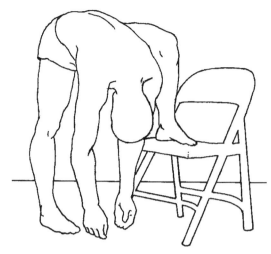

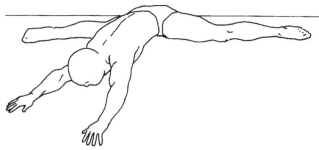

Exercise #16

(Adductors)

1. Sit upright with your legs straddled and straight.
2. Exhale, and slowly lower your chest and belly onto the floor while keeping your back flat.
3. Hold the stretch and relax.
4. You should feel the stretch in the groin (adductors). *Note.* Ideally, your legs should form a straight line when executing a straddle split. People with greater flexibility can roll the hips forward and backward.

Exercise #14

(Adductors)

1. Stand upright with one leg raised and the foot resting on the seat of a chair.
2. Exhale, bend at the hip, and lower your hands toward the floor.
3. Hold the stretch and relax.
4. You should feel the stretch in the groin (adductors).
5. Inhale while raising your upper torso to return to the upright position.

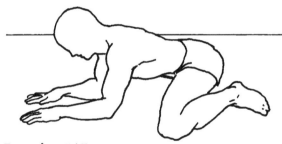

Exercise #15

(Adductors)

1. Kneel on all fours with your toes pointing out to the sides.
2. Bend your arms and rest your elbows on the floor.
3. Exhale, slowly straddle (spread) your knees, and attempt to lower your chest to the floor.
4. Hold the stretch and relax.
5. You should feel the stretch in the groin (adductors). *Caution.* This stretch is one of the most intense exercises for the adductors—it's extremely deceptive.

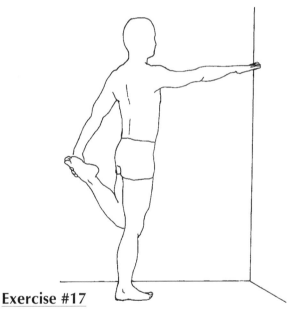

Exercise #17

(Quadriceps)

1. Stand upright with one hand against a surface for balance and support.
2. Flex one knee and raise your heel to your buttocks.
3. Slightly flex the supporting leg.
4. Exhale, reach behind, and grasp your raised foot with one hand.
5. Inhale, and pull your heel toward your buttocks *without* overcompressing the knee.
6. Hold the stretch and relax.
7. You should feel the stretch in the quadriceps.

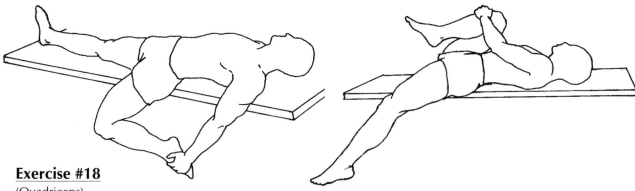

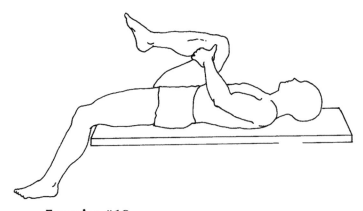

Exercise #18

(Quadriceps)

1. Lie on your back at the edge of a table with one side near the edge.
2. Exhale, slowly lower the outside leg off the table at the hip, and grasp the ankle or foot with the outside hand.
3. Inhale, and slowly pull your heel toward your buttocks.
4. Hold the stretch and relax.
5. You should feel the stretch in the middle to upper thigh. *Note.* This exercise can be an intense stretch. To protect your lower back lift up your head and contract the abdominal muscles.

Exercise #20

(Hip Flexors)

1. Lie on a table near the side, flat on your back.
2. Allow the outside leg to hang over the side of the table at the hip.
3. Inhale, flex the opposite knee, grasp it with your hands, and bring it to your chest.
4. Inhale and compress your thigh to your chest.
5. Hold the stretch and relax.
6. You should feel the stretch in the upper thigh.

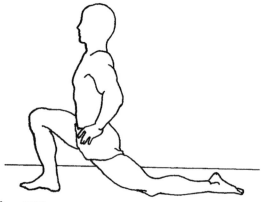

Exercise #19

(Hip Flexors)

1. Lie on a table, flat on your back, with both legs hanging over the edge at the knees.
2. Inhale, flex one hip, and raise the knee toward your chest.
3. Interlock your hands behind the raised knee.
4. Inhale and bring your knee to your chest as you keep the opposite leg hanging over the edge.
5. Hold the stretch and relax.
6. You should feel the stretch in the upper thigh.

Exercise #21

(Hip Flexors)

1. Stand upright with the legs straddled (spread sideways) about 60 cm (2 ft) apart.
2. Flex one knee, lower your body, and place the opposite knee on the floor.
3. Roll the back foot under so that the top of the instep rests on the floor.
4. Place your hands on your hips (some people may prefer placing one hand on the forward knee and one hand on the buttocks) and keep the front knee bent at a 90° angle as much as possible.
5. Exhale, and slowly push the front of the hip of the back leg toward the floor.
6. Hold the stretch and relax.
7. You should feel the stretch in the upper thigh.

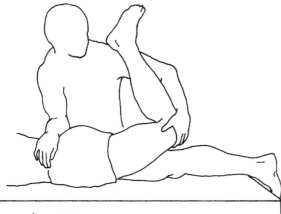

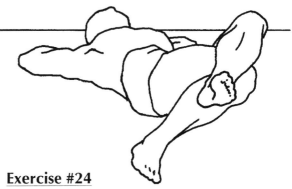

Exercise #22

(Hip Flexors)

1. Lie face down with your body extended and one knee flexed.
2. Your partner is positioned at your side, standing or resting on one knee, with one hand under your knee (on front of thigh) and the other slightly above or on the side of the buttocks.
3. Contract your gluteals (buttocks muscles) as you allow your partner to anchor down the belly to the table or floor with one hand and gently lift your leg higher with the opposite hand.
4. Hold the stretch position and relax.
5. You should feel this stretch in the upper thigh. *Note.* This exercise creates an intense stretch and must be used with extreme caution.

Exercise #24

(Buttocks and Hip)

1. Lie flat on your back, knees flexed, and your hands interlocked underneath your head.
2. Lift your left leg over your right leg and hook your leg.
3. Exhale, and use your left leg to force the inside of your right leg to the floor, while keeping your elbows, head, and shoulders flat on the floor.
4. Hold the stretch and relax.
5. You should feel the stretch in the buttocks and hip.

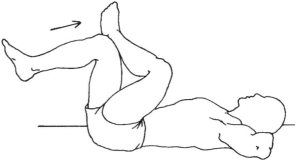

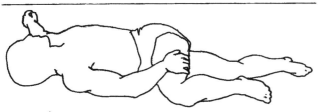

Exercise #23

(Lateral Buttocks and Hip)

1. Lie flat on your back with your legs extended.
2. Flex one knee and raise it to your chest.
3. Grasp your knee or thigh with the opposite hand.
4. Exhale, and pull your knee sideways across your body to the floor, while keeping your elbows, head, and shoulders flat on the floor.
5. Hold the stretch and relax.
6. You should feel the stretch in the lateral buttocks and hip.

Exercise #25

(Buttocks and Hip)

1. Lie flat on your back with your left leg crossed over your right knee.
2. Inhale, flex your right knee, lifting your right foot off the floor, and let it push your left foot toward your face, while keeping your head, shoulders, and back flat on the floor.
3. Hold the stretch and relax.
4. You should feel the stretch in the buttocks and hip.

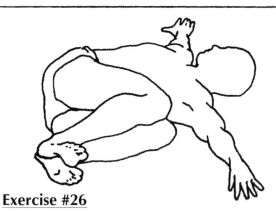

Exercise #26

(Buttocks, Hips, and Trunk)

1. Lie flat on your back, with your knees flexed and arms out to the sides.
2. Exhale, and slowly lower both legs to the floor on the same side, while keeping your elbows, head, and shoulders flat on the floor.
3. Hold the stretch and relax.
4. You should feel the stretch in your buttocks, hip, and lower trunk.

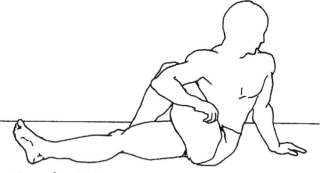

Exercise #28

(Buttocks and Hip)

1. Sit upright on the floor, with the hands behind your hips for support and your legs extended.
2. Flex your left leg, cross your left foot over your right leg, and slide your heel toward your buttocks.
3. Reach over your left leg with your right arm, and place your right elbow on the outside of your left knee.
4. Exhale, and look over your left shoulder while turning your trunk and pushing back on your knee with your right elbow.
5. Hold the stretch and relax.
6. You should feel the stretch in the buttocks and hip.

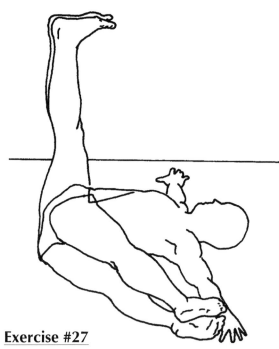

Exercise #27

(Buttocks, Hip, and Trunk)

1. Lie flat on your back, your legs raised and straight, and your arms out to the sides.
2. Exhale, and slowly lower both legs to the floor on the same side, while keeping your elbows, head, and shoulders flat on the floor.
3. Hold the stretch and relax.
4. You should feel the stretch in the buttocks, hip, and lower trunk.

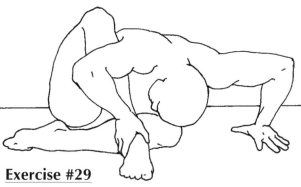

Exercise #29

(Buttocks, Hip, and Trunk)

1. Sit upright on the floor with the outside of your left leg resting on the floor in front of you, with your knee flexed and your foot pointing to your right.
2. Cross your right leg over your left leg and place the foot flat on the floor.
3. Exhale, round your upper torso, and bend forward.
4. Hold the stretch and relax.
5. You should feel the stretch in the buttocks, hip, and trunk.

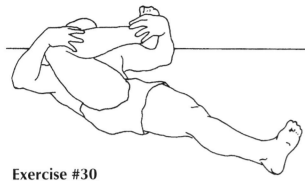

Exercise #30

(Buttocks and Hip)

1. Lie on the floor with your body extended.
2. Flex one leg and slide the heel toward your buttocks.
3. Grasp your knee with the same-side hand and your ankle with the opposite hand.
4. Exhale, and slowly pull your foot to the opposite shoulder, while keeping your head, shoulders, and back flat on the floor.
5. Hold the stretch and relax.
6. You should feel the stretch in the buttocks and hip.

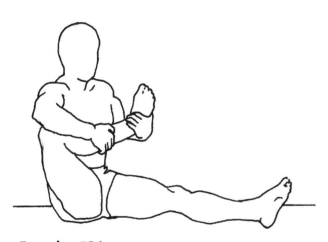

Exercise #31

(Buttocks and Hip)

1. Sit upright on the floor with your back flat against a wall.
2. Flex one leg and slide your heel toward your buttocks.
3. Hook your knee with the same-side elbow and grasp your ankle with the opposite hand.
4. Exhale, and slowly pull your foot to the opposite shoulder.
5. Hold the stretch and relax.

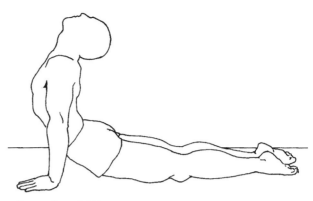

Exercise #32

(Abdomen and Hip Flexors)

1. Lie face down on the floor with your body extended.
2. Place your palms on the floor by your hips with your fingers pointing forward.
3. Exhale, press down on the floor, raise your head and trunk, and arch your back while contracting the gluteals to prevent excessive compression on the lower back.
4. Hold the stretch and relax.
5. You should feel the stretch in the abdomen and upper thighs.

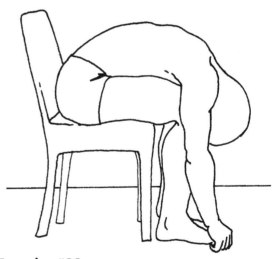

Exercise #33

(Lower Back)

1. Sit upright in a chair with your legs separated slightly.
2. Exhale, extend your upper torso, bend at the hip, and slowly lower your stomach between your thighs.
3. Hold the stretch and relax.
4. You should feel the stretch in your lower back.

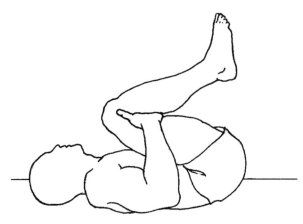

Exercise #34

(Lower Back)

1. Lie flat on your back with your body extended.
2. Flex your knees and slide your feet toward your buttocks.
3. Grasp behind your thighs to prevent hyperflexion of the knees.
4. Exhale, pull your knees toward your chest and shoulders, and elevate your hips off the floor.
5. Hold the stretch and relax.
6. You should feel the stretch in your lower back.
7. Exhale and reextend your legs slowly one at a time to prevent possible pain or spasm.

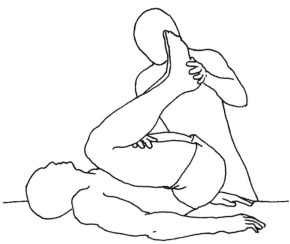

Exercise #35

(Lower Back)

1. Lie flat on your back with your body extended.
2. Flex your knees and slide your feet toward your buttocks.
3. Your partner is positioned to your side, with one hand under your hamstrings and the other grasping your heels.
4. Exhale as you allow your partner to bring your thighs closer to your chest, lifting your buttocks and lower back from the floor.
5. Hold the stretch and relax.
6. You should feel the stretch in the lower back.

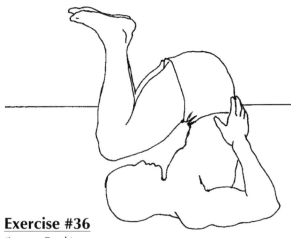

Exercise #36

(Lower Back)

1. Lie flat on your back with your arms at your sides, palms down.
2. Exhale, push down on the floor with your palms, and raise your legs up in a squat position so the knees almost rest on your forehead.
3. Support the weight of your hips with your hands.
4. Hold the stretch and relax.
5. You should feel the stretch in your lower back. *Caution.* Use this controversial stretch with care. Avoid excessive flexion of the neck.

Exercise #37

(Lateral Trunk)

1. Hang from a chin-up bar with your arms straight, hands almost touching, and your body slightly flexed in a C shape (convex toward the front).
2. Exhale, place your chin on your chest, and sink in your shoulders.
3. Hold the stretch and relax.
4. You should feel the stretch in the lateral trunk and upper back.

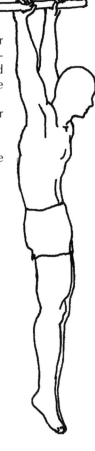

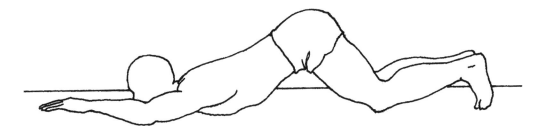

Exercise #38

(Upper Back)

1. Kneel on all fours.
2. Extend your arms forward and lower your chest toward the floor.
3. Exhale, extend your shoulders, and press down on the floor with your arms to produce an arch in your back.
4. Hold the stretch and relax.
5. You should feel the stretch in your upper back.

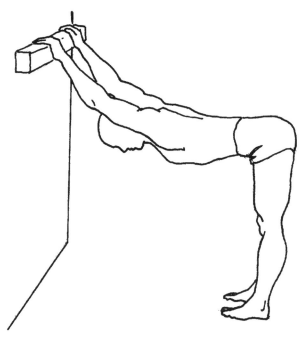

Exercise #39

(Upper Back)

1. Stand upright, feet together, about 1 m (3 ft) from a supporting surface that is approximately waist to shoulder height, and your arms overhead.
2. Exhale, keep your arms and legs straight, flex at the waist, flatten your back, and grasp the supporting surface with both hands.
3. Exhale and press down on the supporting surface to produce an arch in your back.
4. Hold the stretch and relax.
5. You should feel the stretch in your upper back.

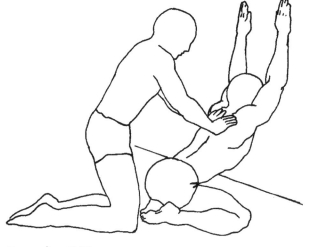

Exercise #40

(Upper Back)

1. Sit upright, knees straddled, facing a wall about an arm's length away.
2. Raise your arms with your elbows straight, lean forward, and place your palms against the wall shoulder-width apart with your fingers pointing upward.
3. Exhale, raise your arms, press down against the wall, open your chest, and produce an arch in your back.
4. Your partner is positioned directly behind with his or her hands placed on the upper portion of your shoulder blades.
5. Exhale, as you allow your partner to gently push down and away from your head. Communicate with your partner and use great care.
6. Hold the stretch and relax.
7. You should feel the stretch in your upper back.

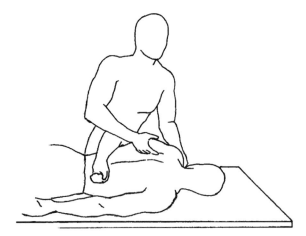

Exercise #41

(Serratus Anterior and Rhomboids)

1. Lie flat on your chest, head turned to the left, with your left elbow flexed and forearm resting on the lower back.
2. Your partner is positioned to your side with his or her left hand grasping the top front portion of your shoulder.
3. Exhale, as you allow your partner to lift up your front shoulder to expose the scapula (shoulder blade).
4. The partner places his or her right hand under your scapula and gently lifts it upward.
5. Hold the stretch and relax.
6. You should feel the stretch in the rhomboids.

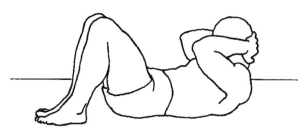

Exercise #42

(Posterior Neck)

1. Lie flat on the floor with both knees flexed.
2. Interlock your hands on the back of your head near the occiputs.
3. Exhale and pull your head off the floor and onto your chest while keeping your shoulder blades flat on the floor.
4. Hold the stretch and relax.
5. You should feel the stretch in the upper back and posterior neck.

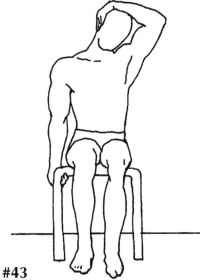

Exercise #43

(Lateral Neck)

1. Sit or stand upright.
2. Place your left hand on the upper right side of your head.
3. Exhale, and slowly pull the left side of your head onto your left shoulder (lateral flexion).
4. Hold the stretch and relax.
5. You should feel the stretch in the lateral side of the neck.

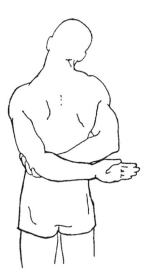

Exercise #44

(Lateral Neck)

1. Sit or stand upright with your left arm flexed behind your back.
2. Grasp the elbow from behind with the opposite hand and pull your elbow across the midline of your back to keep the left shoulder stabilized.
3. Exhale and lower your right ear to the right shoulder.
4. Hold the stretch and relax.
5. You should feel the stretch in the lateral side of the neck.

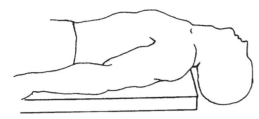

Exercise #45

(Anterior Neck)

1. Lie flat on a table with your head hanging over the edge.
2. Hold the stretch and relax.
3. You should feel the stretch in the anterior part of the neck.

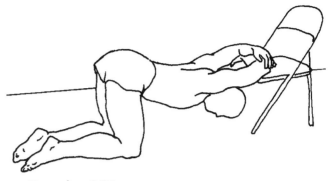

Exercise #47

(Pectorals)

1. Kneel on the floor facing a barre or chair.
2. Interlock your forearms above your head and bend forward to rest them on top of the barre or chair, with your head dropping beneath the supporting surface.
3. Exhale and let your head and chest sink to the floor.
4. Hold the stretch and relax.
5. You should feel the stretch in your upper chest (pectorals).

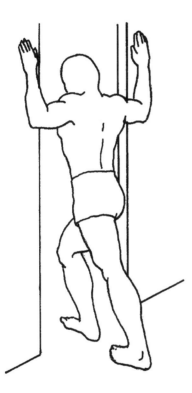

Exercise #46

(Pectorals)

1. Stand upright facing a corner or open doorway.
2. Raise your elbows to shoulder height at your sides, bend your elbows so that your forearms point straight up, and place your palms against the walls or doorframe to stretch the sternal section of the pectoralis muscles on both sides.
3. Exhale and lean your entire body forward.
4. Hold the stretch and relax.
5. You should feel the stretch in your upper chest (pectorals).

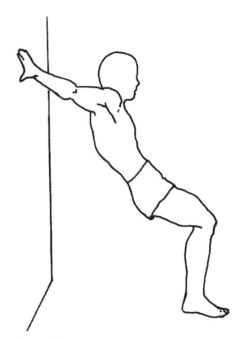

Exercise #48

(Anterior Shoulder)

1. Stand upright, your hands behind you at about shoulder height resting on a wall, and your fingers pointing upward.
2. Exhale and flex your legs to lower your shoulders.
3. Hold the stretch and relax.
4. You should feel the stretch in the anterior shoulder.

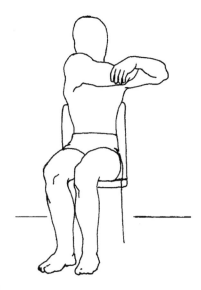

Exercise #49

(Lateral Shoulder)

1. Sit or stand upright with one arm raised to shoulder height.
2. Flex your arm across to the opposite shoulder.
3. Grasp your raised elbow with the opposite hand.
4. Exhale and pull your elbow toward your back.
5. Hold the stretch and relax.
6. You should feel the stretch in the lateral shoulder.

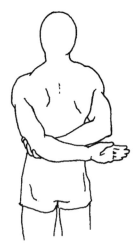

Exercise #51

(Shoulder Abductors)

1. Sit or stand upright with one arm flexed behind your back.
2. Grasp the elbow (or wrist if unable to reach elbow) from behind with the opposite hand.
3. Exhale and pull your elbow across the midline of your back.
4. Hold the stretch and relax.
5. You should feel the stretch in the posterior part of the shoulder.

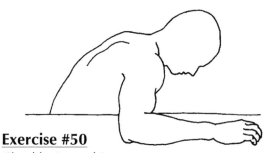

Exercise #50

(Shoulder Internal Rotators)

1. Sit upright with your side next to a table.
2. Rest your forearm along the table edge with your elbow flexed.
3. Exhale, bend forward from the waist, and lower your head and shoulder to table level.
4. Hold the stretch and relax.
5. You should feel the stretch in the upper and medial shoulder.

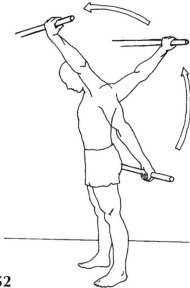

Exercise #52

(Shoulder Internal and External Rotators)

1. Stand upright, feet straddled, and grasp a pole or towel with both hands behind your hips with a wide, reverse grip (your palms facing forward and thumbs on the outside).
2. Inhale and slowly raise your arms overhead, keeping both straight and symmetrical, with no twisting to the side as your arms rotate forward in the shoulder joint and end in an L grip (the palms of the hands face up and the thumbs under the pole).
3. Inhale, then reverse the direction.
4. You should feel this stretch in the shoulders (especially the posterior region).

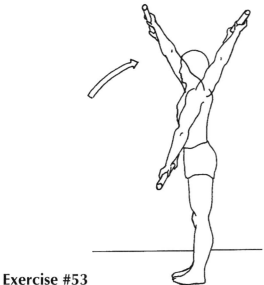

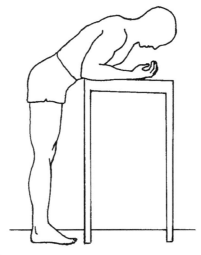

Exercise #53

(Shoulder Internal and External Rotators)

1. Stand upright, feet straddled, and grasp a pole or towel in front of your hips with a wide overgrip (palm facing down).
2. Inhale and slowly raise your arms overhead, keeping them both straight, symmetrical, and with no twisting to the side as they rotate in the shoulder joint and end up behind your head.
3. Exhale, then reverse the direction.
4. You should feel this stretch in the shoulders (especially the anterior region).

Exercise #55

(Triceps Brachii)

1. Stand upright with your forearms resting on a table with the palms facing up.
2. Exhale, bend forward, and bring your shoulders to your wrists.
3. Hold the stretch and relax.
4. You should feel the stretch in the triceps brachii.

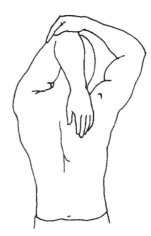

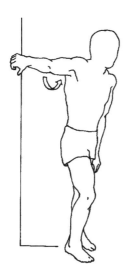

Exercise #54

(Biceps Brachii)

1. Stand upright with your back to a doorframe.
2. Rest one hand against the doorframe with your arm internally rotated at the shoulder, forearm extended, and your hand pronated with your thumb pointing down.
3. Exhale and attempt to roll your biceps so they face upward.
4. Hold the stretch and relax.
5. You should feel this stretch in the biceps brachii.

Exercise #56

(Triceps Brachii)

1. Sit or stand upright with one arm flexed, raised overhead with elbow next to your ear, and your hand resting on your opposite shoulder blade.
2. Grasp your elbow with the opposite hand.
3. Exhale and pull your elbow behind your head.
4. Hold the stretch and relax.
5. You should feel the stretch in the triceps brachii.

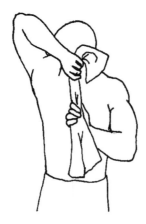

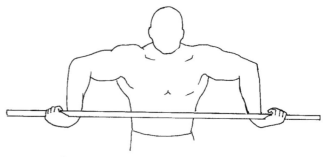

Exercise #59
(Brachioradialis)

1. Hold a pole in front of you in an L grip (the palms of the hands face up and the thumbs on the outside).
2. Exhale and flex your elbows.
3. Hold the stretch and relax.
4. You should feel the stretch in the brachioradialis.

Exercise #57
(Triceps Brachii)

1. Sit or stand upright with one arm behind your lower back, placed as far up on your back as possible.
2. Lift your other arm overhead, while holding a folded blanket or towel, and flex your elbow.
3. Grasp the blanket or towel with your lower hand.
4. Inhale as you slowly pull your hands together.
5. Hold the stretch and relax.
6. You should feel the stretch in the triceps brachii.

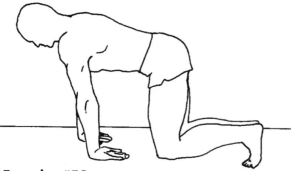

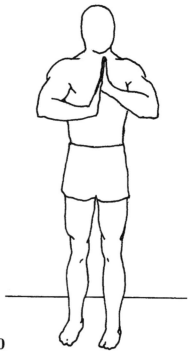

Exercise #58
(Brachioradialis)

1. Kneel on all fours, flex your wrists, and place the tops (dorsa) of your hands against the floor, with fingers pointing toward your knees.
2. Exhale and lean against the floor.
3. Hold the stretch and relax.
4. You should feel the stretch in the brachioradialis.

Exercise #60
(Forearm Flexors)

1. Sit or stand upright on the floor with your wrists hyperextended (bent backwards).
2. Place the heel of one hand against the palmar surface of the fingers of your other hand.
3. Exhale and press the heel of your hand against your fingers.
4. Hold the stretch and relax.
5. You should feel the stretch in the forearm flexors.

References

Aarskog, D., Stoa, K.F., and Thorsen, T. (1966). Urinary oestrogen excretion in newborn infants with congenital dysplasia of the hip joint. *Acta Paediatrica Scandinavica*, 55(4), 394-397.

Aberdeen, D.L., and Joensen, E. (1986). A study of the relevance of handedness to the range of rotation at the glenohumeral joint. *European Journal of Chiropractic*, 34(2), 67-87.

Abraham, W.M. (1977). Factors in delayed muscle soreness. *Medicine and Science in Sports*, 9(1), 11-20.

Abraham, W.M. (1979). Exercise-induced muscular soreness. *The Physician and Sportsmedicine*, 7(10), 57-60.

Abramson, D., Roberts, S.M., and Wilson, P.D. (1934). Relaxation of the pelvic joint in pregnancy. *Surgery, Gynecology, and Obstetrics*, 58(3), 595-613.

ACOG. *See* American College of Obstetricians and Gynecologists.

Adams, M.A., Dolan, P., and Hutton, W.C. (1987). Diurnal variations in the stresses on the lumbar spine. *Spine*, 12(2), 130-137.

Adams, M.A., and Hutton, W.C. (1986). Has the lumbar spine a margin of safety in forward bending? *Clinical Biomechanics*, 1(1), 3-6.

Adams, M.A., Hutton, W.C., and Stott, J.R.R. (1980). The resistance to flexion of the lumbar intervertebral joint. *Spine*, 5(3), 245-253.

Adams, P., and Muir, H. (1976). Qualitative changes with age of proteoglycans of human lumbar discs. *Annals of the Rheumatic Diseases*, 35(4), 289-296.

Adler, S.S., Beckers, D., and Buck, M. (1993). *PNF in practice: An illustrated guide*. New York: Springer-Verlag.

Agre, J.C., Casal, D.C., Leon, A.S., McNally, C., Baxter, T.L., and Serfass, R.C. (1988). Professional ice hockey players: Physiologic, anthropometric, and musculoskeletal characteristics. *Archives of Physical Medicine and Rehabilitation*, 69(3), 188-192.

Agre, J.C., Pierce, L.E., Raab, D.M., McAdams, M., and Smith, E.L. (1988). Light resistance and stretching exercise in elderly women: Effect upon stretch. *Archives of Physical Medicine and Rehabilitation*, 69(4), 273-276.

Akeson, W.H., Amiel, D., and LaViolette, D. (1967). The connective tissue response to immobility: A study of the chondroitin 4-and 6-sulfate and dermatan sulfate changes in periarticular connective tissue of control and immobilized knees of dogs. *Clinical Orthopaedics and Related Research*, 51, 183-197.

Akeson, W.H., Amiel, D., Mechanic, G.L., Woo, S., Harwood, F.L., and Hammer, M.L. (1977). Collagen crosslinking alteration in joint contractures: Changes in reducible crosslinks in periarticular connective tissue collagen after nine weeks of immobilization. *Connective Tissue Research*, 5(1), 15-20.

Akeson, W.H., Amiel, D., and Woo, S. (1980). Immobility effects on synovial joints: The pathomechanics of joint contracture. *Biorheology*, 17(1/2), 95-110.

Akster, H.A., Granzier, H.L.M., and Focant, B. (1989). Differences in I band structure, sarcomere extensibility, and electrophoresis of titin between two muscle fiber types of the perch (*Perca fluviatilis L.*). *Journal of Ultrastructure and Molecular Structure Research*, 102(2), 109-121.

Alabin, V.G., and Krivonosov, M.P. (1987). Excerpts from training aids and specialized exercises in track and field. *Soviet Sports Review*, 22(2), 73-75.

Alexander, M.J.L. (1991). A comparison of physiological characteristics of elite and subelite rhythmic gymnasts. *Journal of Human Movement Studies*, 20(2), 49-69.

Alexander, R.M. (1975). *Biomechanics*. London: Chapman and Hall.

Alexander, R.M. (1988). *Elastic mechanisms in animal movement*. Cambridge: Cambridge University Press.

Allander, E., Björnsson, O., Olafsson, O., Sigfússon, N., and Thorsteinsson, J. (1974). Normal range of joint movements in shoulder, hip, wrist and thumb with special reference to side: A comparison between two populations. *International Journal of Epidemiology*, 3(3), 253-261.

Allen, C.E.L. (1948). Muscle action potentials used in the study of dynamic anatomy. *British Journal of Physical Medicine*, 11, 66-73.

Almekinders, L.C. (1993). Anti-inflammatory treatment of muscular injuries in sports. *Sports Medicine*, 15(3), 139-145.

Alnaqeeb, M.A., Al Zaid, N.S., and Goldspink, G. (1984). Connective tissue changes and physical properties of developing and aging skeletal muscle. *Journal of Anatomy*, 139(4), 677-689.

Al-Rawi, Z.S., Al-Aszawi, A.J., and Al-Chalabi, T. (1985). Joint mobility among university students in Iraq. *British Journal of Rheumatology*, 24(4), 326-331.

Alter, J. (1983). *Surviving exercise*. Boston: Houghton Mifflin.

Alter, J. (1986). *Strength & strengthen*. Boston: Houghton Mifflin.

Alter, J. (1989-1990). Book review. *Kinesiology and Medicine in Dance*, 12(1), 41-43.

Alter, M. (1990). *Sport stretch*. Champaign, IL: Leisure Press.

Alvarez, R., Stokes, I.A.F., Asprino, D.E., Trevino, S., and Braun, T. (1988). Dimensional changes of the feet in pregnancy. *Journal of Bone and Joint Surgery*, 70A(2), 271-274.

American Academy of Orthopaedic Surgeons. (1965). *Joint motion: Method of measuring and recording*. Park Ridge, IL: Author.

American Academy of Orthopaedic Surgeons. (1991). *Athletic training and sports medicine* (2nd ed.). Rosemont, IL: Author.

American Alliance for Health, Physical Education, and Recreation. (1968). *School safety policies with emphasis on physical education, athletics, and recreation*. Washington, DC: Author.

American Chiropractic Association. (1991). *Chiropractic: State of the art 1991-1992*. Arlington, VA: Author.

American College of Obstetricians and Gynecologists [ACOG]. (1985). *Exercise during pregnancy and the postnatal period. ACOG home exercise programs*. Washington, DC: Author.

American College of Obstetricians and Gynecologists [ACOG]. (1994). *Exercise during pregnancy and the postpartum period* (ACOG Technical Bulletin, No. 189). Washington, DC: Author.

The American contortionist. (1882). *Lancet*, 1, 618.

American Medical Association. Subcommittee on Classification of Sports Injuries. (1966). *Standard nomenclature of athletic injuries*. Chicago: Author.

American Orthopaedic Association. (1985). *Manual of orthopaedic surgery*. Chicago: Author.

Anderson, B. (1978). The perfect pre-run stretching routine. *Runners World*, 13(5), 56-61.

Anderson, B. (1980). *Stretching*. Bolinas, CA: Shelter.

Anderson, B. (1985). Stretch: A key to body awareness. *Shape*. 4(3), 37-42.

Anderson, M.B. (1979). Comparison of muscle patterning in the overarm throw and tennis serve. *Research Quarterly* 50(4), 541-553.

Andersson, G.B.J., Herberts, T.N., and Örtengren, R. (1977). Quantitative electromyographic studies of back muscle activity related to posture and loading. *Orthopaedic Clinics of North America*, 8(1), 85-86.

Andren, L., and Borglin, N.E. (1961). Disturbed urinary excretion pattern of oestrogens in newborns with congenital dislocation of the hip. I. The excretion of oestrogen during the first few days of life. *Acta Endocrinologica*, 37(3), 423-433.

Andrews, J.R. (1983). Overuse syndromes of the lower extremity. *Clinics in Sports Medicine*, 2(1), 137-148.

Ansell, B.A. (1972). Hypermobility of joints. In A.G. Apley (Ed.), *Modern trends in orthopaedics* (pp. 25-39). New York: Appleton-Century-Crofts.

Armstrong, C.G., O'Connor, P., and Gardner, D.L. (1992). Mechanical basis of connective tissue disease. In D.L. Gardner (Ed.), *Pathological basis of the connective tissue diseases* (pp. 261-281). Philadelphia: Lea & Febiger.

Armstrong, J.R. (1958). *Lumbar disc lesions*. London: E & S Livingstone.

Armstrong, R.B. (1984). Mechanisms of exercise-induced delayed onset muscle soreness. *Medicine and Science in Sport*, 9(1), 111-26.

Armstrong, R.B., Ogilvie, R.W., and Schwane, J.A. (1983). Eccentric exercise-induced injury to rat skeletal muscle. *Journal of Applied Physiology*, 54(1), 80-93.

Armstrong, R.B., Warren, G.L., and Warren, J.R. (1991). Mechanisms of exercise-induced muscle fibre injury. *Sports Medicine*, 12(3), 184-207.

Arner, O., and Lindholm, A. (1958). What is tennis leg? *Acta Chirurgica Scandinavica*, 116(1), 73-77.

Arnheim, D.D. (1971). Stretching. In L.A. Larson (Ed.), *Encyclopedia of sport sciences and medicine* (pp. 165-166). New York: Macmillan.

Arnheim, D.D. (1989). *Modern principles of athletic training* (7th ed.). St. Louis: Times Mirror/Mosby.

Ashmore, C.R. (1982). Stretch-induced growth in chicken wing muscles: Effects on hereditary muscular dystrophy. *American Journal of Physiology*, 242 (Cell Physiology 11), C178-C183.

Asmussen, E. (1953). Positive and negative work. *Acta Physiologica Scandinavica*, 28(4), 364-382.

Asmussen, E. (1956). Observations on experimental muscle soreness. *Acta Rheumatologica Scandinavica*, 2, 109-116.

Asmussen, E., and Bonde-Petersen, F. (1974). Storage of elastic energy in skeletal muscles in man. *Acta Physiologica Scandinavica*, 91(3), 385-392.

Aspden, R.M. (1988). A new mathematical model of the spine and its relationship to spinal loading in the workplace. *Applied Ergonomics*, 19(4), 319-323.

Asterita, M.F. (1985). *The physiology of stress*. New York: Human Science Press.

Aten, D.W., and Knight, K.T. (1978). Therapeutic exercise in athletic training: Principles and overview. *Athletic Training*, 13(3), 123-126.

Athenstaedt, H. (1970). Permanent longitudinal electric polarization and pyroelectric behaviour of collagenous structures and nervous tissue in man and other vertebrates. *Nature*, 228(5274), 830-834.

Atwater, A.A. (1967, October). What film analysis tells us about movement. Paper presented at the *Annual Meeting of the Midwest Association for Physical Education of College Women*, French Lick, IN.

Atwater, A.A. (1979). Biomechanics of overarm throwing movements and of throwing injuries. *Exercise and Sport Sciences Reviews*, 7, 43-85.

Auber, J., and Couteaux, R. (1962). L'attache des myofilaments secondaires au niveau de la strie y dans les muscles de dipteres. *Comptes Rendus des Seances de L'Academie des Sciences*, 254, 3425-3426.

Auber, J., and Couteaux, R. (1963). Ultrastructure de la strie y dans les muscles de dipteres. *Journal de Microscopie*, 2(3), 309-324.

Aura, O., and Komi, P.V. (1986). Mechanical efficiency of pure positive and pure negative work with special reference to the work intensity. *International Journal of Sports Medicine*, 7(1), 44-49.

Baatsen, P.H., Trombitas, W.K., and Pollack, G.H. (1988). Thick filaments of striated muscle are laterally interconnected. *Journal of Ultrastructure and Molecular Structure Research*, 98(3), 267-280.

Baddeley, S., and Green, S. (1992). Physical education and the pregnant woman: The way forward. *Midwives Chronicle & Nursing Notes*, 105(1253), 144-145.

Badtke, G., Bittmann, F., and Lazik, D. (1993). Changes in the vertebral column in the course of the day. *International Journal of Sports Medicine*, 14(3), 159.

Balaftsalis, H. (1982-1983). Knee joint laxity contributing to footballers' injuries. *Physiotherapy in Sport*, 5(3), 26-27.

Baldissera, F., Hultborn, H., and Illert, M. (1981). Integration in spinal neuronal systems. In *Handbook of physiology. Sec. 1. The nervous system.* (Vol. 2, Part 1, pp. 509-595). Bethesda, MD: American Physiological Society.

Ballantyne, B.T., Reser, M.D., Lorenz, G.W., and Smidt, G.L. (1986). The effects of inversion traction on spinal column configuration, heart rate, blood pressure, and perceived discomfort. *Journal of Orthopaedic and Sports Physical Therapy,* 7(5), 254-260.

Bandy, W.D., and Irion, J.M. (1994). The effect of time on static stretch on the flexibility of the hamstring muscles. *Physical Therapy,* 74(9), 845-850.

Banker, I.A. (1980). The isolated mammalian muscle spindle. *Trends in Neuroscience,* 3(11), 258-265.

Barker, D. (1974). The morphology of muscle receptors. In C.C. Hunt (Ed.), *Handbook of sensory physiology. Muscle receptors* (Vol. 3, Part 2, pp. 1-190). New York: Springer.

Barnard, R.J., Gardner, G.W., Diaco, N.V., McAlpin, R.N., and Kattus, A.A. (1973). Cardiovascular responses to sudden strenuous exercise—Heart rate, blood pressure and ECG. *Journal of Applied Physiology,* 34(6), 833-837.

Barnard, R.J., McAlpin, R., Kattus, A.A., and Buckberg, G.D. (1973). Ischemic response to sudden exercise in healthy men. *Circulation,* 48(5), 936-942.

Barnes, J. (1991). Myofascial release: Its importance to the massage therapy profession. *Massage Message,* 6(1), 4-7.

Barnett, C.H. (1971). The mobility of synovial joints. *Rheumatology and Physical Medicine* 11(February), 20-27.

Barnett, J.G., Holly, R.G., and Ashmore, C.R. (1980). Stretch-induced growth in chicken wing muscles: Biochemical and morphological characterization. *American Journal of Physiology,* Cell Physiology 8, 239, C39-C46.

Barney, V.S., Hirst, C.C., and Jensen, C.R. (1972). *Conditioning exercises: Exercises to improve body form and function* (3rd ed.). St. Louis: Mosby.

Barr, M. (1979). *The human nervous system, an anatomic viewpoint* (3rd ed.). Hagerstown, MD: Harper & Row.

Barrack, R.L., Skinner, H.B., Brunet, M.E., and Cook, S.D. (1983). Joint laxity and proprioception in the knee. *The Physician and Sportsmedicine,* 11(6), 130-135.

Barry, W., Cashman, R., Coote, S., Hastings, B., and Imperatrice, M. (1987). The relationship between lung function and thoracic mobility in normal subjects. *New Zealand Journal of Physiotherapy,* 15(1), 9-11.

Bartelink, D.L. (1957). The role of abdominal pressure in relieving pressure on the lumbar intervertebral discs. *Journal of Bone and Joint Surgery,* 39B(4), 718-725.

Basmajian, J.V. (1963). Control and training of individual motor units. *Science,* 141(3579), 440-441.

Basmajian, J.V. (1967). Control of individual motor units. *American Journal of Physical Medicine,* 46(1), 480-486.

Basmajian, J.V. (1972). Electromyography comes of age. *Science,* 176(4035), 603-609.

Basmajian, J.V. (1975). Motor learning and control. *Archives of Physical Medicine and Rehabilitation,* 58(1), 38-41.

Basmajian, J.V. (1981). Biofeedback in rehabilitation: A review of principles and practices. *Archives of Physical Medicine and Rehabilitation,* 62(10), 469-475.

Basmajian, J.V., Baeza, M., and Fabrigar, C. (1965). Conscious control and training of individual spinal motor neurons in normal human subjects. *Journal of New Drugs,* 5(2), 78-85.

Bassey, E.J., Morgan, K., Dallosso, H.M., and Ebrahim, S.B.J. (1989). Flexibility of the shoulder joint measured as range of abduction in a large representative sample of men and women over 65 years of age. *European Journal of Applied Physiology,* 58(4), 353-360.

Bates, R.A. (1971). *Flexibility training: The optimal time period to spend in a position of maximal stretch.* Unpublished master's thesis, University of Alberta, Edmonton.

Bates, R.A. (1976). Flexibility development: Mind over matter. In J.H. Salmela (Ed.), *The advanced study of gymnastics* (pp. 233-241). Springfield, IL: Charles C Thomas.

Battié, M.C., Bigos, S.J., Fisher, L.D., Spengler, D.M., Hansson, T.H., Nachemson, A.L., and Wortley, M.D. (1990). The role of spinal flexibility in back pain complaints within industry: A prospective study. *Spine,* 15(8), 768-773.

Battié, M.C., Bigos, S.J., Sheehy, A., and Wortley, M.D. (1987). Spinal flexibility and individual factors that influence it. *Physical Therapy,* 67(5), 653-658.

Bauman, P.A., Singson, R., and Hamilton, W.G. (1994). Femoral neck anteversion in ballerinas. *Clinical Orthopaedics and Related Research,* 302(May), 57-63.

Baxter, C., and Reilly, T. (1983). Influence of time of day on all-out swimming. *British Journal of Sports Medicine,* 17(2), 122-127.

Baxter, D.E., and Davis, P.F. (1995). Rehabilitation of the elite athlete. In D.E. Baxter (Ed.), *The foot and ankle in sport* (pp. 379-392). St. Louis: Mosby.

Beauchamp, M., Labelle, H., Grimard, G., Stanciu, C., Poitras, B., and Dansereau, J. (1993). Diurnal variation of cobb angle measurement in adolescent idiopathic scoliosis. *Spine,* 18(12), 1581-1583.

Beaulieu, J.E. (1981). Developing a stretching program. *The Physician and Sportsmedicine,* 9(11), 59-69.

Beccaria, C.W. (1764). *On crimes and punishment* (H. Paolucci, Trans.). New York: Bobbs-Merrill, 1963.

Bechbache, R.R., and Duffin, J. (1977). The entrainment of breathing frequency by exercise rhythm. *Journal of Physiology* (London), 272, 553-561.

Becker, A.H. (1979). Traction for knee-flexion contractures. *Physical Therapy,* 59(9), 1114.

Beekman, S., and Block, B.H. (1975). The relationship of calcaneal varus to hamstring tightening. *Current Podiatry,* 24(11), 7-10.

Beel, J.A., Groswald, D.E., and Luttges, M.W. (1984). Alterations in the mechanical properties of peripheral nerve following crush injury. *Journal of Biomechanics,* 17(3), 185-193.

Beel, J.A., Stodieck, L.S., and Luttges, M.W. (1986). Structural properties of spinal nerve roots: Biomechanics. *Experimental Neurology,* 91(1), 30-40, 1986.

Beighton, P. (1971). How contortionists contort. *Medical Times,* 99(4), 181-187.

Beighton, P., Grahame, R., and Bird, H. (1983). *Hypermobility of joints.* Berlin: Springer-Verlag.

Beighton, P., and Horan, F.T. (1969). Orthopaedic aspects of the Ehlers-Danlos syndrome. *Journal of Bone and Joint Surgery,* 51B(3), 444-453.

Beighton, P., and Horan, F.T. (1970). Dominant inheritance in familial generalized articular hypermobility. *Journal of Bone and Joint Surgery,* 52B(1), 145-147.

Beighton, P.H., Solomon, L., and Soskolne, C.L. (1973). Articular mobility in an African population. *Annals of the Rheumatic Diseases,* 32(5), 413-418.

Bell, R.D., and Hoshizaki, T.B. (1981). Relationship of age and sex with range of motion of seventeen joint actions in humans. *Canadian Journal of Applied Sports Science,* 6(4), 202-206.

Bencke, A. (1897). Zur Lewre von der Spondylitis deformans—Beitrag zur wissenschaftlicher Medizin. *Festschrift an der 59 Versammlung deutscher Naturforscher und Arete,* Braundschweig, Germany.

Benjamin, B.E. (1978). *Are you tense?* New York: Pantheon Books.

Benson, H. (1980). *The relaxation response.* New York: Avon Books.

Berland, T., and Addison, R.G. (1972). *Living with your bad back.* New York: St. Martin's Press.

Bernstein, D.A., and Borkovec, T.D. (1973). *Progressive relaxation training.* Champaign, IL: Research Press.

Bertolasi, L., De Grandis, D., Bongiovanni, L.G., Zanette, G.P., and Gasperini, M. (1993). The influence of muscular lengthening on cramps. *Annals of Neurology,* 33(2), 176-180.

Bick, E.M. (1961). Aging in the connective tissues of the human musculoskeletal system. *Geriatrics,* 16(9), 448-453.

Biesterfeldt, H.J. (1974). Flexibility program. *International Gymnast,* 16(3), 22-23.

Bigland-Ritchie, B., and Woods, J.J. (1976). Integrated electromyogram and oxygen uptake during positive and negative work. *Journal of Physiology* (London), 260(2), 267-277.

Billig, H.E. (1943). Dysmenorrhea: The result of a postural defect. *Archives of Surgery,* 46(5), 611-613.

Billig, H.E. (1951). Fascial stretching. *Journal of Physical and Mental Rehabilitation,* 5(1), 4-8.

Billig, H.E., and Lowendahl, E. (1949). *Mobilization of the human body.* Stanford: Stanford University Press.

Bird, H. (1979). Joint laxity in sport. *MediSport: The Review of Sports Medicine,* 1(5), 30-31.

Bird, H.A., Brodie, D.A., and Wright, V. (1979). Quantification of joint laxity. *Rheumatology and Rehabilitation,* 18, 161-166.

Bird, H.A., Calguneri, M., and Wright, V. (1981). Changes in joint laxity occurring during pregnancy. *Annals of the Rheumatic Diseases,* 40(2), 209-212.

Bird, H.A., Hudson, A., Eastmond, C.J., and Wright, V. (1980). Joint laxity and osteoarthritis: A radiological survey of female physical education specialists. *British Journal of Sports Medicine,* 14(4), 179-188.

Biro, F., Gewanter, H.L., and Baum, J. (1983). The hypermobility syndrome. *Pediatrics,* 72(5), 701-706.

Bissell, M.J., Hall, H.G., and Parry, G. (1982). How does the extracellular matrix direct gene expression? *Journal of Theoretical Biology,* 99(1), 31-68.

Blau, H. (1989). How fixed is the differentiated state? Lessons from heterokaryons. *Trends in Genetics,* 5(8), 268-272.

Block, R.A., Hess, L.A., Timpano, E.V., and Serlo, C. (1985). Physiological changes in foot in pregnancy. *Journal of the American Podiatric Medical Association,* 75(6), 297-299.

Bloom, W., and Fawcett, D.W. (1986). *A textbook of histology* (11th ed.). Philadelphia: W.B. Saunders.

Bloomfield, J., and Blanksby, B.A. (1971). Strength, flexibility and anthropometric measurements. *Australian Journal of Sports Medicine,* 3(10), 8-15.

Bloomfield, J., Blanksby, B.A., Ackland, T.R., and Elliott, B.C. (1985). The anatomical and physiological characteristics of pre-adolescent swimmers, tennis players and non competitors. *The Australian Journal of Science and Medicine in Sport,* 17(3), 19-23.

Bobbert, M.F., Hollander, A.P., and Huijing, P.A. (1986). Factors in delayed onset muscular soreness of man. *Medicine and Science in Sports and Exercise,* 18(1), 75-81.

Bogduk, N. (1984). Applied anatomy of the thoracolumbar fascia. *Spine,* 9(9), 164-170.

Bohannon, R., Gajdovsik, R., and LeVeau, B. (1985). Contribution of pelvic and lower limb motion to increase in the angle of passive straight leg raising. *Physical Therapy,* 65(4), 474-476.

Bompa, T. (1990). *Theory and methodology of training* (2nd ed.). Dubuque, IA: Kendall/Hunt.

Bonci, C.M., Hensal, F.J., and Torg, J.S. (1986). A preliminary study on the measurement of static and dynamic motion at the glenohumeral joint. *The American Journal of Sports Medicine,* 14(1), 12-17.

Boocock, M.G., Garbutt, G., Linge, G., Reilly, T., and Troup, J.D.G. (1990). Changes in stature following drop jumping and post-exercise gravity inversion. *Medicine and Science in Sports and Exercise,* 22(3), 385-390.

Boocock, M.G., Garbutt, G., Reilly, T., Linge, G., and Troup, J.D.G. (1988). The effects of gravity inversion on exercise-induced spinal loading. *Ergonomics,* 31(11), 1631-1637.

Boone, D.C., and Azen, S.P. (1979). Normal range of motion of joints in male subjects. *Journal of Bone and Joint Surgery,* 61A(5), 756-759.

Booth, F.W., and Gould, W. (1975). Training and disuse on connective tissue. In J. Wilmore and J. Keough (Eds.), *Exercise and sports sciences reviews* (Vol. 3, pp. 83-112). New York: Academic Press.

Borg, T.K., and Caulfield, J.B. (1980). Morphology of connective tissue in skeletal muscle. *Tissue & Cell,* 12(1), 197-207.

Borkovec, T.D., and Sides, J.K. (1979). Critical procedural variables related to the physiological effects of progressive relaxation: A review. *Behaviour Research and Therapy,* 17(2), 119-125.

Borms, J., Van Roy, P., Santens, J.P., and Haentjens, A. (1987). Optimal duration of static stretching exercises for improvement of coxo-femoral flexibility. *Journal of Sports Sciences,* 5(1), 39-47.

Bornstein, P., and Byers, P.H. (1980). Collagen metabolism. *Current Concepts.* Kalamazoo: The Upjohn Company.

Boscardin, J.B., Johnson, P., and Schneider, H. (1989). The windup, the pitch, and pre-season conditioning. *SportCare & Fitness,* 2(1), 30-35.

Boscoe, C., Tarkka, I., and Komi, P.V. (1982). Effects of elastic energy and myoelectrical potentiation of triceps surae during stretch-shortening cycle exercise. *International Journal of Sports Medicine,* 3(3), 137-140.

Bosien, W.R., Staples, D.S., and Russell, S.W. (1955). Residual disability following acute ankle sprains. *Journal of Bone and Joint Surgery,* 37A(6), 1237-1243.

Botsford, D.J., Esses, S.I., and Ogilvie-Harris, D.J. (1994). In vivo diurnal variation in intervertebral disc volume and morphology. *Spine,* 19(8), 935-940.

Bowen, W.P. (1934). *Applied kinesiology* (5th ed.). Philadelphia: Lea & Febiger.

Bowker, J.H., and Thompson, E.B. (1964). Surgical treatment of recurrent dislocation of the patella. *Journal of Bone and Joint Surgery,* 46A(7), 1451-1461.

Bozeman, M., Mackie, J., and Kaufmann, D.A. (1986). Quadriceps, hamstring strength and flexibility. *Track Technique,* 96(Summer), 3060-3061.

Brand, R.A. (1986). Knee ligaments: A new view. *Journal of Biomechanical Engineering,* 108(2), 106-110.

Brant, J. (1987). See Dick run: Videotape analysis of your running form can make you a more efficient runner. *Runner's World,* 22(7), 28-35.

Brendstrup, P. (1962). Late edema after muscular exercise. *Archives of Physical Medicine and Rehabilitation,* 43(8), 401-405.

Brewer, B., Wubben, R., and Carrera, G. (1986). Excessive retroversion of the glenoid cavity. *Journal of Bone and Joint Surgery,* 68A(5), 724-731.

Brewer, V., and Hinson, M. (1978). Relationship of pregnancy to lateral knee stability. *Medicine and Science in Sports*, 10(1), 39.

Brincat, M., Versi, E., Moniz, C.F., Magos, A., de Trafford, J., and Studd, J.W.W. (1987). Skin collagen changes in postmenopausal women receiving different regimens of estrogen therapy. *Obstetrics and Gynecology*, 70(1), 123-127.

Brodelius, A. (1961). Osteoarthrosis of the talar joints in footballers and ballet dancers. *Acta Orthopaedica Scandinavica*, 30(4), 309-314.

Brodie, D.A., Bird, H.A., and Wright, V. (1982). Joint laxity in selected athletic populations. *Medicine and Science in Sports and Exercise*, 14(3), 190-193.

Brody, D.M. (1995). Running injuries. In J.A. Nicholas and E.B. Hershman (Eds.), *The lower extremity and spine in sports medicine* (2nd ed., vol. 2, pp. 1475-1507). St. Louis: Mosby.

Broer, M.R. (1966). *Efficiency of human movement* (2nd ed.). Philadelphia: W.B. Saunders.

Broer, M.R., and Gales, N.R. (1958). Importance of various body measurements in performance of toe touch test. *Research Quarterly*, 29(3), 253-257.

Brooks, G.A., and Fahey, T.D. (1987). *Fundamentals of human performance*. New York: Macmillan.

Browne, A.O., Hoffmeyer, P., Tanaka, S., An, K.N., and Morrey, B.F. (1990). Glenohumeral elevation studied in three dimensions. *Journal of Bone and Joint Surgery*, 72B(5), 843-845.

Browse, N.L., Young, A.E., and Thomas, M.L. (1979). The effect of bending on canine and human arterial walls and on blood flow. *Circulation Research*, 45(1), 41-47.

Bryant, S. (1984). Flexibility and stretching. *The Physician and Sportsmedicine*, 12(2), 171.

Bryant, W.M. (1977). Wound healing. *Clinical Symposia*, 29(3), 1-36.

Bryant-Greenwood, G.D., and Schwabe, C. (1994). Human relaxins: Chemistry and biology. *Endocrine Reviews*, 15(1), 5-26.

Buerger, A.A. (1984). A non-redundant taxonomy of spinal manipulative techniques suitable for physiologic explanation. *Manual Medicine*, 1(2), 54-58.

Buller, A.J. (1968). Spinal reflex action. *Physiotherapy*, 54(6), 208-210.

Bunn, J.W. (1972). *Scientific principles of coaching* (2nd ed.). Englewood Cliffs, NJ: Prentice-Hall.

Burgener, M. (1991). How to properly miss with a barbell. *National Strength and Conditioning Journal*, 13(3), 24-25.

Burke, D., Hagbarth, K.E., and Lofstedt, L. (1978). Muscle spindle activity in man during shortening and lengthening contraction. *Journal of Physiology* (London), 277(April), 131-142.

Burke, E.J., and Humphreys, J.H.L. (1982). *Fit to exercise*. London: Pecham Books.

Burke, R.E., and Rudomin, P. (1978). Spinal neurons and synapses. In E.R. Kandel (Ed.), *Handbook of physiology: The nervous system. Cellular biology of neurons* (pp. 877-944). Baltimore, MD: Williams & Wilkins.

Burkett, L.N. (1970). Causative factors in hamstring strain. *Medicine and Science in Sports*, 2(1), 39-42.

Burkett, L.N. (1971). Cause and prevention of hamstring pulls. *Athletic Journal*, 51(6), 34.

Burkett, L.N. (1975). Investigation into hamstring strains: The case of the hybrid muscle. *The Journal of Sports Medicine and Physical Fitness*, 3(5), 228-231.

Burkhardt, S. (1982). The rationale for joint mobilization. In G.W. Bell (Ed.), *Professional preparation in athletic training* (pp. 101-106). Champaign, IL: Human Kinetics.

Burley, L.R., Dobell, H.C., and Farrell, B.J. (1961). Relations of power, speed, flexibility and certain anthropometric measures of junior high school girls. *Research Quarterly*, 32(4), 443-448.

Buroker, K.C., and Schwane, J.A. (1989). Does postexercise static stretching alleviate delayed muscle soreness? *The Physician and Sportsmedicine*, 17(6), 65-83.

Bush, J. (1978). *Dynamic track & field*. Boston: Allyn & Bacon.

Buxton, D. (1957). Extension of the Kraus-Weber test. *Research Quarterly*, 28(3), 210-217.

Byers, P.H., Pyeritz, R.E., and Uitto, J. (1992). Research perspectives in heritable disorders of connective tissue. *Matrix*, 12(4), 333-342.

Byrd, R.J. (1973). The effect of controlled, mild exercise on the rate of physiological aging in rats. *Journal of Sports Medicine and Physical Fitness*, 13(1), 1-3.

Byrd, S.K. (1992). Alterations in the sarcoplasmic reticulum: A possible link to exercise-induced muscle damage. *Medicine and Science in Sports and Exercise*, 24(5), 531-536.

Byrnes, W.C., and Clarkson, P.M. (1986). Delayed onset muscle soreness and training. *Clinics in Sports Medicine*, 5(3), 605-614.

Byrnes, W.C., Clarkson, P.M., White, J.S., Hsieh, S.S., Frykman, P.N., and Maughan, R.J. (1985). Delayed onset muscle soreness following repeated bouts of downhill running. *Journal of Applied Physiology*, 59(3), 710-713.

Cailliet, R. (1966). *Shoulder pain*. Philadelphia: F.A. Davis.

Cailliet, R. (1977). *Soft tissue pain and disability*. Philadelphia: F.A. Davis.

Cailliet, R. (1981). *Low back pain syndrome* (3rd ed.). Philadelphia: F.A. Davis.

Cailliet, R. (1985). Gravity inversion therapy. *Postgraduate Medicine*, 77(6), 270 and 274.

Cailliet, R. (1988). *Low back pain syndrome* (4th ed.). Philadelphia: F.A. Davis.

Cailliet, R. (1991). *Shoulder pain* (3rd ed.). Philadelphia: F.A. Davis.

Cailliet, R., and Gross, L. (1987). *The rejuvenation strategy*. Garden City, NY: Doubleday.

Calais-Germain, B. (1993). *Anatomy of movement*. Seattle: Eastland Press.

Caldwell, W.E., and Moloy, H.C. (1993). Anatomical variations in the female pelvis and their effect in labor with a suggested classification. *American Journal of Obstetrics and Gynecology*, 26(4), 479-505.

Calguneri, M., Bird, H.A., and Wright, V. (1982). Changes in joint laxity occurring during pregnancy. *Annals of the Rheumatic Diseases*, 41(2), 126-128.

Campbell, E.J.M. (1970). Accessory muscles. In E.J.M. Campbell, E. Agostoni, and J.N. Davis (Eds.), *The respiratory muscles mechanics and neural control* (pp. 181-193). Philadelphia: W.B. Saunders.

Cantu, R.C. (1982). *Sports medicine in primary care*. Lexington, MA: Collamore Press.

Cantu, R.I., and Grodin, A.J. (1992). *Myofascial manipulation: Theory and clinical application*. Gaithersburg, MD: Aspen.

Capaday, C., and Stein, R.B. (1987a). Amplitude modulation of the soleus H-reflex in the human during walking and standing. *Journal of Neuroscience Methods*, 21(2-4), 91-104.

Capaday, C., and Stein, R.B. (1987b). Difference in the amplitude of the human soleus H-reflex during walking and running. *Journal of Physiology* (London), 392(November), 513-522.

Carlsen, F., Knappels, G.G., and Buchthal, F. (1961). Ultrastructure of the resting and contracted striated muscle fiber at different degrees of stretch. *Journal of Biophysical and Biochemical Cytology*, 10(1), 95-118.

Carlson, F.D., and Wilkie, D.R. (1974). *Muscle physiology*. Englewood Cliffs, NJ: Prentice-Hall.

Carrico, M. (1986). Yoga with a chair. *Yoga Journal*, 68(May/June), 45-51.

Carter, C., and Sweetnam, R. (1958). Familial joint laxity and recurrent dislocation of the patella. *Journal of Bone and Joint Surgery*, 40B(4), 664-667.

Carter, C., and Sweetnam, R. (1960). Recurrent dislocation of the patella and the shoulder. *Journal of Bone and Joint Surgery*, 42B(4), 721-727.

Carter, C., and Wilkinson, J. (1964). Persistent joint laxity and congenital dislocation of the hip. *Journal of Bone and Joint Surgery*, 46B(1), 40-45.

Cassidy, J.D., Quon, J.A., Lafrance, L.J., and Yong-Hing, K. (1992). The effect of manipulation on pain and range of motion in the cervical spine: A pilot study. *Journal of Manipulative and Physiological Therapeutics*, 15(8), 495-500.

Cassidy, S.S., and Schwiep, F. (1989). Cardiovascular effects of positive end-expiratory pressure. In S.M. Scharf and S.S. Cassidy (Eds.), *Heart-lung interactions in health and disease* (pp. 463-506). New York: Marcel Dekker.

Cavagna, G.A., Dusman, B., and Margaria, R. (1968). Positive work done by a previously stretched muscle. *Journal of Applied Physiology*, 24(1), 21-32.

Cavagna, G.A., Saibene, F.P., and Margaria, R. (1965). Effect of negative work on the amount of positive work performed by an isolated muscle. *Journal of Applied Physiology*, 20(1), 157-160.

Chaitow, L. (1990). *Osteopathic self-treatment*. Rochester, VT: Thorsons.

Chandler, T.J., Kibler, W.B., Uhl, T.L., Wooten, B., Kiser, A., and Stone, E. (1990). Flexibility comparisons of junior elite tennis players to other athletes. *American Journal of Sports Medicine*, 18(2), 134-136.

Chang, D.E., Buschbacher, L.P., and Edlich, R.F. (1988). Limited joint mobility in power lifters. *American Journal of Sports Medicine*, 16(3), 280-284.

Chapman, E.A., de Vries, H.A., and Swezey, R. (1972). Joint stiffness: Effects of exercise on young and old men. *Journal of Gerontology*, 27(2), 218-221.

Chapron, D.J., and Besdine, R.W. (1987). Drugs as obstacle to rehabilitation of the elderly: A primer for therapists. *Topics in Geriatric Rehabilitation*, 2(3), 63-81.

Chatfield, S.J., Byrnes, W.C., Lally, D.A., and Rowe, S.E. (1990). Cross-sectional physiologic profiling of modern dancers. *Dance Research Journal*, 22(1), 13-20.

Cheng, J.C.Y., Chan, P.S., and Hui, P.W. (1991). Joint laxity in children. *Journal of Pediatric Orthopaedics*, 11(6), 752-756.

Cherry, D.B. (1980). Review of physical therapy alternatives for reducing muscle contracture. *Physical Therapy*, 60(7), 877-881.

Child, A.H. (1986). Joint hypermobility syndrome: Inherited disorder of collagen synthesis. *Journal of Rheumatology*, 13(2), 239-243.

Chinn, C.J., Priest, J.D., and Kent, B.E. (1974). Upper extremity range of motion, grip strength, and girth in highly skilled tennis players. *Physical Therapy*, 54(5), 474-483.

Chowrashi, P.K., Pemrick, S.M., and Pepe, F.A. (1989). LC2 involvement in the assembly of skeletal myosin filaments. *Biochemica et Biophysica Acta* (24) 990(2), 216-223.

Christian, G.F., Stanton, G.J., Sissons, D., How, H.Y., Jamison, J., Alder, B., Fullerton, M., and Funder, J.W. (1988). Immunoreactive ACTH, β-endorphin, and cortisol levels in plasma following spinal manipulative therapy. *Spine*, 13(12), 1411-1417.

Christiansen, C., and Baum, C. (1991). Performance deficits as sources of stress. In C. Christiansen and C. Baum (Eds.), *Occupational therapy: Overcoming human performance deficits* (pp. 68-96). Thorofare, NJ: Slack.

Chujoy, A., and Manchester, P.W. (Eds.). (1967). *The dance encyclopedia*. New York: Simon and Schuster.

Ciullo, J.V., and Zarins, B. (1983). Biomechanics of the musculotendinous unit. *Clinics in Sports Medicine*, 2(1), 71-85.

Clark, J.M., Hagerman, F.C., and Gelfand, R. (1983). Breathing patterns during submaximal and maximal exercise in elite oarsmen. *Journal of Applied Physiology*, 55(2), 440-446.

Clarke, H.H. (1975). Joint and body range of movement. *Physical Fitness Research Digest*, 5, 16-18.

Clarkson, P.M., Byrnes, W.C., Gillison, E., and Harper, E. (1987). Adaptation to exercise-induced muscle damage. *Clinical Science*, 73(4), 383-386.

Clarkson, P.M., and Tremblay, I. (1988). Rapid adaptation to exercise induced muscle damage. *Journal of Applied Physiology*, 65(1), 1-6.

Cleak, M.J., and Eston, R.G. (1992). Delayed onset muscle soreness: Mechanisms and management. *Journal of Sports Sciences*, 10(4), 325-341.

Clemente, C.D. (1985). *Anatomy of the human body* (30th ed.). Philadelphia: Lea & Febiger.

Clippinger-Robertson, K. (1988). Understanding contraindicated exercises. *Dance Exercise Today*, 6(1), 57-60.

Cohen, D.B., Mont, M.A., Campbell, K.R., Vogelstein, B.N., and Loewy, J.W. (1994). Upper extremity physical factors affecting tennis serve velocity. *American Journal of Sports Medicine*, 22(6), 746-750.

Colachis, S.C., and Strohm, B.R. (1965). Relationship of time to varied tractive force with constant angle of pull. *Archives of Physical Medicine and Rehabilitation*, 46(11), 815-819.

Committee on the Medical Aspects of Sports of the American Medical Association and the National Federation. (1975). Muscle soreness can be eliminated. *Athletic Training*, 10(1), 42.

Condon, S.A. (1983). *Resistance to muscle stretch induced by volitional muscle contraction*. Unpublished master's thesis, University of Washington, Seattle.

Condon, S.A., and Hutton, R.S. (1987). Soleus muscle electromyographic activity and ankle dorsiflexion range of motion during four stretching procedures. *Physical Therapy*, 67(1), 24-30.

Conroy, R.T.W.L., and Mills, J.N. (1970). *Human circadian rhythms*. London: Churchill.

A contortionist. (1882). *Lancet*, 1, 576.

Cook, E.E., Gray, V.L., Savinar-Nogue, E., and Medeiros, J. (1987). Shoulder antagonistic strength ratios: A comparison between college level baseball pitchers and nonpitchers. *Journal of Orthopaedic and Sports Physical Therapy*, 8(9), 451-461.

Cooke, P. (1985). A periodic cytoskeletal lattice in striated muscle. In J.W. Shay (Ed.), *Cell and muscle mobility* (Vol. 6, pp. 287-313). New York: Plenum Press.

Coplans, C.W. (1978). The conservative treatment of low back pain. In A.J. Heflet and D.M.G. Lee (Eds.), *Disorders of the lumbar spine* (pp. 145-182). Philadelphia: Lippincott.

Corbett, M. (1972). The use and abuse of massage and exercise. *The Practitioner*, 208(1243), 136-139.

Corbin, C.B. (1980). *A textbook of motor development* (2nd ed.). Dubuque, IA: Brown.

Corbin, C.B., Dowell, L.J., Lindsey, R., and Tolson, H. (1978). *Concepts in physical education* (3rd ed.). Dubuque, IA: Brown.

Corbin, C.B., and Noble, L. (1980). Flexibility: A major component of physical fitness. *Journal of Physical Education and Recreation*, 51(6), 23-24, 57-60.

Corlett, E.N., Eklund, J.A.E., Reilly, T., and Troup, J.D.G. (1987). Assessment of workload from measurements of stature. *Applied Ergonomics*, 18(1), 65-71.

Cornelius, W.L. (1983). Stretch evoked EMG activity by isometric contraction and submaximal concentric contraction. *Athletic Training*, 18(2), 106-109.

Cornelius, W.L. (1984). Exercise beneficial to the hip but questionable for the knee. *NSCA Journal*, 6(5), 40-41.

Cornelius, W.L., Hagemann, R.W., and Jackson, A.W. (1988). A study on placement of stretching within a workout. *Journal of Sports Medicine and Physical Fitness*, 28(3), 234-236.

Cornelius, W.L., and Hinson, M.M. (1980). The relationship between isometric contractions of hip extensors and subsequent flexibility in males. *Journal of Sports Medicine and Physical Fitness*, 20(1), 75-80.

Couch, J. (1979). *Runner's World yoga book*. Mountain View, CA: World.

Counsilman, J.E. (1968). *The science of swimming*. Englewood Cliffs, NJ: Prentice-Hall.

Counsilman, J.E. (1977). *The complete book of swimming*. New York: Antheneum.

Cousins, N. (1979). *Anatomy of an illness as perceived by the patient*. New York: Norton.

Coville, C.A. (1979). Relaxation in physical education curricula. *The Physical Educator*, 36(4), 176-181.

Cowan, P.M., McGavin, S., and North, A.C. (1955). The polypeptide chain configuration of collagen. *Nature*, 176(4492), 1062-1064.

Craig, T.T. (Ed.). (1973). *American medical association comments in sports medicine*. Chicago: American Medical Association.

Cramer, L.M., and McQueen, C.H. (1990). Overuse injuries in figure skating. In M.J. Casey, C. Foster, and E.G. Hixson (Eds.), *Winter sports medicine* (pp. 254-268). Philadelphia: Davis.

Crawford, H.J., and Jull, G.A. (1993). The influence of thoracic posture and movement on range of arm elevation. *Physiotherapy Theory and Practice*, 9(3), 143-148.

Crisp, J. (1972). Properties of tendon and skin. In Y.C. Yung, N. Perrone, and M. Anliker (Eds.), *Biomechanics: Its foundation and objectives* (pp. 141-180). Englewood Cliffs, NJ: Prentice-Hall.

Crosman, L.J., Chateauvert, S.R., and Weisberg, J. (1984). The effects of massage to the hamstring muscle group on the range of motion. *Journal of Orthopaedic and Sports Physical Therapy*, 6(3), 168-172.

Cummings, G.S. (1984). Comparison of muscle to other soft tissue in limiting elbow extension. *Journal of Orthopaedic and Sports Physical Therapy*, 5(4), 170-174.

Cummings, G.S., and Tillman, L.J. (1992). Remodeling of dense connective tissue in normal adult tissues. In D.P. Currier and R.M. Nelson (Eds.), *Dynamics of human biologic tissues* (pp. 45-73). Philadelphia: Davis.

Cummings, M.S., Wilson, V.E., and Bird, E.I. (1984). Flexibility development in sprinters using EMG biofeedback and relation training. *Biofeedback and Self-Regulation*, 9(3), 395-405.

Cureton, T.K. (1930). Mechanics and kinesiology of swimming. *Research Quarterly*, 1(4), 87-121.

Cyriax, J. (1978). *Textbook of orthopaedic medicine: Vol. 1. Diagnosis of soft tissue lesions* (8th ed.). London: Bailliere Tindall.

Daleiden, S. (1990). Prevention of falling: Rehabilitative or compensatory interventions? *Topics in Geriatric Rehabilitation*, 5(2), 44-53.

Danforth, D.N. (1967). Pregnancy and labor: From the vantage point of the physical therapist. *American Journal of Physical Medicine*, 46(1), 653-658.

Danforth, D.N., and Ellis, A.H. (1963). Mid-forceps delivery: a vanishing art? *American Journal of Obstetrics and Gynecology*, 86(1), 29-37.

Daniell, H.W. (1979). Simple cure for nocturnal leg cramps. *New England Journal of Medicine*, 301(4), 216.

Davies, C.T.M., and Barnes, C. (1972). Negative (eccentric) work. 1. Effects of repeated exercise. *Ergonomics*, 15(1), 3-14.

Davies, C.T.M., and Young, K. (1983). Effects of training at 30% and 100% maximal isometric force (MVC) on the contractile properties of the triceps surae in man (Abstract). *Journal of Physiology* (London), 336, 31P.

Davies, G.J., Kirkendall, D.T., Leigh, D.H., Lui, M.L., Reinbold, T.R., and Wilson, P.K. (1981). Isokinetic characteristics of professional football players: I. Normative relationships between quadriceps and hamstring muscle group and relative to body weight. *Medicine and Science in Sports and Exercise*, 13(2), 76-77.

Davis, E.C., Logan, G.A., and McKinney, W.C. (1965). *Biophysical values of muscular activity with implications for research* (2nd ed.). Dubuque, IA: Brown.

Davis, L. (1988). Stretching a point. *Hippocrates*, 2(4), 90-92.

Davison, S. (1984). Standing: A good remedy. *Journal of the American Medical Association*, 252(24), 3367.

Davson, H. (1970). *A textbook of general physiology* (4th ed.). Baltimore: Williams & Wilkins.

Day, R.K., Ashmore, C.R., and Lee, Y.B. (1984). The effect of stretch removal on muscle weight and proteolytic enzyme activity in normal and dystrophic chicken muscles. *Muscle & Nerve*, 7(6), 482-485.

Day, R.W., and Wildermuth, B.P. (1988). Proprioceptive training in the rehabilitation of lower extremity injuries. In W.A. Grana (Ed.), *Advances in sports medicine and fitness* (pp. 241-258). Chicago: Year Book Medical.

Dean, E. (1988). Physiology and therapeutic implications of negative work: A review. *Physical Therapy*, 68(2), 233-237.

Debevoise, N.T., Hyatt, G.W., and Townsend, G.B. (1971). Humeral torsion in recurrent shoulder dislocations: A technic of determination by x-ray. *Clinical Orthopaedics and Related Research*, 76(May), 87-93.

de Jong, R.H. (1980). Defining pain terms. *Journal of the American Medical Association*, 244(2), 143.

Delitto, R.S., Rose, S.J., and Apts, D.W. (1987). Electromyographic analysis of two techniques for squat lifting. *Physical Therapy*, 67(9), 1329-1334.

DeLuca, C. (1985). Control properties of motor units. *Journal of Experimental Biology*, 115(March), 125-136.

Denny-Brown, D., and Doherty, M.M. (1945). Effects of transient stretching of peripheral nerve. *Archives of Neurology and Psychiatry*, 54(2), 116-122.

De Puky, P. (1935). The physiological oscillation of the length of the body. *Acta Orthopaedica Scandinavica*, 6(4), 338-347.

De Troyer, A., and Loring, S.H. (1986). Action of the respiratory muscles. In S.R. Geiger (Ed.), *Handbook of physiology: Sec. 3. The respiratory system: Vol. 3. Mechanics of breathing, part 2*. (pp. 443-461). Bethesda, MD: American Physiological Society.

de Vries, H.A. (1961a). Electromyographic observation of the effect of static stretching upon muscular distress. *Research*

Quarterly, 32(4), 468-479.

de Vries, H.A. (1961b). Prevention of muscular distress after exercise. *Research Quarterly, 32*(2), 177-185.

de Vries, H.A. (1962). Evaluation of static stretching procedures for improvement of flexibility. *Research Quarterly, 33*(2), 222-229.

de Vries, H.A. (1963). The "looseness" factor in speed and O_2 consumption of an anaerobic 100-yard dash. *Research Quarterly, 34*(3), 305-313.

de Vries, H.A. (1966). Quantitative electromyographic investigation of the spasm theory of muscle pain. *American Journal of Physical Medicine, 45*(3), 119-134.

de Vries, H.A. (1975). Physical fitness programs: Does physical activity promote relaxation? *Journal of Physical Education and Recreation, 46*(7), 52-53.

de Vries, H.A. (1985). Inversion devices: Potential benefits and precautions. *Corporate Fitness & Recreation, 4*(6), 24-27.

de Vries, H.A. (1986). *Physiology of exercise* (4th ed.). Dubuque, IA: Brown.

de Vries, H.A., and Adams, G.M. (1972). EMG comparison of single doses of exercise and meprobamate as to effects on muscular relaxation. *American Journal of Physical Medicine, 51*(3), 130-141.

de Vries, H.A., and Cailliet, R. (1985). Vagotonic effect of inversion therapy upon resting neuromuscular tension. *American Journal of Physical Medicine, 64*(3), 119-129.

de Vries, H.A., Wiswell, R.A., Bulbulion, R., and Moritani, T. (1981). Tranquilizer effect of exercise. *American Journal of Physical Medicine, 60*(2), 57-66.

Deyo, R.A. (1983). Conservative therapy for low back pain: Distinguishing useful from useless therapy. *Journal of the American Medical Association, 250*(8), 1057-1062.

Deyo, R.A., Walsh, N.E., Martin, D.C., Schoenfeld, L.S., and Ramamurthy, S. (1990). A controlled trial of transcutaneous electrical nerve stimulation (TENS) and exercise for chronic low back pain. *New England Journal of Medicine, 322*(23), 1627-1634.

Dick, F.W. (1980). *Sports training principles*. London: Lepus Books.

Dick, R.W., and Cavanagh, P.R. (1987). An explanation of the upward drift in oxygen uptake during prolonged sub-maximal downhill running. *Medicine and Science in Sports and Exercise, 19*(3), 310-317.

Dickenson, R.V. (1968). The specificity of flexibility. *Research Quarterly, 39*(3), 792-794.

DiMatteo, M.R., and DiNicola, D.D. (1982). *Achieving patient compliance: The psychology of the medical practitioner's role*. New York: Pergamon.

DiMatteo, M.R., Prince, L.M., and Taranta, A. (1979). Patients' perceptions of physicians' behavior: Determinants of patient commitment to the therapeutic relationship. *Journal of Community Health, 4*(4), 280-290.

DiRaimondo, C. (1991). Overuse conditions of the foot and ankle. In G.J. Sammarco (Ed.), *Foot and ankle manual* (pp. 260-275). Philadelphia: Lea & Febiger.

DiTullio, M., Wilczek, L., Paulus, D., Kiriakatis, A., Pollack, M., and Eisenhardt, J. (1989). Comparison of hip rotation in female classical ballet dancers versus female nondancers. *Medical Problems of Performing Artists, 4*(4), 154-158.

Dix, D.J., and Eisenberg, B.R. (1990). Myosin mRNA accumulation and myofibrillogenesis at the myotendinous junction of stretched muscle fibers. *Journal of Cell Biology, 111*(5, Pt. 1), 1885-1894.

Dix, D.J., and Eisenberg, B.R. (1991a). Distribution of myosin

mRNA during development and regeneration of skeletal muscle. *Developmental Biology, 143*(2), 422-426.

Dix, D.J., and Eisenberg, B.R. (1991b). Redistribution of myosin heavy chain mRNA in the midregion of stretched muscle fibers. *Cell and Tissue Research, 263*(1), 61-69.

Dobeln. *See* Allander et al. (1974).

Dobrin, P.B. (1983). Vascular mechanics. In J.T. Shepherd and F.M. Abboud (Eds.), *The handbook of physiology: Sec. 2. The cardiovascular system III: Vol. 3. Peripheral circulation and organ blood flow, Pt. I* (pp. 65-102). Bethesda, MD: American Physiological Society.

Dobson, C.B. (1983). *Stress: The hidden adversary*. Ridgewood, NJ: Bodgen & Son.

Docherty, D., and Bell, R.D. (1985). The relationship between flexibility and linearity measures in boys and girls 6-15 years of age. *Journal of Human Movement Studies, 11*(5), 279-288.

Doherty, K. (1985). *Track and field omnibook* (4th ed.). Swarthmore, PA: Tafmop.

Dominguez, R.H. (1980). Shoulder pain in swimmers. *Physician and Sportsmedicine, 8*(7), 36-42.

Dominguez, R.H., and Gajda, R. (1982). *Total body training*. New York: Warner.

Donatelli, R., and Owens-Burkhart, H. (1981). Effects of immobilization on the extensibility of periarticular connective tissue. *Journal of Orthopaedic and Sports Physical Therapy, 3*(2), 67-72.

Donisch, E.W., and Basmajian, J.V. (1972). Electromyography of deep back muscles in man. *American Journal of Anatomy, 133*(1), 25-36.

DonTigny, R.L. (1985). Function and pathomechanics of the sacroiliac joint. *Physical Therapy, 65*(1), 35-41.

Doran, D.M.L., and Newell, D.J. (1975). Manipulation in the treatment of low back pain: A multicentre study. *British Medical Journal, 2*, 161-164.

Douglas, S. (1980, February-March). *Physical evaluation of the swimmer*. Presented at the First Annual Vail Sportsmedicine Symposium, Vail, CO.

Downer, A.H. (1988). *Physical therapy procedures: Selected techniques* (4th ed.). Springfield, IL: Charles C Thomas.

Dowsing, G.S. (1978). Partner exercise. *Coaching Women's Athletics, 4*(2), 18-20.

Dubrovskii, V.I. (1990). The effect of massage on athletes' cardiorespiratory systems (clinico-physiological research). *Soviet Sports Review, 25*(1), 36-38.

Dummer, G.M., Vaccaro, P., and Clarke, D.H. (1985). Muscular strength and flexibility of two female master swimmers in the eighth decade of life. *Journal of Orthopaedic and Sports Physical Therapy, 6*(4), 235-237.

Dvorak, J., Kranzlin, P., Muhlemann, D., and Walchli, B. (1992). Musculoskeletal complications. In S. Haldeman (Ed.), *Principles and practice of chiropractic* (pp. 549-577). Norwalk, CT: Appleton & Lange.

Dvorkin, L.S. (1986). The young weightlifter: Development of flexibility. *Soviet Sports Review, 21*(3), 153-156.

Dye, A.A. (1939). *The evolution of chiropractic: Its discovery and development*. Philadelphia: Author.

Dyson, G.H.G. (1977). *The mechanics of athletics*. London: Hodder and Stoughton.

Ebbeling, C.B., and Clarkson, P.M. (1989). Exercise-induced muscle damage and adaptation. *Sports Medicine, 7*(4), 207-234.

Ecker, T. (1971). *Track & field dynamics*. Los Altos, CA: Tafnews

Press.

Egan, S. (1984). *Fitness & health: A holistic approach*. Ottawa: Crimcare.

Egelman, E.H., Francis, N., and Derosier, D.J. (1982). F-actin is a helix with a random variable twist. *Nature*, 298(5870), 131-135.

Ehrhart, B. (1976). Thirty Russian flexibility exercises for hurdlers. *Athletic Journal*, 56(7), 38-39, 96.

Einkauf, D.K., Gohdes, M.L., Jensen, G.M., and Jewell, M.J. (1986). Changes in spinal mobility with increasing age in women. *Physical Therapy*, 67(3), 370-375.

Eklund, J.A.E., and Corlett, E.N. (1984). Shrinkage as a measure of the effect of load on the spine. *Spine*, 9(2), 189-194.

Ekman, B., Ljungquist, K.-G., and Stein, U. (1970). Roentgenologic-photometric method for bone mineral determinations. *Acta Radiologica*, 10(July), 305-325.

Ekstrand, J., and Gillquist, J. (1982). The frequency of muscle tightness and injuries in soccer. *American Journal of Sports Medicine*, 10(2), 75-78.

Ekstrand, J., and Gillquist, J. (1983). The avoidability of soccer injuries. *International Journal of Sports Medicine*, 4(2), 124-128.

Eldred, E., Hutton, R.S., and Smith, J.L. (1976). Nature of the persisting changes in afferent discharge from muscle following its contraction. *Progressive Brain Research*, 44, 157-170.

Eldren, H.R. (1968). Physical properties of collagen fibers. In D.A. Hall (Ed.), *International review of connective tissue research* (Vol. 4, pp. 248-283). New York: Academic Press.

Elliott, D.H. (1965). Structure and function of mammalian tendon. *Biological Review*, 40(3), 392-421.

Ellis, C.G., Mathieu-Costello, O., Potter, R.F., MacDonald, I.C., and Groom, A.C. (1990). Effect of sarcomere length on total capillary length in skeletal muscle: In vivo evidence for longitudinal stretching of capillaries. *Microvascular Research*, 40(1), 63-72.

Ellis, J. (1986). Shinsplints too much, too soon. *Runners World*, 21(3), 50-53, 86.

Emmons, M. (1978). *The inner source: A guide to meditative therapy*. San Luis Obispo, CA: Impact.

Ende, L.S., and Wickstrom, J. (1982). Ballet injuries. *The Physician and Sportsmedicine*, 10(7), 101-118.

Engesvik, F. (1993). Leg movements in the breaststroke. *Swimming Technique*, 29(4), 26-27.

Enoka, R.M. (1988). *Neuromechanical basis of kinesiology*. Champaign, IL: Human Kinetics.

Etnyre, B., and Abraham, L. (1984). Effects of three stretching techniques on the motor pool excitability of the human soleus muscle (Abstract). In W. Roll (Ed.), *Abstracts of research papers 1984* (p. 90). Reston, VA: American Alliance of Health, Physical Education, and Recreation.

Etnyre, B.R., and Abraham, L.D. (1986). Gains in range of ankle dorsiflexion using three popular stretching techniques. *American Journal of Physical Medicine*, 65(4), 189-196.

Etnyre, B.R., and Abraham, L.D. (1988). Antagonist muscle activity during stretching: A paradox re-assessed. *Medicine and Science in Sports and Exercise*, 20(3), 285-289.

Etnyre, B.R., and Lee, E.J. (1987). Comments on proprioceptive neuromuscular facilitation stretching techniques. *Research Quarterly for Exercise and Sport*, 58(2), 184-188.

Evans, D.P., Burke, M.S., Lloyd, K.H., Roberts, E.E., and Roberts, G.M. (1978). Lumbar spinal manipulation on trial. 1. Clinical assessment. *Rheumatology and Rehabilitation*, 17(1), 46-53.

Evans, G.A., Harcastle, P., and Frenyo, A.D. (1984). Acute rupture of the lateral ligament of the ankle. *Journal of Bone and Joint Surgery*, 66B(2), 209-212.

Evatt, M.L., Wolf, S.L., and Segal, R.L. (1989). Modification of human spinal stretch reflexes: Preliminary studies. *Neuroscience Letters*, 105(3), 350-355.

Everly, G.S. (1989). *A clinical guide to the treatment of the human stress response*. New York: Plenum Press.

Everly, G.S., Spollen, M., Hackman, A., and Kobran, E. (1987). Undesirable side-effects and self-regulatory therapies. In *Proceedings of the eighteenth annual meeting of the Biofeedback Society of America* (pp. 166-167). Boston.

Evjenth, O., and Hamberg, J. (1984). *Muscle stretching in manual therapy. A clinical manual*. Alfta, Sweden: Alfta Rehab.

Fairbank, J.C.T., Pynsent, P.B., van Poortvliet, J.A., and Phillips, H. (1984). Influence of anthropometric factors and joint laxity in the incidence of adolescent back pain. *Spine*, 9(5), 461-464.

Falkel, J.E. (1988). Swimming injuries. In J.E. Falkel and J.C. Murphy (Eds.), *Shoulder injuries* (pp. 477-503). Baltimore: Williams & Wilkins.

Falls, H.B., and Humphrey, D. (1989). Dr. Falls and Dr. Humphrey reply. *The Physician and Sportsmedicine*, 17(6), 20, 22.

Fardy, P.S. (1981). Isometric exercise and the cardiovascular system. *The Physician and Sportsmedicine*, 9(9), 43-56.

Farfan, H.F. (1973). *Mechanical disorders of the low back*. Philadelphia: Lea & Febiger.

Farfan, H.F. (1978). The biomechanical advantage of lordosis and hip extension for upright activity. *Spine*, 3(4), 336-342.

Farrell, J., and Twomey, L. (1982). Acute low back pain: Comparison of two consecutive treatment approaches. *Medical Journal of Australia*, 1(4), 160-164.

Faucret, B.H. (1980). Biomechanics of the pelvis. In *A collection of monographs on the biomechanics of the pelvis* (pp. 43-75). Des Moines, IA: American Chiropractic Association.

Faulkner, J.A., Brooks, S.V., and Opiteck, J.A. (1993). Injury to skeletal muscle fibers during contractions: Conditions of occurrence and prevention. *Physical Therapy*, 73(12), 911-921.

Fawcett, D.W. (1986). *A textbook of histology* (11th ed.). Philadelphia: W.B. Saunders.

Federation of Straight Chiropractic Organizations (FSCO) (n.d.). *Statement on chiropractic standard of care/patient safety*. Clifton, NJ: Author.

Feit, E.M., and Berenter, R. (1993). Lower extremity tennis injuries: Prevalence, etiology, and mechanisms. *Journal of the American Podiatric Medical Association*, 83(9), 509-522.

Fellabaum, J. (1993). The effect of eye positioning on bodily movement. *Digest of Chiropractic Economics*, 36(1), 14-17.

Ferlic, D. (1962). The range of motion of the "normal" cervical spine. *Bulletin of the Johns Hopkins Hospital*, 110(February), 59-65.

Fick, R. (1911). *Handbuch der Anatomie und Mechanik der Gelenke* (Vol. 3). Jena: Gustav Fischer.

Finkelstein, H. (1916). Joint hypotonia. *New York Medical Journal*, 104(20), 942-944.

Finkelstein, H., and Roos, R. (1990). Ontario study raises doubt about stretching. *The Physician and Sportsmedicine*, 18(1), 48-49.

Finneson, B.E. (1980). *Low back pain*. Philadelphia: Lippincott.

Fisher, A.C., Domm, M.A., and Wuest, D.A. (1988). Adherence to sports-injury rehabilitation programs. *The Physician and Sportsmedicine*, 16(7), 47-51.

Fisk, J.W. (1975). The straight-leg raising test—Its relevance to possible disc pathology. *New Zealand Medical Journal*, 81(542), 557-560.

Fisk, J.W. (1979). A controlled trial of manipulation in a selected group of patients with low back pain favoring one side. *New Zealand Journal of Medicine*, 90(645), 288-291.

Fisk, J.W., and Rose, R.S. (1977). *A practical guide to management of the painful neck and back*. Springfield, IL: Charles C Thomas.

Fitt, S.S. (1988). *Dance kinesiology*. New York: Schirmer Books.

Fitzgerald, J.G. (1972). *Changes in spinal stature following brief periods of static shoulder loading* (IAM Report No. 514). Farnborough: Royal Air Force Institute of Aviation Medicine.

Fixx, J. (1983). Is stretching (yawn) everything you hoped it would be? *Running Times*, 80(September), 66.

Fleischman, E.A. (1964). *The structure and measurement of physical fitness*. Englewood Cliffs, NJ: Prentice-Hall.

Fleisig, G.S., Andrews, J.R., Dillman, C.J., and Escamilla, R.F. (1995). Kinetics of baseball pitching with implication about injury mechanisms. *American Journal of Sports Medicine*, 23(2), 233-239.

Flint, M.M. (1964). Selecting exercises. *Journal of Health, Physical Education, and Recreation*, 35(2), 19-23, 74.

Flintney, F.W., and Hirst, D.G. (1978). Cross-bridge detachment and sarcomere "give" during stretch of active frog's muscle. *Journal of Physiology* (London), 276, 449-465.

Flood, J., and Nauert, J. (1973). Shin splints. *Scholastic Coach*, 42(5), 28, 30, 102-103.

Floyd, W.F., and Silver, P.H.S. (1950). Electromyographic study of patterns of activity of the anterior abdominal wall muscles in man. *Journal of Anatomy*, 84(2), 132-145.

Floyd, W.F., and Silver, P.H.S. (1951). Function of the erectores spinae in flexion of the trunk. *Lancet*, 1, 133-134.

Floyd, W.F., and Silver, P.H.S. (1955). The function of the erectores spinae muscles in certain movements and postures in man. *Journal of Physiology* (London), 129, 184-203.

Follan, L.M. (1981). *Lilias and your life*. New York: Collier Books.

Foreman, T.K., and Linge, K. (1989). The importance of heel compression in the measurement of diurnal stature variation. *Applied Ergonomics*, 20(4), 299-300.

Foreman, T.K., and Troup, J.D.G. (1987). Diurnal variations in spinal loading and the effects on stature: A preliminary study of nursing activities. *Clinical Biomechanics*, 2(1), 48-54.

Forssberg, E. (1899). Om vexlingar i kroppslangden hos kavallerirekryter. *Militar Halsovard*, 24, 19-28.

Fowler, A.W. (1973). Relief of cramp. *Lancet*, 1(7794), 99.

Fowler, P.J., and Messieh, S.S. (1987). Isolated posterior cruciate ligament injuries in athletes. *American Journal of Sports Medicine*, 15(6), 553-557.

Francis, K.T. (1983). Delayed muscle soreness: A review. *Journal of Orthopaedic and Sports Physical Therapy*, 5(1), 10-13.

Frankel, V.H., and Burnstein, A.H. (1974). Biomechanics of the locomotor system. In C. D. Ray (Ed.), *Medical engineering* (pp. 505-515). Chicago: Yearbook Medical.

Frankeny, J.R., Holly, R. G., and Ashmore, C.R. (1983). Effects of graded duration of stretch on normal and dystrophic skeletal muscle. *Muscle & Nerve*, 6(4), 269-277.

Franzblau, C., and Faru, B. (1981). Elastin. In E.D. Hay (Ed.), *Cell biology of extracellular matrix* (pp. 75-78). New York: Plenum Press.

Franzini-Armstrong, C. (1970). Details of the I-band structure revealed by localization of ferritin. *Tissue Cell*, 2(2), 327-338.

Frederick E.C. (1982). Stretching things a bit. *Running*, 8(3), 65.

Freeman, M.A.R., Dean, M.R.E., and Hanham, I.W.F. (1965). The etiology and prevention of functional instability of the foot. *Journal of Bone and Joint Surgery*, 47B(4), 678-685.

Freivalds, A. (1979). *Investigation of circadian rhythms on select psychomotor and neurological functions*. Unpublished doctoral dissertation, University of Michigan, Ann Arbor.

Frekany, G.A., and Leslie, D.K. (1975). Effects of an exercise program on selected flexibility measurements of senior citizens. *The Gerontologist*, 15(2), 182-183.

Friberg, T.R., and Weinreb, R.N. (1985). Ocular manifestations of gravity inversion. *Journal of the American Medical Association*, 253(12), 1755-1757.

Fridén, J. (1984a). Changes in human skeletal muscle induced by long-term eccentric exercise. *Cell Tissue Research*, 236(2), 365-372.

Fridén, J. (1984b). Muscle soreness after exercise: Implications of morphological changes. *International Journal of Sports Medicine*, 5(2), 57-66.

Fridén, J., and Lieber, R.L. (1992). Structural and mechanical basis of exercise-induced muscle injury. *Medicine and Science in Sports and Exercise*, 24(5), 521-530.

Fridén, J., Seger, J., and Ekblom, B. (1988). Sublethal muscle fibre injuries after high-tension anaerobic exercise. *European Journal of Applied Physiology*, 57(3), 360-368.

Fridén, J., Seger, M., Sjöström, M., and Ekblom, B. (1983). Adaptive response in human skeletal muscle subjected to prolonged eccentric training. *International Journal of Sports Medicine*, 4(3), 177-184.

Fridén, J., Sfakianos, P.N., and Hargens, A.R. (1986). Muscle soreness and intramuscular fluid pressure: Comparison between eccentric and concentric load. *Journal of Applied Physiology*, 61(6), 2175-2179.

Fridén, J., Sfakianos, P.N., Hargens, A.R., and Akeson, W.H. (1988). Residual muscular swelling after repetitive eccentric contractions. *Journal of Orthopaedic Research*, 6(4), 493-498.

Fridén, J., Sjöström, M., and Ekblom, B. (1981). A morphological study of delayed muscle soreness. *Experimentia*, 37(5), 506-507.

Fridén, J., Sjöström, M., and Ekblom, B. (1983). Myofibrillar damage following intense eccentric exercise in man. *International Journal of Sports Medicine*, 4(3), 170-176.

Fried, R. (1987). *The hyperventilation syndrome*. Baltimore: Johns Hopkins University Press.

Friedmann, L.W., and Galton, L. (1973). *Freedom from backaches*. New York: Simon and Schuster.

Frost, H.M. (1967). *Introduction to biomechanics*. Springfield, IL: Charles C Thomas.

Fujiwara, M., and Basmajian, J.V. (1975). Electromyographic study of the two-joint muscles. *American Journal of Physical Medicine*, 54(5), 234-242.

Fulton, A.B., and Isaacs, W.B. (1991). Titin: A huge, elastic sarcomeric protein with a probable role in morphogenesis. *BioEssays*, 13(4), 157-161.

Funatsu, T., Higuchi, H., and Ishiwata, S. (1990). Elastic filaments in skeletal muscle revealed by selective removal of titin filaments with plasma gelsolin. *Journal of Cell Biology*, 110(1), 53-62.

Furst, D.O., Osborn, M., Nave, R., and Weber, K. (1988). The organization of titin filaments in the half-sarcomere revealed by monoclonal antibodies in immunoelectron microscopy: A map of ten nonrepetitive epitomes starting at the Z-line extends close to the M line. *Journal of Cell Biology*, 106(5), 1563-1572.

Gabbard, C., and Tandy, R. (1988). Body composition and flexibility among prepubescent males and females. *Journal of Human Movement Studies*, 14(4), 153-159.

Gajda, R. *See* D.R. Murphy (1991).

Gajdosik, R., and Lusin, G. (1983). Hamstring muscle tightness: Reliability of an active-knee-extension test. *Physical Therapy*, 63(7), 1085-1089.

Galin, M.A., McIvor, J.W., and Magruder, G.B. (1963). Influence of position on intraocular pressure. *American Journal of Ophthalmology*, 55(4), 720-723.

Galley, P.M., and Forster, A.L. (1987). *Human movement: An introductory text for physiotherapy students*. Melbourne: Churchill Livingstone.

Garamvölgyi, N. (1971). The functional morphology of muscle. In K. Laki (Ed.), *Contractile proteins and muscle* (pp. 1-96). New York: Marcel Dekker.

Garde, R.E. (1988). Cervical traction: The neurophysiology of lordosis and the rheological characteristics of cervical curve rehabilitation. In D. D. Harrison (Ed.), *Chiropractic: The physics of spinal correction* (pp. 535-659). Sunnyvale, CA: Author.

Garfin, S.R., Tipton, C.M., Mubarak, S.J., Woo, S. L.-Y., Hargens, A.R., and Akeson, W.H. (1981). Role of fascia in maintenance of muscle tension and pressure. *Journal of Applied Physiology*, 51(2), 317-320.

Garhammer, J. (1989a). Principles of training and development. In P.J. Rasch (Ed.), *Kinesiology and applied anatomy* (7th ed., pp. 258-265). Philadelphia: Lea & Febiger.

Garhammer, J. (1989b). Weight lifting and training. In C.L. Vaughan (Ed.), *Biomechanics of sport* (pp. 169-211). Boca Raton, FL: CRC Publishers.

Garrett, W., Bradley, W., Byrd, S., Edgerton, V.R., and Gollnick, P. (1989). Basic science perspectives. In J.W. Frymoyer and S.L. Gordon (Eds.), *New perspectives in low back pain* (pp. 335-372). Park Ridge, IL: American Academy of Orthopaedic Surgeons.

Garu, J. (1986). Exercise do's & don'ts: Side bends. *Dance Exercise Today*, 4(4), 34-35.

Gaskell, W.H. (1877). On the changes of the bloodstream of the muscles through stimulation of their nerves. *Journal of Anatomy and Physiology*, 11, 360-402.

Gathercole, L.J., and Keller, A. (1968). Early development of crimping in rat tail tendon. *Micron*, 89, 83-89.

Gaughran, J.A. (1972). *Advanced swimming*. Dubuque, IA: Brown.

Gaymans, F. (1980). Die Bedeutung der Atemtypen fur Mobilisation der Wirbelsaule. *Manuelle Medizin*, 18, 96.

Gelabert, R. (1966). *Raul Gelabert's anatomy for the dancer*. New York: Danad.

Gelardi, T.A. (n.d.). *What is the difference between CCE and SCASA?* Unpublished paper.

George, G.S. (1980). *Biomechanics of women's gymnastics*. Englewood Cliffs, NJ: Prentice-Hall.

Germain, N.W., and Blair, S.N. (1983). Variability of shoulder flexion with age, activity and sex. *American Corrective Therapy Journal*, 37(6), 156-160.

Giel, D. (1988). Women's weightlifting: Elevating a sport to world-class status. *The Physician and Sportsmedicine*, 16(4), 163-170.

Gifford, L.S. (1987). Circadian variation in human flexibility and grip strength. *Australian Journal of Physiotherapy*, 33(1), 3-9.

Gilliam, T.B., Villanacci, J.F., Freedson, P.S., and Sady, S.P. (1979). Isokinetic torque in boys and girls age 7 to 13: Effect of age, height, and weight. *Research Quarterly*, 50(4), 599-609.

Gladden, M.H. (1986). Mechanical factors affecting the sensitivity of mammalian muscle spindles. *Trends in Neuroscience*, 13(4), 295-297.

Glazer, R.M. (1980). Rehabilitation. In R.B. Happenstall (Ed.), *Fracture treatment and healing* (pp. 1041-1068). Philadelphia: Saunders.

Gold, R. (1987). *Album #1: The philosophy*. Gladwyne, PA: Chiro Products.

Goldspink, G. (1968). Sarcomere length during post-natal growth and mammalian muscle fibres. *Journal of Cell Science*, 3(4), 539-548.

Goldspink, G. (1976). The adaptation of muscle to a new functional length. In D.J. Anderson and B. Matthews (Eds.), *Mastication* (pp. 90-99). Bristol, England: Wright and Sons.

Goldspink, G., Scutt, A., Loughna, P.T., Wells, D.J., Jaenicke, T., and Gerlach, G.F. (1992). Gene expression in skeletal muscle in response to stretch and force generation. *American Journal of Physiology*, 262(31), R356-R363.

Goldspink, G., Tabary, C., Tabary, J.C., Tardieu, C., and Tardieu, G. (1974). Effect of denervation on the adaptation of sarcomere number and muscle extensibility to the functional length of the muscle. *Journal of Physiology* (London), 236(3), 733-742.

Goldspink, G., and Williams, P.E. (1979). The nature of the increased passive resistance in muscle following immobilization of the mouse soleus muscle. *Journal of Physiology* (London), 289, 55P (Proceedings of the Physiological Society December 15-16, 1978).

Goldstein, J.D., Berger, P.E., Windler, G.E., and Jackson, D.W. (1981). Spine injuries in gymnasts and swimmers. An epidemiologic investigation. *American Journal of Sports Medicine*, 19(5), 463-468.

Goldthwait, J.E. (1941). *Body mechanics in health and disease*. Philadelphia: Lippincott.

Golub, L.J. (1987). Exercises that alleviate primary dysmenorrhea. *Contemporary Ob/Gyn*, 29(5), 51-59.

Golub, L.J., and Christaldi, J. (1957). Reducing dysmenorrhea in young adolescents. *Journal of Health, Physical Education, and Recreation*, 28(5), 24-25, 59.

Golub, L.J., Lang, W.R., and Menduke, H. (1958). Dysmenorrhea in high school and college girls: Relationship to sports participation. *Western Journal of Surgery, Obstetrics and Gynecology*, 66(3), 163-165.

Golub, L.J., Menduke, H., and Lang, W.R. (1968). Exercise and dysmenorrhea in young teenagers: A 3-year study. *Obstetrics and Gynecology*, 32(4), 508-511.

Goode, D.J., and Van Hoven, J. (1982). Loss of patellar and achilles tendon reflexes in classical ballet dancers. *Archives of Neurology*, 39(5), 323.

Goode, J.D., and Theodore, B.M. (1983). Voluntary and diurnal variation in height and associated surface contour changes in spinal curves. *Engineering in Medicine*, 12(2), 99-101.

Goodridge, J.P. (1981). Muscle energy technique: Definition, explanation, methods of procedure. *Journal of the American Osteopathic Association*, 81(4), 67-72.

Gordon, A.M., Huxley, A.F., and Julian, F.J. (1966). The variation in isometric tension with sarcomere length in vertebrate muscle fibres. *Journal of Physiology (London)*, 184, 170-192.

Gordon, G.M., and Klein, B.A. (1987). The benefits of weight training for hamstring strains. *Journal of the American Podiatric Medical Association*, 77(10), 567-569.

Gosline, J.M. (1976). The physical properties of elastic tissue. In D.A. Hull and D.S. Jackson (Eds.), *International review of connective tissue research* (Vol. 7, pp. 211-257). New York: Academic Press.

Gotlib, A.C., and Thiel, H. (1985). A selected annotated bibliography of the core biomedical literature pertaining to stroke, cervical spine, manipulation and head/neck movement. *Journal of the Canadian Chiropractic Association*, 29(2), 80-89.

Gould, D. (1987). Understanding attrition in children's sport. In D. Gould and M.R. Weiss (Eds.), *Advances in pediatric sport sciences* (pp. 61-85). Champaign, IL: Human Kinetics.

Gould, G.M., and Pyle, W.L. (1896). *Anomalies and curiosities of medicine*. Philadelphia: Saunders.

Gowitzke, B.A., and Milner, M. (1988). *Understanding the scientific basis of human movement* (2nd ed.). Baltimore: Williams & Wilkins.

Grace, T.G. (1985). Muscle imbalance and extremity injury: A perplexing relationship. *Sports medicine*, 2(2), 77-82.

Gracovetsky, S., Farfan, H.F., and Lamy, C. (1977). A mathematical model of the lumbar spine using an optimized system to control muscles and ligaments. *Orthopaedics Clinics of North America*, 8(1), 135-153.

Gracovetsky, S., Kary, M., Pitchen, I., Levy, S., and Said, R.B. (1989). The importance of pelvic tilt in reducing compression stress in the spine during flexion-extension exercises. *Spine*, 14(4), 412-417.

Graham, C.E. (1987). Plantar fasciitis and the painful heel syndrome. *Medicine and Sport Science*, 23, 99-104.

Graham, G. (1965). Cramp. *Lancet*, 2, 537.

Grahame, R. (1971). Joint hypermobility-clinical aspects. *Proceedings of the Royal Society of Medicine*, 64(June), 692-694.

Grahame, R., and Jenkins, J.M. (1972). Joint hypermobility—Asset or liability? *Annals of the Rheumatic Diseases*, 31(2), 109-111.

Grana, W.A., and Moretz, J.A. (1978). Ligamentous laxity in secondary school athletes. *Journal of the American Medical Association*, 240(18), 1975-1976.

Granit, R. (1962). Muscle tone and postural regulation. In K. Rodahl and S.M. Horvath (Eds.), *Muscle as tissue* (p. 190). New York: McGraw-Hill.

Grant, M.E., Prockop, P.D., and Darwin, J. (1972). The biosynthesis of collagen. *New England Journal of Medicine*, 286(4), 194-199.

Grassino, A., Goldman, M.D., Mead, J., and Sears, T.A. (1978). Mechanisms of the human diaphragm during voluntary contraction statics. *Journal of Applied Physiology*, 44(6), 829-839.

Gray, M.L., Pizzanelli, A.M., Grodzinsky, A.J., and Lee, R.C. (1988). Mechanical and physiochemical determinants of the chondrocyte biosynthetic response. *Journal of Orthopaedic Research*, 6(6), 777-792.

Gray, S.D., and Staub, N.C. (1967). Resistance to blood flow in leg muscles of dog during tetanic isometric contraction. *American Journal of Physiology*, 213(3), 677-682.

Greene, W.B., and Heckman, J.D. (1994). *The clinical measurement of joint motion*. Rosemont, IL: American Academy of Orthopaedic Surgeons.

Greenman, P.E. (1989). *Principles of manual medicine*. Baltimore: Williams & Wilkins.

Greey, G.W. (1955). *A study of the flexibility in five selected joints of adult males ages 18 to 71*. Unpublished doctoral dissertation, University of Michigan, Ann Arbor.

Greipp, J.F. (1986). The flex factor. *Swimming Technique*, 22(3), 17-24.

Grieve, D.W. (1970). Stretching active muscles. *Track Technique*, 42(December), 1333-1335.

Grieve, G.P. (1988). *Common vertebral joint problems* (2nd ed.). London: Churchill Livingstone.

Grieve, G.P. (1991). *Mobilisation of the spine* (5th ed.). Edinburgh: Churchill Livingstone.

Griffith, H.W. (1986). *Complete guide to sport injuries*. Los Angeles: Body Press.

Grob, D. (1983). Common disorders of muscles in the aged. In W. Reichel (Ed.), *Clinical aspects of aging* (2nd ed., pp. 329-343). Baltimore: Williams & Wilkins.

Grodzinsky, A.J. (1983). Electromechanical and physiochemical properties of connective tissue. *CRC Critical Reviews in Biomedical Engineering*, 9(2), 133-199.

Grodzinsky, A.J. (1987). Electromechanical transduction and transport in the extracellular matrix. *Advances in Microcirculation*, 13, 35-46.

Grodzinsky, A.J., Lipshitz, H., and Glimcher, M.J. (1978). Electromechanical properties of articular cartilage during compression and stress relaxation. *Nature*, 275(5679), 448-450.

Gross, J. (1961). Collagen. *Scientific American*, 204(5), 120-133.

Gurewitsch, A.D., and O'Neill, M. (1944). Flexibility of healthy children. *Archives of Physical Therapy*, 25(4), 216-221.

Gurry, M., Pappas, A., Michaels, J., Maher, P., Shakman, A., Goldberg, R., and Rippe, J. (1985). A comprehensive preseason fitness evaluation for professional baseball players. *The Physician and Sportsmedicine*, 13(6), 63-74.

Gustavsen, R. (1985). *Training therapy prophylaxis and rehabilitation*. New York: Thieme.

Gutman, G.M., Herbert, C.P., and Brown, S.R. (1977). Feldenkrais versus conventional exercises for elderly. *Journal of Gerontology*, 32(5), 562-572.

Gutmann, E. (1977). Muscle. In C.E. Finch and L. Hayflick (Eds.), *Handbook of the biology of aging* (pp. 445-469). New York: Van Nostrand Reinhold.

Gutmann, E., Schiaffino, S., and Hanzliková, V. (1971). Mechanism of compensatory hypertrophy in skeletal muscle of the rat. *Experimental Neurology*, 31(3), 451-464.

Gutmann, G. (1983). Injuries to the vertebral artery caused by manual therapy. *Manuelle Medizin*, 21, 2-14.

Haas, M. (1990). The physics of spinal manipulation. Part IV. A theoretical consideration of the physician impact force and energy requirements needed to produce synovial joint cavitation. *Journal of Manipulative and Physiological Therapeutics*, 13(7), 378-383.

Haftek, J. (1970). Stretch injury of peripheral nerve: Acute effects of stretching on rabbit nerve. *Journal of Bone and Joint Surgery*, 52B(2), 354-365.

Halbertsma, J.P.K., and Göeken, L.N.H. (1994). Stretching exercises: Effect on passive extensibility and stiffness in short hamstrings of healthy subjects. *Archives of Physical Medicine and Rehabilitation*, 75(9), 976-981.

Haldeman, S. (1978). The clinical basis for discussion of mechanisms of manipulative therapy. In I.M. Korr (Ed.), *The neurobiologic mechanisms in manipulative therapy* (pp. 53-75). New York: Plenum Press.

Haldeman, S. (1983). Spinal manipulative therapy: A status report. *Clinical Orthopaedics and Related Research*, 179(October), 62-70.

Haley, S.M., Tada, W.L., and Carmichael, E.M. (1986). Spinal mobility in young children: A normative study. *Physical Therapy*, 66(11), 1697-1703.

Hall, A.C., Urban, J.P.G., and Gehl, K.A. (1991). Effects of compression on the loss of newly synthesized proteoglycans and proteins from cartilage explants. *Archives of Biochemistry and Biophysics*, 286, 20-29.

Hall, D.A. (1981). Gerontology: Collagen disease. *Clinical Endocrinology and Metabolism*, 10(1), 23-55.

Halvorson, G.A. (1989). Principles of rehabilitating sports injuries. In C.C. Teitz (Ed.), *Scientific foundations of sports medicine* (pp. 345-371). Philadelphia: Decker.

Hamilton, W.G. (1978a). Ballet and your body: An orthopedist's view. *Dance Magazine*, 52(2), 79.

Hamilton, W.G. (1978b). Ballet and your body: An orthopedist's view. *Dance Magazine*, 52(4), 126-127.

Hamilton, W.G. (1978c). Ballet and your body: An orthopedist's view. *Dance Magazine*, 52(7), 86-87.

Hamilton, W.G. (1978d). Ballet and your body: An orthopedist's view. *Dance Magazine*, 52(8), 84-85.

Hamilton, W.G., Hamilton, L.H., Marshall, P., and Molnar, M. (1992). A profile of the musculoskeletal characteristics of elite professional ballet dancers. *American Journal of Sports Medicine*, 20(3), 267-273.

Hanus, S.H., Homer, T.D., and Harter, D.H. (1977). Vertebral artery occlusion complicating yoga exercises. *Archives of Neurology*, 34(September), 574-575.

Hardaker, W.T., Erickson, L., and Myers, M. (1984). The pathogenesis of dance injury. In C.G. Shell (Ed.), *The dancer as athlete* (pp. 12-13). Champaign, IL: Human Kinetics.

Hardy, L. (1985). Improving active range of hip flexion. *Research Quarterly for Exercise and Sport*, 56(2), 111-114.

Hardy, L., Lye, R., and Heathcote, A. (1983). Active versus passive warm up regimes and flexibility. *Research Papers in Physical Education*, 1(5), 23-30.

Harris, F.A. (1978). Facilitation techniques in therapeutic exercise. In J.V. Basmajian (Ed.), *Therapeutic exercise* (3rd ed., pp. 93-137). Baltimore: Williams & Wilkins.

Harris, H., and Joseph, J. (1949). Variation in extension of the metacarpophalangeal and interphalangeal joints of the thumb. *Journal of Bone and Joint Surgery*, 31B(4), 547-559.

Harris, M.L. (1969a). A factor analytic study of flexibility. *Research Quarterly*, 40(1), 62-70.

Harris, M.L. (1969b). Flexibility. *Physical Therapy*, 49(6), 591-601.

Hartley-O'Brien, S.J. (1980). Six mobilization exercises for active range of hip flexion. *Research Quarterly for Exercise and Sport*, 51(4), 625-635.

Harvey, C., Benedetti, L., Hosaka, L., and Valmassy, R.L. (1983). The use of cold spray and its effect on muscle length. *Journal of the American Podiatry Association*, 73(12), 629-632.

Harvey, V.P., and Scott, F.P. (1967). Reliability of a measure of forward flexibility and its relation to physical dimensions of college women. *Research Quarterly*, 38(1), 28-33.

Hatfield, F.C. (1982). Learning to stretch for strength and safety. *Muscle Fitness*, 43(12), 24-25, 193-194.

Hay, J.G. (1985). *The biomechanics of sports techniques* (3rd ed.). Englewood Cliffs, NJ: Prentice-Hall.

Haywood, K.M. (1980). Strength and flexibility in gymnasts before and after menarche. *British Journal of Sports Medicine*, 14(4), 189-192.

Hebbelinck, M. (1988). Flexibility. In A. Dirix, H.G. Knuttgen, and K. Tittel (Eds.), *The Olympic book of sports medicine* (pp. 213-217). Oxford: Blackwell Scientific.

Heiser, T.M., Weber, J., Sullivan, G., Clare, P., and Jacobs, R.R. (1984). Prophylaxis and management of hamstring muscle injuries in intercollegiate football players. *American Journal of Sports Medicine*, 12(5), 368-370.

Helin, P. (1985). Physiotherapy and electromyography in muscle cramp. *British Journal of Sports Medicine*, 19(4), 230-231.

Hellig, D. (1969). Illustrative points in technique. In J.M. Hoag, W.V. Cole, and S.G. Bradford (Eds.), *Osteopathic medicine* (pp. 197-203). New York: McGraw-Hill.

Heng, M.K., Bai, J.X., Talian, N.J., Vincent, W.J., Reese, S.S., Shaw, S., and Holland, G.J. (1992). Changes in cardiovascular function during inversion. *International Journal of Sports Medicine*, 13(1), 69-73.

Hennessy, L., and Watson, A.W.S. (1993). Flexibility and posture assessment in relation to hamstring injury. *British Journal of Sports Medicine*, 27(4), 243-246.

Henry, J.H. (1986). Commentary. *American Journal of Sports Medicine*, 14(1), 17.

Henry, J.P. (1951). *Studies of the physiology of negative acceleration* (AF Tech. Report #5953). Dayton, OH: U.S. Air Force Air Material Command, Wright-Patterson AFB.

Herbison, G.J., and Graziani, V. (1995). Neuromuscular disease: Rehabilitation and electrodiagnosis. 1. Anatomy and physiology of nerve and muscle. *Archives of Physical Medicine and Rehabilitation*, 76(5), S3-S9.

Hertling, D.M., and Jones, D. (1990). Relaxation. In R.M. Kessler and D. Hertling (Eds.), *Management of common musculoskeletal disorders* (2nd ed., pp. 144-163). Philadelphia: Lippincott.

Herzog, W., Conway, P.J., Kawchuk, G.N., Zhang, Y., and Hasler, E.M. (1993). Forces exerted during spinal manipulative therapy. *Spine*, 18(9), 1206-1212.

Heyward, V.H. (1984). *Designs for fitness*. Minneapolis: Burgess.

Hickok, R.J. (1976). Physical therapy. In F.V. Steinberg (Ed.), *Cowdry's the care of the geriatric patient* (5th ed., pp. 420-432). St. Louis: Mosby.

Highet, W.B., and Sanders, F.K. (1943). The effects of stretching nerves after suture. *British Journal of Surgery*, 30(120), 355-371.

Hill, A.R., Adams, J.M., Parker, B.E., and Rochester, D.F. (1988). Short-term entrainment of ventilation to the walking cycle in humans. *Journal of Applied Physiology* 65(2), 570-578.

Hill, A.V. (1948). The pressure developed in muscle during contraction. *Journal of Physiology* (London), 107, 518-526.

Hill, A.V. (1961). The heat produced by a muscle after the last shock of tetanus. *Journal of Physiology* (London), 159(3), 518-545.

Hill, C., and Weber, K. (1986). Monoclonal antibodies distinguish titins from heart and skeletal muscle. *Journal of Cell Biology*, 102(3), 1099-1108.

Hilyer, J.C., Brown, K.C., Sirles, A.T., and Peoples, L. (1990). A flexibility intervention to reduce the incidence and severity of joint injuries among municipal firefighters. *Journal of Occupational Medicine*, 32(7), 631-637.

Hindle, R.J., and Murray-Leslie, C. (1987). Diurnal stature variation in ankylosing spondylitis. *Clinical Biomechanics*, 2(3), 152-157.

Hinrichs, R.N. (1990). Whole body movement: Coordination of arms and legs in walking and running. In J.M. Winters and S.L.-Y. Woo (Eds.), *Multiple muscle systems: Biomechanics and movement organization* (pp. 694-705). New York: Springer-Verlag.

Hinrichs, R.N. (1992). Case studies of asymmetrical arm action in running. *International Journal of Sport Biomechanics*, 8(2), 111-128.

Hinterbuchner, C. (1980). Traction. In J.B. Rogoff (Ed.), *Manipulation, traction, and massage* (2nd ed., pp. 184-210). Baltimore: Williams & Wilkins.

Hirche, H., Raff, W.K., and Grün, D. (1970). The resistance to blood flow in the gastrocnemius of the dog during sustained and rhythmical isometric and isotonic contractions. *European Journal of Physiology*, 314, 97-112.

Hoeger, W.W.K. (1991). *Principles and labs for physical fitness and wellness*. Englewood, CO: Morton.

Hoeger, W.W.K., and Hopkins, D.R. (1992). A comparison of the sit and reach and the modified sit and reach in the measurement of flexibility in women. *Research Quarterly for Exercise and Sport*, 63(2), 191-195.

Hoeger, W.W.K., Hopkins, D.R., Button, S., and Palmer, T.A. (1990). Comparing the sit and reach with the modified sit and reach in measuring flexibility in adolescents. *Pediatric Exercise Science*, 2(2), 156-162.

Hoeger, W.W.K., Hopkins, D.R., and Johnson, L.C. (1991). *Muscular flexibility: Test protocols and national flexibility norms for the modified sit-and-reach test, total body rotation test, and shoulder rotation test*. Addison, IL: Novel Products Figure Finder Collection.

Hoehler, F.K., and Tobis, J.S. (1982). Low back pain and its treatment by spinal manipulation: Measures of flexibility and asymmetry. *Rheumatology and Rehabilitation*, 21, 21-26.

Hoehler, F.K., Tobis, J.S., and Buerger, A.A. (1981). Spinal manipulation for low back pain. *Journal of the American Medical Association*, 245(18), 1836-1838.

Hoen, T.I., and Brackett, C.E. (1970). Peripheral nerve lengthening. I. Experimental. *Journal of Neurosurgery*, 13(1), 43-62.

Hoeve, C.A.J., and Flory, P.J. (1974). The elastic properties of elastin. *Biopolymers*, 13(4), 677-686.

Holland, G.J. (1968). The physiology of flexibility. A review of the literature. *Kinesiology Review*, 1, 49-62.

Holland, G.J., and Davis, E.L. (1975). *Values of physical activity* (3rd ed.). Dubuque, IA: Brown.

Holly, R.G., Barnett, J.G., Ashmore, C.R., Taylor, R.G., and Mole, P.A. (1980). Stretch-induced growth in chicken wing muscles: A new model of stretch hypertrophy. *American Journal of Physiology*, 238(Cell Physiology 7), C62-C71.

Holmer, I., and Gullstrand, L. (1980). Physiological responses to swimming with a controlled frequency of breathing. *Scandinavian Journal of Sports Sciences*, 2(1), 1-6.

Holt, L.E. (n.d.). *Scientific stretching for sport (3-s)*. Halifax, Nova Scotia: Sport Research.

Holt, L.E., and Smith, R.K. (1983). The effects of selected stretching programs on active and passive flexibility. In J. Terauds (Ed.), *Biomechanics in sport* (pp. 54-67). Del Mar, CA: Research Center for Sports.

Holt, L.E., Travis, T.M., and Okita, T. (1970). Comparative study of three stretching techniques. *Perceptual and Motor Skills*, 31(2), 611-616.

Hooper, A.C.B. (1981). Length, diameter and number of ageing skeletal muscle fibres. *Gerontology*, 27(3), 121-126.

Hoover, H.V. (1958). Functional technic. *Academy of Applied Osteopathy Yearbook 1958*, 47-51.

Hopkins, D.R. (1981). *The relationship between selected anthropometric measures and sit-and-reach performance*. Paper presented at the American Alliance for Health, Physical Education, Recreation and Dance National Measurement Symposium, Houston, TX.

Hopkins, D.R., and Hoeger, W.W.K. (1986). The modified sit and reach test. In Hoeger, W.W.K. (Ed.), *Lifetime physical fitness and wellness: A personalized program* (pp. 47-48). Englewood, CO: Morton.

Hopkins, D.R., Murrah, B., Hoeger, W.W., and Rhodes, R.C.

(1990). Effects of low-impact aerobic dance on the functional fitness of elderly women. *The Gerontologist*, 30(2), 189-192.

Horowits, R. (1992). Passive force generation and titin isoforms in mammalian skeletal muscle. *Biophysical Journal*, 61(2), 392-398.

Horowits, R., Kempner, E.S., Bisher, M.E., and Podolsky, R.J. (1986). A physiological role for titin and nebulin in skeletal muscle. *Nature*, 323(6084), 160-163.

Horowits, R., and Podolsky, R.J. (1987a). The positional stability of thick filaments in activated skeletal muscle depends on sarcomere length: Evidence for the role of titin filaments. *Journal of Cell Biology*, 105(5), 2217-2223.

Horowits, R., and Podolsky, R.J. (1987b). Thick filament movement and the effect of titin filaments in activated skeletal muscle. (Abstract). *Biophysical Journal*, 51(2, Pt. 2), 219a.

Hossler, P. (1989). To bend or not to bend. *The Physician and Sportsmedicine*, 17(6), 20.

Hough, T. (1902). Ergographic studies in muscular soreness. *American Journal of Physiology*, 7(1), 76-92.

Houk, J.C., and Henneman, E. (1967). Responses of Golgi tendon organs to forces applied to muscle tendon. *Journal of Neurophysiology*, 30, 466-481.

Houk, J.C., Singer, J.J., and Goldman, M.R. (1971). Adequate stimulus for tendon organs with observations on mechanics of ankle joint. *Journal of Neurophysiology*, 34(6), 1051-1065.

Howell, J.N., Chila, A.G., Ford, G., David, D., and Gates, T. (1985). An electromyographic study of elbow motion during postexercise muscle soreness. *Journal of Applied Physiology*, 58(5), 1713-1718.

Howse, A.J. (1972). Orthopedist's aide ballet. *Clinical Orthopaedics and Related Research*, 89, 52-63.

Hsieh, C., Walker, J.M., and Gillis, K. (1983). Straight-leg raising test: Comparison of three instruments. *Physical Therapy*, 63(9), 1429-1433.

Hu, D.H., Kimura, S., and Maruyama, K. (1986). Sodium dodecyl sulfate gel electrophoretic studies of connectin-like high molecular weight proteins of various types of vertebrate and invertebrate muscles. *Journal of Biochemistry* (Tokyo), 99, 1485-1492.

Hubley-Kozey, C.L. (1991). Testing flexibility. In E.D. MacDougall, H.A. Wenger, and H.J. Green (Eds.), *Physiological testing of the high-performance athlete* (2nd ed., pp. 309-359). Champaign, IL: Human Kinetics.

Hubley-Kozey, C.L., and Stanish, W.D. (1990). Can stretching prevent athletic injuries? *Journal of Musculoskeletal Medicine*, 7(3), 21-31.

Hull, M. (1990-1991). Flexible ankles: Faster swimming. *Swimming Technique*, 27(3), 23-24.

Hunt, T.K., and Winkle, W.V. (1979). Normal repair. In T.K. Hunt and J.E. Dunphy (Eds.), *Fundamentals of wound management* (pp. 2-67). New York: Appleton-Century-Crofts.

Hupprich, F.L., and Sigerseth, P.O. (1950). The specificity of flexibility in girls. *Research Quarterly*, 21(1), 25-33.

Hussain, S.N.A., Rabinovitch, B., Macklem, P.T., and Pardy, R.L. (1985). Effects of separate rib cage and abdominal restriction on exercise performance in normal humans. *Journal of Applied Physiology*, 58(6), 2020-2026.

Huxley, A.F. (1984). Response to "Is stepwise sarcomere shortening an artifact?" *Nature*, 309(5970), 713-714.

Huxley, A.F. (1986). Comments on quantal mechanisms in cardiac contraction. *Circulation Research*, 59, 9-14.

Huxley, A.F., and Niedergerke, R. (1954). Structural changes in muscle during contraction: Interference microscopy of living muscle fibres. *Nature*, 173(4412), 971-973.

Huxley, A.F., and Peachey, L.D. (1961). The maximum length for contraction in vertebrate striated muscle. *Journal of Physiology*, 156(1), 150-165.

Huxley, H.E. (1957). The double array of filaments in cross-striated muscle. *Journal of Biophysics and Biochemical Cytology*, 3(5), 631-648.

Huxley, H.E. (1967). Muscle cells. In J. Brachet and A. Mirsky (Eds.), *The cell* (pp. 367-481). New York: Academic Press.

Huxley, H.E., and Hanson, J. (1954). Changes in the cross-striations of muscle during contraction and stretch and their structural interpretation. *Nature*, 173(4412), 973-976.

Iashvili, A.V. (1983). Active and passive flexibility in athletes specializing in different sports. *Soviet Sports Review*, 18(1), 30-32.

Ice, R. (1985). Long-term compliance. *Physical Therapy*, 65(12), 1832-1839.

Ikai, M., and Fukunaga, T. (1970). A study on training effect on strength per unit cross-sectional area of muscle by means of ultrasonic measurement. *European Journal of Applied Physiology*, 28, 173-180.

Ingber, D.E., Prusty, D., Frangioni, J.V., Cragoe, E.J., Lechene, C., and Schwartz, M.A. (1990). Control of intracellular pH and growth by fibronectin in capillary endothelial cells. *Journal of Cell Biology*, 110(5), 1803-1811.

Inglis, B.D., Fraser, B., and Penfold, B.R. (1979). *Commission of inquiry into chiropractic #62, Royal Commission of Inquiry*, Wellington, New Zealand: Hasselberg Government Printers.

Inman, V.T., Saunders, J.B., and Abbot, L.C. (1944). Observations on the functions of the shoulder joint. *The Journal of Bone and Joint Surgery*, 26(1), 1-30.

Inoue, S., and Leblond, C.P. (1986). The microfibrils of connective tissue: I. Ultrastructure. *American Journal of Anatomy*, 176(2), 121-138.

International Anatomical Nomenclature Committee (1983). *Nomina anatomica* (5th ed.). Philadelphia: Williams & Wilkins.

International Chiropractors Association. (1993). *Policy handbook & code of ethics*. Arlington, VA: Author.

International Dance-Exercise Association. (n.d.). *Guidelines for convention presenters*. San Diego: Author.

Irrgang, J.J. (1993). Rehabilitation. In F.H. Fu and D.A. Stone (Eds.), *Sports injuries: Mechanisms, prevention, treatment* (2nd ed., pp. 81-95). Baltimore: Williams & Wilkins.

Itay, S., Ganel, A., Horoszowski, H., and Farine, I. (1982). Clinical and functional status following lateral ankle sprains. *Orthopaedic Review*, 11(5), 73-76.

Itoh, Y., Susuki, T., Kimura, S., Ohashi, K., Higuchi, H., Sawada, H., Shimizu, T., Shibata, M., and Maruyama, K. (1988). Extensible and less-extensible domains of connectin filaments in stretched vertebrate skeletal muscle as detected by immunofluorescence and immunoelectron microscopy using monoclonal antibodies. *Journal of Biochemistry* (Tokyo), 104, 504-508.

Iyengar, B.K.S. (1979). *Light on yoga*. New York: Schocken Books.

Jackman, R.V. (1963). Device to stretch the Achilles tendon. *Journal of the American Physical Therapy Association*, 43(10), 729.

Jackson, A.W., and Baker, A.A. (1986). The relationship of the sit and reach test to criterion measures of hamstring and back flexibility in young females. *Research Quarterly for Exercise and Sport*, 57(3), 183-186.

Jackson, A.W., and Langford, N.J. (1989). The criterion-related validity of the sit and reach test: Replication and extension of previous findings. *Research Quarterly for Exercise and Sport*, 60(4), 384-385.

Jackson, C.P., and Brown, M.D. (1983). Is there a role for exercise in the treatment of patients with low back pain? *Clinical Orthopedics and Related Research*, 179(October), 39-45.

Jackson, D.W., Wiltse, L.L., and Cirincione, R.J. (1976). Spondylolysis in the female gymnast. *Clinical Orthopaedics and Related Research*, 117, 68-73.

Jacobs, M. (1976). Neurophysiological implications of slow, active stretching. *American Corrective Therapy Association*, 30(8), 151-154.

Jacobs, S.J., and Berson, B.L. (1986). Injuries to runners: A study of entrants to a 10,000 meter race. *American Journal of Sports Medicine*, 14(2), 151-155.

Jacobson, E. (1929). *Progressive relaxation*. Chicago: University of Chicago Press.

Jacobson, E. (1938). *Progressive relaxation* (2nd ed.). Chicago: University of Chicago Press.

Jahss, S.A. (1919). Joint hypotonia. *New York Medical Journal*, 109(2106), 638-639.

Jami, L. (1992). Golgi tendon organs in mammalian skeletal muscle: Functional properties and central actions. *Physiological Reviews*, 72(3), 623-666.

Janse, J. (1975). History of the development of chiropractic concepts; chiropractic terminology. In M. Goldstein (Ed.), *The research status of spinal manipulative therapy* (DHEW Publication No. [NIH] 76-998, pp. 25-42). Bethesda, MD: U.S. Department of Health, Education, and Welfare.

Janse, J., Houser, R.H., and Wells, B.F. (1947). *Chiropractic principles and technic*. Chicago: National College of Chiropractic.

Jaskoviak, P.A. (1980). Complications arising from manipulation of the cervical spine. *Journal of Manipulative and Physiological Therapeutics*, 3, 213-219.

Jaskoviak, P.A., and Schafer, R.C. (1986). *Applied physiotherapy*. Arlington, VA: The American Chiropractic Association.

Javurek, I. (1982). Experience with hypermobility in athletes. *Theorie A Praxe Telesne Vychovy*, 30(3), 185.

Jay, I., and Rappaport, S. (1983). *Hanging out, the upside down exercise book*. Mill Valley, CA: Jay Ra Productions.

Jayson, M., Sims-Williams, H., Young, S., Baddeley, H., and Collins, E. (1981). Mobilization and manipulation for the low back pain. *Spine*, 6(4), 409-416.

Jenkins, R., and Little, R.W. (1974). A constitutive equation for parallel-fibered elastic tissue. *Journal of Biomechanics*, 7(5), 397-402.

Jervey, A.A. (1961). *A study of the flexibility of selected joints in specified groups of adult females*. Unpublished doctoral dissertation, University of Michigan, Ann Arbor.

Jesse, E.F., Owen, D.S., and Sagar, K.B. (1980). The benign hypermobile joint syndrome. *Arthritis Rheumatism*, 23(9), 1053-1056.

Jobbins, B., Bird, H.A., and Wright, V. (1979). A joint hyperextensometer for the quantification of joint laxity. *Engineering in Medicine*, 8(2), 103-104.

Johns, R.J., and Wright, V. (1962). Relative importance of various tissues in joint stiffness. *Journal of Applied Physiology*, 17(5), 824-828.

Johnson, J.E., Sim, F.H., and Scott, S.G. (1987). Musculoskeletal injuries in competitive swimmers. *Mayo Clinic Proceedings*, 62(4), 289-304.

Johnson, R.J. (1991). Help your athletes heal themselves. *The Physician and Sportsmedicine*, 19(5), 107-110.

Jones, A. (1975). Flexibility and metabolic condition. *Athletic Journal*, 56(2), 56-61, 80-81.

Jones, D.A., and Newham, D.J. (1985). The effect of training on human muscle pain and damage. *Journal of Physiology* (London), 365, 76P.

Jones, D.A.., Newham, D.J., and Clarkson, P.M. (1987). Skeletal muscle stiffness and pain following eccentric exercise of the elbow flexors. *Pain*, 30(2), 233-242.

Jones, D.A., Newham, D.J., Obletter, G., and Giamberardino, M.A. (1987). Nature of exercise-induced muscle pain. *Advances in Pain and Therapy*, 10, 207-218.

Jones, D.A., and Rutherford, O.M. (1987). Human muscle strength training: The effects of three different training regimes and the nature of the resultant changes. *Journal of Physiology* (London), 391, 1-11.

Jones, H.H. (1965). The Valsalva procedure. *Journal of the American Physical Therapy Association*, 45(6), 570-572.

Jones, L.H. (1964). Spontaneous release by positioning. *The DO*, 4, 109-116.

Jones, L.H. (1981). *Strain and counterstrain*. Colorado Springs: American Academy of Osteopathy.

Jones, M.A., Buis, J.M., and Harris, I.D. (1986). Relationship of race and sex to physical and motor measures. *Perceptual and Motor Skills*, 63(1), 169-170.

Jones, R.E. (1970). A kinematic interpretation of running and its relationship to hamstrings injury. *Journal of Health, Physical Education and Recreation*, 41(8), 83.

Journal of Clinical Chiropractic Editorial Advisory Board. (1969). Exercises. *Journal of Clinical Chiropractic*, 2(4), 10-15.

Jungueira, L.C., Carneiro, J., and Long, J.A. (1989). *Basic histology* (6th ed.). Los Altos, CA: Lange Medical.

Kabat, H., McLeod, M., and Holt, C. (1959). The practical application of proprioceptive neuromuscular facilitation. *Physiotherapy*, 45(4), 87-92.

Kalenak, A., and Morehouse, C. (1975). Knee stability and knee ligament injuries. *Journal of the American Medical Association*, 234(11), 1143-1145.

Kaltenborn, F.M. (1989). *Manual mobilization of the extremity joints* (4th ed.). Oslo, Norway: Olaf Norlis Bokhandel.

Kanamaru, A., Sibuya, M., Nagai, T., Inoue, K., and Homma, I. (1990). Stretch gymnastics training in asthmatic children. In M. Kaneko (Ed.), *International series on sport sciences: Vol. 20. Fitness for the aged, disabled, and industrial worker* (pp. 178-181). Champaign, IL: Human Kinetics.

Kandel, E.R., and Swartz, J.H. (1981). *Principles of neural science*. New York: Elsevier.

Kane, M.D., Karl, R.D., and Swain, J.H. (1985). Effects of gravity-facilitated traction on intervertebral dimensions of the lumbar spine. *Journal of Orthopaedic and Sports Physical Therapy*, 6(5), 281-288.

Kapandji, I.A. (1974). *The physiology of the joints: Vol. 3. The trunk and the vertebral column* (2nd ed.). Edinburgh: Churchill Livingstone.

Kapandji, I.A. (1982). *The physiology of the joints: Vol. 1. Upper limb* (2nd ed.). Edinburgh: Churchill Livingstone.

Kapandji, I.A. (1987). *The physiology of the joints: Vol. 2. Lower limb* (5th ed.). Edinburgh: Churchill Livingstone.

Karpovich, P.V., and Sinning, W.E. (1971). *Physiology of muscular activity* (7th ed.). Philadelphia: Saunders.

Karvonen, J. (1992). Importance of warm-up and cool-down on exercise performance. *Medicine in Sport Science*, 35, 189-214.

Kasteler, J., Kane, R.L., Olse, D.M., and Thetford, C. (1976). Issues underlying prevalence of "doctor-shopping" behavior. *Journal of Health and Social Behavior*, 17(4), 328-339.

Kastelic, J., Galeski, A., and Baer, E. (1978). The multicomposite structure of tendon. *Connective Tissue Research*, 6(1), 11-23.

Kauffman, T. (1987). Posture and age. *Topics in Geriatric Rehabilitation*, 2(4), 13-28.

Kauffman, T. (1990). Impact of aging-related musculoskeletal and postural changes on fall. *Topics in Geriatric Rehabilitation*, 5(2), 34-43.

Kazarian, L.E. (1974). Unpublished data. NASA.

Kazarian, L.E. (1975). Creep characteristics of the spinal column. *Orthopedic Clinics of North America*, 6(1), 3-18.

Keating, J.C. (1995). Purpose-straight chiropractic: Not science, not health care. *Journal of Manipulative and Physiological Therapeutics*, 18(6), 416-418.

Kellett, J. (1986). Acute soft tissue injuries—A review of the literature. *Medicine and Science in Sports and Exercise*, 18(5), 489-500.

Kelley, D.L. (1971). *Kinesiology fundamentals of motion description*. Englewood Cliffs, NJ: Prentice-Hall.

Kendall, H.O., and Kendall, F.P. (1948). Normal flexibility according to age groups. *Journal of Bone and Joint Surgery*, 30A(3), 690-694.

Kendall, H.O., Kendall, F.P., and Boynton, D.A. (1970). *Posture and pain*. New York: Krieger.

Kendall, H.O., Kendall, F.P., and Wadsworth, G.E. (1971). *Muscles testing and function*. Baltimore: Williams & Wilkins.

Kerner, J.A., and D'Amico, J.C. (1983). A statistical analysis of a group of runners. *Journal of the American Podiatry Association*, 73(3), 160-164.

Keskinen, K.L., and Komi, P.V. (1991). Breathing patterns of elite swimmers in aerobic/anaerobic loading. *Journal of Biomechanics*, 215(7), 709.

Key, J.A. (1927). Hypermobility of joints as a sex linked hereditary characteristic. *Journal of the American Medical Association*, 88(22), 1710-1712.

Khalil, T.M., Asfour, S.S., Martinez, L.M., Waly, S.M., Rosomoff, R.S., and Rosomoff, H.L. (1992). Stretching in rehabilitation of low-back pain patients. *Spine*, 17(3), 311-317.

Kim, P.S., Santos, D.D., O'Neill, G., Julien, S., Kelm, D., and Dube, M. (1992). The effect of single chiropractic manipulation on sagittal mobility of the lumbar spine in symptomatic low back pain patients. In *Proceedings of the 1992 International Conference on Spinal Manipulation*. Chicago.

Kim, Y.-J., Sah, R.L.Y., Grodzinsky, A.J., Plaas, A.H.K., and Sandy, J.D. (1994). Mechanical regulation of cartilage biosynthetic behavior: Physical stimuli. *Archives of Biochemistry and Biophysics*, 311(1), 1-12.

Kimberly, P.E. (1980). Formulating a prescription for osteopathic manipulative treatment. *Journal of the American Osteopathic Association*, 79(8), 146-152.

King, J.W., Brelsford, H.J., and Tullos, H.S. (1969). Analysis of the pitching arm of the professional baseball pitcher. *Clinical Orthopaedics and Related Research*, 67(November-December), 116-123.

King, N.J. (1980). The therapeutic utility of abbreviated progressive relaxation: A critical review with implications for clinical practice. In M. Hersen, R. Eisler, and P. Miller (Eds.), *Progress in behavior modification* (Vol. 10). New York: Academic Press.

Kippers, V., and Parker, A.W. (1984). Posture related to myoelectric silence of erectores spinae during trunk flexion. *Spine*, 9(7), 740-745.

Kirk, J.A., Ansell, B.M., and Bywaters, E.G.L. (1967). The hypermobility syndrome. *Annals of the Rheumatic Diseases*, 26(5), 419-425.

Kirkebø, A., and Wisnes, A. (1982). Regional tissue fluid pressure in rat calf muscle during sustained contraction or stretch. *Acta Physiologica Scandinavica*, 114(4), 551-556.

Kirstein, L. (1939). *Ballet alphabet; A primer for laymen*. New York: Kamin.

Kisner, C., and Colby, L.A. (1990). *Therapeutic exercise foundations and techniques* (2nd ed.). Philadelphia: Davis.

Klatz, R.M., Goldman, R.M., Pinchuk, B.G., Nelson, K.E., and Tarr, R.S. (1983). The effects of gravity inversion procedures on systemic blood pressure, and central retinal arterial pressure. *Journal of American Osteopathic Association*, 82(11), 111-115.

Klein, K.K. (1961). The deep squat exercise as utilized in weight training for athletics and its effect on the ligaments of the knee. *Journal of the Association for Physical and Mental Rehabilitation*, 15(1), 6-11.

Klein, K.K., and Allman, F.L. (1969). *The knee in sports*. Austin, TX: Pemberton Press.

Klein, K.K., and Roberts, C.A. (1976). Mechanical problems of marathoners and joggers: Cause and solution. *American Corrective Therapy Journal*, 30(6), 187-191.

Klemp, P., and Learmonth, I.D. (1984). Hypermobility and injuries in a professional ballet company. *British Journal of Sports Medicine*, 19(3), 143-148.

Klemp, P., Stevens, J.E., and Isaacs, S. (1984). A hypermobility study in ballet dancers. *Journal of Rheumatology*, 11(5), 692-696.

Kleynhans, A.M. (1980). Complications and contraindications to spinal manipulative therapy. In S. Haldeman (Ed.), *Modern developments in the principles and practice of chiropractic* (pp. 359-384). New York: Appleton-Century-Crofts.

Knapp, M.E. (1990). Massage. In J.F. Lehmann and B.J. de Lateur (Eds.), *Krusen's handbook of physical medicine and rehabilitation* (4th ed., pp. 433-435). Philadelphia: Saunders.

Knight, E.L., and Davis, J.B. (1984). *Flexibility: The concept of stretching and exercise*. Dubuque, IA: Kendall/Hunt.

Knight, K.L. (1995). *Cryotherapy in sport injury management*. Champaign, IL: Human Kinetics.

Knott, M., and Voss, D.E. (1968). *Proprioceptive neuromuscular facilitation*. New York: Harper & Row.

Knuttgen, H.G. (1986). Human performance in high-intensity exercise with concentric and eccentric muscle contractions. *International Journal of Sports Medicine*, 7(Suppl. 1), 6-9.

Knuttgen, H.G., Patton, J.F., and Vogel, J.A. (1982). An ergometer for concentric and eccentric muscular exercise. *Journal of Applied Physiology*, 53(3), 784-788.

Kobet, K.A. (1985). Retinal tear associated with gravity boot use. *Annals of Ophthalmology*, 17(4), 308-310.

Koceja, D.M., Burke, J.R., and Kamen, G. (1991). Organization of segmental reflexes in trained dancers. *International Journal of Sports Medicine*, 12(3), 285-289.

Koeller, W., Funke, F., and Hartman, F. (1984). Biomechanical behavior of human intervertebral discs subjected to long lasting axial loading. *Biorheology*, 21(5), 675-686.

Kokjohn, K., Schmid, D.M., Triano, J.J., and Brennan, P.C. (1992). The effect of spinal manipulation on pain and prostaglandin levels in women with primary dysmenorrhea. *Journal of Manipulative and Physiological Therapeutics*, 15(5), 279-285.

Komi, P.V. (1986). Training of muscle strength and power: Interaction of neuromotoric, hypertrophic, and mechanical factors. *Journal of Sports Medicine*, 7(1), 10-15.

Komi, P.V., and Boscoe, C. (1978). Utilization of stored elastic energy in men and women. *Medicine and Science in Sport*, 10(4), 261-265.

Komi, P.V., and Buskirk, E.R. (1972). Measurement of eccentric and concentric conditioning on tension and electrical activity in human muscle. *Ergonomics*, 15(July), 417-434.

Kopell, H.P. (1962). The warm-up and autogenic injury. *New York State Journal of Medicine*, 62(20), 3255-3258.

Kornberg, L., and Juliano, R.L. (1992). Signal transduction from the extracellular matrix: The integrin-tyrosine kinase connection. *Trends in Pharmacological Sciences*, 13(3), 93-95.

Korr, I.M. (1975). Proprioceptors and somatic dysfunction. *Journal of the American Osteopathic Association*, 74(7), 638-650.

Koslow, R.E. (1987). Bilateral flexibility in the upper and lower extremities as related to age and gender. *Journal of Human Movement Studies*, 13(9), 467-472.

Kottke, F.J., Pauley, D.L., and Ptak, K.A. (1966). Prolonged stretching for correction of shortening of connective tissue. *Archives of Physical Medicine and Rehabilitation*, 47(6), 345-352.

Kraeger, D.R. (1993). Foot injuries. In W.A. Lillegard and K.S. Rucker (Eds.), *Handbook of sportsmedicine: A symptom-oriented approach* (pp. 159-171). Boston: Andover Medical.

Krahenbuhl, G.S., and Martin, S.L. (1977). Adolescence body size and flexibility. *Research Quarterly*, 48(4), 797-799.

Kramer, A.M., and Schrier, R.W. (1990). Demographic, social, and economic issues. In R.W. Schrier (Ed.), *Geriatric medicine* (pp. 1-11). Philadelphia: Saunders.

Kranz, K.C. (1988). Chiropractic treatment of low-back pain. *Topics in Acute Care and Trauma Rehabilitation*, 2(4), 47-62.

Kraus, H. (1965). *Backache stress and tension: Their cause, prevention and treatment*. New York: Simon and Schuster.

Kraus, H. (1970). *Clinical treatment of back and neck pain*. New York: McGraw-Hill.

Kreighbaum, E., and Barthels, K.M. (1985). *Biomechanics: A qualitative approach for studying human movement* (2nd ed.). Minneapolis: Burgess.

Krejci, V., and Koch, P. (1979). *Muscle and tendon injuries in athletes*. Stuttgart: Georg Thieme.

Krieglstein, G.K., and Langham, M.E. (1975). Influence of body position on the intraocular pressure of normal and glaucomatous eyes. *Ophthalmologica*, 171(2), 132-145.

Krissoff, W.B., and Ferris, W.D. (1979). Runners' injuries. *The Physician and Sportsmedicine*, 7(12), 55-64.

Kronberg, M., Brostrom, L-A., and Soderlund, V. (1990). Retroversion of the humeral head in the normal shoulder and its relationship to the normal range of motion. *Clinical Orthopaedics and Related Research*, 253(April), 113-117.

Kuchera, W.A., and Kuchera, M.L. (1992). *Osteopathic principles in practice*. Kirksville, MO: Kirksville College of Osteopathic Medicine.

Kudina, L. (1980). Reflex effects of muscle afferents on antagonists studies on single firing motor units in man. *Electroencephalography and Clinical Neurophysiology*, 50(3-4), 214-221.

Kuipers, H.J., Drukker, P.M., Frederik, P.M., Guerten, P., and Kranenburg, G.V. (1983). Muscle degeneration after exercise in rats. *International Journal of Sports Medicine*, 4(1), 45-51.

Kulakov, V. (1989). The harmony of training: The training of long-distance runners. *Soviet Sport Review*, 24(4), 164-168.

Kulund, D.N. (1980). The foot in athletics. In A.J. Helfet and D.M.G. Lee (Eds.), *Disorders of the foot* (pp. 58-79). Philadelphia: Lippincott.

Kulund, D.N., Dewey, J.B., Brubaker, C.E., and Roberts, J.R. (1978). Olympic weight-lifting injuries. *The Physician and Sportsmedicine*, 6(11), 111-119.

Kulund, D.N., and Töttössy, M. (1983). Warm-up, strength, and power. *Orthopaedic Clinics of North America*, 14(2), 427-448.

Kunz, H., and Kaufmann, D. A. (1980). How the best sprinters differ. *Track & Field Quarterly Review*, 80(2).

Kuprian, W., Ork, H., and Meissner, L. (1982). Spinal column and torso. In W. Kuprian (Ed.), *Physical therapy for sports* (pp. 262-286). Philadelphia: Saunders.

Kurzban, G.P., and Wang, K. (1988). Giant polypeptides of skeletal muscle titin: Sedimentation equilibrium in guanidine hydrochloride. *Biochemical and Biophysical Research Communications*, 150, 1155-1161.

Kushner, S., Saboe, L., Reid, D., Penrose, T., and Grace, M. (1990). Relationship of turnout to hip abduction in professional ballet dancers. *American Journal of Sports Medicine*, 18(3), 286-291.

Laban, M.M. (1962). Collagen tissue: Implications of its response to stress in vitro. *Archives of Physical Medicine and Rehabilitation*, 43(9), 461-465.

Ladermann, J.P. (1981). Accidents of spinal manipulations. *Annals of the Swiss Chiropractic Association*, 7, 161-208.

LaFreniere, J.G. (1979). *The low back patient: Procedures for treatment by physical therapy.* New York: Mason.

Larson, L.A., and Michelman, H. (1973). *International guide to fitness and health.* New York: Crown.

Larsson, L.-G., Baum, J., Mudholkar, G.S., and Kollia, G. (1993). Benefits and disadvantages of joint hypermobility among musicians. *New England Journal of Medicine*, 329(15), 1079-1082.

Lasater, J. (1983). Asana triang mukhaikapada paschimottanasana. *Yoga Journal*, 52(September-October), 9-11.

Lasater, J. (1986). Supta virasana: Reclining hero pose. *Yoga Journal*, 67(March-April), 23-24.

Lasater, J. (1988a). Janu Sirsasana: Head of the knee pose. *Yoga Journal*, 83(November-December), 35-40.

Lasater, J. (1988b). Uttanasana intense stretch pose. *Yoga Journal*, 79(March-April), 30-35.

Laubach, L.C., and McConville, J.T. (1966a). Muscle strength, flexibility, and bone size of adult males. *Research Quarterly*, 37(3), 384-392.

Laubach, L.C., and McConville, J.T. (1966b). Relationship between flexibility, anthropometry, and somatotype of college men. *Research Quarterly*, 37(2), 241-251.

Lawton, R.W. (1957). Some aspects of research in biological elasticity. In J.W. Remington (Ed.), *Tissue elasticity* (pp. 1-11). Washington DC: American Physiological Society.

Laxton, A.H. (1990). Practical approaches to the normalization of muscle tension. *Journal of Manual Medicine*, 5(3), 115-120.

Leard, J.S. (1984). Flexibility and conditioning in the young athlete. In L.J. Micheli (Ed.), *Pediatric and adolescent sports medicine* (pp. 194-210). Boston: Little, Brown.

Leatt, P., Reilly, T., and Troup, J.G.D. (1986). Spinal loading during circuit weight-training and running. *British Journal of Sports Medicine*, 20(3), 119-124.

Leboeuf, C., Ames, R.A., Budich, C.W., and Vincent, A.F. (1987). Changes in blood pressure and pulse rate following exercise in the inverted position. *Journal of the Australian Chiropractic Association*, 17(2), 60-62.

Lee, D. (1989). *The pelvic girdle.* Edinburgh: Churchill Livingstone.

Lee, G.C. (1980). Finite element analysis in soft tissue mechanics. In B.R. Simon (Ed.), *Vol. 1. International conference on finite elements in biomechanics* (pp. 27-37). Tucson, AZ: National Science Foundation and the University of Arizona College of Engineering.

Lee, M.A., and Kleitman, N. (1923). Studies on the physiology of sleep. II. Attempts to demonstrate functional changes in the nervous system during experimental insomnia. *American Journal of Physiology*, 67(1), 141-152.

Lehmann, J.F., Masock, A.J., Warren, C.G., and Koblanski, J.N. (1970). Effect of therapeutic temperature on tendon extensibility. *Archives of Physical Medicine and Rehabilitation*, 51(8), 481-487.

Lehmann, J.P., and de Lateur, B.J. (1990). Diathermy and superficial heat, laser, and cold therapy. In J.F. Lehmann and B.J. de Lateur (Eds.), *Krusen's handbook of physical medicine and rehabilitation* (4th ed., pp. 285-367). Philadelphia: Saunders.

Lehrer, P.M., and Woolfolk, R.L. (1984). Are stress reduction techniques interchangeable, or do they have specific effects? A review of the comparative empirical literature. In R.L. Woolfolk and P.M. Lehrer (Eds.), *Principles and practices of stress management.* New York: Guilford Press.

Leighton, J.R. (1956). Flexibility characteristics of males ten to eighteen years of age. *Archives of Physical and Mental Rehabilitation*, 37(8), 494-499.

Leighton, J.R. (1960). On the significance of flexibility for physical education. *Journal of Health, Physical Education, and Recreation*, 31(8), 27-28.

Le Marr, J.D., Golding, I.A., and Adler, J.G. (1984). Intraocular pressure responses to inversion. *American Journal of Optometry and Physiological Optics*, 61(11), 679-682.

Leonard, T.J.K., Muir, M.G., Kirkby, G.R., and Hitchings, R.A. (1983). Ocular hypertension and posture. *British Journal of Ophthalmology*, 67(6), 362-366.

Lepique, G., and Sell, G. (1962). Der Gelenk binnendruck im normalen und geshadigten Gelenk [Internal pressure in the normal and pathological joint]. *Zeitschrift Orthopaedie und Ihre Grenzgebiete*, 96(July), 235-238.

Levarlet-Joye, H. (1979). Relaxation and motor capacity. *Journal of Sports Medicine*, 19(2), 151-156.

Levin, R.M., and Wolf, S.L. (1987). Preliminary analysis on conditioning of exaggerated triceps surae stretch reflexes among stroke patients. *Biofeedback and Self-Regulation*, 12(2), 153.

Levine, M.G., and Kabat, H. (1952). Cocontraction and reciprocal innervation in voluntary movement in man. *Science*, 116(3005), 115-118.

Levtov, V.A., Shushtova, N.Y., Regirer, S.A., Shadrina, N.K., Maltsev, N.A., and Levkovich, Y.I. (1985). Topographic and hydrodynamic heterogeneity of the terminal bed of the cat gastrocnemius muscle vessel. *Fiziologicheski Zhurnal SSR Imeni I.M. Sechenova*, 71(9), 1105-1111. (In *Biological Abstracts*, 81(9), AB-164, #79767.)

Lewin, G. (1979). *Swimming.* Berlin: Sportverlag.

Lewit, K. (1991). *Manipulative therapy in rehabilitation of the locomotor system* (2nd ed.). Oxford: Buttersworth-Heinmann.

Lewit, K. (1992). An assessment of the different treatment techniques in manipulative medicine. *Journal of Manual Medicine*, 6(6), 194-197.

Ley, P. (1977). Psychological studies of doctor-patient communication. In S. Rachman (Ed.), *Contributions to medical psychology.* Oxford: Pergamon.

Ley, P. (1988). *Communicating with patient: Improving communication, satisfaction and compliance.* London: Croom Helm.

Liberson, W.T., and Asa, M.M. (1959). Further studies of brief isometric exercises. *Archives of Physical Medicine*, 40(8), 330-336.

Lichtor, J. (1972). The loose-jointed young athlete. *American Journal of Sports Medicine*, 1(1), 22-23.

Liemohn, W. (1978). Factors related to hamstring strains. *Journal of Sports Medicine and Physical Fitness*, 18(1), 71-75.

Liemohn, W. (1988). Flexibility and muscular strength. *Journal of Physical Education, Recreation and Dance*, 59(7), 37-40.

Light, K.E., Nuzik, S., Personius, W., and Barstrom, A. (1984). A low-loading prolonged stretch vs. high-low brief stretch in treating knee contractures. *Physical Therapy*, 64(3), 330-333.

Lindner, E. (1971). The phenomenon of the freedom of lateral deviation in throwing (Wurfseitenfreiheit). In J. Vredenbregt and J. Wartenwiller (Eds.), *Medicine and sport: Vol. 6. Biomechanics II* (pp. 240-245), Basel: Karger.

Livingston, M.C.P. (1968). Spinal manipulation in medical practice: A century of ignorance. *Medical Journal of Australia*, 2(13), 552-555.

Livingston, M.C.P. (1971). Spinal manipulation causing injury. *Clinical Orthopaedics and Related Research*, 81, 82-86.

Locke, J.C. (1983). Stretching away from back pain, injury. *Occupational Health and Science*, 52(7), 8-13.

Locker, R.H., Daines, G.J., and Leet, N.G. (1976). Histology of highly-stretched beef muscle. III. Abnormal contraction patterns in ox muscle, produced by overstretching during prerigor blending. *Journal of Ultrastructure Research*, 55(2), 173-181.

Locker, R.H., and Leet, N.G. (1975). Histology of highly-stretched beef muscle. I. The fine structure of grossly stretched single fibers. *Journal of Ultrastructure Research*, 52(1), 64-75.

Locker, R.H., and Leet, N.G. (1976a). Histology of highly-stretched beef muscle. II. Further evidence on the location and nature of gap filaments. *Journal of Ultrastructure Research*, 55(2), 157-172.

Locker, R.H., and Leet, N.G. (1976b). Histology of highly-stretched beef muscle. IV. Evidence for movement of gap filaments through the Z-line. Using the N2-line and M-line as markers. *Journal of Ultrastructure Research*, 56(1), 31-38.

Loeper, J. (1985). *Range of motion exercise*. Minneapolis: Sister Kenny Institute.

Logan, G.A., and Egstrom, G.H. (1961). Effects of slow and fast stretching on the sacro-femoral angle. *Journal Association for Physical and Mental Rehabilitation*, 15(3), 85-89.

Long, C. (1974). Physical medicine and rehabilitation. In C.D. Ray (Ed.), *Medical engineering* (pp. 516-541). Chicago: Yearbook Medical.

Long, P.A. (1971). *The effects of static, dynamic, and combined stretching exercise programs on hip joint flexibility*. Unpublished master's thesis, University of Maryland.

Longworth, J.C. (1982). Psychophysiological effects of slow stroke back massage on normotensive females. *Advances in Nursing Science*, 4(4), 44-61.

Louttit, C.M., and Halford, J.F. (1930). The relationship between chest girth and vital capacity. *Research Quarterly*, 1(4), 34-35.

Low, F.N. (1961a). The extracellular portion of the human blood-air barrier and its relation to tissue space. *Anatomical Record*, 139(2), 105-122.

Low, F.N. (1961b). Microfibrils, a small extracellular component of connective tissue. *Anatomical Record*, 139(2), 250.

Low, F.N. (1962). Microfibrils, fine filamentous components of the tissue space. *Anatomical Record*, 142(2), 131-137.

Lowther, D.A. (1981). Molecular aspects of connective tissue remodeling. In G.D. Bryant-Greenwood, H.D. Niall, and F.C. Greenwood (Eds.), *Relaxin* (pp. 277-291). New York: Elsevier.

Lubell, A. (1989). Potentially dangerous exercises: Are they harmful to all? *The Physician and Sportsmedicine*, 17(1), 187-192.

Luby, S., and St. Onge, R.A. (1986). *Bodysense*. Winchester, MA: Faber and Faber.

Lucas, R.C., and Koslow, R. (1984). Comparative study of static, dynamic, and proprioceptive neuromuscular facilitation stretching techniques on flexibility. *Perceptual and Motor Skills*, 58(2), 615-618.

Lund, J.P., Donga, R., Widmer, C.G., and Stohler, C.S. (1991). The pain-adaptation model: A discussion of the relationship between chronic musculoskeletal pain and motor activity. *Canadian Journal of Physiological Pharmacology*, 69(5), 683-694.

Lundberg, A. (1975). Control of spinal mechanisms from the brain. In D.B. Tower (Ed.), *The nervous system. The basic neurosciences* (Vol. 1, pp. 253-265). New York: Raven Press.

Lundborg, G. (1975). Structure and function of the intraneural microvessels as related to trauma, edema formation and nerve function. *Journal of Bone and Joint Surgery*, 57A(7), 938-948.

Lundborg, G. (1993). Peripheral nerve injuries: Pathophysiology and strategies for treatment. *Journal of Hand Therapy*, 6(3), 179-188.

Lundborg, G., and Brånemark, P.-I. (1968). Microvascular structure and function of peripheral nerves. *Advances in Microcirculation*, 1, 68-88.

Lundborg, G., and Rydevik, B. (1973). Effects of stretching the tibial nerve of the rabbit. *Journal of Bone and Joint Surgery*, 55B(2), 390-401.

Lunde, B.K., Brewer, W.D., and Garcia, P.A. (1972). Grip strength of college women. *Archives of Physical Medicine and Rehabilitation*, 53(10), 491-493.

Luthe, W. (1969). *Psychosomatic medicine*. New York: Harper & Row.

Lutter, L.D. (1983). Problems in the foot and ankle in runners. In R.H. Kiene and K.A. Johnson (Eds.), *American Academy of Orthopaedic Surgeons symposium on the foot and ankle* (pp. 15-20). St. Louis: Mosby.

MacDonald, J. (1985). Falls in the elderly: The role of drugs in the elderly. *Clinical Geriatric Medicine*, 1, 621-636.

MacDonald, J.B., and MacDonald, E.T. (1977). Nocturnal femoral fracture and continuing widespread use of barbiturate hypnotics. *British Medical Journal*, 2(6085), 483-485.

Macintosh, J.E., Bogduk, N., and Pearcy, M.J. (1993). The effects of flexion on the geometry and actions of the lumbar erector spinae. *Spine*, 18(7), 884-893.

Maclennan, S.E., Silvestri, G.A., Ward, J., and Mahler, D.A. (1994). Does entrainment breathing improve the economy of rowing? *Medicine and Science in Sport and Exercise*, 26(5), 610-614.

Madden, J.W., and Arem, A.J. (1986). Wound healing: Biological and clinical features. In D.C. Sabiston (Ed.), *Textbook of surgery* (13th ed., pp. 193-213). Philadelphia: Saunders.

Madding, S.W., Wong, J.G., Hallum, A., and Medeiros, J.M. (1987). Effects of duration of passive stretch on hip abduction range of motion. *Journal of Orthopaedic Sports Physical Therapy*, 8(8), 409-416.

Magder, R., Baxter, M.L., and Kassam, Y.B. (1986). Does a diuretic improve morning stiffness in rheumatoid arthritis? *British Journal of Rheumatology*, 25(3), 318-319.

Magid, A., Ting-Beall, H.P., Carvell, M., Kontis, T., and Lucaveche, C. (1984). Connecting filaments, core filaments, and side struts: A proposal to add three new load bearing structures to the sliding filament model. In G.H. Pollack and H. Sugi (Eds.), *Contractile mechanisms in muscle* (pp. 307-323). New York: Plenum.

Magnusson, M., Hult, E., Lindstrom. I., Lindell, V., Pope, M., and Hansson, T. (1990). Measurement of time-dependent height-loss during sitting. *Clinical Biomechanics,* 5(3), 137-142.

Magnusson, S.P., Gleim, G.W., and Nicholas, J.A. (1994). Shoulder weakness in professional baseball pitchers. *Medicine and Science in Sports and Exercise,* 26(1), 5-9.

Mahler, D.A., Hunter, B., Lentine, T., and Ward, J. (1991). Locomotor-respiratory coupling develops in novice female rowers with training. *Medicine and Science in Sports and Exercise,* 23(12), 1362-1366.

Maitland, G.D. (1979). *Peripheral manipulation.* Boston: Buttersworth.

Malina, R.M. (1988). Physical anthropology. In T.G. Lohman, A.F. Roche, and R. Martorell (Eds.), *Anthropometric standardization reference manual* (pp. 99-102). Champaign, IL: Human Kinetics.

Mallik, A.K., Ferrell, W.R., McDonald, A.G., and Sturrock, R.D. (1994). Impaired proprioceptive acuity at the proximal interphalangeal joint in patients with the hypermobility syndrome. *British Journal of Rheumatology,* 33(7), 631-637.

Maltz, M. (1970). *Psycho-Cybernetics.* New York: Simon and Schuster.

Manheim, C.J., and Lavett, D.K. (1989). *The myofascial release manual.* Thorofare, NJ: Slack.

Mann, R.A., Baxter, D.E., and Lutter, L.D. (1981). Running symposium. *Foot and Ankle,* 1(4), 190-224.

Marino, M. (1984). Profiling swimmers. *Clinics in Sports Medicine,* 3(1), 211-229.

Markee, J.E., Logue, J.T., Williams, M., Stanton, W.B., Wrenn, R.N., and Walker, L.B. (1955). Two-joint muscles of the thigh. *Journal of Bone and Joint Surgery,* 37A(1), 125-145.

Marras, W.S., and Wongsam, P.E. (1986). Flexibility and velocity of the normal and impaired lumbar spine. *Archives of Physical Medicine and Rehabilitation,* 67(4), 213-217.

Marshall, J.L., Johanson, N., Wickiewicz, T.L., Tischler, H.M., Koslin, B.L., Zeno, S., and Meyers, A. (1980). Joint looseness: A function of the person and the joint. *Medicine and Science in Sports and Exercise,* 12(3), 189-194.

Martin, D., and Coe, P. (1991). *Training distance runners.* Champaign, IL: Human Kinetics.

Martin, R.M. (1982). *The gravity guiding system.* Pasadena, CA: Gravity Guidance.

Maruyama, K. (1976). Connectin, an elastic protein from myofibrils. *Journal of Biochemistry,* 80(2), 405-407.

Maruyama, K. (1986). Connectin, an elastic filamentous protein of striated muscle. *International Review of Cytology,* 104, 81-115.

Maruyama, K., Kimura, S., Ohashi, K., and Kuwano, Y. (1981). Connectin, an elastic protein of muscle. Identification of "titin" with connectin. *Journal of Biochemistry* (Tokyo), 89(3), 701-709.

Maruyama, K., Kimura, S., Yoshidomi, H., Sawada, H., and Kikuchi, M. (1984). Molecular size and shape of B-connectin, an elastic protein of striated muscle. *Journal of Biochemistry* (Tokyo), 95(5), 1423-1433.

Maruyama, K., Matsubara, S., Natori, R., Nonomura, Y., Kimura, S., Ohashi, K., Murakami, F., Handa, S., and Eguchi, G. (1977). Connectin, an elastic protein of muscle. *Journal of Biochemistry* (Tokyo), 82(2), 317-337.

Maruyama, K., Natori, R., and Nonomura, Y. (1976). New elastic protein from muscle. *Nature,* 262(5563), 58-60.

Marvey, D. (1887). Recherces experimentales sur la morphologie

de muscles [Experimental research on the morphology of muscles]. *Comptes Rendus Hebdomadaires du Seances de l'Academie des Sciences* (Paris), 105, 446-451.

Mason, T., and Rigby, B.J. (1963). Thermal transition in collagen. *Biochemica et Biophysica Acta,* 79(PN1254), 448-450.

Massey, B.A., and Chaudet, N.L. (1956). Effects of systematic, heavy resistance exercise on range of joint movement in young adults. *Research Quarterly,* 27(1), 41-51.

Massie, W.K., and Howarth, M.B. (1951). Congenital dislocation of the hip. *Journal of Bone and Joint Surgery,* 33A, 171-198.

Matchanov, A.T., Levtov, V.A., and Orlov, V.V. (1983). Changes of the blood flow in longitudinal stretch of the cat gastrocnemius muscle. *Fiziologicheskii Zhurnal SSSR Imeni I.M. Sechenova,* 69(1), 74-83. (In *Biological Abstracts,* 77(9), p. 7196 #65430, May 1984.)

Matchanov, A.T.N., Shustova, N.Y., Shuvaeva, V.N., Vasil'eva, L.I., and Levtov, V.A. (1983). Effects of stretch of the cat gastrocnemius muscle on its tetani, postcontraction hyperemia and parameters of energy metabolism. *Fiziologicheskii Zhurnal SSSR Imeni I.M. Sechenova,* 69(2), 210-219. (In *Biological Abstracts,* 77(6), p. 4883, #44673, March 1984.)

Mathews, D.K., Shaw, V., and Bohnen, M. (1957). Hip flexibility of college women as related to body segments. *Research Quarterly,* 28(4), 352-356.

Mathews, D.K., Shaw, V., and Woods, J.W. (1959). Hip flexibility of elementary school boys as related to body segments. *Research Quarterly,* 31(3), 297-302.

Mathews, D.K., Stacy, R.W., and Hoover, G.N. (1964). *Physiology of muscular activity and exercise.* New York: Ronald Press.

Matsumura, K., Shimizu, T., Nonaka, I., and Mannen, T. (1989). Immunochemical study of connectin (titin) in neuromuscular diseases using a monoclonal antibody: Connectin is degraded extensively in Duchenne muscular dystrophy. *Journal of the Neurological Sciences,* 93(2-3), 147-156.

Matthews, P.B.C. (1972). *Mammalian muscle receptors and their central actions.* Baltimore: Williams & Wilkins.

Matveyev, L. (1981). *Fundamentals of sports training.* Moscow: Progress.

Matvienko, L.A., and Kartasheva, M.V. (1990). Treating calf-muscle cramps with a simple physical exercise. *Soviet Sport Review* 25(4), 162-163.

May, B.J. (1990). Principles of exercise for the elderly. In J.V. Basmajian and S.L. Wolf (Eds.), *Therapeutic exercise* (5th ed., pp. 279-298). Baltimore: Williams & Wilkins.

Mayer, T.G., Gatchel, R.J., Kishino, N., Keeley, N., Capra, P., Mayer, H., Barnett, J., and Mooney, V. (1985). Objective assessment of spine function following industrial injury. A prospective study with comparison group and one-year follow-up. *Spine,* 10(6), 482-493.

Mayer, T.G., Gatchel, R.J., Mayer, H., Kishino, N.D., and Keeley, J. (1987). A prospective two-year study of functional restoration in industrial low back injury. An objective assessment procedure. *Journal of the American Medical Association,* 258(13), 1763-1767.

Mayhew, T.P., Norton, B.J., and Sahrmann, S.A. (1983). Electromyographic study of the relationship between hamstring and abdominal muscles during unilateral straight leg raise. *Physical Therapy,* 63(11), 1769-1773.

McAtee, R.E. (1993). *Facilitated stretching.* Champaign, IL: Human Kinetics.

McCue, B.F. (1963). Flexibility measurements of college women. *Research Quarterly,* 24(3), 316-324.

McCutcheon, L.J., Byrd, S.K., and Hodgson, D.R. (1992). Ultrastructural changes in skeletal muscle after fatiguing exercise. *Journal of Applied Physiology*, 72(3), 1111-1117.

McDonagh, M.J.N., and Davies, C.T.M. (1984). Adaptive response of mammalian skeletal muscle to exercise with high loads. *European Journal of Applied Physiology*, 52(2), 139-155.

McDonagh, M.J.N., Hayward, C.M., and Davies, C.T.M. (1983). Isometric training in human elbow flexor muscles: The effects on voluntary and electrically evoked forces. *Journal of Bone and Joint Surgery*, 65B(3), 355-358.

McDonough, A.L. (1981). Effects of immobilization and exercise on articular cartilage—A review of the literature. *The Journal of Orthopaedic and Sports Physical Therapy*, 3(1), 2-5.

McFarlane, A.C., Kalucy, R.S., and Brooks, P.M. (1987). Psychological predictor of disease course in rheumatoid arthritis. *Journal of Psychosomatic Research*, 31(6), 757-764.

McFarlane, B. (1987). A look inside the biomechanics and dynamics of speed. *NSCA Journal*, 9(5), 35-41.

McGee, S.R. (1990). Muscle cramps. *Archives of Internal Medicine*, 150(3), 511-518.

McGeorge, S. (1989). Warming up and warming down. *Health and Physical Education Project Newsletter*, No. 22.

McGill, S.M., and Brown, S. (1992). Creep response of the lumbar spine to prolonged full flexion. *Clinical Biomechanics*, 7(1), 43-46.

McGlynn, G.H., Laughlin, N.T., and Rowe, V. (1979). Effect of electromyographic feedback and static stretching on artificially induced muscle soreness. *American Journal of Physical Medicine*, 58(3), 139-148.

McKenzie, R. (1981). *Mechanical diagnosis and treatment of the lumbar spine*. New Zealand: Spinal.

McKenzie, R. (1983). *Treat your own neck*. New Zealand: Spinal.

McKusick, V.A. (1956). *Heritable disorders of connective tissue*. St. Louis: Mosby.

McNeil, P.A., and Hoyle, G. (1967). Evidence for super thin filaments. *American Zoologist*, 7(3), 483-503.

McNitt-Gray, J.L. (1991). Biomechanics related to exercise and pregnancy. In R.A. Mittelmark, R.A. Wiswell, and B.L. Drinkwater (Eds.), *Exercise in pregnancy* (2nd ed., pp. 133-140). Philadelphia: Williams & Wilkins.

McPoil, T.G., and McGarvey, T.C. (1995). The foot in athletics. In G.C. Hunt and T.G. McPoil (Eds.), *Physical therapy of the foot and ankle* (2nd ed., pp. 207-236). New York: Churchill Livingstone.

Mead, N. (1994). Eating for flexibility. *Yoga Journal*, 117 (July-August), 91-98.

Meal, G.M., and Scott, R.A. (1986). Analysis of the joint crack by simultaneous recording of sound and tension. *Journal of Manipulative and Physiological Therapeutics*, 9(3), 189-195.

Medeiros, J.M., Smidt, G.L., Burmeister, L.F., and Soderberg, G.L. (1977). The influence of isometric exercise and passive stretch on hip joint motion. *Physical Therapy*, 57(5), 518-523.

Meeker, W.C. (1991). Designing research on spinal manipulation. *ABS Newsletter*, 7(2), 19-21.

Mellerowicz, H., and Hansen, G. (1971). Conditioning. In L.A. Larson (Ed.), *Encyclopedia of sport sciences and medicine* (pp. 1586-1587). New York: Macmillan.

Mellin, G. (1985). Physical therapy for chronic low back pain: Correlations between spinal mobility and treatment outcome. *Scandinavian Journal of Rehabilitation Medicine*, 17(4), 163-166.

Mennell, J. (1960). *Back pain*. Boston: Little, Brown.

Merletti, R., Repossi, F., Richetta, E., Mathis, C., Saracco, C.R. (1986). Size and x-ray density of normal and denervated muscles of the human legs and forearms. *International Rehabilitation Medicine*, 8(2), 82-89.

Merni, F., Balboni, M., Bargellini, S., and Menegatti, G. (1981). Differences in males and females in joint movement range during growth. *Medicine and Sport*, 15, 168-175.

Merskey, H. (1979). Pain terms: A list with definitions and notes on usage. Recommended by the ISAP Subcommittee on Taxonomy. *Pain*, 6(3), 249-252.

Metheny, E. (1952). *Body dynamics*. New York: McGraw-Hill.

Michaud, T. (1990). Biomechanics of unilateral overhand throwing motion: An overview. *Chiropractic Sports Medicine*, 4(1), 13-26.

Michele, A.A. (1971). *Orthotherapy*. New York: Evans.

Micheli, L.J. (1983). Overuse injuries in children's sport: The growth factor. *Orthopaedic Clinics of North America*, 14(2), 337-360.

Michelson, L. (1987). Cognitive-behavioral assessment and treatment of agoraphobia. In L. Michelson and L.M. Ascher (Eds.), *Anxiety and stress disorders* (pp. 213-279). New York: Guilford Press.

Mikawa, Y., Watanabe, R., Yamano, Y., and Miyake, S. (1988). Stress fracture of the body of pubis in a pregnant woman. *Archives of Orthopaedic and Traumatic Surgery*, 107(3), 193-194.

Milberg, S., and Clark, M.S. (1988). Moods and compliance. *British Journal of Social Psychology*, 27(Pt. I, March), 79-90.

Miller, E.H., Schneider, H.J., Bronson, J.L., and McClain, D. (1975). The classical ballet dancer: A new consideration in athletic injuries. *Clinical Orthopaedics and Related Research*, 111, 181-191.

Miller, G., Boster, F., Roloff, M., and Seibold, D. (1977). Compliance-gaining message strategies: A typology and some findings concerning effects of situational differences. *Communication Monographs*, 44(1), 37-51.

Miller, G., Wilcox, A., and Schwenkel, J. (1988). The protective effect of a prior bout of downhill running on delayed onset muscular soreness (DOMS). *Medicine and Science in Sports and Exercise*, 20(2 Suppl.), S75.

Miller, M.D., and Major, M.D. (1994). Posterior cruciate ligament injuries: History, examination, and diagnostic testing. *Sports Medicine and Arthroscopy Review*, 2(2), 100-105.

Miller, W.A. (1977). Rupture of the musculotendinous juncture of the medial head of the gastrocnemius muscle. *American Journal of Sports Medicine*, 5(5), 191-193.

Milne, C., Seefeldt, V., and Reuschlein, P. (1976). Relationship between grade, sex, race, and motor performance in young children. *Research Quarterly*, 47(4), 726-730.

Milne, R.A., and Mierau, D.R. (1979). Hamstring distensibility in the general population: Relationship to pelvic and low back stresses. *Journal of Manipulative and Physiological Therapeutics*, 2(1), 146-150.

Milne, R.A., Mierau, D.R., and Cassidy, J.D. (1981). Evaluation of sacroiliac joint movement and its relationship to hamstring distensibility (Abstract). *International Review of Chiropractic*, 35(2), 40.

Milner-Brown, H.S., Stein, R.B., and Lee, R. G. (1975). Synchronization of human motor units: Possible roles of exercise and supraspinal reflexes. *Electroencephalography and Clinical Neurophysiology*, 38(3), 245-254.

Mironov, V.M. (1969a). Correlation of breathing and movement in male gymnasts during execution of routines on the apparatus. *Theory and Practice of Physical Culture*, 7, 23-26. (In *Yessis Review*, 5(1), 14-19, 1970.)

Mironov, V.M. (1969b). The relationship between breathing and movement in masters of sport in gymnastics. *Theory and Practice of Physical Culture*, 7, 14-16. (In *Yessis Review*, 4(2), 35-40, 1969.)

Mitchell, F.L., and Pruzzo, N.A. (1971). Investigation of voluntary and primary respiratory mechanisms. *Journal of the American Osteopathic Association*, 70(June), 149-153.

Mittelmark, R.A., Wiswell, R.A., Drinkwater, B.L., and St. Jones-Repovich, W.E. (1991). Exercise guidelines for pregnancy. In R.A. Mittelmark, R.A. Wiswell, and B.L. Drinkwater (Eds.), *Exercise in pregnancy* (2nd ed., pp. 299-312). Philadelphia: Williams & Wilkins.

Modis, L. (1991). *Organization of the extracellular matrix: A polarization microscopic approach*. Boca Raton, FL: CRC Press.

Mohan, S., and Radha, E. (1981). Age related changes in muscle connective tissue: Acid mucopolysaccharides and structural glycoprotein. *Experimental Gerontology*, 16(5), 385-392.

Möller, M., Ekstrand, J., Öberg, B., and Gillquist, J. (1985). Duration of stretching effect on range of motion in lower extremities. *Archives of Physical Medicine and Rehabilitation*, 66(3), 171-173.

Möller, M.H.L., Öberg, B.E., and Gillquist, J. (1985). Stretching exercise and soccer: Effect of stretching on range of motion in the lower extremity in connection with soccer training. *International Journal of Sports Medicine*, 6(1), 50-52.

Moore, J.C. (1984). The Golgi tendon organ: A review and update. *American Journal of Occupational Therapy*, 38(4), 227-236.

Moore, J.S. (1993). *Chiropractic in America: The history of a medical alternative*. Baltimore: Johns Hopkins University Press.

Moore, M.A. (1979). *An electromyographic investigation of muscle stretching techniques*. Unpublished masters thesis, University of Washington, Seattle.

Moore, M.A., and Hutton, R.S. (1980). Electromyographic investigation of muscle stretching techniques. *Medicine and Science in Sports and Exercise*, 12(5), 322-329.

Moos, R.H. (1974). Coping with physical illness. In R.H. Moss and V.D. Tsu (Eds.), *The crisis of physical illness: An overview* (pp. 3-21). New York: Plenum Press.

Mora, J. (1990). Dynamic stretching. *Triathlete*, 84, 28-31.

Morehouse, L.E., and Miller, A.T. (1971). *Physiology of exercise*. St. Louis: Mosby.

Morelli, M., Seaborne, D.E., and Sullivan, S.J. (1989). Motoneurone excitability changes during massage of the triceps sura (Abstract). *Canadian Journal of Sport Sciences*, 14(4), 129P.

Moretz, A.J., Walters, R., and Smith, L. (1982). Flexibility as a predictor of knee injuries in college football players. *The Physician and Sportsmedicine*, 10(7), 93-97.

Morey, M.C., Cowper, P.A., Feussner, J.R., Dipasquale, R.C., Croeley, G.M., Kitzman, D.W., and Sullivan, R.J. (1989). Evaluation of a supervised exercise program in a geriatric population. *Journal of the American Geriatrics Society*, 37(4), 348-354.

Morgan, W.P., and Horstman, D.H. (1976). Anxiety reduction following acute physical activity. *Medicine and Science in Sports*, 8(1), 62.

Moritani, T., and de Vries, H.A. (1979). Neural factors versus hypertrophy in time course of muscle strength gain. *American Journal of Physical Medicine*, 58(3), 115-130.

Morris, J.M., Brenner, G., and Lucas, D.B. (1962). An electromyographic study of the intrinsic muscles of the back in man. *Journal of Anatomy*, 96(4), 509-520.

Moss, F.P., and Leblond, C.P. (1971). Satellite cells as the source of nuclei in muscles of growing rats. *Anatomical Record*, 170(4), 421-436.

Mottice, M., Goldberg, D., Benner, E.K., and Spoerl, J. (1986).

Soft tissue mobilization. N.p.: JEMD.

Mountcastle, V.B. (1974). *Medical physiology*. St. Louis: Mosby.

Muckle, D.S. (1982). Associated factors in recurrent groin and hamstring injuries. *British Journal of Sports Medicine*, 16(1), 37-39.

Mühlemann, D., and Cimino, J.A. (1990). Therapeutic muscle stretching. In W.I. Hammer (Ed.), *Functional soft tissue examination and treatment by manual methods. The extremities* (pp. 251-275). Gaithersburg, MD: Aspen.

Muir, H. (1983). Proteoglycans as organizers of the intercellular matrix. *Biochemical Society Transactions*, 11(6), 613-622.

Munns, K. (1981). Effects of exercise on the range of joint motion in elderly subjects. In E.L. Smith and R.C. Serfass (Eds.), *Exercise and aging: The scientific basis* (pp. 167-178). Hillsdale, NJ: Enslow.

Munroe, R.A., and Romance, T.J. (1975). Use of the leighton flexometer in the development of a short flexibility test battery. *American Corrective Therapy Journal*, 29(1), 22-25.

Murphy, D.R. (1991). A critical look at static stretching: Are we doing our patients harm? *Chiropractic Sports Medicine*, 5(3), 67-70.

Murphy, P. (1986). Warming up before stretching advised. *Physician and Sportsmedicine*, 14(3), 45.

Murray, M.P., and Sepic, S.B. (1968). Maximum isometric torque of hip abductor and adductor muscles. *Physical Therapy*, 48(12), 1327-1335.

Myers, E.R., Armstrong, C.G., and Mow, V.C. (1984). Swelling, pressure, and collagen tension. In D.W.L. Hukin (Ed.), *Connective tissue matrix* (pp. 161-186). Deerfield Beach, FL: Verlag Chemie.

Myers, M. (1983). Stretching. *Dance Magazine*, 57(6), 66-68.

Myklebust, B.M., Gottlieb, G.L., and Agarwal, G.C. (1986). Stretch reflexes of the normal human infant. *Developmental Medicine and Child Neurology*, 28(4), 440-449.

Mysorekar, V.R., and Nandedkar, A.N. (1986). Surface area of the atlanto-occipital articulations. *Acta Anatomica*, 126(4), 223-225.

Nagler, W. (1973a). Mechanical obstruction of vertebral arteries during hyperextension of neck. *British Journal of Sports Medicine*, 7(1-2), 92-97.

Nagler, W. (1973b). Vertebral artery obstruction by hyperextension of the neck: Report of three cases. *Archives of Physical Medicine and Rehabilitation*, 54(5), 237-240.

National Institute for Occupational Safety and Health (1981). *Work practices guide for manual lifting* (DHHS [NIOSH] Publication No. 81:122). Cincinnati: U.S. Department of Health, Education and Welfare.

Neff, C. (1987). He ran a crooked 26 miles, 385 yards. *Sports Illustrated*, 67(21), 18.

Neilsen, P.D., and Lance, J.W. (1978). Reflex transmission characteristics during voluntary activity in normal man and patients with movement disorders. In J.E. Desmont (Ed.), *Cerebral motor control in man: Long loop mechanisms. Progress in neurophysiology* (Vol 4. pp. 263-299). Basel, Switzerland: S. Kagar AG Medical and Scientific.

Nelson, J.K., Johnson, B.L., and Smith, G.C. (1983). Physical characteristics, hip, flexibility and arm strength of female gymnasts classified by intensity of training across age. *Journal of Sports Medicine and Physical Fitness*, 23(1), 95-100.

Neu, H.N., and Dinnel, H.R. (1957). The shoulder girdle in the chronic respirator patient. *Physical Therapy Review*, 37(6), 373-375.

Neumann, D.A. (1993). Arthrokinesiologic considerations in the aged adult. In A.A. Guccione (Ed.), *Geriatric Physical Therapy* (pp. 47-71). St. Louis: Mosby.

Newham, D.J. (1988). The consequences of eccentric contraction and their relationships to delayed onset muscle pain. *European Journal of Applied Physiology*, 57(3), 353-359.

Newham, D.J., McPhail, G., Mills, K.R., and Edwards, R.H.T. (1983). Ultrastructural changes after concentric and eccentric contractions of human muscle. *Journal of Neurological Sciences*, 61(1), 109-122.

Newham, D.J., Mills, K.R., Quigley, B.M., and Edwards, R.H.T. (1982). Muscle pain and tenderness after exercise. *Australian Journal of Sports Medicine*, 14(4), 129-131.

Newham, D.J., Mills, K.R., Quigley, B.M., and Edwards, R.H.T. (1983). Pain and fatigue after concentric and eccentric muscle contractions. *Clinical Science*, 64(1), 55-62.

Nicholas, J.A. (1970). Injuries to the knee ligaments: Relationship to looseness and tightness in football players. *Journal of the American Medical Association*, 212(13), 2236-2239.

Nielsen, A.J. (1981). Case study: Myofascial pain of the posterior shoulder relieved by spray and stretch. *Journal of Orthopaedic and Sports Physical Therapy*, 3(1), 21-26.

Nielsen, J., Crone, C., and Hultborn, H. (1993). H-reflexes are smaller in dancers from the Royal Danish Ballet than in well-trained athletes. *European Journal of Applied Physiology*, 66, 116-121.

Nieman, D.C. (1990). *Fitness and sports medicine: An introduction*. Palo Alto, CA: Bull.

Nikolic, V., and Zimmermann, B. (1968). Functional changes of the tarsal bones of ballet dancers. *Radovi Fakulteta u Zagrebu*, 16, 131-146.

Nimmo, M.A., and Snow, D.H. (1982). Time course of ultrastructural changes in skeletal muscle after two types of exercise. *Journal of Applied Physiology*, 52(4), 910-913.

Nimmo, R.L. (1958). *The Receptor*. 1(3), 1-4.

Nimz, R., Radar, U., Wilke, K., and Skipka, W. (1988). The relationship of anthropometric measures to different types of breaststroke kicks. In B.E. Ungerechts, K. Wilke, and K. Reischle (Eds.), *Swimming science V* (pp. 115-119). Champaign, IL: Human Kinetics.

Nirschl, R.P. (1973). Good tennis—good medicine. *The Physician and Sportsmedicine*, 1(1), 26-36.

Norback, C.R., and Demarest, R.J. (1981). *The human nervous system* (3rd ed.). New York: McGraw-Hill.

Nordschow, M., and Bierman, W. (1962). Influence of manual massage on muscle relaxation. *Journal of the American Physical Therapy Association*, 42(10), 653-657.

Norris, F.H., Gasteiger, E.L., and Chatfield, P.O. (1957). An electromyographic study of induced and spontaneous muscle cramps. *Electroencephalography and Clinical Neurophysiology*, 9(1), 139-147.

Northrip, J.W., Logan, G.A., and McKinney, W.C. (1983). *Analysis of sport motion: Anatomic and biomechanic perspectives* (3rd ed.). Dubuque, IA: Brown.

Nosse, L.J. (1978). Inverted spinal traction. *Archives of Physical Medicine and Rehabilitation*, 59(8), 367-370.

Noverre, J.G. [1782-1783]. (1978). *The works of Monsieur Noverre* (Vol. II). Reprint, New York: AMS.

Nwuga, V.C. (1982). Relative therapeutic efficiency of vertebral manipulation and conventional treatment in back pain management. *American Journal of Physical Medicine*, 61(6), 273-278.

Nyberg, R. (1993). Manipulation: Definition, types, application. In J.V. Basmajian and R. Nyberg (Eds.), *Rational manual therapies* (pp. 21-47). Baltimore: Williams & Wilkins.

Oakes, B.W. (1981). Acute soft tissue injuries: Nature and management. *Australian Family Physician*, 13(Suppl.), 3-16.

Öberg, B. (1993). Evaluation and improvement of strength in competitive athletes. In K. Harms-Ringdahl (Ed.), *Muscle strength* (pp. 167-185). Edinburgh: Churchill Livingstone.

Ochs, A., Newberry, J., Lenhardt, M., and Harkins, S.W. (1985). Neural and vestibular aging associated with falls. In J.E. Birren and K.W. Schaie (Eds.), *Handbook of the psychology of aging* (2nd ed., pp. 378-399). New York: Van Nostrand Reinhold.

O'Donoghue, D.H. (1984). *Treatment of injuries to athletes* (4th ed.). Philadelphia: Saunders.

O'Driscoll, S.L., and Tomenson, J. (1982). The cervical spine. *Clinical Rheumatic Diseases*, 8(3), 617-630.

Ogata, K., and Naito, M. (1986). Blood flow of peripheral nerve effects of dissection, stretching and compression. *Journal of Hand Surgery*, 11B(1), 10-14.

Ohshiro, T. (1991). *Low reactive-level laser therapy*. New York: Wiley.

Okada, M. (1970). Electromyographic assessment of muscular load in forward bending postures. *Journal of Faculty Science* (University of Tokyo), 8, 311-336.

Olcott, S. (1980). Partner flexibility exercises. *Coaching Women's Athletics*, 6(2), 10-14.

O'Malley, E.F., and Sprinkle, R.L. (1986). Stretching exercises for pretibial periostitis. *Current Podiatric Medicine*, 35(7), 22-23.

O'Neil, R. (1976). Prevention of hamstring and groin strain. *Athletic Training*, 11(1), 27-31.

Oppliger, R., Clark, B.A., Mayhew, J.L., and Haywood, K.M. (1986). Strength, flexibility, and body composition differences between age-group swimmers and non-swimmers. *Australian Journal of Science and Medicine in Sport*, 18(2), 14-16.

Oseid, S., Evjenth, G., Evjenth, O., Gunnari, H., and Meen, D. (1974). Lower back troubles in young female gymnasts. Frequency, symptoms and possible causes. *Bulletin of Physical Education*, 10, 25-28.

Osolin, N.G. (1952). *Das Training des Leichtathleten*. Berlin: Sportverlag.

Osolin, N.G. (1971). *Sovremennaia systema sportnnoi trenirovky* [Athlete's training system for competitions]. Moscow: Phyzkultura i sport.

Osternig, L.R., Robertson, R.N., Troxel, R.K., and Hansen, P. (1990). Differential responses to proprioceptive neuromuscular facilitation (PNF) stretch techniques. *Medicine and Science in Sports and Exercise*, 22(1), 106-111.

Owen, E. (1882). Notes on the voluntary dislocations of a contortionist. *British Medical Journal*, 1, 650-653.

Ozkaya, N., and Nordin, M. (1991). *Fundamentals of biomechanics, equilibrium, motion and deformation*. New York: Van Nostrand Reinhold.

Pachter, B.R., and Eberstein, A. (1985). Effects of passive exercise on neurogenic atrophy in rat skeletal muscle. *Experimental Neurology*, 90(2), 467-470.

Page, S.G., and Huxley, H.E. (1963). Filament lengths in striated muscle. *Journal of Cell Biology*, 19(2), 369-390.

Panagiotacopulos, N.D., Knauss, W.G., and Bloch, R. (1979). On the mechanical properties of human intervertebral disc material. *Biorheology*, 16(4-5), 317-330.

Pang. See Barker (1974).

Pardini, A. (1984). Exercise, vitality and aging. *Aging*, 344, 19-29.

Paris, S.V. (1990). Cervical symptoms of forward head posture. *Topics in Geriatric Rehabilitation*, 5(4), 11-19.

Parker, M.G., Ruhling, R.O., Holt, D., Bauman, E., and Drayna,

M. (1983). Descriptive analysis of quadriceps and hamstrings muscle torque in high school football players. *Journal of Orthopaedic and Sports Physical Therapy, 5*(1), 2-6.

Parry, L.A. (1975). *The history of torture in England.* Muntclair, NJ: Patterson Smith.

Partridge, S.M. (1966). Elastin. In E.J. Briskey, R.G. Cassens, and J.C. Trautman (Eds.), *The physiology and biochemistry of muscle as food* (pp. 327-337). Madison, WI: University of Wisconsin Press.

Pate, R.R., Pratt, M., Blair, S.N., Haskell, W.L., Macera, C.A., Bouchard, C., Buchner, D., Ettinger, W., Health, G.W., King, A.C., Kriska, A., Leon, A.S., Marcus, B.H., Morris, J., Paffenbarger, R.S., Patrick, K., Pollock, M.L., Rippe, J.M., Sallis, J., and Wilmore, J.H. (1995). Physical activity and public health: A recommendation from the Centers for Disease Control and Prevention and the American College of Sports Medicine. *Journal of the American Medical Association, 273*(5), 402-407.

Patel, D.J., and Fry, D.L. (1964). In situ pressure-radius-length measurements in ascending aorta of anesthetized dogs. *Journal of Applied Physiology, 19*(3), 413-416.

Patel, D.J., Greenfield, J.C., and Fry, D.L. (1963). In vivo pressure-length-radius relationship of certain blood vessels in man and dog. In E.O. Attinger (Ed.), *Pulsatile blood flow* (pp. 293-306). Philadelphia: McGraw-Hill.

Pauly, J.E. (1966). An electromyographic analysis of certain movements and exercises. I. Some deep muscles of the back. *Anatomical Record, 155*(2), 223-234.

Pearcy, M., Portek, I., and Shepherd, J. (1985). The effect of low-back pain on lumbar spinal movements measured by three-dimensional x-ray analysis. *Spine, 10*(2), 150-153.

Pechinski, J.M. (1966). *The effects of interval running and breath-holding on cardiac intervals.* Unpublished master's thesis, University of Illinois, Champaign.

Pechtl, V. (1982). Fundamentals and methods for the development of flexibility. In D. Harre (Ed.), *Principles of sports training* (pp. 146-152). Berlin: Sportverlag.

Perez, H.R., and Fumasoli, S. (1984). Benefit of proprioceptive neuromuscular facilitation on the joint mobility of youth-aged female gymnasts with correlations for rehabilitation. *American Corrective Therapy Journal, 38*(6), 142-146.

Peters, J.M., and Peters, H.K. (1983). *The flexibility manual.* Berwyn, PA: Sports Kinetics.

Peterson, L., and Renstrom, P. (1986). *Sports injuries: Their prevention and treatment.* Chicago: Year Book Medical.

Pheasant, S. (1986). *Bodyspace—Anthropometry, ergonomics and design.* London: Taylor and Francis.

Pheasant, S. (1991). *Ergonomics, work and health.* Gaithersburg, MD: Aspen.

Phillips, C.G. (1969). The ferrier lecture, 1968. Motor apparatus of the baboons. *Proceedings of the Royal Society* (Biology), 173, 141-174.

Phillips, R.B., and Mootz, R.D. (1992). Contemporary chiropractic philosophy. In S. Haldeman (Ed.), *Principles and practice of chiropractic* (2nd ed.) (p. 45-52), Norwalk, Ct: Appleton & Lange.

Ploucher, D.W. (1982). Inversion petechiae. *New England Journal of Medicine, 307*(22), 1406-1407.

Pollack, G.H. (1983). The cross-bridge theory. *Physiological Review, 63*(3), 1049-1113.

Pollack, G.H. (1986). Quantal mechanisms in cardiac contraction. *Circulation Research,* 59, 1-8.

Pollack, G.H. (1990). *Muscles & molecules: Uncovering the principles of biological motion.* Seattle: Ebner & Sons.

Pollack, G.H., Iwazumi, T., ter Keurs, H.E.D.J., and Shibata, E.F. (1977). Sarcomere shortening in striated muscle occurs in stepwise fashion. *Nature, 268*(5622), 757-759.

Pollock, M.L., and Wilmore, J.H. (1990). *Exercise in health and disease: Evaluation and prescription for prevention and rehabilitation.* Philadelphia: Saunders.

Pope, M.H., Andersson, G.B.J., Frymoyer, J.W., and Chaffin, D.B. (1991). *Occupational low back pain: Assessment, treatment and prevention.* Chicago: Mosby Yearbook.

Pope, M.H., and Klingenstierna, U. (1986). Height changes due to autotraction. *Clinical Biomechanics, 1*(4), 191-195.

Portenfield, J.A., and De Rosa, C. (1991). *Mechanical low back pain perspectives in functional anatomy.* Philadelphia: Saunders.

Portnoy, H., and Morin, F. (1956). Electromyographic study of postural muscles in various positions and movements. *American Journal of Physiology, 186*(1), 122-126.

Pountain, G. (1992). Musculoskeletal pain in Omanis, and the relationship to joint mobility and body mass index. *British Journal of Rheumatology, 31*(2), 81-85.

Pratt, M. (1989). Strength, flexibility, and maturity in adolescent athletes. *American Journal of Diseases of Children, 143*(5), 560-563.

Prentice, W.E. (1982). An electromyographic analysis of the effectiveness of heat or cold and stretching for inducing relaxation in injured muscle. *Journal of Orthopaedic and Sports Physical Therapy, 3*(3), 133-140.

Prentice, W.E. (1983). A comparison of static stretching and PNF stretching for improving hip joint flexibility. *Athletic Training, 18*(1), 56-59.

Prentice, W.E. (1990). *Rehabilitation techniques in sports medicine.* St. Louis: Times Mirror/Mosby.

Price, M.G. (1991). In *Advances in structural biology* (Vol. 1, pp. 175-207). New York: JAI Press.

Prichard, B. (1984, January). *Lower extremity injuries in runners induced by upper body torque (UBT).* Presented at the Biomechanics and Kinesiology in Sports U.S. Olympic Sports Medicine Conference, Colorado Springs, CO.

Priest, J.D. (1989). A physical phenomenon: Shoulder depression in athletes. *SportCare & Fitness, 2*(2), 20-25.

Priest, J.D., Jones, H.H., Tichenor, C.J., and Nagel, D.A. (1977). Arm and elbow changes in expert tennis players. *Minnesota Medicine, 60*(5), 399-404.

Priest, J.D., and Nagel, D.A. (1976). Tennis shoulder. *American Journal of Sports Medicine, 4*(1), 28-42.

Pringle, J.W.S. (1967). The contractile mechanism of insect fibrillar muscle. *Progress in Biophysics and Molecular Biology,* 17, 1-60.

Prockop, D.J. and Guzman, N.A. (1977). Collagen diseases and the biosynthesis of collagen. *Hospital Practice, 12*(2), 61-68.

Puschel, J. (1930). Der Wassergehalt voraler un degenerieter Zwischenwirbelschiben. *Beitrage zur Pathologischen Anatomie und zur Allgemeinen Pathologie,* 84, 123-130.

Quebec Task Force on Spinal Disorders (1987). Scientific approach to the assessment and management of activity-related spinal disorders: A monograph for clinicians. *Spine, 12*(7), S1-S55.

Raab, D.M., Agre, J.C., McAdam, M., and Smith, E.L. (1988). Light resistance and stretching exercise in elderly women: Effect upon flexibility. *Archives of Physical Rehabilitation, 69*(4), 268-272.

Radin, E.L. (1989). Role of muscles in protecting athletes from injury. *Acta Medica Scandinavica.* 711(Suppl.), 143-147.

Ramachandran, G.W. (1967). Structure of collagen at the molecular level. In G.W. Ramachandran (Ed.), *Treatise of collagen* (Vol. 1, pp. 103-179). New York: Academic Press.

Ramacharaka, Y. (1960). *The hindu-yogi science of breath*. London: L.N. Fowler.

Rankin, J.M., and Thompson, C.B. (1983). Isokinetic evaluation of quadriceps and hamstrings function: Normative data concerning body weight and sport. *Athletic Training*, 18(2), 110-114.

Rao, V. (1965). Reciprocal inhibition: Inapplicability to tendon jerks. *Journal of Postgraduate Medicine*, 11(July), 123-125.

Rasch, P.J., and Burke, J. (1989). *Kinesiology and applied anatomy* (7th ed.). Philadelphia: Lea & Febiger.

Rasmussen, G.G. (1979). Manipulation in low back pain: A randomized clinical trial. *Manual Medicine*, 1(1), 8-10.

Rath, W.W. (1984). Cervical traction, a clinical perspective. *Orthopaedic Review*, 13(8), 29-48.

Rathbone, J.L. (1971). Relaxation. In L.A. Larson (Ed.), *Encyclopedia of sport sciences and medicine* (pp. 1312-1313). New York: Macmillan.

Ray, W.A., and Griffin, M.R. (1990). Prescribed medications and the risk of falling. *Topics in Geriatric Rehabilitation*, 5(2), 12-20.

Read, M. (1989). Over stretched. *British Journal of Sports Medicine*, 23(4), 257-258.

Reedy, M.K. (1971). Electron microscope observations concerning the behavior of the cross-bridge in striated muscle. In R.J. Podolsky (Ed.), *Contractility of muscle cells and related processes* (pp. 229-246). Englewood Cliffs, NJ: Prentice-Hall.

Reid, D.C. (1992). *Sports injury assessment and rehabilitation*. London: Churchill Livingstone.

Reilly, T., Tyrrell, A., and Troup, J.D.G. (1984). Circadian variation in human stature. *Chronobiology International*, 1(2), 121-126.

Renstrom, P., and Roux, C. (1988). Clinical implications of youth participation in sports. In A. Dirix, H.G. Knuttgen, and K. Tittel (Eds.), *The Olympic book of sports medicine* (Vol. 1, pp. 469-488). London: Blackwell Scientific.

Rhodin, J.A.G. (1988). Architecture of the vessel wall. In S.R. Geiger (Ed.), *Handbook of physiology: Sec. 2: The cardiovascular system* (Vol. 2, pp. 1-31). Bethesda, MD: American Physiological Society.

Riddle, K.S. (1956). *A comparison of three methods for increasing flexibility of the trunk and hip joints*. Unpublished doctoral dissertation, University of Oregon.

Rigby, B. (1964). The effect of mechanical extension under thermal stability of collagen. *Biochimica et Biophysica Acta*, 79 (SC 43008), 634-636.

Rigby, B.J., Hirai, N., Spikes, J.D., and Eyring, J. (1959). The mechanical properties of rat tail tendon. *Journal of General Physiology*, 43(2), 265-283.

Rikkers, R. (1986). *Seniors on the move*. Champaign, IL: Human Kinetics.

Rikli, R., and Busch, S. (1986). Motor performance of women as a function of age and physical activity. *Journal of Gerontology*, 41(5), 645-649.

Rippe, J.M. (1990). Staying loose. *Modern Maturity*, 33(3), 72-77.

Ritchen, P. (1975). A way to stay loose. *Runner's World*, 10(2), 32-33.

Roaf, R. (1977). *Posture*. New York: Academic Press.

Robertson, D.F. (1960). *Relationship of strength of selected muscle groups and ankle flexibility to flutter kick in swimming*. Unpublished master's thesis, Iowa State University, Ames.

Robison, C., Jensen, C., James, S., and Hirschi, W. (1974). *Prevention, evaluation, management & rehabilitation*. New Jersey: Prentice-Hall.

Rochcongar, P., Dassonville, J., and Le Bars, R. (1979). Modifications of the Hoffmann reflex in function of athletic training. *European Journal of Applied Physiology*, 40(3), 165-170.

Rockstein, M., and Sussman, M. (1979). *Biology of aging*. Belmont, CA: Wadsworth.

Rodenburg, J.B., Steenbeek, D., Schiereck, P., and Bar, P.R. (1994). Warm-up, stretching and massage diminish harmful effects of eccentric exercise. *International Journal of Sports Medicine*, 15(7), 414-419.

Rodeo, S. (1984). Swimming the breaststroke—A kinesiological analysis and considerations for strength straining. *NSCA Journal*, 6(4), 4-6, 74-76, 80.

Rodeo, S. (1985a). The butterfly: A kinesiological analysis and strength training program. *NSCA Journal*, 7(4), 4-10, 74.

Rodeo, S. (1985b). The butterfly: Physiologically speaking. *Swimming Technique*, 21(4), 14-19.

Roland, P.E., and Ladegaard-Pedersen, H. (1977). A quantitative analysis of sensations of tension and of kinesthesia in man. Evidence for a peripherally originating muscular sense and for a sense of effort. *Brain*, 100(4), 671-692.

Rose, B.S. (1985). The hypermobility syndrome loose-limbed and liable. *New Zealand Journal of Physiotherapy*, 13(2), 18-19.

Rose, D.L., Radzyminski, S.F., and Beatty, R.R. (1957). Effect of brief maximal exercise on strength of the quadriceps femoris. *Archives of Physical Medicine and Rehabilitation*, 38(3), 157-164.

Rosenberg, B.S., Cornelius, W.L., Jackson, A.W., and Czubakowski, S. (1985). The effects of proprioceptive neuromuscular facilitation (PNF) flexibility techniques with local cold application on hip joint range of motion in 55-84 year old females. In *Abstracts research papers 1977* (p. 110). Washington, DC: AAHPER.

Rosenbloom, J., Abrams, W.R., and Mecham, R. (1993). Extracellular matrix 4: The elastic fiber. *The FASEB Journal*, 7(13), 1208-1218.

Roston, J.B., and Haines, R.W. (1947). Cracking in the metacarpophalangeal joint. *Journal of Anatomy*, 81(2), 165-173.

Round, J.M., Jones, D.A., and Cambridge, G. (1987). Cellular infiltrates in human skeletal muscle: Exercise induced damage as a model for inflammatory disease? *Journal of the Neurological Sciences*, 82(1), 1-11.

Rowe, R.W.D. (1981). Morphology of perimysial and endomysial connective tissue in skeletal muscle. *Tissue & Cell*, 13(4), 681-690.

Rowinski, M.J. (1985). Afferent neurobiology of the joint. In J.A. Gould and G.J. Davies (Eds.), *Orthopaedic and sports physical therapy* (pp. 50-64). St. Louis: Mosby.

Roy, S., and Irwin, R. (1983). *Sports medicine: Prevention, evaluation, management, and rehabilitation*. Englewood Cliffs, NJ: Prentice-Hall.

Rubin, E., and Farber, J.L. (1994). *Pathology* (2nd ed.). Philadelphia: Lippincott.

Rusk, H.A. (1977). *Rehabilitation medicine* (4th ed.). St. Louis: C.V. Mosby.

Russell, B., and Dix, D.J. (1992). Mechanisms for intracellular distribution of mRNA: In situ hybridization studies in muscle. *American Journal of Physiology*, 262 (31:1), C1-C8.

Russell, B., Dix, D.J., Haller, D.L., and Jacobs-El, J. (1992). Repair of injured skeletal muscle: A molecular approach. *Medicine and Science in Sports and Exercise*, 24(2), 189-196.

Russell, G.S., and Highland, T.R. (1990). *Care of the low back*. Columbia, MO: Spine.

Russell, P., Weld, A., Pearcy, M.J., Hogg, R., and Unsworth, A. (1992). Variation in lumbar spine mobility measured over a 24-hour period. *British Journal of Rheumatology*, 31(5), 329-332.

Ryan, A.J. (Moderator). (1976). Ballet dancers pose sports medicine challenge. *The Physician and Sportsmedicine*, 4(11), 44-57.

Rydevik, B.L., Kwan, M.K., Myers, R.R., Brown, R.A., Triggs, K.J., Woo, S. L-Y., and Garfin, S.R. (1990). An in vitro mechanical and histological study of acute stretching on rabbit tibial nerve. *Journal of Orthopaedic Research*, 8(5), 694-701.

Rydevik, B., Lundborg, G., and Skalak, R. (1989). Biomechanics of peripheral nerves. In M. Nordin and V.H. Frankel (Eds.), *Basic biomechanics of the musculoskeletal system* (pp. 76-87). Philadelphia: Lea & Febiger.

Rymer, W.Z., Houk, J.C., and Crago, P.E. (1979). Mechanisms of the clasp-knife reflex studied in an animal model. *Experimental Brain Research*, 37(1), 93-113.

Saal, J.S. (1987). Flexibility training. *Physical Medicine and Rehabilitation: State of the Art Reviews*, 1(4), 537-554.

Sachse, J., and Berger, M. (1989). Cervical mobilization induced by eye movement. *Journal of Manual Medicine*, 4(4), 154-156.

Sackett, D.L., and Snow, J.C. (1979). The magnitude of compliance and noncompliance. In R.B. Haynes, D.W. Taylor, and D.L. Sackett (Eds.), *Compliance in health care* (pp. 11-22). Baltimore: Johns Hopkins Press.

Sady, S.P., Wortman, M., and Blanke, D. (1982). Flexibility training: Ballistic, static or proprioceptive neuromuscular facilitation. *Archives of Physical Medicine and Rehabilitation*, 63(6), 261-263.

Sage, G.H. (1971). *Introduction to motor behavior. A neurophysiological approach*. Reading, MA: Addison-Wesley.

Sah, R.L., Doong, J.Y.H., Grodzinsky, A.J., Plaas, A.H.K., and Sandy, J.D. (1991). Effects of compression on the loss of newly synthesized proteoglycans and proteins from cartilage explants. *Archives of Biochemistry and Biophysics*, 286, 20-29.

Sah, R.L., Grodzinsky, A.J., Plaas, A.H.K., and Sandy, J.D. (1992). Effects of static and dynamic compression on matrix metabolism in cartilage explants. In K.E. Kuettner, R. Schleyerbach and J.G. Peyron (Eds.), *Articular cartilage and osteoarthritis* (pp. 373-391). New York: Raven Press.

Sale, D.G. (1986). Neural adaptation in strength and power training. In N.L. Jones, N. McCartney, and A.J. McComas (Eds.), *Human muscle power* (pp. 289-307). Champaign, IL: Human Kinetics.

Sale, D.G., MacDougall, J.D., Upton, A.R.M., and McComas, A.J. (1983). Effect of strength training upon motorneuron excitability in man. *Medicine and Science in Sports and Exercise*, 15(1), 57-62.

Sale, D.G., McComas, A.J., MacDougall, J.D., and Upton, A.R.M. (1982). Neuromuscular adaptation in human thenar muscles following strength training and immobilization. *Journal of Applied Physiology*, 53(2), 419-424.

Sale, D.G., Upton, A.R.M., McComas, A.J., and MacDougall, J.D. (1983). Neuromuscular function in weight-trainers. *Experimental Neurology*, 82(3), 521-531.

Salminen, J.J., Oksanen, A., Maki, P., Pentti, J., and Kujala, U.M. (1993). Leisure time physical activity in the young. Correlation with low-back pain, spinal mobility and trunk muscle strength in 15-year-old school children. *International Journal of Sports Medicine*, 14(7), 406-410.

Sanders, G.E., Reinert, O., Tepe, R., and Maloney, P. (1990). Chiropractic adjustive manipulation on subjects with acute lowback pain: Visual analog pain scores and plasma β-endorphin levels. *Journal of Manipulative and Physiological Therapeutics*, 13(7), 391-395.

Sandoz, R. (1969). The significance of the manipulative crack and of other articular noises. *Annals of the Swiss Chiropractic Association*, 4, 47-68.

Sandoz, R. (1976). Some physical mechanisms and effects of spinal adjustments. *Annals of the Swiss Chiropractic Association*, 6, 91-141.

Sands, B. (1984). *Coaching women's gymnastics*. Champaign, IL: Human Kinetics.

Sandstead, H.L. (1968). *The relationship of outward rotation of the humerus to baseball throwing velocity*. Unpublished master's thesis, Eastern Illinois University, Charleston.

Sapega, A.A., Quedenfeld, T.C., Moyer, R.A., and Butler, R.A. (1981). Biophysical factors in range-of-motion exercise. *The Physician and Sportsmedicine*, 9(12), 57-65.

Saunders, H.D. (1986). Lumbar traction. In G.P. Grieve (Ed.), *Modern manual therapy of the vertebral column* (pp. 787-795). Edinburgh: Churchill Livingstone.

Schiaffino, S. (1974). Hypertrophy of skeletal muscle induced by tendon shortening. *Experimentia*, 30, 1163-1164.

Schiaffino, S., and Hanzlikova, V. (1970). On the mechanisms of compensatory hypertrophy in skeletal muscle. *Experimentia*, 26, 152-153.

Schneider, H.J., King, A.Y., Bronson, J.L., and Miller, E.H. (1974). Stress injuries and developmental change of lower extremities in ballet dancers. *Radiology*, 113(3), 627-632.

Schneiderman, R., Kevet, D., and Maroudas, A. (1986). Effects of mechanical and osmotic pressure on the rate of glycosaminoglycan synthesis in the human adult femoral head cartilage: An in vivo study. *Journal of Orthopaedic Research*, 4, 393-408.

Schnitt, J.M., and Schnitt, D. (1989). Psychological issues in a dancer's career. In A.J. Ryan and R.E. Stephens (Eds.), *The healthy dancer*. Princeton, NJ: Princeton Book.

Schottelius, B.A., and Senay, L.C. (1956). Effect of stimulation-length sequence on shape of length-tension diagram. *American Journal of Physiology*, 186(1), 127-130.

Schubert, M., and Hammerman, D. (1968). *A primer on connective tissue biochemistry*. Philadelphia: Lea & Febiger.

Schultz, A.B., Andersson, G.B., Haderspeck, K., Ortengren, R., Nordin, M., and Bjork, R. (1982). Analysis and measurement of lumbar trunk loads in tasks involving bends and twists. *Journal of Biomechanics*, 15(9), 669-675.

Schultz, A.B., Haderspeck-Grib, K., Sinkora, G., and Warwick, D.N. (1985). Quantitative studies of the flexion-relaxation phenomenon in the back muscles. *Journal of Orthopaedic Research*, 3(2), 189-197.

Schultz, P. (1979). Flexibility: Day of the static stretch. *The Physician and Sportsmedicine*, 7(11), 109-117.

Schuster, D.F. (1988). Exploring backbends. *Yoga Journal*, 80(May-June), 55-60.

Schuster, R.O. (1978). Shin splints. *Running Review*, 2(5), 20-21.

Schwane, J.A., and Armstrong, R.B. (1983). Effect of training on skeletal muscle injury from downhill running in rats. *Journal of Applied Physiology*, 55(3), 969-975.

Schwane, J.A., Williams, J.S., and Sloan, J.H. (1987). Effects of training on delayed muscle soreness and serum creatine kinase activity after running. *Medicine and Science in Sports and Exercise*, 19(6), 584-590.

Schweitzer, G. (1970). Laxity of the metacarpo-phalangeal joints of the finger and interphalangeal joint of the thumb in comparative inter-racial studies. *South African Medical Journal*, 44(9), 246-249.

Scott, A.B. (1994). Change of eye muscle sarcomeres according to eye position. *Journal of Pediatric Ophthalmology and Strabismus*, 31(2), 85-88.

Scott, D., Bird, H.A., and Wright, V. (1979). Joint laxity leading to osteoarthrosis. *Rheumatology and Rehabilitation*, 18, 167-169.

Scott, J.T. (1960). Morning stiffness in rheumatoid arthritis. *Annals of the Rheumatic Diseases*, 19(4), 361-368.

Sechrist, W.C., and Stull, G.A. (1969). Effects of mild activity, heat applications, and cold applications on range of joint movement. *American Corrective Therapy Journal*, 23(4), 120-123.

Segal, D.D. (1983). An anatomic and biomechanical approach to low back health: A preventive approach. *Journal of Sports Medicine and Physical Fitness*, 23(4), 411-421.

Segal, R.L., and Wolf, S.L. (1994). Operant conditions of spinal stretch reflexes in patients with spinal cord injuries. *Experimental Neurology* 130(2), 202-213.

Seimon, L.P. (1983). *Low back pain: Clinical diagnosis and management*. Norwalk, CT: Appleton-Century-Crofts.

Seliger, V., Dolejs, L., and Karas, V. (1980). A dynamometric comparison of maximum eccentric, concentric and isometric contraction using EMG and energy expenditure measurements. *European Journal of Applied Physiology*, 45(2-3), 235-244.

Seno, S. (1968). The motion of the spine and the related electromyogram of the patient suffering from lumbago. *Electromyography*, 8(2), 185-186.

Sermeev, B.V. (1966). Development of mobility in the hip joint in sportsmen. *Yessis Review*, 2(1), 16-17.

Shambaugh, P. (1987). Changes in electrical activity in muscles resulting from chiropractic adjustment: A pilot study. *Journal of Manipulative and Physiological Therapeutics*, 10(6), 300-304.

Shamos, M.H., and Lavine, L.S. (1967). Piezoelectricity as a fundamental property of biological tissues. *Nature*, 213(5073), 267-269.

Sharratt, M.T. (1984). Wrestling profile. *Clinics in Sports Medicine*, 3(1), 273-289.

Shellock, F.G., and Prentice, W.E. (1985). Warming-up and stretching for improved physical performance and prevention of sports-related injuries. *Sports Medicine*, 2(4), 267-278.

Shephard, R.J. (1978). *The fit athlete*. Oxford: Oxford University Press.

Shephard, R.J. (1982). *Physiology and biochemistry of exercise*. New York: Praeger.

Shephard, R.J., Berridge, M., and Montelpare, W. (1990). On the generality of the "sit and reach" test: An analysis of flexibility data for an aging population. *Research Quarterly for Exercise and Sport*, 61(4), 326-330.

Sherrington, C.S. (1906). *Integrative action of the nervous system*. Reprint. Cambridge: Cambridge University Press, 1947.

Shestack, R., and Ditto, E.W. (1964). *Physician's physical therapy manual*. Englewood Cliffs, NJ: Prentice-Hall.

Shirado, O., Ito, T., Kaneda, K., and Strax, T.E. (1995). Flexion-relaxation phenomenon in the back muscles. *American Journal of Physical Medicine and Rehabilitation*, 74(2), 139-144.

Shuman, D., and Staab, G.R. (1960). *Your aching back and what you can do about it*. New York: Gramery.

Shustova, N.Y., Maltsev, N.A., Levkovich, Y.I., and Levtov, V.A. (1985). Postelongation hyperemia in gastrocnemius muscle capillaries. *Fiziologicheskii Zhurnal SSR Imeni I.M. Sechenova*, 71(5), 599-608. (In *Biological Abstract*, 81(4), p. 169. No. 30857, Feb. 1986.)

Shustova, N.Y., Matchanov, A.T., and Levtov, V.A. (1985). Effect of the compression of gastrocnemius muscle vessels on the muscle blood supply in stretching. *Fiziologicheskii Zhurnal SSSR Imeni I.M. Sechenova*. 71(9), 1105-1111. (In *Biological Abstract*, 81(9), p. 164. No. 79766, May 1986.)

Shyne, K. (1982). Richard H. Dominguez, M.D.: To stretch or not to stretch? *The Physician and Sportsmedicine*, 10(9), 137-140.

Sigerseth, P.C. (1971). Flexibility. In L.A. Larson (Ed.), *Encyclopedia of sport sciences and medicine* (pp. 280-281). New York: Macmillan.

Sihvonen, T., Partanen, J., Hanninen, O., and Soimakallio, S. (1991). Electric behavior of low back muscles during lumbar pelvic rhythm in low back pain patients and healthy controls. *Archives of Physical Medicine and Rehabilitation*, 72, 1080-1087.

Silman, A.J., Haskard, D., and Day, S. (1986). Distribution of joint mobility in a normal population: Results of the use of fixed torque measuring devices. *Annals of the Rheumatic Diseases*, 45(1), 27-30.

Simard, T.G., and Basmajian, J.V. (1967). Methods in training conscious control of motor units. *Archives of Physical Medicine and Rehabilitation*, 48(1), 12-19.

Sime, W.E. (1977). A comparison of exercise and meditation in reducing physiological response to stress. *Medicine and Science in Sports*, 9(1), 55.

Simpson, D.G., Carver, W., Borg, T.K., and Terracio, L. (1994). Role of mechanical stimulation in the establishment and maintenance of muscle cell differentiation. *International Review of Cytology*, 150, 69-94.

Sing, R.F. (1984). *The dynamics of the javelin throw*. Cherry Hill, NJ: Reynolds.

Sjostrand, F.S. (1962). The connection between A- and I-band filaments in striated frog muscle. *Journal of Ultrastructure Research*, 7(3-4), 225-246.

Slocum, D.B., and James, S.L. (1968). Biomechanics of running. *Journal of the American Medical Association*, 205(11), 97-104.

Smith, C.A. (1994). The warm-up procedure: To stretch or not to stretch. A brief review. *Journal of Orthopaedic Sports Physical Therapy*, 19(1), 12-17.

Smith, C.F. (1977). Physical management of muscular low back pain in the athlete. *Canadian Medical Association Journal*, 117(September 17), 632-635.

Smith, J.L., Hutton, R.S., and Eldred, E. (1974). Post contraction changes in sensitivity of muscle afferents to static and dynamic stretch. *Brain Research*, 78(September-October), 193-202.

Smith, J.W. (1966). Factors influencing nerve repair. I. Blood supply of peripheral nerves. *Archives of Surgery*, 93(2), 335-341.

Smith, R.E. (1986). Toward a cognitive-affective model of athletic burnout. *Journal of Sport Psychology*, 8(1), 36-50.

Snell, R.S. (1992). *Clinical anatomy for medical students* (4th. ed.). Boston: Little, Brown and Company.

Solomonow, M., and D'Ambrosia, R. (1991). Neural reflex arcs and muscle control of knee stability and motion. In W.N. Scott (Ed.), *Ligament and extensor mechanism injuries of the knee* (pp. 389-400). St. Louis: Mosby-Year Book.

Song, T.M.K. (1979). Flexibility of ice hockey players and comparison with other groups. In J. Terauds and H.J. Gros (Eds.), *Science in skiing, skating and hockey* (pp. 117-125). Del Mar, CA: Academic.

Song, T.M., and Garvie, G.T. (1976). Wrestling with flexibility. *Canadian Journal for Health, Physical Education and Recreation*, 43(1), 18-26.

Song, T.M.K., and Garvie, G.T. (1980). Anthropometric, flexibility, strength, and physiological measures of Canadian and Japanese Olympic wrestlers. *Canadian Journal of Applied Sport Science*, 5(1), 1-8.

Sontag, S., and Wanner, J.N. (1988). The cause of leg cramps and knee pains: A hypothesis and effective treatment. *Medical Hypotheses*, 25(1), 35-41.

Soussi-Yanicostas, N., Hamida, C.B., Butler-Browne, G.S., Hentati, F., Bejaoui, K., and Hamida, M.B. (1991). Modification in the expression and location of contractile and cytoskeletal proteins in Schwartz-Jampel syndrome. *Journal of the Neurological Sciences*, 104(1), 64-73.

Souza, T.A. (1994). General treatment approaches for shoulder disorder. In T.A. Souza (Ed.), *Sports injuries of the shoulder: Conservative management* (pp. 487-508). Edinburgh: Churchill Livingstone.

Spence, A.P., and Mason, E.B. (1987). *Human anatomy and physiology* (3rd ed.). Menlo Park, CA: Benjamin/Cummings.

Spindler, K.P., and Benson, E.M. (1994). Natural history of posterior cruciate ligament injury. *Sports Medicine and Arthroscopy Review*, 2(2), 73-79.

Stafford, M., and Grana, W. (1984). Hamstring/quadriceps ratios in college football players: A high velocity evaluation. *American Journal of Sports Medicine*, 12(3), 209-211.

Stainsby, W.N., Fales, J.T., and Lilienthal, J.L. (1956). Effect of stretch on oxygen consumption of dog skeletal muscle in situ. *Bulletin of the Johns Hopkins Hospital*, 99(5), 249-261.

Stamford, B. (1981). Flexibility and stretching. *The Physician and Sportsmedicine*, 12(2), 171.

Stanitski, C.L. (1995). Articular hypermobility and chondral injury in patients with acute patellar dislocation. *The American Journal of Sports Medicine*, 23(2), 146-150.

Stauber, W.T. (1989). Eccentric action of muscles: Physiology, injury, and adaptation. In K. Pandolf (Ed.), *Exercise and sports sciences reviews* (pp. 157-185). Baltimore: Williams & Wilkins.

Steban, R.E., and Bell, S. (1978). *Track & field: An administrative approach to the science of coaching*. New York: Wiley & Sons.

Steinacker, J.M., Both, M., and Whipp, B.J. (1993). Pulmonary mechanics and entrainment of respiration and stroke rate during rowing. *International Journal of Sports Medicine*, 14(Suppl. 1), S15-S19.

Steindler, A. (1977). *Kinesiology of the human body*. Springfield, IL: Charles C Thomas.

Stevens, A., Stijns, H., Rosselle, N., and Decock, F. (1977). Litheness and hamstring muscles. *Electromyography and Clinical Neurophysiology*, 17(6), 507-511.

Stevens, A., Stijns, H., Rosselle, N., Stappaerts, K., and Michels, A. (1974). Slowly stretching the hamstrings and compliance. *Electromyography and Clinical Neurophysiology*, 14(5-6), 495-496.

Stewart, R.B. (1987). Drug use and adverse drug reactions in the elderly: An epidemiological perspective. *Topics in Geriatric Rehabilitation*, 2(3), 1-11.

Stiles, E.G. (1984). Manipulation: A tool for your practice? *Patient Care*, 18(9), 16-42.

Stockton, I.D., Reilly, T., Sanderson, F.H., and Walsh, T.J. (1980). Investigations of circadian rhythm in selected components of sports performance. *Bulletin of the Society of Sports Sciences*, 1(1), 14-15.

Stoddart, A. (1979). *The back, relief from pain*. New York: Arco.

Stokes, I.A., Wilder, D.G., Frymoyer, J.W., and Pope, M.H. (1981). Assessment of patients with low back pain by biplanar radiographic measurement of intervertebral motion. *Spine*, 6(3), 233-238.

Stone, W.J., and Kroll, W.A. (1986). *Sports conditioning and weight training programs for athletic competition* (2nd ed.). Boston: Allyn and Bacon.

Stonebrink, R.D. (1990). *Evaluation and manipulative management of common musculo-skeletal disorders*. Portland: Author.

Strauss, J.B. (1993). *Chiropractic philosophy*. Levittown, PA: Foundation for the Advancement of Chiropractic Education.

Strickland, A.L., and Shearin, R.B. (1972). Diurnal height variation in children. *Journal of Pediatrics*, 80(6), 1023-1025.

Strickler, T., Malone, T., and Garrett, W.E. (1990). The effects of passive warming on muscle injury. *American Journal of Sports Medicine*, 18(2), 141-145.

Strocchi, R., Leonardi, L., Guizzardi, S., Marchini, M., and Ruggeri, A. (1985). Ultrastructural aspects of rat tail tendon sheaths. *Journal of Anatomy*, 140(1), 57-67.

Stroebel, C.F. (1979). *Non-specific effects and psychodynamic issues in self-regulatory techniques*. Paper presented at the Johns Hopkins Conference on Clinical Biofeedback, Baltimore, MD.

Sturkie, P.D. (1941). Hypermobile joints in all descendants for two generations. *Journal of Heredity*, 32(7), 232-234.

Subotnick, S.I. (1979). Podiatric aspects of children in sports. *Journal of the American Podiatric Association*, 69(7), 443-453.

Sullivan, M.K., Dejulia, J.J., and Worrell, T.W. (1992). Effect of pelvic position and stretching method on hamstring muscle flexibility. *Medicine and Science in Sports and Exercise*, 24(12), 1383-1389.

Sullivan, P.D., Markos, P.E., and Minor, M.D. (1982). *An integrated approach to therapeutic exercise theory and clinical application*. Reston, VA: Reston.

Sunderland, S. (1978). Traumatized nerves, roots and ganglia: Musculoskeletal factors and neuropathological consequences. In I.M. Korr (Ed.), *The neurobiologic mechanism in manipulative therapy* (pp. 137-166). New York: Plenum Press.

Sunderland, S. (1991). *Nerve injuries and their repair: A critical appraisal* (3rd ed.). London: Churchill Livingstone.

Sunderland, S., and Bradley, K.C. (1961). Stress-strain phenomena in human spinal nerve roots. *Brain*, 84(1), 102-119.

Surburg, P.R. (1981). Neuromuscular facilitation techniques in sportsmedicine. *The Physician and Sportsmedicine*, 18(1), 114-127.

Surburg, P.R. (1983). Flexibility exercise re-examined. *Athletic Training*, 18(1), 37-40.

Sutcliffe, M.C., and Davidson, J.M. (1990). Effect of static stretching on elastin production by porcine aortic smooth muscle cells. *Matrix*, 10(3), 148-153.

Sutro, C.J. (1947). Hypermobility of bones due to "overlengthened" capsular and ligamentous tissues. *Surgery*, 21(1), 67-76.

Sutton, G. (1984). Hamstrung by hamstring strains: A review of the literature. *Journal of Orthopaedic and Sports Physical Therapy*, 5(4), 184-195.

Suzuki, S., and Hutton, R.S. (1976). Postcontractile motorneuron discharge produced by muscle afferent activation. *Medicine and Science in Sports*, 8(4), 258-264.

Suzuki, S., and Pollack, G.H. (1986). Bridge-like interconnections between thick filaments in stretched skeletal muscle fibers observed by the freeze-fractured method. *Journal of Cell Biology*, 102(3), 1093-1098.

Sward, L., Eriksson, B., and Peterson, L. (1990). Anthropometric characteristics, passive hip flexion, and spinal mobility in relation to back pain in athletes. *Spine*, 15(5), 376-382.

Swezey, R.L. (1978). *Arthritis: Rational therapy and rehabilitation*. Philadelphia: Saunders.

Szmelskyj, A.O. (1990). The difference between holistic osteopathic practice and manipulation. *Holistic Medicine*, 5(2), 67-79.

Tabary, J.C., Tabary, C., Tardieu, C., Tardieu, G., and Goldspink, G. (1972). Physiological and structural changes in the cat's soleus muscle due to immobilization at different lengths by plaster casts. *Journal of Physiology* (London), 224(1), 231-244.

Talag, T. (1973). Residual muscle soreness as influenced by concentric, eccentric, and static contractions. *Research Quarterly*, 44(4), 458-469.

Tamkun, J.W., DeSimone, D.W., Fonda, D., Patel, R.S., Buck, C., Horwitz, A.F., and Hynes, R.O. (1986). Structure of integrin, a glycoprotein involved in the transmembrane linkage between fibronectin and actin. *Cell*, 46(2), 271-282.

Tanigawa, M.C. (1972). Comparison of the hold-relax procedure and passive mobilization on increasing muscle length. *Physical Therapy*, 52(7), 725-735.

Taunton, J.E. (1982). Pre-game warm-up and flexibility. *New Zealand Journal of Sports Medicine*, 10(1), 14-18.

Taylor, D.C., Dalton, J.D., Seaber, A.V., and Garrett, W.E. (1990). Viscoelastic properties of muscle-tendon units: The biomechanical effects of stretching. *American Journal of Sports Medicine*, 18, 300-309.

Teitz, C.C. (1982). Sports medicine concerns in dance and gymnastics. *Pediatric Clinics of North America*, 29(6), 1399-1421.

Terracio, L., Gullberg, D., Rubin, K., Craig, S., and Borg, T.K. (1989). Expression of collagen adhesion proteins and their association with the cytoskeleton in cardiac myocytes. *Anatomical Record*, 223(1), 62-71.

Terrett, A.G.J. (1987). Vascular accidents from cervical spine manipulation: Report on 107 cases. *Journal of the Australian Chiropractors' Association*, 17, 15-24.

Terrett, A.G.J. (1988). Vascular accidents from cervical spine manipulation: Report on 107 cases. *ACA Journal of Chiropractic*, 25(4), 63-72.

Terrett, A.G.J. (1990). It is more important to know when not to adjust. *Chiropractic Technique*, 2(1), 1-9.

Terrett, A.G.J. (1995). Misuse of the literature by medical authors in discussing spinal manipulative therapy injury. *Journal of Manipulative and Physiological Therapeutics*, 18(4), 203-210.

Terrett, A.G.J., and Kleynhans, A.M. (1992). Complications from manipulation of the low back. *Chiropractic Journal of Australia*, 22(4), 129-139.

Terrett, A.G.J., and Vernon, H. (1984). Manipulation and pain tolerance. *American Journal of Physical Medicine*, 63(5), 217-225.

Terrier, J.C. (1959). Umriss und Grundlagen der manipulativen Therapie. *WS in Forschung und Praxis*, 13, 56-68.

Terrier, J.C. (1963). Betrachtungen zur manipulativen WS Therapie. *WS in Forschung und Praxis*, 26, 62-67.

Tesch, P.A., Hjort, H., and Balldin, U.I. (1983). Effects of strength training on G tolerance. *Aviation Space and Environmental Medicine*, 54(8), 691-695.

Tesh, K.M., Evans, J.H., Dunn, J.S., and O'Brien, J.P. (1985). The contribution of skin, fascia, and ligaments to resisting flexion of the lumbar spine. In W. Whittle and D. Harris (Eds.), *Biomechanical measurement in orthopaedic practice* (pp. 179-187). Oxford: Clarendon Press.

Tessman, J.R. (1980). *My back doesn't hurt anymore*. New York: Quickfox.

Thieme, W.T., Wynne-Davis, R., Blair, H.A.F., Bell, E.T., and Joraine, J.A. (1968). Clinical examination and urinary oestrogen assays in newborn children with congenital dislocation of the hip. *The Journal of Bone and Joint Surgery*, 50B(3), 546-550.

Thigpen, L.K. (1984). Neuromuscular variation in association with static stretching (Abstract). In W. Kroll (Ed.), *Abstracts of research papers 1984* (p. 28). American Alliance for Health, Physical Education and Recreation. Washington, DC.

Thigpen, L.K., Moritani, T., Thiebaud, R., and Hargis, J.L. (1985). The acute effects of static stretching on alpha motoneuron excitability. In D.A. Winter, R.W. Norman, R.P. Wells, K.C. Hayes, and A.E. Patla (Eds.), *Biomechanics IX-A. International series on biomechanics* (Vol. 5A, pp. 352-357). Champaign, IL: Human Kinetics.

Thompsen, P., and Luco, J.V. (1944). Changes of weight and neuromuscular transmission in muscles of immobilized joints. *Journal of Neurophysiology*, 7, 245-251.

Tideiksaar, R. (1986). Preventing falls: Home hazard checklists to help older patients protect themselves. *Geriatrics*, 41(5), 26-28.

Tillman, L.J., and Cummings, G.S. (1992). Biologic mechanisms of connective tissue mutability. In D.P. Currier and R.M. Nelson (Eds.), *Dynamics of human biologic tissues* (pp. 1-44). Philadelphia: Davis.

Tilney, F., and Pike, F.H. (1925). Muscular coordination experimentally studied in its relation to the cerebellum. *Archives of Neurology and Psychiatry*, 13(3), 289-334.

Tinker, D., and Rucker, R.B. (1985). Role of selected nutrients in synthesis, accumulation, and chemical modification of connective tissue proteins. *Physiological Reviews*, 65(3), 607-657.

Tippett, S.R. (1986). Lower extremity strength and active range of motion in college baseball pitchers: A comparison between stance leg and kick leg. *Journal of Orthopaedic and Sports Physical Therapy*, 8(1), 10-14.

Tobias, M., and Stewart, M. (1985). *Stretch and relax*. Tucson, AZ: Body Press.

Toft, E., Espersen, G.T., Kålund, S., Sinkjaer, T., and Hornemann, B.C. (1989). Passive tension of the ankle before and after stretching. *American Journal of Sports Medicine*, 17(4), 489-494.

Tolsma, B. (1985). Flexibility and velocity. *Track & Field Quarterly Review*, 84(3), 44-47.

Torg, J.S., Vegso, J.J., and Torg, E. (1987). *Rehabilitation of athletic injuries: An atlas of therapeutic exercise*. Chicago: Year Book Medical.

Torgan, C.J. (1985). *The effects of static stretching upon muscular distress*. Unpublished master's thesis, University of Massachusetts.

Toufexis, A. (1974). The price of an art. *Physician's World*, 2(4), 44-50.

Travell, J.G., and Simmons, D.G. (1983). *Myofascial pain and dysfunction: The trigger point manual*. Baltimore: Williams & Wilkins.

TRECO. (n.d.). *Power stretch*. Newport News, VA: TRECO Products.

Trinick, J., Knight, P., and Whiting, A. (1984). Purification and properties of native titin. *Journal of Molecular Biology*, 180(2), 331-356.

Troels, B. (1973). Achilles tendon rupture. *Acta Orthopaedica Scandinavica*, 152(Suppl.), 1-126.

Trombitas, K., Pollack, G.H., Wright, J., and Wang, K. (1993). Elastic properties of titin filaments demonstrated using a "freeze-break" technique. *Cell Motility and the Cytoskeleton*, 24(4), 274-283.

Troup, J.D.G., Hood, C.A., and Chapman, A.E. (1968). Measurement of the sagittal mobility of the lumbar spine and hips. *Annals of Physical Medicine*, 9(8), 308-321.

Tsai, L., and Wredmark, T. (1993). Spinal posture, sagittal mobility, and subjective rating of back problems in former elite gymnasts. *Spine*, 18(7), 872-875.

Tucker, C. (1990). *The mechanics of sports injuries: An osteopathic approach*. Oxford: Blackwell Scientific.

Tullos, H.S., and King, J.W. (1973). Throwing mechanism in sport. *Orthopedic Clinics of North America*, 4(3), 709-720.

Tullson, P., and Armstrong, R.B. (1968). Exercise induced muscle inflammation. *Federation Proceeding*, 37(3), 663.

Tullson, P., and Armstrong, R.B. (1981). Muscle hexose monophosphate shunt activity following exercise. *Experimentia*, 37(12), 1311-1312.

Tumanyan, G.S., and Dzhanyan, S.M. (1984). Strength exercises as a means of improving active flexibility of wrestlers. *Soviet Sports Review*, 19(3), 146-150.

Turek, S.L. (1984). *Orthopaedics principles and their application* (4th ed.). Philadelphia: Lippincott.

Turner, A.A. (1977). *The effects of two training methods on flexibility.* Unpublished master's thesis, Lakehead University.

Tuttle, W.W. (1924). The effect of sleep upon the patellar tendon reflex. *American Journal of Physiology*, 68(2), 345-348.

Tweitmeyer, T.A. (1974). *A comparison of two stretching techniques for increasing and retaining flexibility.* Unpublished master's thesis, University of Iowa.

Twomey, L., and Taylor, J. (1982). Flexion creep deformation and hysteresis in the lumbar vertebral column. *Spine*, 7(2), 116-122.

Tyne, P.J., and Mitchell, M. (1983). *Total stretching.* Chicago: Contemporary Books.

Tyrance, H.J. (1958). Relationships of extreme body types to ranges of flexibility. *Research Quarterly*, 29(3), 349-359.

Tyrer, P.J., and Bond, A.J. (1974). Diurnal variation in physiological tremor. *Electroencephalography and Clinical Neurophysiology*, 37(1), 35-40.

Tyrrell, A.R., Reilly, T., and Troup, J.D.G. (1985). Circadian variation in stature and the effects of spinal loading. *Spine*, 10(2), 161-164.

Ulmer, R.A. (1989). The past, present, and predicted future of the patient compliance field. [Editorial] *Journal of Compliance in Health Care*, 4(2), 89-93.

Unsworth, A., Dowson, D., and Wright, V. (1971). Cracking joints: A bioengineering study of cavitation in the metacarpophalangeal joint. *Annals of the Rheumatic Diseases*, 30(4), 348-358.

Upton, A.R.M., and Radford, P.F. (1975). Motoneuron excitability in elite sprinters. In P.V. Komi (Ed.), *Biomechanics* (pp. 82-87). Baltimore, MD: University Park.

Uram, P. (1980). *The complete stretching book.* Mountain View, CA: Anderson World.

Urban, J.P.G., and Bayliss, M.T. (1989). Regulation of proteoglycan synthesis rate in cartilage in vitro: Influence of extracellular ionic composition. *Biochemica et Biophysica Acta*, 992, 59-65.

Urban, J., Maroudas, A., Bayliss, M., and Dillon, J. (1979). Swelling pressures of proteoglycans at the concentration found in cartilagenous tissues. *Biorheology*, 16(6), 447-464.

Urban, L.M. (1981). The straight-leg-raising test: A review. *The Journal of Orthopaedic and Sports Physical Therapy*, 2(3), 117-134.

Urry, D.W. (1984). Protein elasticity based on conformations of sequential polypeptides: The biological elastic fiber. *Journal of Protein Chemistry*, 3(5-6), 403-436.

Vallbo, A.B. (1974a). Afferent discharge from human muscle spindles in non-contracting muscles. Steady state impulse frequency as a function of the joint angle. *Acta Physiologica Scandinavica*, 90(2), 303-318.

Vallbo, A.B. (1974b). Human muscle spindle discharge during isometric voluntary contractions. Amplitude relations between spindle frequency and torque. *Acta Physiologica Scandinavica*, 90(2), 319-336.

Vandenburgh, H.H. (1987). Motion into mass: How does tension stimulate muscle growth? *Medicine and Science in Sports*

and Exercise, 19(5), S142-S149.

Vandenburgh, H.H. (1992). Mechanical forces and their second messengers in stimulating cell growth in vitro. *American Journal of Physiology*, 31(3), R350-R355.

Vandenburgh, H.H., and Kaufman, S. (1979). In vitro model for stretch-induced hypertrophy of skeletal muscle. *Science*, 203(4377), 265-268.

Vander, A.J., Sherman, J.H., and Luciano, D.S. (1975). *Human physiology: The mechanics of body function* (2nd. ed.). New York: McGraw-Hill.

Van der Meulin, J.H.C. (1982). Present state of knowledge on processes of healing in collagen structures. *International Journal of Sports Medicine*, 3(Suppl. 1), 4-8.

Vandervoort, A.A., Chesworth, B.M., Cunningham, D.A., Patterson, D.H., Rechnitzer, and Koval, J.J. (1992). Age and sex effects on mobility of the human ankle. *Journal of Gerontology*, 47(1), M17-M21.

Van Deusen, J., and Harlowe, D. (1987). A comparison of the ROM dance home exercise rest program with traditional routines. *Occupational Therapy Journal of Research*, 7(6), 349-361.

van Dieën, J.H., and Toussaint, H.M. (1993). Spinal shrinkage as a parameter of functional load. *Spine*, 18(11), 1504-1514.

van Mechelen, W., Hlobil, H., Kemper, H.C.G., Voorn, W.J., and de Jongh, R. (1993). Prevention of running injuries by warm-up, cool-down, and stretching exercises. *American Journal of Sports Medicine*, 21(5), 711-719.

Van Wjimen, P.M. (1986). The management of recurrent low back pain. In G.P. Grieve (Ed.), *Modern manual therapy of the vertebral column* (pp. 756-776). Edinburgh: Churchill Livingstone.

Vasu, S.C. (1933). *The Gheranda Samhita: A treatise on hatha yoga.* Adyar, Madras, India: Theosophical.

Vernon, H.T., Dhami, M.S.I., Howley, T.P., and Annett, R. (1986). Spinal manipulation and beta-endorphin: A controlled study of the effect of a spinal manipulation on plasma beta-endorphin levels in normal males. *Journal of Manipulative and Physiological Therapeutics*, 9(2), 115-123.

Vernon, H., Meschino, J., and Naiman, J. (1985). Inversion therapy: A study of physiological effects. *Journal of the Canadian Chiropractic Association*, 29(3), 135-140.

Verzar, F. (1963). Aging of collagen. *Scientific American*, 208(4), 104-117.

Verzar, F. (1964). Aging of collagen fiber. In D.A. Hall (Ed.), *International review of connective tissue research* (Vol. 2, pp. 244-300). New York: Academic Press.

Viidik, A. (1973). Functional properties of collagenous tissue. *International Review of Connective Tissue Research*, 6, 127-217.

Viidik, A., Danielson, C.C., and Oxlund, H. (1982). On fundamental and phenomenological models, structure and mechanical properties of collagen, elastin and glycoasaminolycan complexes. *Biorheology*, 19(3), 437-451.

Volkov, V.M., and Milner, E.G. (1990). Running and injuries. *Soviet Sports Review*, 25(2), 95-98.

Voluntary power of dislocation. (1882). *The British Medical Journal*, 1, 515.

Volz, R.G., Lieb, M., and Benjamin, J. (1980). Biomechanics of the wrist. *Clinical Orthopaedics and Related Research*, 149(June), 112-117.

Vorobiev, A.N. (Ed.). (1987). Weightlifting: Development of physical qualities. *Soviet Sports Review*, 22(2), 62-68.

Voss, D.E., Ionta, M.J., and Myers, B.J. (1985). *Proprioceptive neuromuscular facilitation* (3rd ed.). New York: Harper & Row.

Vujnovich, A.L., and Dawson., N.J. (1994). The effect of therapeutic muscle stretch on neural processing. *Journal of Ortho-*

paedic and Sports Physical Therapy, 20(3), 145-153.

Wahl, L.M., Blandau, R.J., and Page, R. (1977). Effect of hormones on collagen metabolism and collagenase activity in the pubic symphysis ligament of the guinea pig. *Endocrinology*, 100(2), 571-579.

Walcott, B., and Ridgeway, E.B. (1967). The ultrastructure of myosin-extracted striated muscle fibers. *American Zoologist*, 7(3), 499-503.

Walker, J.M. (1981). Development, maturation and aging of human joints: A review. *Physiotherapy Canada*, 33(3), 153-160.

Walker, S.M. (1961). Delay of twitch relaxation induced by stress and stress-relaxation. *Journal of Applied Physiology*, 16(5), 801-806.

Wall, E.J., Massie, J.B., Kwan, M.K., Rydevik, B.J., Myers, R.R., and Garfin, S.R. (1992). Experimental stretch neuropathy: Changes in nerve conduction under tension. *Journal of Bone and Joint Surgery*, 74B(1), 126-129.

Wallensten, R., and Eklund, B. (1983). Intramuscular pressures and muscle metabolism after short-term and long-term exercise. *International Journal of Sports Medicine*, 4(4), 231-235.

Wallis, E.L., and Logan, G.A. (1964). *Figure improvement and body conditioning through exercise*. Englewood Cliffs, NJ: Prentice-Hall.

Walsh, M. (1985). Review. In F.J. Novakovski, *Trainer-assisted isolated stretching (TAIS)* (pp. ii). Lorton, VA: American Canoe Association.

Walter, S.D., Hart, L.E., McIntosh, J.M., and Sutton, J.R. (1989). The Ontario cohort study of running-related injuries. *Archives of Internal Medicine*, 149(11), 2561-2564.

Walter, S.D., Hart, L.E., Sutton, J.R., McIntosh, J.M., and Gauld, M. (1988). Training habits and injury experience in distance runners: Age- and sex-related factors. *The Physician and Sportsmedicine*, 16(6), 101-113.

Walther, D.S. (1981). *Applied kinesiology: Vol. 1. Basic procedures and muscle testing*. Pueblo, CO: Systems DC.

Wang, K. (1984). Cytoskeletal matrix in striated muscle: The role of titin, nebulin and intermediate filaments. In G.H. Pollack and H. Sugi (Eds.), *Contractile mechanisms in muscle* (pp. 285-306). New York: Plenum Press.

Wang, K. (1985). Sarcomere-associated cytoskeletal lattices in striated muscle. In J.W. Shay (Ed.), *Cell and muscle motility* (Vol. 6, pp. 315-369). New York: Plenum.

Wang, K., Ash, J.G., and Singer, S.J. (1975). Filamin, a new high molecular weight protein of smooth muscle and non-muscle cells. *Proceedings of the National Academy of Science* (USA), 72, 4483-4486.

Wang, K., McCarter, R., Wright, J., Beverly, J., and Ramirez-Mitchell, R. (1991). Regulation of skeletal muscle stiffness and elasticity by titin isoforms: A test of the segmental extension model of resting tension. *Proceedings of the National Academy of Science* (USA), 88(6), 7101-7105.

Wang, K., McClure, J., and Tu, A. (1979). Titin: Major myofibrillar components of striated muscle. *Proceedings of the National Academy of Science* (USA), 76(8), 3698-3702.

Wang, K., Ramirez-Mitchell, R., and Palter, D. (1984). Titin is an extraordinarily long, flexible, and slender myofibrillar protein. *Proceedings of the National Academy of Science* (USA), 81(12), 3685-3689.

Wang, K., and Wright, J. (1988). Architecture of the sarcomere matrix of skeletal muscle: Immunoelectron microscopic evidence that suggests a set of parallel inextensible nebulin filaments anchored at the Z-line. *Journal of Cell Biology*, 107(6, Pt. 1), 2199-2212.

Wang, K., Wright, J., and Ramirez-Mitchell, R. (1985). Architecture of the titin/nebulin containing cytoskeletal lattice of the striated muscle sarcomere: Evidence of elastic and inelastic domains of the bipolar filaments (Abstract). *Biophysical Journal*, 47, 349a.

Ward, R.C. (1985). *Principles of myofascial release*. East Lansing, MI: Michigan State University.

Ward, R.C. (1993). Myofascial release concepts. In J.V. Basmajian and R. Nyberg (Eds.), *Rational manual therapies* (p. 223-241). Baltimore: Williams & Wilkins.

Warren, A. (1968). Mobilization of the chest wall. *Physical Therapy*, 48(6), 582-585.

Warren, C.G., Lehmann, J.F., and Koblanski, J.N. (1971). Elongation of rat tail tendon: Effect of load and temperature. *Archives of Physical Medicine and Rehabilitation*, 57(3), 122-126.

Warren, C.G., Lehmann, J.F., and Koblanski, J.N. (1976). Heat and stretch procedures: An evaluation using rat tail tendon. *Archives of Physical Medicine and Rehabilitation*, 57(3), 122-126.

Warren, G.W. (1989). *Classical ballet technique*. Tampa, FL: University of South Florida Press.

Wasserstrom, R. (1977). Some problems with theories of punishment. In J.B. Cederblom and W.L. Blizek (Eds.), *Justice and punishment* (pp. 173-196). Cambridge, MA: Ballinger.

Waterman-Storer, C.M. (1991). The cytoskeleton of skeletal muscle: Is it affected by exercise? A brief review. *Medicine and Science in Sports and Exercise*, 23(11), 1240-1249.

Watkins, A., Woodhull-McNeal, A.P., Clarkson, P.M., and Ebbeling, C. (1989). Lower extremity alignment and injury in young, preprofessional, college, and professional ballet dancers. *Medical Problems of Performing Artists*, 4(4), 148-153.

Watts, N. (1968). Improvement of breathing patterns. *Physical Therapy*, 48(6), 563-581.

Wear, C.R. (1963). Relationship of flexibility measurements to length of body segments. *Research Quarterly*, 34(3), 234-238.

Weaver, D. (1979). Weight-lifting advice: Flexibility the key to better lifting. *Strength Health*, 47(4), 50-53.

Webber, C.E., and Garnett, E.S. (1976). Density of os calcis and limb dominance. *Journal of Anatomy*, 121(1), 203-205.

Weber, S., and Kraus, H. (1949). Passive and active stretching of muscles: Spring stretch and control group. *Physical Therapy Review*, 29(9), 407-410.

Webster, D. (1986). *Preparing for competition weightlifting*. Huddershfield, England: Springfield Books.

Weiner, I.H., and Weiner, H.L. (1980). Nocturnal leg muscle cramps. *Journal of the American Medical Association*, 244(20), 2332-2333.

Weinreb, R.N., Cook, J., and Friberg, T.R. (1984). Effect of inverted body position on intraocular pressure. *American Journal of Ophthalmology*, 98(6), 784-787.

Weis-Fogh, T., and Anderson, S.O. (1970a). In E.A. Balazs (Ed.), *Chemistry and molecular biology of the intracellular matrix* (Vol. 1, pp. 671-684). London: Academic Press.

Weis-Fogh, T., and Anderson, S.O. (1970b). New molecular model for the long-range elasticity of elastin. *Nature*, 213(5259), 718-721.

Weiss, L., and Greep, R.O. (1983). *Histology* (5th ed.). New York: Elsevier Biomedical.

Weiss, R. (1993). Bones of contention. *Health*, 7(4), 44-52.

Wessling, K.C., DeVane, D.A., and Hylton, C.R. (1987). Effects of static stretch versus static stretch and ultrasound combined on triceps surae muscle extensibility in healthy women. *Physical Therapy*, 67(5), 674-679.

Whipple, R.H., Wolfson, L.I., and Amerman, P.M. (1987). The relationship of knee and ankle weakness to falls in nursing home residents: An isokinetic study. *Journal of the American Geriatric Society*, 35(1), 13-20.

White, A.A., and Panjabi, M.M. (1978). *Clinical biomechanics of the spine*. Philadelphia: Lippincott.

White, A.H. (1983). *Back school and other conservative approaches to low back pain*. St. Louis: Mosby.

Whiting, A., Wardale, J., and Trinick, J. (1989). Does titin regulate the length of muscle thick filaments? *Journal of Molecular Biology*, 205(1), 263-268.

Wickstrom, R.L. (1963). Weight training and flexibility. *Journal of Health, Physical Education and Recreation*, 34(2), 61-62.

Wieman, H.M., and Calkins, E. (1986). Falls. In E. Calkins, P.J. Davis, and A.B. Ford (Eds.), *The practice of geriatrics* (pp. 272-280). Philadelphia: Saunders.

Wigley, F.M. (1984). Osteoarthritis: Practical management in older patients. *Geriatrics*, 39(3), 101-120.

Wiktorssohn-Möller, M., Öberg, B., Ekstrand, J., and Gillquist, J. (1983). Effects of warming up, massage, and stretching on range of motion and muscle strength in the lower extremity. *American Journal of Sports Medicine*, 11(4), 249-252.

Wilby, J., Linge, K., Reilly, T., and Troup, J.D.G. (1987). Spinal shrinkage in females: Circadian variation and the effects of circuit weight-training. *Ergonomics*, 30(1), 47-54.

Wiles, P. (1935). Movements of the lumbar vertebrae during flexion and extension. *Proceedings of the Royal Society of London*, 28(5), 647-651.

Wilkinson, H.A. (1983). *The failed back syndrome: Etiology and therapy*. New York: Harper & Row.

Williams, J.C.P., and Sperryn, G. (1976). *Sports medicine* (2nd ed.). Baltimore: Williams & Wilkins.

Williams, P.C. (1977). *Low back and neck pain: Causes and conservative treatments*. Springfield, IL: Charles C Thomas.

Williams, P.E. (1988). Effect of intermittent stretch on immobilized muscle. *Annals of the Rheumatic Diseases*, 47(12), 1014-1016.

Williams, P.E., Catanese, T., Lucey, E.G., and Goldspink, G. (1988). The importance of stretch and contractile activity in the prevention of connective tissue accumulation in muscle. *Journal of Anatomy*, 158(June), 109-114.

Williams, P.E., and Goldspink, G. (1971). Longitudinal growth of striated muscle fibres. *Journal of Cell Science*, 9(3), 751-767.

Williams, P.E., and Goldspink, G. (1973). The effect of immobilization on the longitudinal growth of striated muscle fibres. *Journal of Anatomy*, 116(1), 45-55.

Williams, P.E., and Goldspink, G. (1976). The effect of denervation and dystrophy on the adaptation of sarcomere number to the functional length of the muscle in young and adult mice. *Journal of Anatomy*, 122(2), 455-465.

Williams, P.E., and Goldspink, G. (1984). Connective tissue changes in immobilised muscle. *Journal of Anatomy*, 138(2), 343-350.

Williams, P.L., Warwick, R., Dyson, M., and Bannister, L.H. (1989). *Gray's anatomy* (37th ed.). Philadelphia: Saunders.

Williford, H.N., East, J.B., Smith, F.H., and Burry, L.A. (1986). Evaluation of warm-up for improvement in flexibility. *American Journal of Sports Medicine*, 14(4), 316-319.

Wilmore, J.H. (1982). *Training for sport and activity* (2nd ed.). Boston: Allyn and Bacon.

Wilmore, J.H. (1991). The aging of bone and muscle. *Clinics in Sports Medicine*, 10(2), 231-244, 1991.

Wilmore, J., Parr, R.B., Girandola, R.N., Ward, P., Vodak, P.A., Pipes, T.V., Romerom, G.T., and Leslie, P. (1978). Physiological alterations consequent to circuit weight training. *Medicine and Science in Sports*, 10(2), 79-84.

Wilson, V.E., and Bird, E.I. (1981). Effects of relation and/or biofeedback training upon hip flexion in gymnasts. *Biofeedback and Self-Regulation*, 6(1), 25-34.

Winget, C.M., DeRoshia, C.W., and Holley, D.C. (1985). Circadian rhythms and athletic performance. *Medicine and Science in Sports and Exercise*, 17(5), 498-516.

Winterstein, J.F. (1989). In what way would a graduate of a SCASA college practice differently from a graduate of a CCE college? *Dynamic Chiropractic*, 7(15), 1.

Wirhed, R. (1984). *Athletic ability: The anatomy of winning*. New York: Harmony Books.

Wisnes, A., and Kirkebø, A. (1976). Regional distribution of blood flow in calf muscles of rat during passive stretch and sustained contraction. *Acta Physiologica Scandinavica*, 96(2), 256-266.

Wolf, M.D. (1983). Stretching a point. *Women's Sports*, 5(8), 53.

Wolf, S.L., and Segal, R.L. (1990). Conditioning of the spinal stretch reflex: Implication for rehabilitation. *Physical Therapy*, 70(10), 652-656.

Wolff, H.D. (1967). Bemerkungen zur Theorie der manuellen Therapie. *Manuelle Medizin*, 1, 13-20.

Wolpaw, J.R. (1983). Adaptive plasticity in the primate spinal stretch reflex: Reversal and redevelopment. *Brain Research*, 278(1-2), 299-304.

Wolpaw, J.R., Braitman, D.J., and Seegal, R.F. (1983). Adaptive plasticity in the primate spinal stretch reflex: Initial development. *Journal of Neurophysiology*, 50(6), 1296-1311.

Wolpaw, J.R., and Carp, J.S. (1990). Memory traces in spinal cord. *Trends in Neuroscience*, 13(4), 137-142.

Wolpaw, J.R., and Lee, C.L. (1989). Memory traces in primate spinal cord produced by operant conditioning of H-reflex. *Journal of Neurophysiology*, 61(3), 563-572.

Wolpaw, J.R., Lee, C.L., and Carp, J.S. (1991). Operantly conditioned plasticity in spinal cord. *Annals of the New York Academy of Sciences*, 627, 338-348.

Wolpaw, J.R., Noonan, P.A., and O'Keefe, J.A. (1984). Adaptive plasticity and diurnal rhythm in the primate spinal stretch reflex are independent phenomenon. *Brain Research*, 33(2), 385-391.

Wolpaw, J.R., and Seegal, R.F. (1982). Diurnal rhythm in the spinal stretch reflex. *Brain Research*, 244(2), 365-369.

Wolpe, J. (1958). *Psychotherapy by reciprocal inhibition*. Stanford: Stanford University Press.

Woo, S.L.-Y., Gomez, M.A., and Akeson, W.H. (1985). Mechanical behaviors of soft tissues: Measurements, modifications, injuries, and treatments. In A.M. Nahum and J. Melvin (Eds.), *The biomechanics of trauma*. Norwalk, CT: Appleton-Century-Crofts.

Woo, S., Matthews, J.V., Akeson, W.H., Amiel, D., and Convery, R. (1975). Connective tissue response to immobility: Correlative study of biomechanical and biologic measurements of normal and immobilized rabbit knees. *Arthritis Rheumatology*, 18(3), 257-264.

Wood, P.H.N. (1971). Is hypermobility a discrete entity? *Proceedings of the Royal Society of Medicine*, 64(6), 690-692.

Woods, J.H. (1914). *The yoga-system of Patanjali*. Boston: Harvard University Press.

Wordsworth, P., Ogilvie, D., Smith, R., and Sykes, B. (1987). Joint mobility with particular reference to racial variation and inherited connective tissue disorders. *British Journal of Rheumatology, 26*(1), 9-12.

World Chiropractic Alliance (1993). *Practice guidelines for straight chiropractic.* Chandler, AZ: Author.

Wright, V., and Johns, R.J. (1960). Physical factors concerned with the stiffness of normal and diseased joints. *Bulletin of the Johns Hopkins Hospital, 106,* 215-231.

Wyke, B. (1967). The neurology of joints. *Annals of the Royal College of Surgeons of England, 41,* 25-50.

Wyke, B. (1972). Articular neurology—A review. *Physiotherapy, 58*(3), 94-99.

Wyke, B. (1979). Neurology of the cervical spinal joints. *Physiotherapy, 65*(3), 72-76.

Wyke, B. (1985). Articular neurology and manipulative therapy. In E.F. Glasgow, L.T. Twomey, E.R. Scull, and A.M. Kleynhans (Eds.), *Aspects of manipulative therapy* (2nd ed., pp. 72-77). London: Churchill Livingstone.

Wynne-Davies, R. (1971). Familial joint laxity. *Proceedings of the Royal Society of Medicine, 64,* 689-690.

Yagi, N., and Matsubara, I. (1984). Cross-bridge movements during a slow length change of active muscle. *Biophysical Journal, 45*(3), 611-614.

Yamamoto, T. (1993). Relationship between hamstring strains and leg muscle strength. *Journal of Sports Medicine and Physical Fitness, 33*(2), 194-199.

Yanicostas, N.S., Hamida, C.B., Butler-Browne, G.S., Hentati, F., Bejaoui, K., and Hamida, M.B. (1991). Modification in the expression and localization of contractile and cytoskeletal proteins in Schwartz-Jampel syndrome. *Journal of the Neurological Sciences, 104*(1), 64-73.

Yates, J. (1990). *A physician's guide to therapeutic massage: Its physiological effects and their application to treatment.* Vancouver: Massage Therapists' Association of British Columbia.

Yeomans, S.G. (1992). The assessment of cervical intersegmental mobility before and after spinal manipulative therapy. *Journal of Manipulative and Physiological Therapeutics, 15*(2), 106-114.

Yessis, M. (1986). A flexible spine: How you can develop one. *Muscle & Fitness, 47*(5), 60-63, 203-204.

Yogendra, J. (1988). *Cyclopedia yoga* (Vol. 1). Bombay, India: Yoga Institute.

Yoshioka, T., Higuchi, H., Kimura, S., Ohashi, K., Umazume, Y., and Maruyama, K. (1986). Effects of mild trypsin treatment on the passive tension generation and connectin splitting in stretched skinned fibers from frog skeletal muscle. *Biomedical Research, 7,* 181-186.

Yu, S.H., and Blumenthal, H. (1967). The calcification of elastic tissue. In B.M. Wagner and D.E. Smith (Eds.), *The connective tissue* (pp. 17-49). Baltimore: Williams & Wilkins.

Zacharkow, D. (1984). *The healthy lower back.* Springfield, IL: Charles C Thomas.

Zachazewski, J.E. (1990). Flexibility for sports. In B. Sanders (Ed.), *Sports physical therapy* (pp. 201-238). Norwalk, CT: Appleton & Lange.

Zajonc, R.B. (1965). Social facilitation. *Science, 149*(3681), 269-274.

Zarins, B., Andrews, J.R., and Carson, W.G. (Eds.). (1985). *Injuries to the throwing arm.* Philadelphia: Saunders.

Zebas, C.J., and Rivera, M.L. (1985). Retention of flexibility in selected joints after cessation of a stretching exercise program. In C.O. Dotson and J.H. Humphrey (Eds.), *Exercise physiology. Current selected research I* (pp. 181-191). New York: AMS Press.

Zernicke, R.F., and Salem, G.J. (1991). Flexibility training. In B. Reider (Ed.), *Sports medicine: The school-age athlete* (pp. 40-51). Philadelphia: Saunders.

Zierler, K.L. (1974). Mechanisms of muscular contraction and its energetics. In V.B. Mountcastle (Ed.), *Medical physiology* (12th ed., Vol. 2, pp. 1128-1171). St. Louis: Mosby.

Zulak, G. (1991). Fascial stretching. The ignored exercise technique. *Flex, 9*(1), 94, 107-108.

Author Index

Subject Index

About the Author

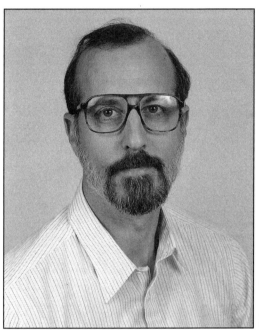

© Lenny Furman

A former gymnast, coach, and nationally certified men's gymnastics judge, Michael J. Alter is an expert on the subject of stretching. The first edition of his book, *Science of Stretching*, as well as the how-to book *Sport Stretch*, received rave reviews from athletes, coaches, trainers, and sports medicine professionals.

Michael earned his MS in health education from Florida International University in 1976. He taught high school physical education and coached gymnastics for several years prior to his current position in Miami as a high school teacher of history.

Michael has been a guest lecturer at annual meetings across the country, including the 1994 Chiropractic Sports Science Symposium and the 1992 Scientific Meeting of the North American Society of Pediatric Exercise Medicine.

In his leisure time, Michael enjoys bicycling, listening to classical music, working out with weights, and studying sports medicine.

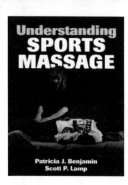
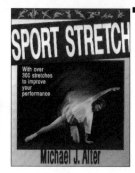
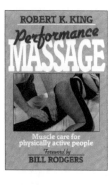